Diagnostic Approaches to Presenting Syndromes

Diagnostic Approaches to Presenting Syndromes

EDITED BY

JEREMIAH A. BARONDESS, M.D.

CLINICAL PROFESSOR OF MEDICINE,
CORNELL UNIVERSITY MEDICAL COLLEGE;
ATTENDING PHYSICIAN,
THE NEW YORK HOSPITAL, NEW YORK

The Williams & Wilkins Company BALTIMORE

MADE IN THE UNITED STATES OF AMERICA

LIBRARY OF CONGRESS CATALOG CARD NUMBER 77-141764

SBN 683-00418-2

COMPOSED AND PRINTED AT THE

WAVERLY PRESS, INC.

MT. ROYAL AND GUILFORD AVES.

BALTIMORE, MD. 21202, U.S.A.

Preface

Diagnosis is the foundation on which all clinical activity rests. While the contributions of the various clinical laboratories, departments of radiology, electrocardiographic stations, and all the other ancillary services are steadily expanding in sophistication and in their capacity to help illuminate clinical problems, the central constellation in diagnosis has not changed over the centuries since the Hippocratic method was first evolved. Fundamentally this constellation consists of a patient with a set of complaints and a physician who attempts to understand and identify the disease process responsible for them. Diagnostic effort consists of the business of translating the syndrome with which the patient presents into identification of his disease.

The diagnostic procedure begins at the bedside. It is there that the salient facts are gathered by elicitation of the patient's medical history and performance of a physical examination. It is at the bedside that appreciation of the nature and dimensions of the patient's presenting syndrome is largely accomplished and the physician begins to assemble in his mind the specific diagnostic possibilities which might underlie it.

In this volume an effort has been made to examine this process in relation to a number of common complex presenting syndromes germane to internal medicine. The emphasis in each chapter is on the main clinical features of the various diagnostic possibilities, and on those techniques of organization of thought which the authors have found useful. At the same time there is some variation from chapter to chapter in the manner in which the material is presented, by virtue of the fact that some topics lend themselves best to one approach, and others to another.

The group of syndromes considered is not intended by any means to encompass all of internal medicine. Rather, they have been selected by the editor because they appear with considerable frequency in every internist's experience, and because each may be produced by a large number of specific disease processes. Each, therefore, is a common source of diagnostic perplexity.

My grateful thanks go to the contributors to the book, each of whom made room in an extraordinarily busy schedule to write for it. Additional thanks go to Dr. Walsh McDermott, old friend and wise counselor, for his advice and encouragement, to Dr. Richard Fleming, for his help with the selection of some of the x-ray figures, and to my wife and son, for their patience and forbearance during the many months the book was in work.

JEREMIAH A. BARONDESS

Contributors

Thomas P. Almy, M.D. Nathan Smith Professor and Chairman, Department of Medicine, Dartmouth Medical School, and Director of Medicine, Dartmouth-Hitchcock Affiliated Hospitals, Hanover, New Hampshire

Jeremiah A. Barondess, M.D. Clinical Professor of Medicine, Cornell University Medical College; Attending Physician, New York Hospital, New York

Lawrence S. Cohen, M.D. Professor of Medicine and Chief, Section of Cardiology, Yale University School of Medicine, New Haven, Connecticut

James S. Forrester, M.D. Scientific Director, Myocardial Infarction Research Unit, Cedars of Lebanon Hospital, and Assistant Professor of Medicine, UCLA School of Medicine, Los Angeles, California

James H. Gault, M.D. Chief, Cardiology Division and Associate Professor of Medicine, Pennsylvania State College of Medicine, Hershey, Pennsylvania

Jay S. Goodman, M.D. Assistant Professor of Medicine, Vanderbilt University School of Medicine, Nashville, Tennessee

Richard Gorlin, M.D. Chief, Cardiovascular Division, Peter Bent Brigham Hospital, and Associate Professor of Medicine, Harvard Medical School, Boston, Massachusetts

David Grob, M.D. Director, Department of Medicine, Maimonides Medical Center, and Professor of Medicine, State University of New York, Downstate Medical Center, Brooklyn, New York

Edward W. Hook, M.D. Henry B. Mulholland Professor and Chairman, Department of Medicine, University of Virginia School of Medicine, Charlottesville, Virginia

Harvey G. Kemp, Jr., M.D. Director, Division of Cardiology, St. Luke's Hospital Center, and Assistant Clinical Professor of Medicine, College of Physicians and Surgeons, Columbia University, New York

Thomas Killip III, M.D. Roland Harriman Professor of Medicine, Cornell University Medical College, and Attending Physician, New York Hospital, New York

John E. Lee, M.D. Clinical Associate Professor of Neurology, Cornell University Medical College, and Associate Attending Neurologist, New York Hospital, New York

Morton H. Maxwell, M.D. Chief, Nephrology and Hypertension Service, Cedars-Sinai Medical Center, and Clinical Professor of Medicine, UCLA Medical Center, Los Angeles, California

W. P. Laird Myers, M.D. Professor of Medicine, Cornell University Medical College, and Chairman, Department of Medicine, Memorial Hospital for Cancer and Allied Diseases, New York

Ralph L. Nachman, M.D. Associate Professor of Medicine and Chief, Division of Hematology, Department of Medicine, Cornell University Medical College, New York

Robert G. Petersdorf, M.D. Professor and Chairman, Department of Medicine, University of Washington School of Medicine, and Physician-in-Chief, University of Washington Hospital, Seattle, Washington

Fred Plum, M.D. Anne Parrish Titzell Professor and Chairman, Department of Neurology, Cornell University Medical College, New York

David E. Rogers, M.D. Professor of Medicine, Dean, and Vice President (Medicine), The Johns Hopkins University School of Medicine, and Medical Director, The Johns Hopkins Hospital, Baltimore, Maryland

John Ross, Jr., M.D. Professor of Medicine and Director, Cardiovascular Division, University of California at San Diego School of Medicine, La Jolla, California

Paul D. Saville, M.D. Professor of Medicine, Creighton University School of Medicine, Omaha, Nebraska

Richard T. Silver, M.D. Clinical Associate Professor of Medicine and Director, Chemotherapy Service, Division of Hematology, Cornell University Medical College; Associate Attending Physician, New York Hospital, New York; Member of the Polycythemia Vera National Study Group under the auspices of the National Cancer Institute

James F. Wallace, M.D. Assistant professor of Medicine and Head, Division of Ambulatory Medicine, University of Washington School of Medicine, Seattle, Washington

Contents

Mitral Regurgitation

LAWRENCE S. COHEN, JAMES H. GAULT, and JOHN ROSS, JR.

The concept that mitral valve disease might be a cause of cardiac disability has been attributed to Vieussens, the eighteenth-century physician.[42,57,58] A century later Corvisart[15] and Laënnec[28] pointed out that the malformed mitral valve could be the source of a cardiac murmur. Over the next 100 years there were active shifts of opinion concerning the pathophysiological importance of mitral regurgitation. Although it is now generally agreed that many patients with minor degrees of mitral regurgitation may tolerate this lesion for many years without developing significant symptoms, left ventricular failure is the expected outcome if mitral regurgitation is of major proportions.

The approach to the patient with mitral regurgitation resolves itself into two general lines of investigation. The diagnosis of mitral regurgitation first must be established and, once established, the specific etiology then must be sought. Since a systolic murmur is almost always a constant accompaniment of mitral regurgitation, the differential diagnosis initially becomes that of the patient with a systolic murmur. Table 1 lists the major congenital and acquired cardiac lesions causing systolic murmurs, each of which might be confused with mitral regurgitation.

THE CLINICAL DIAGNOSIS OF MITRAL REGURGITATION

Ventricular septal defect, aortic stenosis (subvalvular, valvular, supravalvular), pulmonic stenosis, congenital tricuspid regurgitation, and idiopathic hypertrophic subaortic stenosis are the congenital lesions most likely to be confused with mitral regurgitation. The most common acquired lesions which enter into the differential diagnosis are rheumatic valvular aortic stenosis, tricuspid regurgitation, and rupture of the ventricular septum due to myocardial infarction. The history, physical examination, electrocardiogram, chest roentgenogram, and special laboratory tests[22] may all be useful in establishing the diagnosis of mitral regurgitation.

History

The incidence of congenital mitral regurgitation is lower than that of ventricular septal defect or aortic stenosis, and the history of a murmur

LAWRENCE S. COHEN, M.D. Professor of Medicine and Chief, Section of Cardiology, Yale University School of Medicine, New Haven, Connecticut. JAMES H. GAULT, M.D. Associate Professor of Medicine and Chief, Cardiology Division, Pennsylvania State College of Medicine Hershey Medical Center, Hershey, Pennsylvania. JOHN ROSS, JR., M.D. Professor of Medicine and Director, Cardiovascular Division, University of California at San Diego School of Medicine, La Jolla, California

TABLE 1

Differential Diagnosis of the Systolic Murmur. The physical findings in both congenital and acquired lesions may simulate mitral regurgitation.

Congenital
  1. Ventricular septal defect
  2. Aortic stenosis
     a. Subvalvular membrane
     b. Valvular
     c. Supravalvular
  3. Pulmonic stenosis
  4. Tricuspid regurgitation
  5. Idiopathic hypertrophic subaortic stenosis
Acquired
  1. Rheumatic valvular aortic stenosis
  2. Rheumatic tricuspid regurgitation
     a. Primary
     b. Secondary to left-sided valvular lesions
  3. Ventricular septal defect secondary to myocardial infarction

---

since birth would favor one of the latter diagnoses. Since half the patients with idiopathic hypertrophic subaortic stenosis represent the familial form of the disease,[11,20] a family history of cardiac disease is often a clue to this diagnosis. It must be remembered, however, that rheumatic fever with mitral valve involvement may also be present in more than one member of a family, since rheumatic heart disease also tends to cluster in families.

In considering the acquired diseases which may be confused with mitral regurgitation the patient's symptoms are often helpful in approaching the differential diagnosis. Angina pectoris and syncope, frequent concomitants of significant aortic stenosis, are unusual in mitral regurgitation, in which fatigue is the prime symptom. In an individual whose heart murmur can be dated to the onset of a myocardial infarction rupture of the interventricular septum must be excluded. This lesion, however, is much less common than papillary muscle dysfunction or rupture with consequent mitral regurgitation.

Physical Examination

The physical examination is of major importance in establishing the diagnosis of mitral regurgitation.

THE PULSE

The pulse in patients with mitral regurgitation characteristically has a water-hammer quality, abrupt and collapsing.[60] The distinctive arterial pulse of mitral regurgitation is attributed to a combination of overfilling of the left ventricle and a systolic leak into the left atrium. Although the rate of upstroke is rapid, the pulse is unsustained and of poor volume because of the large fraction of blood that is regurgitated into the left atrium instead of entering the aorta. The pulse in a patient with ventricular septal defect is similar to that in mitral regurgitation. Thus, with ventricular septal defect, the left ventricle is overfilled at end diastole, and with the onset of ventricular contraction the stroke volume is diverted in two directions, part of the cardiac output entering the aorta and part entering the right ventricle. The pulse in patients with idiopathic hypertrophic subaortic stenosis (IHSS) also may simulate the pulse of patients with mitral regurgitation, the upstroke time being rapid and the volume often small. Frequently, however, one can palpate a double systolic impulse, and this finding should alert the examiner to the possibility of IHSS. Diminution in the amplitude of the pulse in the beat following a premature contraction also should raise the possibility of IHSS. In adults the nature of the pulse in aortic stenosis is a major means of differentiating this lesion from mitral regurgitation. In aortic stenosis the carotid pulse has a slow upstroke, an anacrotic notch, and a delayed peak, although in children with congenital aortic stenosis and in elderly patients the pulse may be rather brisk in spite of marked stenosis.

THE JUGULAR VENOUS PULSE

The jugular venous pulse is valuable in differentiating regurgitation at the tricuspid valve from mitral regurgitation. Large V waves with a rapid Y descent are very suggestive of tricuspid regurgitation, as is an augmentation of the holosystolic murmur with inspiration.[29,46] In the absence of these findings a holosystolic murmur is more likely to be mitral than tricuspid in origin.

PALPATION OF THE PRECORDIUM

Palpation of the precordium will help to focus down upon the etiology of a systolic murmur. In mitral regurgitation a systolic thrill at the apex is commonly present, and is often quite widely transmitted. Patients with valvular aortic stenosis frequently have a palpable thrill in the second right intercostal space at the sternal border, and the thrill often radiates to the neck vessels. However, a thrill in this area may also be found in patients with mitral regurgitation. Regurgitation through the posterior leaflet of the mitral valve can often be heard best along the left or right upper sternum, and is frequently associated with a thrill. The explanation for this physical sign appears related to the direction of the regurgitant jet, which strikes the interatrial septum near the aortic root.[18] A systolic thrill in the third, fourth, or fifth intercostal space to the left of the sternum is characteristic of ventricular septal defect, and a thrill in the second left intercostal space and suprasternal notch is often present with pulmonic stenosis.

Because of the increased volume load imposed upon the left ventricle, the apex beat in patients with mitral regurgitation is often displaced laterally, and commonly it is quite diffuse. In the patient with severe aortic stenosis and concentric hypertrophy of the left ventricle, the apex impulse is small but forceful, and is sustained throughout systole. The impulse generally is not particularly displaced and may even be located within the midclavicular line. A palpable outward movement in early diastole, coincident with the peak of the rapid filling phase, is extremely common in mitral regurgitation. This event is simultaneous with a ventricular filling sound (third heart sound) and reflects the large flow across the mitral valve in early diastole. The presence of an atrial impulse at the cardiac apex late in diastole is distinctly unusual in patients with mitral regurgitation. An atrial impulse presupposes a sinus mechanism, and the majority of patients with long-standing mitral regurgitation have atrial fibrillation. However, patients with mitral regurgitation of recent onset secondary to ruptured chordae tendineae are usually in sinus rhythm and may demonstrate an atrial impulse.[14] This finding is extremely uncommon in patients with mitral regurgitation of rheumatic origin, even in the presence of sinus rhythm. Thus, it is likely that the acute nature of mitral regurgitation resulting from a ruptured chorda brings the patient to medical attention before the left atrium has become dilated and incapable of a forceful contraction.

Before leaving the subject of precordial palpation it should be pointed out that patients with severe mitral regurgitation often develop pulmonary hypertension, and the prominent features of the physical examination may be related to the pulmonary hypertension. In most instances patients who demonstrate the findings of a right ventricular heave, a palpable pulmonary outflow tract, and an increased pulmonic component of the second heart sound will have pulmonary hypertension. However, this constellation of findings may also be found in patients with marked mitral regurgitation without pulmonary hypertension, in whom an enlarged left atrium may force the anterior surface of the heart (comprising the right ventricle and pulmonary outflow tract) against the chest wall, thereby simulating the physical findings of pulmonary hypertension. This occurrence was noted in 22 out of a series of 125 patients with mitral regurgitation and normal pulmonary artery pressures.[32]

AUSCULTATORY FINDINGS

The auscultatory findings in the patient with mitral regurgitation are 1) a soft first heart sound at the apex, 2) wide splitting of the second heart sound at the base, 3) a loud third heart sound or ventricular knock, 4) a holosystolic apical murmur, and 5) a short mid-diastolic rumble.[34,60] It is generally considered that the first heart sound is related to closure and tensing of the atrioventricular valve leaflets during isovolumetric contraction. The presence of mitral regurgitation may prevent tensing of the valve leaflets, and may therefore cause diminution of the first heart sound. Other factors also may contribute to the muffling of the first heart sound. Diastasis, equilibration of the atrial and ventricular pressure pulses, has generally been achieved in pure mitral regurgitation at the outset of ventricular contraction. The valve leaflets have therefore had an opportunity to float toward apposition, and the excursion coincident with valve closure is less than that found normally or in patients with pure mitral stenosis. Mitral regurgitation is often associated with some degree of leaflet destruction, and this anatomic abnormality may also contribute to the attenuation of the first heart sound.[23] Lastly, mitral valve calcification may produce marked limitation of mobility.

The second heart sound at the base may be widely split, and sometimes it does not vary discernibly with respiration. Two explanations have been advanced to explain these findings. The aortic component of the second heart sound may occur early, the systolic runoff into the left atrium leading to a shortened ejection period. In addition, in patients with pulmonary hypertension and right ventricular decompensation, the duration of right ventricular ejection may be prolonged and may vary little with respiration. The delay in pulmonic valve closure thus contributes to wide splitting of the second heart sound.

Nixon and associates[39] have described an opening snap in some patients with pure mitral regurgitation. They ascribe this sound to the rapid opening of the mitral valve leaflets at the onset of ventricular filling.

The diagnosis of significant mitral regurgitation must be questioned if a ventricular filling gallop (third heart sound) is not heard. This sound occurs during the early phase of rapid ventricular filling and originates either in the ventricular muscle or in mitral cusps and chordae. A "ventricular knock sound"[30] produced by the impact of an enlarged left ventricle against the anterior chest wall may have the same timing as a ventricular gallop sound, but is often louder.

An atrial gallop (fourth heart sound) is a rare finding in patients with mitral regurgitation. It has been described in patients with ruptured mitral chordae tendineae or ruptured papillary muscles[14,38] (Fig. 1). In both these lesions the onset of regurgitation is generally of recent origin, and symptoms progress rapidly and bring the patient to medical attention early in the course of the disease. The left atrium is either of normal size or only slightly dilated, and is therefore able to produce a contraction of sufficient strength to contribute significantly to ventricular filling. In contrast, in patients with mitral valve disease of rheumatic origin, the course tends to be more chronic and the left atrium is often dilated and incapable of forceful contractions. In addition, atrial fibrillation is common in patients with mitral regurgitation secondary to rheumatic heart disease, whereas normal sinus rhythm is the usual finding in patients with ruptured chordae or papillary muscles.

The hallmark of mitral regurgitation is the systolic murmur. In general this murmur commences with the first heart sound and continues up to or slightly beyond the aortic component of the second heart sound. The murmur is due to the turbulence caused by retrograde flow of blood across the incompetent mitral valve, from ventricle to atrium, occurring during the systolic and early diastolic phases of the cardiac cycle when ventricular pressure exceeds that in the left atrium. The radiation of the murmur

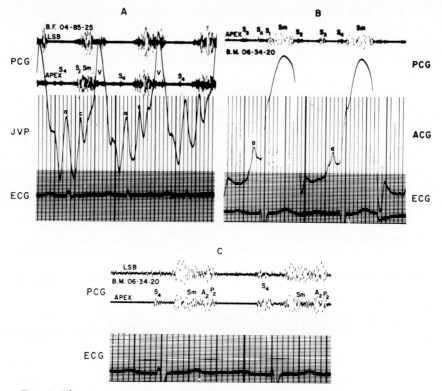

FIG. 1. The occurrence of an atrial gallop sound (S₄) in patients with ruptured mitral chordae tendineae. Panel A, patient B. F. PCG = phonocardiogram; JVP = jugular venous pulse; a, c, and v = component waves of jugular venous pulse; ECG = electrocardiogram; LSB = left sternal border; SM = systolic murmur. Panels B and C, patient B. M. ACG = apex cardiogram. (Reprinted, with permission, from Circulation 35:112, 1967.)

generally is to the left axilla, and it is often heard at the angle of the left scapula and in the lower interscapular area. Because of transmission along the bony skeleton it may be heard in any region from the occiput to the lumbar spine.[56] Mitral regurgitant murmurs that radiate well to the back are generally due to incompetence of the anterior leaflet, in which the regurgitant stream is directed posterolaterally into the atrium. Jet lesions on the posterior atrial wall have been correlated with this type of regurgitation.

In recent years the syndrome of mitral regurgitation simulating aortic stenosis has been recognized with increasing frequency.[36,40,50,53] In this variety of mitral regurgitation the jet of blood from the insufficient posterior leaflet is directed toward the atrial septum, where it is adjacent to the aortic valve and aortic root. This murmur will often simulate the murmur of aortic stenosis, both in its location and in its ejection quality.

The syndrome of mitral valve regurgitation due to papillary muscle dysfunction is also associated with an atypical regurgitant murmur.[12,43]

This murmur characteristically begins in mid- to late systole, well after the termination of the first heart sound. It is most often recognized in patients with ischemic heart disease in whom papillary muscle function has been compromised. As pressure develops in the ventricle during ejection the papillary muscles normally have the function of maintaining mitral valve competency, but when the papillary muscles are fibrotic, they cannot maintain the tension necessary to keep the valve leaflets from prolapsing, and mitral regurgitation occurs. In this syndrome the papillary muscles can usually maintain mitral valve leaflet position early in systole, but as the intraventricular pressure rises during systole valvular regurgitation develops, explaining the late onset of the systolic murmur. At necropsy or at operation the papillary muscles in these patients are often totally replaced by fibrous tissue. The posteromedial papillary muscle is affected more often than the anterolateral papillary muscle; this relative incidence no doubt reflects the better collateral circulation to the anterolateral muscle.[19]

Although the murmur of mitral regurgitation is usually blowing in quality, in certain patients the murmur has muscial components. Calcific deposits in the mitral annulus and leaflets, a ruptured chorda, or ballooning of the mitral valve into the left atrium are the usual causes of musical mitral murmurs. It is often quite difficult to distinguish a musical mitral murmur from the musical murmur of aortic stenosis, which may be transmitted to the cardiac apex. At the bedside an examination of the carotid pulse is a useful maneuver in differentiating valvular aortic stenosis from mitral regurgitation. In the former condition the upstroke time is delayed, and there is often an accompanying carotid thrill, while in the latter condition the carotid pulse is brisk.

A short, early to mid-diastolic rumble is also frequently present in patients with severe mitral regurgitation. The rumble occurs during the phase of rapid ventricular filling, and is assumed to be due to torrential flow across the mitral valve.

Drugs that influence hemodynamics will modify auscultatory findings and help to identify the source of cardiac murmurs. The two agents used most frequently for this purpose are amyl nitrite[4,59] and phenylephrine.[1] The inhalation of amyl nitrite produces a biphasic hemodynamic response. In the initial 20 seconds after inhalation systemic vasodilation, hypotension, and tachycardia occur; in the second phase, approximately 45 seconds after inhalation, there is an increase in venous return to the right side of the heart and an increase in cardiac output. The initial fall in pressure in the left ventricle and systemic arterial bed has the following effects on murmurs: 1) the murmur of mitral regurgitation decreases because of a decrease in the left ventricular–left atrial pressure gradient and a consequent reduction in regurgitant flow; 2) the murmur of ventricular septal defect is diminished on account of the fall in left ventricular pressure and the reduction of the pressure gradient and flow across the interventricular septum; and 3) the murmur of patent ductus arteriosus decreases as the pressure gradient and flow from aorta to pulmonary artery diminish. During the second phase after amyl nitrite inhalation, which reaches a maximum approximately 45 seconds after inhalation, there is an increased venous return and an augmentation of cardiac output. Thus, any murmur resulting from flow across a stenotic orifice will be augmented. Therefore 1) the murmur of isolated pulmonary stenosis increases in intensity, 2) the murmur of aortic stenosis increases, and 3) the murmur of tricuspid regurgitation also increases, as the enhanced venous return augments right ventricular filling. These differing effects on cardiac murmurs of diverse origin make amyl nitrite a most useful adjunct to the physical examination of the patient with a systolic murmur. The major drawback to its use is its unpleasant odor, but this can be lessened by prompt disposal of the ampoule after the patient has inhaled from it deeply two or three times. Crushing the ampoule often produces a loud noise, and this should not be performed in close proximity to the patient's face.

Elevation of the blood pressure with vasopressors may also be of benefit in assessing the origin of a systolic murmur. The drugs which have been used most often for this purpose are methoxamine and phenylephrine, as both these agents increase systemic vascular resistance without directly stimulating the heart. Generally a rise in systemic arterial blood pressure of between 40 and 50 mm Hg is produced, with the following effects: 1) The murmur of mitral regurgitation increases, owing to an increase in the left ventricular to left atrial pressure gradient and an augmentation of regurgitant flow per beat. 2) The murmur of ventricular septal defect or patent ductus arteriosus increases because of augmented flow secondary to the enhanced pressure gradient between the left and right sides of the heart. 3) The murmurs of tricuspid regurgitation and aortic stenosis are usually unaffected. The major drawback of the pressor amine infusion is the frequent occurrence of transient headache during the acute elevation of blood pressure.

Electrocardiogram

The electrocardiogram yields limited information in the differential diagnosis of mitral regurgitation.[6] Evidence of left or right ventricular hypertrophy may be present. In patients with sinus rhythm evidence of left atrial enlargement is likely to be found, but the majority of patients with mitral regurgitation have atrial fibrillation.

Chest X-ray

The chest x-ray is of some assistance, but is often not diagnostic of the presence of mitral regurgitation.[44] The left ventricle and left atrium are frequently enlarged, the latter often to gigantic proportions (Fig. 2). The presence of a huge left atrium, at times filling the right chest out to the lateral chest wall, is strong evidence of mitral regurgitation. The syndrome of giant left atrium with normal left atrial pressure[10] has been increasingly

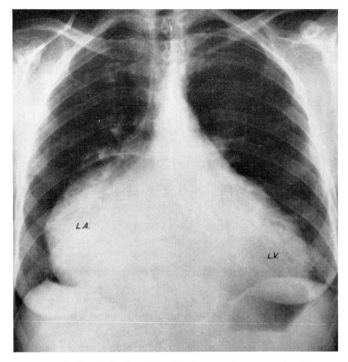

Fig. 2. Patient L. P., with chronic mitral regurgitation. The left atrium (LA) is markedly enlarged, almost filling the entire right chest. LV = left ventricle.

recognized. Symptoms in patients with this syndrome progress slowly over many years, and the major manifestations appear to be those of low cardiac output. Because of the increased compliance of the left atrium, these patients do not develop significant pulmonary hypertension and may not display the usual signs of left heart failure, i.e., pulmonary edema, paroxysmal nocturnal dyspnea, hemoptysis, dyspnea, and orthopnea.

If the diagnosis of mitral regurgitation or an estimation of its severity cannot be made by clinical means, it may be necessary to perform cardiac catheterization studies and left ventricular cineangiography. These special laboratory measures may also be required to distinguish among the various causes of mitral regurgitation.

Catheterization Laboratory Studies

Hemodynamic studies in the majority of patients with mitral regurgitation have shown that the left atrial or pulmonary artery wedge pressures generally exceed the values observed in normal individuals.[48] The V wave is the most prominent wave in the left atrial pressure pulse, and this wave may at times be recognized in the pulmonary artery pressure pulse.[55] Following the opening of the mitral valve there is a rapid Y descent, reflecting the rapid emptying of the overdistended left atrium. In spite of a normal-sized mitral orifice there is frequently a left atrial to left ventricular gradient during the first 100 to 200 milliseconds following mitral valve opening. The left ventricular end diastolic pressure may be normal, but as the course of the disease progresses it is common for the end diastolic pressure to become elevated. Early in the course of the disease the cardiac output at rest may be normal and may increase appropriately with moderate exercise. Later, as the left ventricle fails, the cardiac output may become subnormal, even at rest.

Indicator dilution curves are helpful in establishing the diagnosis of mitral regurgitation. Prompt appearance of dye in the left atrium following left ventricular injection denotes leakage at the mitral valve. When sampling is performed from the brachial artery the indicator dilution curve characteristically ascends rapidly but exhibits a gradual descending limb as indicator is washed back and forth between the left ventricle and left atrium.

Angiography with injection of contrast medium into the left ventricle is the most effective means of establishing the diagnosis.

ETIOLOGY OF MITRAL REGURGITATION

Once the diagnosis of mitral regurgitation is established an investigation into its etiology is of importance. In a number of congenital and acquired cardiac diseases mitral regurgitation is the major pathophysiologic disturbance. Table 2 lists many of these conditions. Since the prognosis and the therapy in many of these diseases are different, a definition of the etiology of mitral regurgitation is of more than academic interest.

Congenital Mitral Regurgitation[25]

Congenital mitral regurgitation occurs most frequently as part of a more complex cardiac lesion. Thus, it occurs frequently with endocardial cushion defect, endocardial fibroelastosis, the Marfan syndrome, or as a secondary phenomenon in patients with an anomalous origin of the left coronary artery from the pulmonary artery. Although these lesions are usually recognized in the pediatric age group, occasionally mitral regurgitation due to one of these etiologies may be first recognized in a young adult. If mitral regurgitation is the major hemodynamic abnormality the clinical picture may be indistinguishable from that of rheumatic mitral regurgitation.

Isolated Congenital Mitral Regurgitation

Congenital mitral regurgitation may occur as an isolated lesion. In this setting several anomalies of the mitral valve have been described, such as cleft leaflets, fused and fixed valve leaflets, anomalous insertion of the chordae tendineae, perforated valve leaflet, shortened or defective valve tissue, double orifice of the mitral valve, and an Ebstein type of valve anomaly.[9]

TABLE 2

Etiology of Mitral Regurgitation. There are a large number of disease states in which mitral regurgitation is a prominent feature.

Congenital
  1. Congenital mitral regurgitation
      a. Isolated lesion
      b. As part of atrioventricular canal
  2. Endocardial fibroelastosis
  3. The Marfan syndrome
  4. Anomalous left coronary artery from the pulmonary artery
  5. The Ehlers-Danlos syndrome
  6. Corrected transposition of the great arteries with Ebstein's anomaly of the left atrioventricular valve
  7. Idiopathic hypertrophic subaortic stenosis
Acquired
  1. Rheumatic valvulitis
  2. Bacterial endocarditis
  3. Ruptured mitral chordae tendineae
  4. Papillary muscle rupture or dysfunction
  5. Calcified mitral annulus fibrosus
  6. Secondary to left ventricular dilation

Atrioventricular Canal

Mitral regurgitation may at times be the most prominent feature of an endocardial cushion defect. In the complete form of endocardial cushion defect the complex of an atrial septal defect, a ventricular septal defect, a common atrioventricular valve, and often subaortic stenosis due to anomalous chordae tendineae may be present. More commonly only a part of this complex exists, and an atrial septal defect with cleft anterior mitral valve leaflet may be the sole anatomic abnormalities. The finding of a holosystolic murmur at the apex radiating to the axilla in a patient with fixed splitting of the second heart sound suggests this diagnosis. An electrocardiogram showing left axis deviation, deep S waves in leads II, III, and AVF, partial bundle branch block, and a long P-R interval provides supporting evidence. The QRS vector in the frontal plane usually describes a counterclockwise loop above the isoelectric point, or a figure-of-eight loop in the horizontal plane.[13] The precise diagnosis of atrioventricular canal is important in dealing with mitral regurgitation in childhood. Thus, in partial atrioventricular canal, the surgeon has only to correct a cleft anterior leaflet of the mitral valve and an interatrial communication. This operation is most often curative and can be performed at a very acceptable risk. However, operation in the complete form of atrioventricular canal carries a much higher risk. An interventricular communication is often present, and the bundle of His runs along the upper margin of the defect. Heart block is an acknowledged complication of operation under these circumstances. It is also important to identify the abnormal chordae tendineae which may be present in atrioventricular canal.[17] These must be divided, or the chordae may restrict the motion of the mitral valve, prohibiting complete closure during ventricular systole. Cardiac catheterization with angiography remains the most useful means of assessing these anatomic abnormalities.

Endocardial Fibroelastosis and Mitral Regurgitation

The etiology of endocardial fibroelastosis is not known. Moller et al.[37] found evidence of mitral regurgitation in each of their cases of fibroelastosis in which associated anomalies of the aortic valve, coronary arteries, or aorta were absent. In this disease the endocardium is made up of collagen and elastic fibers and the opaque gray layer is sufficiently thick to be identified readily. The left ventricle may be either dilated or hypoplastic. Mitral regurgitation is usually associated with abnormal placement of the papillary muscles high on the left ventricular wall. The development of tension in these muscles tends to keep the mitral valve leaflets open, and mitral regurgitation is common. In general this is a disease of infants, and few patients survive into the second decade of life.

The Marfan Syndrome[52]

The manifestations of the Marfan syndrome are skeletal, ocular, and cardiovascular, associated clinical features being arachnodactyly, high arched palate, iridodonesis, and long thin habitus. The characteristic cardiovascular malformations in this syndrome include aortic regurgitation, fusiform dilation of the aorta, dissecting aneurysm, rupture of the aorta, and histologic abnormalities of the pulmonary artery and the large systemic arteries. The most common valvular lesion associated with the Marfan syndrome is aortic regurgitation, but mitral regurgitation has been recognized with increasing frequency. In some of these patients mitral regurgitation is due to myxomatous transformation of the mitral valve (floppy valve syndrome),[45] while in others long mitral chordae tendineae are present. It now appears to be relatively common for patients with histologically proven Marfan syndrome not to conform to the prototype of a tall, thin "Abe Lincoln" physique. Recognition of this syndrome is of particular importance, since the operative risk is relatively high, the generalized disease of the connective tissues resulting in delayed healing and postoperative complications.

Anomalous Left Coronary Artery from Pulmonary Artery[8,24]

In this anomaly abnormal partitioning of the fetal truncus causes the left coronary artery to be included in that portion destined to be the pulmonary artery. Early in fetal life the left ventricular myocardium is perfused by the anomalous vessel and receives unsaturated blood from the high-pressure pulmonary artery. After birth, as the pulmonary arterial pressure falls, the perfusion pressure to the myocardium also diminishes. This neonatal stage is very critical, and survival of the infant depends largely upon the development of adequate collateral channels from the right coronary artery. It is common at this stage of the disease for electro-cardiographic signs of subendocardial ischemia to be apparent. The papillary muscles are quite susceptible to ischemic damage, since their blood supply is derived from terminal branches of the coronary arteries. The onset of mitral regurgitation due to papillary muscle damage is a frequent occurrence during this period of prolonged ischemia. If a sizable collateral network between right coronary artery and anomalous left coronary artery does form, the anomalous coronary vessel may then carry blood retrograde into the pulmonary artery and act as a left-to-right shunt. Although it is uncommon, patients with anomalous left coronary artery at times survive into adulthood. In such individuals mitral regurgitation may be due both to papillary muscle damage and to ventricular dilation. In a young individual with mitral regurgitation, evidence of myocardial damage, and sometimes a continuous murmur in addition to the murmur of mitral regurgitation, anomalous left coronary artery must be considered.

Ehlers-Danlos Syndrome

The most striking feature of this disease is related to the cutis, although its manifestations involve different organ systems. Characteristically the skin is velvety in appearance and to the touch; it is hyperelastic and often redundant. Wound healing is very slow and bruising is common. The joints are hyperextensible, often to an incredible degree, and these individuals are frequently the "India rubber men" in circus sideshows.[35] The internal organs are often affected; aneurysm of the aorta has been reported, and mitral regurgitation also has been described[31] in a patient with this disease. At postmortem examination in the latter patient the mitral valve showed a decrease in the number of elastic fibers and an increase in the ground substance and vascularity. Although the number of documented cases of this syndrome is relatively small, the true incidence is probably higher. In patients with mild degrees of the syndrome it can easily be overlooked, and this entity should enter into the differential diagnosis of any patient with mitral regurgitation of unknown etiology.

Corrected Transposition of the Great Arteries with Ebstein's Anomaly of the Left Atrioventricular Valve

This anomaly is also quite rare, but regurgitation at the left-sided atrioventricular valve is common in corrected transposition, and therefore this condition deserves mention in any discussion of mitral regurgitation.[16] Although the systemic atrioventricular valve is tricuspid, it is located between the left atrium and the systemic ventricle, and is displaced downward into the systemic ventricle. The altered embryologic development of the heart with corrected transposition predisposes to abnormalities of this valve. Although the diagnosis is most often confirmed at cardiac catheterization, there are certain clinical points which suggest the diagnosis. Since the pulmonic valve is located further to the right and is more distant from the anterior chest wall than normally, the second component of the second heart sound is often soft. The aortic valve is more superficially located and is displaced further to the left than normally. Therefore, the aortic closure sound is well heard in the third left intercostal space, and the erroneous conclusion that pulmonary hypertension is present may be reached. First-degree heart block is very common, and second- or third-degree heart block also occurs. Because of the reversal in direction of ventricular septal depolarization the right precordial electrocardiographic leads often show a qR or qRs pattern, while the left precordial leads demonstrate an rS or RS pattern. The absence of a Q wave in V_5 or V_6 should also raise suspicion of this lesion. In a patient with a known apical murmur from birth and the clinical and electrocardiographic findings noted, corrected transposition with Ebstein's anomaly of the mitral valve should be considered.

Idiopathic Hypertrophic Subaortic Stenosis

Mitral regurgitation occurs in at least half of all patients with idiopathic hypertrophic subaortic stenosis. It is therefore not surprising that many patients with this entity are diagnosed as having rheumatic mitral regurgitation. Certain clinical features, however, should raise the suspicion of IHSS even if there is concomitant mitral regurgitation. The patient is very often in the third decade or younger and has no history of rheumatic fever. Angina pectoris or syncope may be present, and both these symptoms are unusual in rheumatic mitral regurgitation. The carotid arteries have a brisk upstroke and may even have a bisferiens quality. The jugular venous pulse has a large A wave. There is frequently a double apical impulse in the left lateral position. The second heart sound may be paradoxically split, and a ventricular diastolic gallop and an atrial gallop may be present. Although the murmur may be holosystolic at the apex, generally it takes on an ejection quality along the left sternal border. The electrocardiogram is often bizarre, with Q waves in the standard or precordial leads, and normal sinus rhythm is usually present.

Angiographic studies[51] have suggested that the protrusion of the inferior portion of the septal mass causes an angulation of the left ventricular cavity and a change of axis of the papillary muscles. The papillary muscles are displaced and cause abnormal traction on the chordae tendineae, and hence on the mitral valve leaflets, during systole. Thus, the leaflets do not complete their normal excursion from the outflow tract during systole and contribute to the posterior component of the obstruction. This restricted motion of the mitral leaflets may also cause mitral regurgitation. The complete elimination of severe mitral regurgitation in a patient with IHSS who underwent an outflow tract and septal myomectomy at the National Heart Institute tends to support the hypothesis that the mitral regurgitation is related to restricted motion of the valve leaflets.

Acquired Mitral Regurgitation

Rheumatic Valvulitis

By far the most common cause of mitral regurgitation is rheumatic valvulitis. This lesion, in contrast to mitral stenosis, occurs more commonly in males. The murmur characteristically develops at the time of the acute episode of rheumatic fever or chorea. This is in contrast to the murmur of mitral stenosis, which is often not detected until some time after the acute episode. The frequency with which a history of acute rheumatic fever or chorea can be elicited depends upon the acuity of both the physician and the patient. A careful history will elicit an episode of rheumatic fever in over half of patients with rheumatic mitral valvulitis. Concurrent involvement of the aortic valve favors a rheumatic etiology. In general rheumatic mitral regurgitation is well tolerated, patients often remaining symptom-free for up to 20 years after the establishment of mitral regurgitation. Once symptoms do occur, they are often rapidly progressive, and patients may become severely incapacitated over the course of only a few years.

As outlined previously, the cardinal features of the physical examination are a systolic thrill at the apex, a hyperdynamic left ventricular heave, and the holosystolic murmur which is the hallmark of the lesion. A low-pitched third heart sound is invariably present 0.12 to 0.17 second after the aortic component of the second sound, and it often initiates a rumbling mid-diastolic murmur.

The clinical and hemodynamic picture in the patient with acquired mitral regurgitation is largely dependent upon the size and compliance characteristics of the left atrium and the pulmonary venous bed.[10] On this basis three major groups of patients with mitral regurgitation can be identified (Fig. 3):

1. Patients with marked elevation of atrial pressure leading to significant elevation of pulmonary vascular resistance and pulmonary hypertension. Symptoms of right-sided congestive heart failure are common in these patients. In general this picture is seen more frequently in patients who have a sudden onset of mitral regurgitation.

2. Patients who demonstrate modest increases in left atrial pressures and moderate to massive enlargement of the left atrium. This is by far the most common picture, and while these patients may at times have signs of right-sided failure, more often they complain of fatigue and exhaustion, reflecting low cardiac output.

3. Patients who develop compliant, massively enlarged left atria. These patients may have normal pressures in the left atrium and pulmonary venous bed, but invariably they exhibit the signs and symptoms of low cardiac output. Right ventricular hypertrophy is extremely rare.[7]

The rheumatic process produces deformity of the valve cusps as well as shortening of the chordae tendineae. It should be further emphasized that

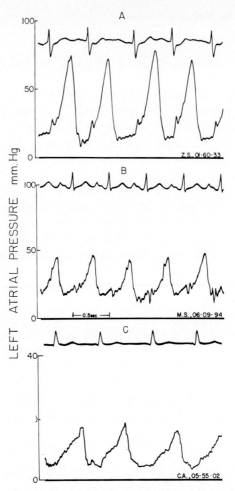

Fig. 3. The spectrum of left atrial pressure in patients with mitral regurgitation. Panel *A*, patient Z. S., showing markedly elevated V waves to 80 mm Hg, reflecting severe mitral regurgitation into a noncompliant atrium. Panel *B*, patient M. S. There is left atrial hypertension with V waves of 50 mm Hg. Panel *C*, patient C. A. In spite of severe mitral regurgitation, V waves are 18 mm Hg. This low pressure in spite of marked mitral regurgitation reflects a very compliant left atrium.

mitral regurgitation tends to be a gradually progressive disease, since enlargement of the left atrium places tension on the posterior mitral leaflet, pulling it away from the mitral orifice and thereby aggravating and augmenting the leakage. Similarly, the dilation of the left ventricle increases the regurgitation, which in turn further enlarges the left atrium and ventricle.

Bacterial Endocarditis

Bacterial endocarditis seems to have a predilection for patients with mild mitral regurgitation, and its occurrence may change a mild leak into massive regurgitation. In addition to the development of specific therapy, recent years have witnessed modification of the picture of bacterial endocarditis in several ways: 1) The treatment of streptococcal pharyngitis has resulted in a decline in rheumatic fever and rheumatic valvulitis; therefore the incidence of bacterial endocarditis has declined, since its most common antecedent is prior damage to a valve. 2) The increased life expectancy of the population has brought a clear shift in the age incidence of bacterial endocarditis. The average patient who develops bacterial endocarditis is now 10 years older than he was generation ago.[26] In elderly patients special difficulties have been encountered in making an early diagnosis. Thus, many of the subtle signs and symptoms of bacterial endocarditis may be attributed in these individuals to the aging process and concomitant degenerative phenomena. Low-grade fever, anemia, anorexia, weight loss, arthritis, unexplained uremia, mild cerebrovascular accident, personality changes, or optic neuritis in the elderly are often attributed to other processes. 3) With the advent of open heart surgery and the placement of prosthetic valves or patches, eradication of bacterial endocarditis is extremely difficult once the infection implants on the prosthetic foreign material.

The mitral and aortic valves are affected by bacterial endocarditis with about equal frequency, and the appearance of the murmur of mitral regurgitation may be the first clue to the presence of bacterial endocarditis. In any patient, therefore, with either a new murmur of mitral regurgitation or a changing murmur, multiple blood cultures should be drawn. Changing murmurs are a poor prognostic sign, as they usually indicate progressive valvular destruction, a sign of a well-established infection. It must be recognized that some patients with bacterial endocarditis may have consistently negative blood cultures, and antibiotic therapy must often be initiated and continued if the clinical picture strongly suggests endocarditis.

Ruptured Chordae Tendineae

Although the majority of ruptured chordae have been considered to be due to rheumatic fever,[21] trauma,[3] or bacterial endocarditis,[41] several reports have pointed out the frequency with which spontaneous rupture of normal mitral chordae tendineae occurs.[2,21,33,47,49] In cases in which blunt trauma to the chest initiates a systolic murmur in a previously healthy individual the diagnosis of mitral regurgitation is fairly secure. When during the course of acute bacterial endocarditis a new murmur at the cardiac apex occurs, a ruptured mitral chorda may be responsible, even though perforation of a valve leaflet leads to the same clinical picture. Although the etiology may be infection, trauma, or spontaneous, the clinical picture of acute mitral regurgitation differs from that of chronic rheumatic mitral regurgitation. Certain features, especially in the physical examination, point to the acute nature of the lesion.

1. Sinus rhythm is extremely common, and, in addition, an atrial gallop sound is frequently heard. Of 51 patients with severe mitral regurgitation,

only 6 of 40 with a rheumatic etiology were in sinus rhythm while all 11 with ruptured chordae were in sinus rhythm. Of the 6 patients with a rheumatic etiology who were in sinus rhythm, none had atrial gallop sounds. Nine of the 11 patients with ruptured mitral chordae tendineae had atrial gallop sounds.[14] At least a part of the explanation for the occurrence of an atrial gallop sound in patients with ruptured chordae tendineae may be found in the shorter time course of their disease. In patients with chronic rheumatic mitral regurgitation the left atrium is distended slowly but persistently. It is likely that the atrial gallop sound is dependent upon a vigorous atrial contraction, and the chronically diseased, thin-walled, dilated atrium may not be capable of generating a contraction of sufficient force to produce a fourth heart sound.

2. The murmur associated with sudden rupture of mitral chordae tendineae often radiates to the second right intercostal space in the usual distribution of the murmur of aortic stenosis. There appears to be a predilection for rupture of posterior leaflet chordae, and the regurgitant jet causes vibration and turbulence along the septal wall of the left atrium. This location is immediately posterior to the aorta, and the sound is transmitted to the chest wall in the aortic area.

3. Generally there is only mild cardiomegaly, and the left atrium is of normal size or only mildly enlarged.

4. Abrupt onset of congestive heart failure is much more common in acute mitral regurgitation than in cases of chronic rheumatic valvular disease.

5. A systolic murmur ending in midsystole has been described in a case of severe acute mitral regurgitation.[54] In association with the markedly elevated left atrial V wave there is equilibration of left atrial and left ventricular pressures in midsystole, and no further regurgitation occurs.

6. A picture mimicking constrictive pericarditis has been reported in four patients with acute mitral regurgitation.[5] The findings were felt to reflect constriction of the heart by the pericardium when a volume load was acutely imposed. The nearly identical diastolic pressure curves in the two ventricles as well as in the atria were considered evidence that a common membrane, the pericardium, was limiting diastolic expansion.

Although these features may not be present in each instance of acute mitral regurgitation, recognition of one or two of them may lead to the correct diagnosis. The differentiation of acute from chronic mitral regurgitation may be important, as the operative approach in the acute cases may at times be through repair of chordae rather than valve replacement.

Papillary Muscle Rupture or Dysfunction

Rupture of a left ventricular papillary muscle is an uncommon but well-recognized complication of acute myocardial infarction.[38] The papillary muscles, being subendocardial structures, are supplied by terminal branches of the coronary arteries. Posteromedial papillary muscle rupture is approximately 6 times as common as anterolateral papillary muscle rupture. In the majority of hearts the blood supply of the posteromedial papillary muscle is derived from the posterior descending branch of the right coronary artery. The collateral circulation is generally poor, and occlusion of the right coronary artery may lead to severe acute ischemia of this muscle. The anterolateral papillary muscle is usually supplied by one or more branches from the left anterior descending artery and by marginal tributaries from the circumflex branch of the left coronary artery. Collateral circulation to the anterolateral muscle is generally more abundant.

Each left ventricular papillary muscle usually originates as a single belly, then divides into a variable number of apical heads, from which chordae tendineae of the first order arise. It is likely that rupture of the central muscle belly is incompatible with survival in any patient, since approximately half the support to each valve leaflet is destroyed, and regurgitation of overwhelming severity results. The regurgitant flow which follows rupture of one or more apical heads is often of lesser magnitude, and although regurgitation may be severe, immediate survival is dependent upon the degree to which the function of the left ventricle has been impaired by the infarct (Fig. 4). Although the prognosis must remain guarded in any patient who develops papillary muscle rupture, early recognition of this complication, vigorous supportive therapy, and operative intervention may alter the outcome.

The development of a late systolic murmur with a diamond-shaped configuration in a patient with a recent myocardial infarction suggests papillary muscle dysfunction.[12,43] The murmur is usually not holosystolic, in that the papillary muscles are able to maintain sufficient tension during

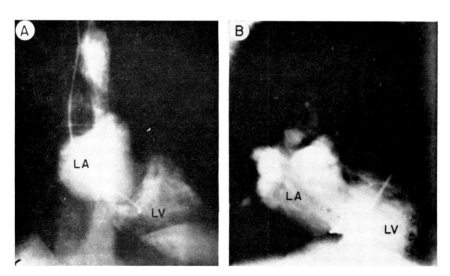

Fig. 4. Left ventriculogram in patient P. I. The injection into the left ventricle (LV) demonstrates massive regurgitation into the left atrium (LA) and pulmonary veins. This patient had rupture of an apical head of a papillary muscle.

ventricular isovolumetric contraction to keep the mitral valve competent. As pressure builds up within the ventricle the fibrotic papillary muscle cannot maintain adequate tension, and the valve leaflets balloon into the atrium. The lesion is generally well tolerated, but, as in papillary muscle rupture, the impairment of the left ventricle that results from underlying ischemic heart disease often determines the clinical outcome.

Calcified Mitral Annulus Fibrosus

A minor degree of calcification of the mitral annulus can be found at routine autopsy examinations in approximately 10 per cent of adult patients. Massive calcification of the annulus without any evidence of previous rheumatic inflammatory disease was found in 0.2 per cent of an autopsy population 51 years of age and older.[27] This entity is more common in women, and although often an incidental autopsy finding, it may be the cause of significant mitral regurgitation or stenosis.

If carefully sought, a characteristic J or U shape can be identified radiographically (Fig. 5). In an elderly woman with no previous history of rheumatic disease this finding is almost diagnostic of this condition. Although the etiology is not certain, it is likely that the calcification process is related to aging and to local degenerative changes in the valve skeleton.

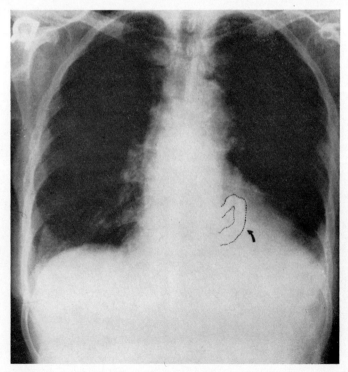

FIG. 5. Patient C. H. The area indicated by the dots is a heavily calcified mitral valve annulus.

Secondary to Ventricular Dilation

A wide variety of disorders leading to left ventricular dilation will result in varying degrees of mitral regurgitation. The ventricular dilation leads to disordered alignment of the papillary muscles and chordae tendineae, resulting in an abnormal mitral valve mechanism. Aortic valve disease, particularly aortic regurgitation, cardiomyopathy, coronary artery disease, hypertension, and anemia are but a few of the many causes of ventricular dilation which may lead to mitral regurgitation. In general the degree of mitral regurgitation caused by ventricular dilation is not severe, and the manifestations of the underlying heart disease are more prominent.

CONCLUSION

As indicated previously, the approach to the patient with mitral regurgitation resolves itself into two general lines of investigation. A variety of conditions other than mitral regurgitation may cause a systolic murmur (Table 1). In general cardiac catheterization is carried out in order to establish a diagnosis, or in preparation for operation.

In patients with established mitral regurgitation of congenital origin (Table 2) cardiac catheterization is usually indicated in order to define fully the extent of the associated cardiac lesion. In patients with acquired mitral regurgitation it has been our practice to defer cardiac catheterization until symptoms become sufficiently severe to warrant operative intervention. The approach to the patient with suspected or proved mitral regurgitation must be flexible, as the natural history of mitral regurgitation in different patients may be extremely variable.

REFERENCES

1. Abrams, W. B., Bernstein, A., and Pocelinko, R. The effects of drugs on heart sounds and murmurs. In *The Theory and Practice of Auscultation*, B. Segal, W. Likoff, and J. Moyer, Eds., p. 545. F. A. Davis Co., Philadelphia, 1964.
2. Bailey, O. T., and Hickam, J. B. Rupture of mitral chordae tendineae. Clinical and pathologic observations on seven cases in which there was no bacterial endocarditis. Amer. Heart J. 28:578, 1944.
3. Barber, H. The effects of trauma, direct and indirect, on the heart. Quart. J. Med. 13:137, 1944.
4. Barlow, J., and Shillingford, J. The use of amyl nitrite in differentiating mitral and aortic systolic murmurs. Brit. Heart J., 20:162, 1958.
5. Bartle, S. H., and Hermann, H. J. Acute mitral regurgitation in man. Hemodynamic evidence and observations indicating an early role for the pericardium. Circulation 36:839, 1967.
6. Bentivoglio, L. G., Uricchio, J. F., Waldow, A., Litsoff, W., and Goldberg, H. An electrocardiographic analysis of 65 cases of mitral regurgitation. Circulation 18:572, 1958.
7. Best, P. V., and Heath, D. The right ventricle and small pulmonary arteries in aneurysmal dilatation of the left atrium. Brit. Heart J. 26:312, 1964.
8. Bland, E. F., White, P. D., and Garland, J. Congenital anomalies of the coronary arteries: report of an unusual case associated with cardiac hypertrophy. Amer. Heart J. 8:787, 1933.
9. Braunwald, E., Ross, R. S., Morrow, A. G., and Roberts, W. C. Differential diagnosis of mitral regurgitation in childhood. Ann. Intern. Med. 54:1223, 1961.

10. Braunwald, E., and Awe, W. C. The syndrome of severe mitral regurgitation with normal left atrial pressure. Circulation 27:29, 1963.
11. Braunwald, E., Lambrew, C. T., Rockoff, S. D., Ross, J., Jr., and Morrow, A. G. Idiopathic hypertrophic subaortic stenosis. I. Description of the disease based upon an analysis of 64 patients. Circulation 30(Suppl. IV): 1964.
12. Burch, G. E., DePasquale, N. P., and Phillips, J. H. Clinical manifestations of papillary muscle dysfunction. Arch. Intern. Med. 112:112, 1963.
13. Burchell, H. B., DuShane, J. W., and Brandenburg, R. O. Electrocardiogram of patients with atrioventricular cushion defects (defects of atrioventricular canal). Amer. J. Cardiol. 6:575, 1960.
14. Cohen, L. S., Mason, D. T., and Braunwald, E. Significance of an atrial gallop sound in mitral regurgitation. Circulation 35:112, 1967.
15. Corvisart, J. N. An Essay on the Organic Diseases and Lesions of the Heart and Great Vessels. Bradford and Reed, Boston, 1812.
16. Edwards, J. E. Differential diagnosis of mitral stenosis: a clinicopathologic review of simulating conditions. Lab. Invest. 3:89, 1954.
17. Edwards, J. E. The problems of mitral insufficiency caused by accessory chordae tendineae in persistent common atrio-ventricular canal. Proc. Staff Meet. Mayo Clin. 35:299, 1960.
18. Edwards, J. E., and Burchell, H. B. Endocardial and intimal lesions (jet impact) as possible sites of origin of murmurs. Circulation 18:946, 1958.
19. Estes, E. H., Jr., Dalton, F. M., Entman, M. L., Dixon, H. B., and Hackel, D. B. The anatomy and blood supply of the papillary muscles of the left ventricle. Amer. Heart J. 71:356, 1966.
20. Frank, S., and Braunwald, E. Idiopathic hypertrophic subaortic stenosis. A clinical analysis of 126 patients with emphasis on the natural history. Circulation 37:759, 1968.
21. Frothingham, C., and Hass, G. Rupture of normal chordae tendineae of the mitral valve. Amer. Heart J. 9:492, 1934.
22. Harvey, W. P. Heart sounds and murmurs. Circulation 30:262, 1964.
23. Harvey, W. P., Corrado, M., and Perloff, J. Some newer or poorly recognized auscultatory findings of the heart. Circulation 16:414, 1957.
24. Kaunitz, P. E. Origin of left coronary artery from pulmonary. Review of the literature and report of two cases. Amer. Heart. J. 33:182, 1947.
25. Keith, J. D. Congenital mitral insufficiency. Progr. Cardiovasc. Dis. 5:264, 1962.
26. Kerr, A., Jr. Bacterial endocarditis revisited. Mod. Concepts Cardiovasc. Dis. 33:831, 1964.
27. Korn, D., DeSanctis, R. W., and Sell, S. Massive calcification of the mitral annulus. New Engl. J. Med. 267:900, 1962.
28. Laënnec, R. T. H. A Treatise on Diseases of the Chest and on Mediate Auscultation. James Webster, Philadelphia, 1823.
29. Leon, D. F., Leonard, J. J., Lancaster, J. F., Kroetz, F. W., and Shaver, J. A. Effect of respiration on pansystolic regurgitant murmurs as studied by biatrial intracardiac phonocardiography. Amer. J. Med. 39:429, 1965.
30. Levine, S. A., and Harvey, W. P. Clinical Auscultation of the Heart, 2nd ed., p. 542. W. B. Saunders Co., Philadelphia, 1959.
31. Madison, W. M., Jr., Bradley, E. J., and Castillo, A. J. Ehlers-Danlos syndrome with cardiac involvement. Amer. J. Cardiol. 11:689, 1963.
32. Manchester, G. H., Block, P., and Gorlin, R. Misleading signs in mitral insufficiency. J.A.M.A. 191:99, 1965.
33. Marchand, P., Barlow, J. B., DuPlessis, L. A., and Webster, I. Mitral regurgitation with rupture of normal chordae tendineae. Brit. Heart J. 28:746, 1966.
34. McKusick, V. Cardiovascular Sound in Health and Disease, p. 316. The Williams & Wilkins Co., Baltimore, 1958.
35. McKusick, V. A. Heritable Disorders of Connective Tissue, 2nd ed., p. 143. The C. V. Mosby Co., St. Louis, 1960.
36. Miller, R., Jr., and Pearson, R. J., Jr. Mitral insufficiency simulating aortic stenosis. New Engl. J. Med. 260:1210, 1959.
37. Moller, J. H., Lucas, R. V., Jr., Adams, P. A., Jr., Anderson, R. C., Jorgens, J., and Edwards, J. E. Endocardial fibroelastosis. A clinical and anatomic study of 47 patients with emphasis on its relationship to mitral insufficiency. Circulation 30:759, 1964.

38. Morrow, A. G., Cohen, L. S., Roberts, W. C., Braunwald, N. S., and Braunwald, E. Severe mitral regurgitation following acute myocardial infarction and ruptured papillary muscle. Circulation 37(Suppl. II):124, 1968.

39. Nixon, P., Wooler, G., and Radigan, L. The opening snap in mitral incompetence. Brit. Heart J. 22:395, 1960.

40. Osmundson, P. J., Callahan, J. A., and Edwards, J. E. Mitral insufficiency from ruptured chordae tendineae simulating aortic stenosis. Proc. Staff Meet. Mayo Clin. 35:235, 1958.

41. Osmundson, P. J., Callahan, J. A., and Edwards, J. E. Ruptured mitral chordae tendineae. Circulation 23:42, 1961.

42. Perloff, J. K., and Harvey, W. P.: Auscultatory and phonocardiographic manifestations of pure mitral regurgitation. Progr. Cardiovasc. Dis. 5:172, 1962.

43. Phillips, J. H., Burch, G. E., and DePasquale, N. P. The syndrome of papillary muscle dysfunction. Its clinical recognition. Ann. Intern. Med. 59:508, 1963.

44. Priest, E. A., Finlayson, J. K., and Short, D. S. The x-ray manifestations in the heart and lungs of mitral regurgitation. Progr. Cardiovasc. Dis. 5:219, 1962.

45. Read, R. C., Thal, A. P., and Wendt, V. E. Symptomatic valvular myxomatous transformation (the floppy valve syndrome). A possible forme fruste of the Marfan syndrome. Circulation 32:897, 1965.

46. Rivero Carvallo, J. M. Signo para el diagnostico de las insuficiencias tricuspideas. Arch. Inst. Cardiol. Mex. 16:531, 1946.

47. Roberts, W. C., Braunwald, E., and Morrow, A. G. Acute severe mitral regurgitation secondary to ruptured chordae tendineae. Circulation 33:58, 1966.

48. Ross, J., Jr., Braunwald, E., and Morrow, A. G. Clinical and hemodynamic observations in pure mitral insufficiency. Amer. J. Cardiol. 2:11, 1958.

49. Selzer, A., Kelly, J. J. Jr., Vannitamby, M., Walker, P., Gerbode, F., and Kerth, W. J. The syndrome of mitral insufficiency due to isolated rupture of the chordae tendineae. Amer. J. Med. 43:822, 1967.

50. Shapiro, H. A., and Weiss, D. R. Mitral insufficiency due to ruptured chordae tendineae simulating aortic stenosis. New Engl. J. Med. 261:272, 1959.

51. Simon, A. L. Ross, J., Jr., and Gault, J. H. Angiographic anatomy of the left ventricle and mitral valve in idiopathic hypertrophic subaortic stenosis. Circulation 36:852, 1967.

52. Sinclair, R. The Marfan syndrome. Quart. J. Med. 29:19, 1960.

53. Sleeper, J. C., Orgain, E. S., and McIntosh, H. D. Mitral insufficiency simulating aortic stenosis. Circulation 26:428, 1962.

54. Sutton, G. C., and Craige, E. Clinical signs of severe acute mitral regurgitation. Amer. J. Cardiol. 20:141, 1967.

55. Tatooles, C. J., Gault, J. H., Mason, D. T., and Ross, J., Jr. Reflux of oxygenated blood into the pulmonary artery in severe mitral regurgitation. Amer. Heart J. 75:102, 1968.

56. Turrettini, G. De la propagation insolite et lointaine du souffle de l'insuffisance mitrale. Arch. Mal Coeur Vaisseaux 15:489, 1922.

57. Vander Veer, J. B. Mitral insufficiency, historical and clinical aspects. Amer. J. Cardiol. 2:5, 1958.

58. Vieussens, R. Traité nouveau de la structure et des causes. Mouvement naturel du coeur. Jean Guillemette, Toulouse, 1715 (quoted by White, P. D., Heart Disease, 4th ed. The Macmillan Co., New York, 1951).

59. Vogelpoel, L., Nellen, M., Swanepoel, A. and Schire, V., The use of amyl nitrite in the diagnosis of systolic murmurs. Lancet 2:810, 1959.

60. Wood, P. Diseases of the Heart and Circulation, 2nd ed., p. 506. J. B. Lippincott Co., Philadelphia, 1956.

Aortic Regurgitation

JEREMIAH A. BARONDESS

Aortic regurgitation, a common type of valvular heart disease which may be found at any age, may be caused by a number of underlying pathologic processes. The physiologic effects may be profound, and are often life-limiting. With significant and increasing frequency, however, the process affecting the aortic valve may be treated effectively, with resultant arrest or elimination of a hemodynamic abnormality which may otherwise be progressive. Specific diagnosis of the etiologic basis of the valve lesion thus assumes therapeutic importance. This is in addition to its evident relation to clinical competence, and its value in aiding understanding of a number of congenital and acquired disorders associated with aortic valve disease.

Cowper[31] first called clinical attention to aortic regurgitation in 1705, and noted that ". . . these valves give that assistance to the heart in its office that it cannot be without, and . . . it gradually suffers according to their indisposition." Hodgkin[70] noted cusp eversion and laceration as causes of aortic incompetence in 1829; he described the *bruit de scie*, or musical murmur, and commented upon the occurrence of angina pectoris and the relative infrequency of cardiac irregularity in these patients. Corrigan's communication,[30] in 1832, pointed out various types of valvular lesions that may be associated with aortic regurgitation, including cusp fenestration or perforation and cusp rupture, as well as relative incompetence of the valve due to dilation of the root of the aorta. He noted the associated visible bounding pulsations of major superficial arteries and the characteristics of the peripheral arterial pulse with which his name has since been linked. Flint's description of an apical murmur simulating that of mitral stenosis in cases of aortic regurgitation was published in 1862[43] and amplified in 1883[44] and 1886.[45]

Studies in recent years have helped to develop understanding of many of the clinical, physiologic, and pathologic features of aortic regurgitation, and have strengthened consideration of this process as a more or less discrete presenting syndrome. Diagnostic analysis of the disorder was aided by Hamman's arrangement of the causes into eight categories, namely rheumatic, syphilitic, bacterial, calcific, congenital, arteriosclerotic, relative, and traumatic.[61] This approach was developed further by Harvey and Bordley.[62] Clinical and pathologic studies in recent years have defined new and previously unrecognized etiologic relationships in aortic regurgitation, and an effort has been made in the present chapter to include these in an expanded categorization of the causes of this disorder.

JEREMIAH A. BARONDESS, M.D. Clinical Professor of Medicine, Cornell University Medical College; Attending Physician, New York Hospital, New York

THE DIAGNOSIS OF AORTIC REGURGITATION

The diagnosis of aortic regurgitation is based primarily on the finding of a diastolic murmur, usually of characteristic quality and location, and often, but not invariably, associated with other evidence of central diastolic runoff of blood from the arterial tree. The signs of this lesion may vary considerably, however. In addition, murmurs identical with those of aortic regurgitation may be produced by pulmonic insufficiency and some other conditions. The peripheral circulatory signs suggesting aortic regurgitation may also be noted in a variety of disorders characterized by widening of the pulse pressure. Included in this group are such structural defects as aortico-pulmonary communications, communications between the aorta and various cardiac chambers, arteriovenous fistulae, and conditions such as high fever, anemia, pregnancy, hyperthyroidism, and other states characterized by high stroke volume and/or peripheral vasodilation. Hence, the diagnosis of aortic regurgitation must be based on a thoughtful evaluation of all the evidence available, especially that derived from the physical examination. The physical signs of this valvular abnormality will therefore be considered in some detail.

Physical Examination

Inspection and Palpation of the Precordium

Precordial inspection and palpation in aortic regurgitation may yield reliable information concerning the heart size and suggestive clues to the presence of associated or underlying lesions or heart failure. Thus, the location and character of the apex impulse, typically broadened in area, increased in forcefulness, and displaced caudally and laterally toward or into the axilla, may permit an estimate of the degree of left ventricular dilation and hypertrophy present. Visible pulsations may be present in the aortic area, suggesting associated dilation of the ascending aorta. Slight, quick pulsations of either sternoclavicular joint in the presence of aortic regurgitation suggest associated disease of the aorta, including atherosclerotic or syphilitic aneurysm and especially aortic dissection; this sign, when found in association with aortic regurgitation, hypertension, and dilation of the aorta, has been regarded as highly suggestive of dissecting aneurysm.[86, 87] Occasionally a precordial lift may be palpated in aortic regurgitation; it is usually a sign of heart failure, the lift being produced by right ventricular hypertension due to disease on the left side of the heart.

A double outward movement of the left ventricle in diastole may be visible and palpable when aortic regurgitation is severe.[141] The initial outward movement of the ventricular wall is thought to be due to rapid ventricular filling from the left atrium and the aorta. This is followed by a diastolic inward movement of the cardiac apex, readily demonstrated on apex cardiograms, and occurring at the time when left ventricular pressure exceeds left atrial pressure during diastole, that is, at the time of diastolic closure of the mitral valve; this may be accompanied by an early diastolic sound, as will be noted below. The second outward movement appears to be related to the continuing aortic insufficiency following the premature mitral valve closure.

Arterial Pulses and Associated Peripheral Signs

The increased amplitude of the arterial pulse in aortic regurgitation provides the basis for some of the most time-honored signs available to the clinician, though it is to be emphasized that several of them may be seen with marked widening of the pulse pressure generally, and hence are not specific to the valvular lesion. The pulse pressure widening in aortic regurgitation reflects high stroke volume and rapid diastolic runoff of blood from the aorta, and is abetted by peripheral vasodilation. Among the more florid signs of widening of the pulse pressure are visibly exaggerated pulsations in the epigastrium and in the carotid arteries. Aortic regurgitation is the commonest organic cause of exaggerated carotid pulses in adults.[48] Flagrant pulsations of the temporal, brachial, and radial arteries may also be seen. The classical pulse described by Corrigan[30] has proven to be a reasonably reliable indicator of pulse pressure widening, though this must be considerable in degree to produce the sign. Head-bobbing synchronous with the heart beat (de Musset's sign) is uncommon, and more of a bedside curiosity than a useful diagnostic aid. It is seen when aortic regurgitation is severe.

Pistol-shot or water-hammer sounds over the larger superficial arteries are commonly heard in aortic regurgitation and in other conditions which result in increased pulse pressure. In all these conditions there is a change in the shape of the arterial pressure curve, which becomes steeper in both its anacrotic and catacrotic limbs with higher peak pressure and a generally narrower contour. The pistol-shot sound is produced by the impact of this sharp pulse wave on the peripheral arteries. The immediate mode of production of the sound is in doubt; McKusick[93] has summarized some of the views currently held, including sudden expansion and vibration of the vessel wall, sudden changes in flow, fluttering of the vessel wall due to the Bernoulli effect, and sudden changes from one velocity profile to another.

Similarly, the to-and-fro or double murmur of Duroziez, noted on light or moderate compression of superficially placed peripheral arteries with the stethoscope bell, is a frequent finding. The systolic component may be heard in normal individuals, though it may be exaggerated with pulse pressure widening of mild or moderate degree. The second, or diastolic, component appears to be due to backflow past the site of arterial narrowing.[47]

The sign of Traube is a double sound (not a double murmur), also heard over peripheral arteries in the presence of increased pulse pressure, but without compression by the stethoscope. It is uncommon compared with the Duroziez sign, but probably of similar mechanism.[93] Quincke's capillary pulse may usually be demonstrated with marked widening of the pulse pressure, particularly if transillumination of the nail bed is combined with varying pressure on the tip of the nail so as to produce pallor of the distal nail bed, thus providing more marked contrast with the ebb and flow of blood in the proximal portion. Peripheral vasodilation, common in aortic regurgitation, is part of the basis for this phenomenon.

Pulsus bisferiens is a useful sign in aortic valve disease, and usually reflects substantial regurgitation associated with mild or moderate stenosis. It is most readily appreciated on palpation of the carotid artery as a twin-peaked impulse in systole. It has been suggested that the notch between the peaks of this pulse wave is due to the suction effect of the high-velocity flow across the valve.[42] On occasion this pulse abnormality may be noted with aortic regurgitation alone.

Gorlin and Goodale[58] have pointed out the typically warm, flushed state of the patient with aortic regurgitation as a reflection of associated vasodilation. As left ventricular failure supervenes peripheral vasoconstriction occurs, as is usual in congestive heart failure; diastolic blood pressure then rises and the patient is likely to become cool and pallid. Peripheral signs of aortic regurgitation may ameliorate. With digitalization reversal of these changes is likely to occur, with fall in the diastolic pressure, return of warmth and flushing of the skin, and accentuation of peripheral signs.

Heart Sounds

The second sound in the aortic region may be increased or decreased in intensity. Increase in this sound may reflect cusp stiffening due to fibrosis as well as rapid fall in aortic pressure, with accelerated aortic valve closure.[93] In syphilitic aortic valve disease the sound may be especially ringing in quality, perhaps in part because of preservation to some extent of flexibility of the cusps. In advanced aortic valve disease with cusp thickening and fixation, the second sound in the aortic area may be strikingly diminished.

The first sound at the apex may be considerably reduced in intensity or absent. This has been attributed by Meadows et al.[97] and by Wigle and Labrosse[141] to premature mitral valve closure related to rapid and severe elevation of left ventricular pressure exceeding left atrial pressure during diastole, and possibly enhanced by increased left ventricular impedance. Meadows and his co-workers have noted this especially in the more rapidly developing forms of aortic regurgitation, such as occurs in bacterial endocarditis, in aortic valve rupture, or after some types of aortic valve surgery, and believe that the sign is of ominous prognostic import.

Aortic ejection sounds, or early systolic clicks, are usually of pathologic significance and may be heard in a variety of circumstances associated with dilation of the aortic root, including aortic regurgitation; they have been related by Leatham[81] to accentuated ejection vibrations in the aorta. Aortic clicks are usually heard best at the apex, but may also be loud at the base; at the apex such a click may be difficult to distinguish from splitting of the first sound. In contrast to pulmonic systolic clicks, those of aortic origin do not show expiratory accentuation.

An early diastolic sound may be heard at the apex when aortic regurgitation is severe, and may be due to premature diastolic closure of the mitral valve.[97, 109, 141]

Murmurs

Four murmurs are to be found in patients with aortic regurgitation, though not all may be found in every instance.

AORTIC DIASTOLIC MURMUR

Certainly the most important single sign of the lesion is the aortic diastolic murmur; it is the *sine qua non* of the diagnosis. This murmur, reflecting high-velocity flow, is the highest-pitched of all cardiac murmurs, and may also be the lowest in intensity and therefore the most easily missed despite the high frequency being optimal for the human ear. Typically the murmur is heard best at Erb's point, in the third left interspace parasternally, sometimes the fourth or second, and is usually pandiastolic. Occasionally a brief silent period may be noted immediately after semilunar valve closure and before the murmur begins; the basis for this is unclear. On occasion the murmur has a crescendo-decrescendo quality, peaking early in diastole, because of changes in the gradient between the aorta and the left ventricular cavity with consequent fluctuations in rate of flow across the incompetent valve. Occasionally this reflects the coexistence of first-degree heart block.[105] Very soft murmurs of aortic regurgitation may be confined to early diastole, when the gradient is greatest. In very severe aortic regurgitation the murmur may disappear before diastole ends, as the gradient narrows because of rapid falloff in aortic pressure and the rising intracavitary pressure in the left ventricle.[83]

Murmurs of moderate intensity may be obvious with the patient recumbent, and are sometimes better heard in this position; frequently, however, the murmur is better heard in the sitting position with the patient leaning forward; occasionally it can be heard only with the patient on all fours. In any position fully held expiration is helpful, as the frequencies of respiratory noises extend into the range occupied by aortic diastolic murmurs. On occasion the murmur may not be well heard with any of these maneuvers; in such instances Besterman[10] has reported that phenylephrine in a dose of 0.25 mg given intravenously may bring out the murmur of aortic regurgitation within 2 to 3 minutes, and that the murmur may remain audible for 15 to 25 minutes. Phenylephrine in this dose predictably induces a pressor response and reflex bradycardia, conditions which might be expected to enhance reflux through a slightly incompetent aortic valve.

Sometimes the murmur of aortic regurgitation is heard only in the first right interspace, or may be loudest or heard only at the apex or in the axilla; the latter distribution has been referred to as the Cole-Cecil murmur.[29] McKusick[93] has emphasized that murmurs of aortic regurgitation are transmitted to the apex rather as a rule, and that in transmission these murmurs often acquire a rather rumbling quality, making confusion with the murmur of mitral stenosis or with the Austin Flint murmur readily

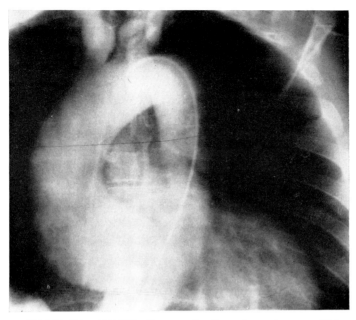

Fig. 6. (N.Y.H. No. 1111455). Retrograde thoracic aortogram. Male, age 54. Aortic regurgitation of recent onset in a patient with long-standing mild hypertension. Aortic diastolic murmur heard best down right sternal border. There is marked dilation of the aortic root and ascending aorta and lesser dilation of the arch and descending portion and of the proximal portions of the brachiocephalic vessels. No evidence of aortic dissection. Underlying aortic disease unknown.

possible. The fact that the murmur of aortic regurgitation usually begins immediately with the second sound helps in its identification.

Harvey, Corrado, and Perloff[64] have pointed out the occasional occurrence of murmurs of aortic regurgitation transmitted down the right sternal border rather than the left. In general this has been seen with relatively uncommon causes of aortic regurgitation, and has generally been associated with dilation and rightward displacement of the aortic root (Fig. 6); on occasion this transmission pattern has also been noted with deformity of the aortic valve alone. Proximal aortic lesions which have been involved include aneurysm, dissection, syphilitic aortitis, cystic medial necrosis with the Marfan syndrome, sinus of Valsalva aneurysm, and others less readily categorized. Among the causes of aortic valve deformity associated with rightward transmission of the diastolic murmur are bacterial endocarditis, syphilis, trauma, interventricular septal defect with aortic regurgitation, and perhaps atherosclerosis. It is to be noted that with these valvular lesions left-sided transmission of the murmur is more common. It is worthy of emphasis that rheumatic aortic regurgitation very rarely produces this pattern of murmur transmission.

That the murmur of aortic regurgitation may on occasion demonstrate musical qualities was pointed out, as noted above, by Hodgkin.[70] In recent years the musical aortic diastolic murmur has again been studied.[55, 93, 128]

These murmurs are rare, sometimes very loud, and generally associated with eversion of a cusp with creation of a lip which is free to vibrate in the regurgitant stream; such cusp eversion is usually due to syphilitic changes, but occasionally occurs in rheumatic disease. Occasionally the musical murmur is found with cusp rupture, spontaneous or traumatic, or with bacterial endocarditis. Overall, however, this murmur is more often associated with syphilitic aortic regurgitation than any other cause; this was true in 75 per cent of 48 cases collected from the literature by Stembridge and associates.[128] Most often the right anterior (right coronary) cusp is the one involved, perhaps because the aorta receives less support from contiguous structures in this region. McKusick[93] has noted that the musical qualities of the murmur may be less pure when a cause other than cusp eversion underlies it.

AORTIC EJECTION MURMUR

This is found in most patients with aortic regurgitation, and may be so intense as to be accompanied by a systolic thrill. This murmur is related to high stroke volume and high velocity of flow across the deformed valve, and may be contributed to by any aortic root dilation that may be present, e.g., in syphilis or the Marfan syndrome; it may be of great intensity even in the absence of anatomic aortic stenosis. Diagnosis of the coexistence of true stenosis may be difficult; marked widening of the pulse pressure makes this highly unlikely. In addition, the later in systole the peak intensity of the murmur occurs, the more likely is it that true stenosis is present. Generally the ejection murmur of aortic regurgitation is less harsh than that heard in patients with predominant aortic stenosis.

APICAL DIASTOLIC RUMBLING MURMUR

The apical diastolic rumbling murmur described by Austin Flint[43] is a common finding in marked aortic regurgitation, and was present in 63 per cent of Thayer's cases of aortic regurgitation with an anatomically normal mitral valve.[131] The clinical features helpful in distinguishing the Austin Flint murmur from that of true mitral stenosis have been well summarized by Segal, Harvey, and Corrado.[122] The patient with the Austin Flint murmur is more likely to be male, less likely to have marked exertional dyspnea or hemoptysis, and is more likely to be in normal sinus rhythm. The second sound over the pulmonic area is normal or only slightly accentuated, and the first sound at the apex is likely to be faint, in contrast with the findings in mitral stenosis. A systolic ejection sound is frequently heard, and an apical ventricular gallop is a common finding. The opening snap of mitral stenosis is not heard. The low-pitched diastolic murmur is usually early and mid-diastolic in aortic regurgitation, rather than mid-diastolic with presystolic accentuation, as in mitral stenosis. On occasion it may be helpful to note the auscultatory changes following inhalation of amyl nitrite, as described by Kiger;[78] patients with mitral stenosis, with or without aortic regurgitation, show an increase in the intensity of the diastolic murmur, while the intensity of the Flint murmur diminishes.

APICAL HOLOSYSTOLIC MURMUR

The fourth murmur to be heard in aortic regurgitation is an apical holosystolic murmur, which is due to functional mitral regurgitation. It is seen in patients with considerable left ventricular dilation, and is transmitted into the axilla.

Several other diastolic murmurs are to be distinguished from the high-pitched, basal diastolic murmur originating at the aortic valve. Chief among these is the murmur of pulmonic regurgitation. Regurgitation of blood at the pulmonic valve is almost always secondary to pulmonary hypertension, and reflects dilation of the valve ring. In patients with mitral stenosis evaluation of basal diastolic murmurs may be exceedingly difficult. In the past the Graham Steell murmur of relative pulmonic regurgitation was frequently invoked in this setting, but recent studies have indicated that such murmurs are much more often due to aortic regurgitation. Thus, in the series studied by Runco and his associates, 10 of 13 patients with mitral stenosis thought to have the Graham Steell murmur were found by aortic valvulography to have aortic regurgitation, and in 8 of 12 additional patients with no definite clinical conclusion regarding the origin of the basal diastolic murmur, aortic regurgitation was similarly documented.[117] It is of note that none of the patients had low diastolic pressures on routine sphygmomanometry; none had peripheral signs of aortic regurgitation, few had striking left ventricular enlargement on cardiac fluoroscopy, and all demonstrated increased intensity of the second sound in the pulmonic area. Thus, clinical criteria were not useful in making the distinction between pulmonic and aortic regurgitation in this setting. Others have commented on this difficulty;[51, 82] the essential point is that relative pulmonic regurgitation is an uncommon cause of basal diastolic murmurs in patients with mitral stenosis.

The murmur of organic pulmonic regurgitation differs from the typical decrescendo murmur of aortic or relative pulmonic regurgitation. This murmur is characteristically short, low in pitch, and separated from the second sound by a short interval. Typically it is crescendo-decrescendo in shape, and is heard only in early diastole, when the pulmonary artery–right ventricular gradient is maximal.[13] Such murmurs are heard most commonly after surgery for pulmonic stenosis or as a result of bacterial endocarditis; occasionally congenital malformations of the pulmonic valve or pulmonary artery, or perhaps syphilitic or rheumatic changes in the pulmonic valve, may be responsible.

An additional interesting diastolic murmur has been described by Dock and Zoneraich[35] in a patient with marked stenosis of the anterior descending branch of the left coronary artery; the heart valves were normal at autopsy. This murmur was sharply localized to the third left interspace, was heard only with the patient in the sitting position, and was high-pitched, with striking early and late (presystolic) accentuation. The murmur was attributed to the coronary artery stenosis.

Diastolic murmurs have been described in patients with ventricular aneurysm.[119,134] In some instances these have been musical and have been noted especially in early diastole, though in some reports they have lasted through diastole or have shown presystolic accentuation; they have almost always been accompanied by systolic murmurs and have been loudest over the abnormal pulsation or bulge of the aneurysm. It is to be noted that in most of these cases autopsy demonstration of normal cardiac structures, especially the valves, has been lacking, and that other studies of ventricular aneurysm have not revealed diastolic murmurs.[59] Nevertheless, it is likely that on occasion patterns of flow and turbulence within ventricular aneurysms may give rise to diastolic murmurs which might be confused with the murmur of aortic regurgitation.

THE CAUSES OF AORTIC REGURGITATION

The causes of aortic regurgitation are numerous; several additions to the list of potential underlying lesions have been made in recent years. The causes may be arranged as in Table 3, and in general fall into nine more or less discrete categories, while a miscellaneous group of rare causes makes up a tenth.

The majority of cases of aortic regurgitation are caused by rheumatic heart disease and bacterial endocarditis, though the relative frequency of the various causes is changing. Thus, in an autopsy series of 258 cases at The New York Hospital–Cornell Medical Center, experience in the past 35 years has been as indicated in Table 4. It is to be noted that throughout this experience rheumatic heart disease, syphilis, calcific disease of the aortic valve, and bacterial endocarditis have accounted for more than 90 per cent of all aortic regurgitation seen at autopsy, and that rheumatic heart disease alone was responsible for 78 per cent of cases seen in the past decade. While some diagnostic bias is unquestionably introduced in an autopsy study, the preponderance of rheumatic heart disease as a cause of aortic incompetence in this series was closely similar to the experience in living patients described by Segal, Harvey, and Hufnagel;[123] 80 per cent of their cases were rheumatic in origin.

Of additional interest is the persistence of syphilis as an important cause of aortic regurgitation, despite a drop of 66 per cent in relative frequency at autopsy from the 1932–1945 period to 1958–1967. A further drop in the incidence of syphilitic aortic valve disease in the next few years is likely.

The autopsy incidence of calcific disease of the aortic valve has not increased appreciably in frequency with the years. Congenital lesions causing aortic regurgitation, on the other hand, have probably increased somewhat in relative frequency, and now occur at autopsy about as often as syphilitic aortic incompetence. This incidence is sufficient to make careful diagnostic

TABLE 3

The Causes of Aortic Regurgitation

1. Rheumatic heart disease
2. Bacterial endocarditis
3. Calcific disease of the aortic valve
4. Syphilis
5. Aortic dilation or distortion
    a. Aortic dissection
    b. Sinus of Valsalva aneurysm
    c. Marfan syndrome
    d. Idiopathic cystic medial necrosis of the aorta
    e. Takayasu's arteritis
    f. Relapsing polychondritis
    g. Chronic aortitis of unknown cause
    h. Ehlers-Danlos syndrome
    i. Systemic arterial hypertension
    j. Other causes
6. Congenital causes
    a. Bicuspid aortic valve
    b. Ventricular septal defect
    c. Coarctation of the aorta
    d. Subaortic stenosis
    e. Coronary arteriovenous fistula
    f. Quadricuspid aortic valve
7. Atherosclerosis
8. Trauma and rupture
9. Causes related to aortic valve surgery
    a. Following aortic valvulotomy
    b. Regurgitation around margins of valve prosthesis
    c. Changes in Silastic poppet in valve prosthesis
    d. Bacterial endocarditis
10. Other causes
    a. Rheumatoid disease
    b. Systemic lupus erythematosus
    c. Osteogenesis imperfecta
    d. Cusp fenestrations
    e. Morquio-Ullrich syndrome
    f. Scheie's syndrome
    g. Hurler syndrome
    h. Reiter's syndrome
    i. Progressive systemic sclerosis (scleroderma)
    j. Pseudoxanthoma elasticum
    k. Valvular myxomatous change
    l. Cogan's syndrome

consideration of this group of causes mandatory in relation to the individual case. Surgical procedures on the aortic valve represent a new and expanding basis of aortic regurgitation which will likely become increasingly important. Miscellaneous causes, categorized as "other" in Table 4, have not changed significantly in occurrence at autopsy in the past $3\frac{1}{2}$ decades. This group consists largely of elderly patients with relative aortic incompetence.

TABLE 4

Causes of Aortic Regurgitation at Autopsy, 1932–1967*

Interval	RHD† Only	RHD, BE‡	Total RHD	BE Only	Syphilis	Calcific	Congenital	Other
1932–1943 (73	43%	26%	69%	8%	15%	3%	1%	4%
cases)	(31)§	(19)	(50)	(6)	(11)	(2)	(1)	(3)
1944–1955 (59	54%	15%	69%	2%	19%	2%	2%	7%
cases)	(32)	(9)	(41)	(1)	(11)	(1)	(1)	(4)
1956–1967 (126	78%	2%	80%	2%	5%	3%	5%	6%
cases)	(98)	(2)	(100)	(2)	(7)	(4)	(6)	(7)
Totals	62%	12%	74%	4%	11%	3%	3%	4%
	(161)	(30)	(191)	(9)	(29)	(7)	(8)	(14)

* Reprinted, by permission, from Transactions of the American Clinical and Climatological Association 80: 23, 1968.

† Rheumatic heart disease.

‡ Bacterial endocarditis.

§ Numbers in parentheses represent numbers of cases.

General Clinical Features of the Various Causes of Aortic Regurgitation

Rheumatic Aortic Regurgitation

Although the diagnostic dilemma is made somewhat easier by the fact that rheumatic fever is the commonest cause of aortic regurgitation, this probability, like so many others, is difficult to apply to the individual patient. A frank and well-documented history of acute rheumatic fever, especially in childhood, is most helpful, particularly if there have been recurrences. Segal's group found histories of prior frank rheumatic fever in 80 per cent of their series of patients with severe aortic regurgitation,[123] and such a history was elicited in 69 per cent in our experience.[4] Hamann[61] has pointed out the necessity for critical appraisal of histories of prior rheumatic manifestations, and has emphasized the fact that rheumatic heart disease is frequently seen in the total absence of a history of prior rheumatic equivalents of any variety.

An additional historical point that is helpful in suggesting the presence of rheumatic heart disease is the prior occurrence of bacterial endocarditis. While this infection may be superimposed on any type of valvular disease as well as on normal valves, such a history may be regarded as relatively more suggestive of underlying rheumatic heart disease than of other types, particularly if a viridans type of streptococcus is known to have been the infecting organism.

The importance of the age at which aortic valve disease is discovered or at which congestive heart failure first occurs has been emphasized.[11] Generally speaking, aortic regurgitation of significant degree due to rheumatic heart disease is established early in life and tends to progress over a 7- to 10-year period, so that the patient is likely to have substantial valvular disease by the time he is in his early twenties.[24] Conversely, the first appearance of clinical evidence of the disease after the age of 40 makes rheumatic heart disease relatively less likely as the cause.[123]

Once congestive heart failure supervenes in the course of aortic regurgitation, the evolution of this process may be diagnostically helpful. In rheumatic heart disease the symptoms and signs may resolve to a remarkable degree with appropriate therapy, and the patient may then be relatively well for months or even years before heart failure recurs. Thus, as Hamman pointed out some years ago,[61] multiple episodes of failure may occur over a period of several years, separated from each other by intervals of relatively good compensation. Such a sequence is perhaps less often seen in aortic regurgitation due to other causes, though recent advances in the treatment of congestive heart failure make this distinction less useful than it formerly was.

The presence of disease involving other heart valves or the concomitant presence of aortic stenosis may be helpful in assigning a rheumatic basis to aortic regurgitation. As the Austin Flint murmur is a common finding in this setting, signs suggesting coexisting mitral stenosis must be interpreted with care unless the aortic regurgitation is of mild degree. As noted above, however, the distinction between the murmur of organic mitral stenosis and the Austin Flint murmur can often be made with reasonable assurance at the bedside; in addition, x-ray demonstration of marked left atrial enlargement is helpful as supporting evidence for the presence of mitral valve disease, as is roentgenographic demonstration of calcification in the region of the mitral valve. On occasion angiocardiography and/or cardiac catherization may be required to establish the presence of multivalvular disease or concomitant aortic stenosis (Fig. 7).

Coexistent aortic stenosis may be difficult to diagnose at the bedside unless stenosis is hemodynamically the predominant lesion. When it is clearly present and hemodynamically significant the likelihood is that the aortic valve lesion is due to rheumatic heart disease or to a congenital cause, or, in the older patient, to calcific disease of the aortic valve. Thus, for all practical purposes, the presence of significant aortic stenosis makes highly unlikely the rarer causes of aortic regurgitation.

Although the mitral valve is the one usually involved when rheumatic heart disease involves a single valve, solitary involvement of the aortic valve is not uncommon, and is not a reliable basis for excluding rheumatic heart disease as the underlying process.

Bacterial Aortic Regurgitation

In general aortic regurgitation due to or contributed to by bacterial endocarditis has a relatively poor prognosis, particularly if congestive heart failure supervenes. This fact, together with the ominous outlook for patients with unrecognized bacterial endocarditis generally, makes it wise to consider the diagnosis of bacterial endocarditis in every patient with aortic regurgitation which is newly discovered, or increases in degree, or becomes associated with congestive heart failure.

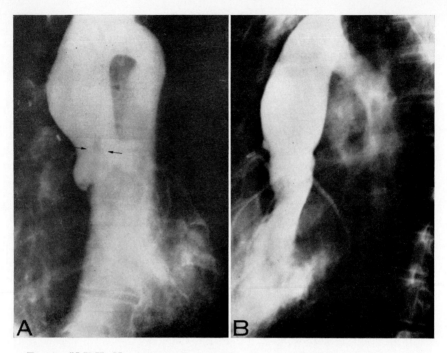

Fig. 7. (N.Y.H. No. 717093). Retrograde thoracic aortogram. Female, age 41. Aortic stenosis and regurgitation due to rheumatic heart disease. *A.* Posteroanterior view in systole; arrows indicate lucent jet due to unopacified left ventricular blood. *B.* Lateral view in diastole, demonstrating regurgitation of dye into the left ventricle.

The nature of the aortic valve lesion in bacterial endocarditis is usually complex, consisting of a mixture of the effects of the underlying valvular lesion which is usually present and the changes due to the superimposed bacterial infection. The latter include varying mixtures of valve retraction and ulceration, interference with cusp closure by vegetations, cusp perforation, damage to the aortic ring and sinuses of Valsalva, tearing or rupture of the valve, and sagging of fibrotic cusps after healing.[50] Usually when aortic regurgitation occurring during bacterial endocarditis is severe, aortic cusp perforation is the chief underlying lesion.

Since the development of effective antimicrobial therapy for bacterial endocarditis, congestive heart failure has become the chief cause of death in this disease. Perforation of heart valves has been found to underly this in almost 65 per cent of cases,[113] and perforation of the aortic valve has been noted in half the cases of aortic regurgitation found at autopsy in late deaths due to bacterial endocarditis.[99]

In patients with acute bacterial endocarditis the clinical picture is generally dominated by evidence of overt sepsis. The diagnosis is frequently not made during life, either because the patients do not survive long enough after hospital admission to permit a diagnosis to be made, or, more often, because the systemic nature of the infection is masked by signs of overwhelming infection elsewhere, notably pneumonia, meningitis, or peritonitis; in this setting the evidence of valvular disease may be misinterpreted or dismissed.[62] It is to be noted, however, that in some cases evidence of severe aortic regurgitation may appear rapidly, as a result of fulminating valve destruction.

In addition to the fulminant course typical of acute bacterial endocarditis, the features that may be seen include other metastatic foci of infection, the occasional presence of Janeway lesions on the palms or soles, and perhaps a higher frequency of Roth spots in the optic fundi than in the subacute form of the disease. On occasion evidence of atrioventricular block or arrhythmias may be seen; this is likely related to involvement of the conducting system in the inflammatory process. In general, however, aortic regurgitation per se does not dominate the clinical course or determine the outcome in acute bacterial endocarditis.

Although a wide variety of microorganisms may cause acute bacterial endocarditis, *Staphylococcus aureus* is the commonest offender, and was responsible for 60 per cent of the cases of Morgan and Bland.[99] This organism, like the pneumococci and β-hemolytic streptococci, may produce particularly fulminant disease. The gonococcus is an uncommon cause, but may occasionally be suspected in patients demonstrating double daily temperature spikes or presenting a history of any venereal disease or of treatment for such.

By contrast, aortic regurgitation due to subacute bacterial endocarditis is associated with a much more indolent erosion of general health. Although the disease is notably protean, fever and heart murmurs are virtually constant features. In addition to these and other familiar features of the disease, purpura, mental depression or dementia, weight loss, cough, shifting unexplained pains, and intercurrent phenomena suggesting embolic episodes may be seen. The combination of any of these or of anemia, azotemia, or urinary abnormalities with evidence of aortic regurgitation is a clinical constellation suggesting subacute bacterial endocarditis, and should be investigated with blood cultures.

In further contrast to acute bacterial endocarditis, aortic regurgitation associated with the subacute disease is usually evident; its severity may increase sharply during the course of the disease, and congestive heart failure may be a prominent or dominating feature during the active phase or after bacteriologic cure.

As noted above, when aortic regurgitation is associated with bacterial endocarditis, valve perforation is frequently the mechanism, and may account for 50 per cent of such instances in which regurgitation is severe.[99] It presents as the sudden appearance or worsening of regurgitation, with classical signs of severe valve incompetence. Although the degree of regurgitation produced is related to the size of the valve lesion, it does not correlate well with the intensity of the murmur.[50] Generally the aortic diastolic murmur does not present unique features on auscultation, though occasionally it has a musical quality. On rare occasions it may disappear.

In Cecil's case this was associated with amelioration of severe heart failure.[22] At autopsy it was found that increase in the size of the vegetations had occluded two perforations in the aortic cusps.

An additional clinical peculiarity that may be observed on rare occasions is the association of bacterial endocarditis with systemic arteriovenous fistulae. The endocarditis may involve the aortic valve. An animal counterpart has been described by Lillehei et al.[84]

Calcific Disease of the Aortic Valve

This lesion seems clearly to be caused by a variety of antecedent processes, including rheumatic fever, atherosclerosis or other "degenerative" processes, syphilis, and healed bacterial endocarditis. In addition, congenital bicuspid aortic valves may calcify, as may valves involved in congenital aortic stenosis.[93] Other causes will undoubtedly be described in time.

The disorder occurs with increasing frequency with advancing age, and is uncommon before the age of 50. Hultgren[73] found the peak incidence between 60 and 70 years of age, with no particular difference in sex incidence.

Evidence of aortic stenosis almost always predominates in these patients; aortic regurgitation as an associated feature is not uncommon, however, and was present in 35 per cent of the series studied by Dry and Willius.[37] In the typical case hemodynamic evidence of high-grade obstruction or regurgitation at the aortic valve is uncommon. While the thrill and murmur typical of aortic stenosis are usually striking, the accompanying murmur of aortic regurgitation is soft. Widening of the pulse pressure is often present, but usually reflects systolic hypertension due to decrease in aortic elasticity, rather than decrease in diastolic pressure due to aortic regurgitation.

In an appropriate clinical setting the diagnosis can usually be confirmed by roentgenographic demonstration of calcium in the aortic annulus or cusps. This is best visualized by fluoroscopy with image intensification or by tomography of the aortic valve region.

Syphilitic Aortic Regurgitation

This type of aortic regurgitation, once one of the commonest causes, has become a great deal less frequent in recent years, as noted in Table 4. Syphilis accounted for 12 of the 100 cases of severe aortic regurgitation collected by Segal, Harvey, and Hufnagel in the early 1950s,[123] and for 5 per cent of the New York Hospital autopsy series for the same period.[4]

It is clear that this type of valvular disease is associated with a relatively long asymptomatic period, which may extend to 6 to 10 years or more.[91] Considerable longevity is not infrequent among these patients; thus, in one series, 43 per cent of patients were alive at the end of 10 years after the diagnosis of aortic regurgitation was made, and 30 per cent were living after 15 years.[137] The same study demonstrated that survival is related to the presence or absence of symptoms, and hence to the severity of the valvular lesion. Once congestive heart failure develops these patients do poorly, with fewer and less satisfactory remissions after appropriate treatment than those with some other types of aortic regurgitation, although it is to be noted that this clinical experience was largely gathered before modern diuretic therapy was developed; the extent to which such a difference in response to therapy still obtains is unclear.

On the average these patients have their primary syphilitic lesions at about age 20, though the range is obviously wide. The murmur is noted, again on the average, at about age 36, or 15 to 16 years after the average murmur of rheumatic aortic regurgitation is found; the onset of symptoms of heart failure and/or angina pectoris occurs around 7 or 8 years later, at an average age of 43, contrasted with an average age of 29 for rheumatic patients.

In addition to these general clinical features, certain aspects of the physical examination are suggestive of a syphilitic basis for aortic regurgitation in the individual patient. Evidence of late syphilis elsewhere is the first of these, and should be sought particularly in relation to the central nervous system. Thus, Argyll Robertson pupils, diminution of ankle jerks, impaired position and vibratory sense and deep sensation, and abnormalities of gait may be present. A very occasional patient shows perforation of the nasal septum or hepar lobatum.

As noted previously, diastolic murmurs of aortic origin which are musical are more often caused by syphilitic change in the valve than by any other type. In addition, radiation of the aortic diastolic murmur down the right sternal border rather than the left tends to be associated with dilation of the aortic root, and is sometimes due to syphilis, as described above.

Calcification of the ascending aorta on x-ray examination of the chest is highly suggestive of syphilitic aortitis, and may be seen in up to 40 per cent of cases.[75, 132] Among patients with advanced atherosclerosis in the absence of syphilis such calcification is present in only 2 to 3 per cent. Patients with this roentgen finding have positive routine serologic tests for syphilis in the blood, spinal fluid, or both in about 60 per cent of cases,[75] and have associated aortic regurgitation in 45 per cent of cases.[132] Thus, the finding of linear calcification of the ascending aorta in association with aortic regurgitation points strongly to a syphilitic etiology of the latter. Roentgen evidence of aortic aneurysm involving the thoracic aorta is an additional finding highly suggestive of aortic syphilis, as is calcification of the sinuses of Valsalva.[127]

The proportion of patients with syphilitic aortic regurgitation who have positive serologic tests for syphilis cannot be estimated with accuracy at the present time. Older figures were accumulated largely in the years prior to World War II, at a time when the sensitivity of the reagin tests was changing. Further, the impact of the widespread use of penicillin and other antimicrobial drugs, given for other reasons to patients with early syphilis, may well be considerable; such courses of therapy may be inadequate to eradicate the syphilitic infection, though the appearance of positive reagin-type serologic tests may be prevented. Thus, the meaning of a negative serologic test may be unclear, though both reagin-based and treponemal antigen-based tests should be drawn.[2, 107] Recent studies indicate that the fluorescent treponemal antibody absorption test is positive in more than 93 per cent of cases of late syphilis.[28]

Aortic Regurgitation Due to Aortic Dilation or Distortion (Relative Aortic Regurgitation)

AORTIC DISSECTION

Aortic regurgitation appears in 10 to 15 per cent of patients with aortic dissection.[69] It may be due, in this setting, to dilation and distortion of the valve ring or the valve itself by the medial hematoma or by underlying changes in the aortic wall reflecting the presence of an underlying disease, such as hypertensive disease, the Marfan syndrome,[93] idiopathic cystic medial necrosis, or, on occasion, rheumatic,[77] tuberculous,[98] or so-called giant cell aortitis.[39]

From a clinical point of view, the commonest setting in which aortic dissection appears is in patients 40 to 60 years of age, often with prior long-standing hypertension. It has also been reported a number of times in pregnancy, in myxedema, and in association with aortic coarctation or aortic stenosis. It is common in patients with the Marfan syndrome. In general it is more common in males. Pain is a nearly constant feature, and is usually intense and frequently described as tearing in quality. It is likely to be substernal in location, but may be felt prominently in the back. Its location may shift, e.g., to the low back or legs, as the dissection progresses. Bizarre neurologic signs are not infrequent, and asymmetry of carotid or other pulses may be seen, owing to obstruction of aortic branches by the process.

Pulsation of a sternoclavicular joint may be seen on either side, and, though not specific for aortic dissection, this sign is highly suggestive.[86, 87] Increased pulsation of an involved carotid artery may be found.[85]

Systolic murmurs, sometimes musical, are not infrequent, and are usually heard over the upper anterior chest or in the base of the neck; they may reflect vibrations produced by the aortic distortions associated with the dissection, or by associated changes in involved arterial structures in the neck. The aortic diastolic murmur may radiate down the right sternal border, rather than the left, because of dilation of the aortic root.

Aortic dissection as the basis for aortic regurgitation should be suspected particularly when the valvular lesion appears abruptly, especially in hypertensive patients or others with predisposing conditions, or in patients giving a history of antecedent episodes of pain consistent with dissection. The diagnosis may be confirmed by aortography (Fig. 8).

SINUS OF VALSALVA ANEURYSM

Aneurysmal dilations of the aortic sinuses of Valsalva are uncommon and may affect cardiac structure and function in a variety of ways. Congenital aneurysms are somewhat more common than acquired ones,[77] but may not come to clinical attention until adult life; in the group studied by Steinberg and Finby the age range on clinical presentation was 7 to 47 years.[127] These aneurysms usually involve the right coronary sinus or adjacent portions of the noncoronary sinus, and are frequently associated with other congenital anomalies, especially anomalies of the aortic cusps (bicuspid aortic valves, enlarged or rudimentary cusps, thickened, calcified, or fenestrated cusps) and interventricular septal defect. Occasionally subaortic stenosis, coarctation of the aorta, pulmonary conus stenosis, or other malformations may be associated.[77] On occasion these aneurysms are associated with the Marfan syndrome.

Congenital aortic sinus aneurysms are rarely more than 4 cm in diameter and usually are markedly thin-walled; as a result of the latter feature they frequently rupture, with the production of cardioaortic fistulae, usually communicating between the right coronary sinus and the right ventricle, or the noncoronary sinus and the right atrium. These aneurysms do not affect extracardiac structures or rupture outside the heart. They frequently interfere with intracardiac structures, however, notably the pulmonary and tricuspid valves.[77] Aortic regurgitation associated with these aneurysms may be due to associated anomalies of the aortic valve, to distortion of the valve produced by the aneurysm itself, or to bacterial endocarditis,

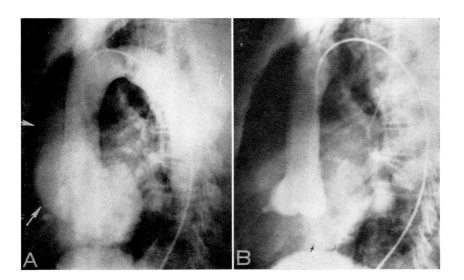

Fig. 8. (N.Y.H. No. 903096). Retrograde thoracic aortogram. Male, age 47; hypertensive. Aortic regurgitation due to aortic dissection. Cystic medial necrosis of the aorta. Sudden precordial pain lasting 6 hours. Grade 3/6 diastolic murmur loudest to right of lower sternum. At operation 75 per cent of circumference of proximal aorta dissected. Aortic cusps normal but prolapsed into left ventricular cavity; when the dissected intima was elevated, aortic cusps coapted and the valve appeared competent. A. Systole. Arrows indicate false lumen. B. Diastole. Arrow indicates regurgitant puff of dye.

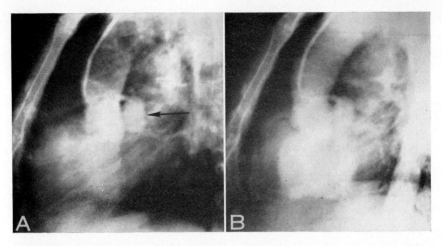

FIG. 9. (N.Y.H. No. 1070770). Retrograde thoracic aortogram. Female, age 66. Aortic regurgitation due to sinus of Valsalva aneurysm resulting from subacute bacterial endocarditis 18 months previously. At operation there was a ragged defect at the commissure between the left and noncoronary cusps due to erosion of the cusps, permitting reflux of blood into the diverticular pocket, which lay just proximal and posterior to this point. A. Systole. Arrow indicates sinus of Valsalva aneurysm projecting posteriorly. B. Diastole. Marked regurgitation of dye into left ventricle.

which may become superimposed on the aneurysmal sac or on associated anomalies.

Congenital sinus of Valsalva aneurysms are rarely productive of symptoms unless they have ruptured. Rupture produces a clinical picture that varies, depending on the cavity into which perforation has occurred. This is most commonly the right ventricle, next most often the right atrium, and occasionally the left ventricle or pulmonary artery. Chest pain, shock, and the rapid development of the picture of severe right heart failure are usually produced, often with systolic pulsations in the distended neck veins and liver. Concomitantly harsh systolic and diastolic murmurs appear; these often have a superficial rasping quality and may be loudest in the third and fourth interspaces to the left of the sternum. The diastolic murmur may radiate down the right sternal border. The murmurs are similar whether the fistula leads to the right atrium or right ventricle.[77] Evidence of marked central diastolic runoff of blood from the aorta occurs, and simulates free aortic valvular regurgitation. Examination may reveal evidence of associated aortic coarctation or other anomalies, or of coexistent bacterial endocarditis. Evidence of right ventricular "strain" or hypertrophy may appear in the electrocardiogram; the combination of this finding with physical signs of free aortic regurgitation should suggest cardioaortic fistula involving the right heart.[68] Supraventricular arrhythmias or heart block may be seen. Although conventional chest x-rays are not especially helpful, angiocardiograms are diagnostic.[127]

Acquired aneurysms of the sinuses of Valsalva are usually due to syphilis or bacterial endocarditis (Fig. 9), occasionally to aortic dissection (Fig. 10)

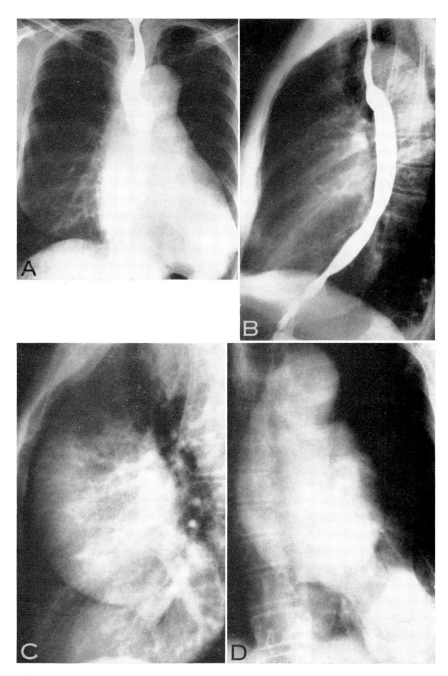

FIG. 10. (N.Y.H. No. 632709). Intravenous aortogram. Female, age 56. Aortic regurgitation due to huge sinus of Valsalva aneurysm with involvement of the entire ascending aorta and probably the arch as well; cause uncertain, possibly aortic dissection. *A* and *B*. Posteroanterior and lateral plain films with barium swallow. Although there is evidence of left ventricular enlargement, these films give no evidence of the huge sinus aneurysm revealed by the dye injection, as seen in *C* and *D*. Note the marked diastolic regurgitation of dye in *D*.

or atherosclerosis. Any sinus may be involved. These aneurysms are frequently large, and for this reason extend upward, often becoming extracardiac and rupturing outside the heart, e.g., into the pericardial sac or pleural cavity.[77] Associated aortic regurgitation is usually due to syphilis or bacterial endocarditis, though the clinical picture associated with rupture of the aneurysm may, as in congenital aneurysms, be marked by evidence of free aortic regurgitation. Heart failure may be present in advance of rupture.

The patients with syphilitic aneurysms of the aortic sinuses tend to be older than those with congenital aneurysms, averaging 54 years in one series.[127] Chest x-rays may show linear calcification of the ascending aorta, a finding highly suggestive of syphilitic aortitis, as noted above. On occasion calcification of the intracardiac origin of the aorta and of the aortic sinuses may be noted; in these circumstances the diagnosis of syphilitic aneurysm of a sinus of Valsalva becomes highly likely.[127]

THE MARFAN SYNDROME

The basic structural lesion in the Marfan syndrome, cystic medial necrosis of the aorta, provides a substrate that permits aortic regurgitation to develop in several ways. Thus, diffuse dilation of the proximal aorta may be associated with dilation of the aortic valve ring; aortic dissection may occur; aneurysm of the sinuses of Valsalva may develop; or deformities of the aortic valve cusps themselves may be present, associated with myxomatous change in the valve.[108] On rare occasions an aortic cusp or commissure may tear, allowing sagging of a cusp or even free vibration of a cusp fragment in the regurgitant stream of blood. Any of these mechanisms may result in greater or lesser degrees of aortic regurgitation. In addition, the myxomatous valve change of the Marfan syndrome can on occasion provide a basis for the development of bacterial endocarditis with resultant aortic regurgitation.[108]

The aortic diastolic murmur in these patients may occasionally be musical, as a result of either cusp eversion or tearing, though it is usually of conventional type;[93] it may be heard preferentially along the right sternal border rather than or better than along the left, as the aortic root is frequently dilated.

Systolic murmurs at the apex are common, and may likewise be musical; they may reflect involvement of the mitral cusps or their chordae tendineae, or similar changes in the tricuspid valve.[72]

Systolic clicks are heard with some frequency in the Marfan syndrome, and have been attributed by McKusick[93] to the frequently associated chest deformities, notably pectus excavatum and pectus carinatum ("pigeon breast"). The dilation of the aorta frequently present in these patients may play a role in the genesis of some of these clicks, which may be prominent both in the aortic area and at the apex.

The associated features that suggest the Marfan syndrome are well known, and include a gracile habitus, arachnodactyly, kyphoscoliosis, ectopia lentis, often with iris tremor, dolichocephaly, high arched palate, flat feet, "double-jointedness," and lack of a normal amount of subcutaneous fat. A family history of some of these abnormalities may sometimes be elicited. In some patients, however, the cardiovascular abnormalities may predominate, and associated findings suggesting the presence of the Marfan syndrome may be difficult or impossible to distinguish. Read and his associates[108] have emphasized some of these difficulties in relation to patients with myxomatous transformation of the aortic or mitral valves; in general most of these individuals appear to represent either overt instances or *formes frustes* of the Marfan syndrome, but the lesion is also occasionally seen as an isolated one in patients not to be distinguished by external appearance from the normal population. Contrariwise, many of the general physical features which are common clinical findings in patients with the Marfan syndrome may be seen with no apparent relation to this disorder in other patients, thus compounding the diagnostic difficulties.

Aortic regurgitation may exist for years in these patients in the absence of evident dilation of the aorta; in some cases the latter may never occur. Aortic dissection may be the first aortic complication of the disease to come to clinical attention, or may be superimposed on antecedent diffuse dilation of the proximal aorta. It has been estimated that more than 17 per cent of aortic dissections in patients under the age of 40 years are associated with the Marfan syndrome.[94] In addition to the generally younger age of these patients with dissection, they are more likely than those unrelated to the Marfan syndrome to demonstrate aortic regurgitation, and are less often hypertensive. As in other instances of aortic dissection, peculiar systolic and occasionally diastolic murmurs may be heard.

Angina pectoris may occur in the Marfan syndrome, as in other types of aortic regurgitation. Once this symptom complex or congestive heart failure appears, survival for more than 2 years is uncommon.

The diagnosis of the Marfan syndrome in a patient with suggestive evidence of its presence is best made when ectopia lentis and a positive family history are demonstrable. In the absence of these features it is difficult to be certain, even though a sporadic case may be encountered.[94]

IDIOPATHIC CYSTIC MEDIAL NECROSIS OF THE AORTA

This aortic wall lesion may occur in the absence of other features suggesting the Marfan syndrome, aortic coarctation, relapsing polychondritis, aortic stenosis, or other specific associations. Its cause and significance are obscure; some have felt that the lesion sometimes represents a nonspecific response of the aortic wall to mechanical and hydraulic stress.[96]

The process may be associated with aortic regurgitation based on diffuse aortic dilation that involves the aortic valve ring, on aortic dissection with resultant aortic regurgitation, or on weakening and tearing of aortic cusps.[67] The presence of cystic medial necrosis of the aorta as the underlying lesion in these circumstances cannot be more than suspected on clinical grounds; the diagnosis must be made histologically.

TAKAYASU'S ARTERITIS

This peculiar type of arteritis involving the aorta and its main branches was described by a Japanese ophthalmologist 60 years ago. Vinijchaikul[135] has described eight autopsied cases in two of which aortic regurgitation was noted, as a result of dilation of the aortic root, including the aortic valve ring.

The disease affects females primarily, especially those under the age of 30. The underlying lesion consists of intimal fibrosis, disruption of elastic fibers in the media associated with scarring and vascularization, and round cell infiltration in the media and adventitia. Rarely, giant cells may be seen. Involvement of the major branches of the aortic arch is common, with partial stenosis or thrombosis, producing the "pulseless disease" soubriquet by which the disorder has been known. Saccular aneurysms of the aorta, frequently multiple, are common; these may reach great size, especially in the abdomen; rupture of abdominal aneurysms caused death in two of Vinijchaikul's eight cases. Hypertension is common, and usually reflects involvement of the renal arteries, frequently with the production of unilateral renal atrophy. Anomalies of the major aortic arch branches have been observed, and have caused some speculation about possible congenital defects in the structure of the aortic wall as a factor in the pathogenesis of the disease.

Clinical features relate primarily to poor perfusion of the head, and include convulsions, transient ischemic attacks with hemiparesis, headache, and attacks of amaurosis. Ophthalmologic findings may include iris atrophy, optic atrophy, presenile cataracts, and retinal abnormalities. Masseter claudication may occur, as may atrophy of facial muscles and perforation of the nasal septum. Absence of palpable arterial pulses in the neck and upper extremities is associated with strikingly diminished or absent blood pressure in the arms. This feature, together with normal or elevated blood pressure in the lower extremities, has led to use of the term "reversed coarctation" to describe the syndrome. The analogy is furthered by the frequent presence of palpable collateral arteries about the neck and intercostal spaces, and rib notching on x-rays of the chest. Prognosis is poor; blindness and death from cerebral infarction are common.

In this country, as Ross and McKusick[115] have pointed out, occlusion of the ostia of aortic arch branches may be due to a number of causes, including syphilitic aortitis with superimposed atheroma, chronic dissection, polyarteritis nodosa, and Buerger's disease. These must be considered in the differential diagnosis of Takayasu's disease.

Marquis and his group[89] have concluded that the aortic and arterial lesions in Takayasu's disease are identical with those described in rheumatoid disease, scleroderma, Reiter's syndrome, giant cell arteritis, and granulomatous aortitis, and refer to the pathologic process as idiopathic medial aortopathy and arteriopathy. Thus, the specificity of a number of these lesions is in some doubt. Nevertheless, the clinical pictures produced permit their separation for diagnostic purposes.

RELAPSING POLYCHONDRITIS

More than 50 cases of this protean syndrome have been reported. The clinical picture has been well described by Dolan et al.[36] and by Pearson and associates.[103] Typically a disease of the middle decades with equal distribution between the sexes, it tends to follow an episodic and multi-focal course over several years. Acute episodes of painful, tender swelling of the external ear reflect the commonest location of cartilaginous inflammation. The overlying skin becomes deeply violaceous; the external auditory meatus narrows, and serous discharge from it may be noted. The portion of the ear lobe containing no cartilage is never involved. With subsidence the ear shrinks, the sharp cartilaginous margins are blunted, and the ear falls forward for lack of support. Similar events may result in a saddle nose deformity. Arthralgias or rheumatoid-type arthropathies may be seen, as may episcleritis, iridocyclitis, keratitis, fever, and involvement of the costal cartilages. Laryngotracheal involvement with tracheal stenosis or collapse may be life-threatening. Cardiovascular involvement has included associated cystic medial necrosis of the aorta[124] and aortic regurgitation due to dilation of the valve ring.[103, 124] The valve cusps have been normal. Some cases have required aortic valvuloplasty or prosthetic valves because of the severity of the progressive aortic incompetence and the rapid course of the ensuing heart failure. In general, however, aortic regurgitation has not been a prominent feature, occurring only in about 10 per cent of recorded cases. The clinical course has generally been dominated by involvement of the ears and airway.

CHRONIC AORTITIS OF UNKNOWN CAUSE

A number of reports have described varieties of aortitis which do not readily fit established clinical entities. McGuire and his co-workers[92] have described five patients with severe aortic regurgitation and rapidly fatal congestive heart failure, with death in a few months. The patients ranged in age from 15 to 37 years; three were females and two males. Anterior chest pain of a burning or aching quality was noted in three cases. At autopsy the aortic cusps were thickened and scarred, and there was commissural separation. The proximal aorta, as far as the diaphragm, showed destruction of elastica with diffuse dilation of moderate degree, and medial, intimal, and adventitial scarring and round cell infiltration; in two cases there were areas of coagulation necrosis just above the aortic ring. No giant cells were seen. There was no clinical or pathologic evidence of syphilis or rheumatoid disease.

Gouley and Sickel[60] have described a group of patients, largely elderly males, with long-standing murmurs of aortic regurgitation in the absence of peripheral signs of the lesion. Most had systolic hypertension. Dilation of the aortic ring and the root of the aorta was present in most cases, associated with a peculiar, fibrous, nodular replacement of the corpora Arantii of the aortic valve cusps; the latter changes were thought to be secondary to the aortic ring dilation. In some cases rolling and lipping of the free margins of the cusps were noted. Commissural separation was frequent. These patients died of congestive heart failure; atrial fibrillation was noted in 5 of 11 patients. Unfortunately, histologic studies of the aortic wall were not included in this report; for this reason appropriate categorization of these cases is difficult.

Bedford and Caird[7] found isolated aortic incompetence in 4.4 per cent of admissions to a geriatric unit. In these cases the valve dysfunction could not be ascribed to rheumatic heart disease, syphilis, diastolic hypertension, or other specific causes. It was as common as aortic stenosis in their experience, as common as all forms of rheumatic heart disease combined, and more common than syphilitic aortic regurgitation in this group of patients, all of whom were more than 65 years of age. The condition was slightly more common in men than in women, and its incidence increased with age. The characteristics of the aortic diastolic murmur were not unusual. Aortic ejection murmurs were heard in 85 per cent. Marked diastolic hypotension was infrequent, though systolic hypertension of more than 200 mm Hg was seen in 41 per cent. Rhythm disturbances were uncommon. The aortic regurgitation in these patients was attributed to dilation of the aortic ring and ascending aorta due to diminution in elastic tissue with advancing age. Atheroma was thought to be of only trivial importance in this aortic lengthening and dilation of the elderly.

The relation of so-called "giant cell aortitis"[21] to other types of chronic aortitis of unknown cause is unclear; as noted previously, Marquis[89] believes that the lesion is common to a number of clinical entities. Varying degrees of aortic regurgitation may be seen, as may aneurysm formation,[3] aortic dissection, and cusp lesions.

EHLERS-DANLOS SYNDROME

Serious cardiac disease is uncommon in the Ehlers-Danlos syndrome, but an occasional case has demonstrated a diastolic murmur compatible with aortic regurgitation. Harsh systolic murmurs at the apex or at the base, the latter transmitted into the neck, have also been seen. Some of the described murmurs have been bizarre and scratchy in quality, simulating pericardial friction rub. Massive cardiomegaly has also been observed. The specific nature of the valvular pathology is unknown.[94] Aortic dissection and sinus of Valsalva aneurysm have been reported.[94, 133]

The classical associated signs include velvety, fragile skin, easy bruising, paper-thin scars, cutaneous hyperelasticity and pseudotumors, protuberant and abnormally angulated ears, hyperextensibility of the joints with frequent luxations, epicanthal folds, and kyphoscoliosis. Intracranial aneurysms, spontaneous rupture of large arteries, spontaneous mediastinal emphysema, gastrointestinal bleeding, and bowel perforation may occur.

Although clinical manifestations usually appear in childhood, they may not be apparent until adult life. Additional affected family members may be found. The disease is ordinarily transmitted as an autosomal dominant, though an X-linked variety has been described.[8]

SYSTEMIC ARTERIAL HYPERTENSION

Diastolic murmurs characteristic of aortic regurgitation are occasionally heard in hypertensive patients and, though usually soft, may be surprisingly intense. Although many of these patients can be demonstrated to have other causes for aortic regurgitation, in a small number this is not the case. In these instances the murmur may be apparent only at considerable levels of diastolic pressure, e.g., 110 mm Hg or more, disappearing when lower levels obtain. Free aortic regurgitation is not a feature of the hypertensive cases unless a complication, such as aortic dissection or cusp rupture, supervenes. In some instances of severe and long-standing hypertensive disease with congestive heart failure, dilation of the aortic ring and normal aortic valve leaflets have been demonstrated at autopsy. In Garvin's[54] series of 200 consecutive autopsied cases of hypertensive heart disease 7 per cent had relative aortic regurgitation. The incidence among hypertensives not sick enough to die of their disease is almost certainly much lower. All of Garvin's patients had been in congestive heart failure for varying periods of time, and marked cardiac dilation was a constant feature; the average aortic ring circumference in his cases was 8.25 cm, whereas the average calculated normal value was 7.3 cm. The valve cusps themselves were normal.

Bedford and Caird[7] concluded from their study that hypertension may increase the aortic root dilation frequently seen in old age, which they attribute to loss of medial elastic fibers, as noted previously.

In our own experience[4] aortic insufficiency was ascribed to arterial hypertension in 5 of 258 autopsied cases. In general the aortic leak seemed to be small and the levels of diastolic pressure considerable, 112 to 124 mm Hg. Three of these patients had severe kidney disease underlying the hypertension and were uremic when the aortic diastolic murmur was noted. In all these patients the aortic valves were normal.

OTHER CAUSES

On occasion relative aortic regurgitation develops on the basis of marked dilation of the left ventricle. In our series of autopsied cases there were three such instances. In two others dilation of the aortic valve ring appeared to be related to advanced atheromatous disease of the aorta. The degree of aortic incompetence was small in all these patients, and clinical findings in general did not allow accurate etiologic diagnosis of the cause of the aortic valve leak.

Congenital Aortic Regurgitation

CONGENITAL BICUSPID AORTIC VALVE

This lesion cannot be diagnosed definitively at the bedside, but may be suspected on occasion by virtue of its association with other cardiac anomalies. Its clinical importance is heightened by its susceptibility to the development of superimposed bacterial endocarditis. A congenital bicuspid aortic valve may be associated with no murmur or may present only with the murmur of aortic regurgitation. The murmur is usually soft, but may on occasion be quite loud, even though there is no hemodynamic evidence of a high-grade diastolic leak at the aortic valve; it is usually typical in quality, location, and radiation. Many of these valves appear to function competently until atheromatous or calcific change occurs. A systolic murmur at the aortic area is common, as these valves do not open normally and tend to produce some degree of obstruction to the forward movement of blood through the orifice.[93]

These valves have a tendency to undergo degeneration, fibrosis, and calcification, perhaps because of tissue defects in the cusps themselves as well as abnormal mechanical stresses related to their shape and disposition. In such circumstances features of aortic stenosis may become more prominent, chiefly in terms of accentuation of the systolic ejection murmur.

Although the anomaly itself is uncommon (0.5 to 1.0 per cent of the general population), it was the most common single cardiac anomaly in Koletsky's series,[79] surpassing coarctation of the aorta, patent interventricular septum, transposition of the great vessels, and patent ductus arteriosus, which followed in that order. Abbott[1] has pointed out that anomalies associated with congenital bicuspid aortic valve tend to be "minor" ones, on the left side of the circulation, in the acyanotic or cyanose tardive groups, such as coarctation of the aorta, patent ductus arteriosus, and interventricular septal defect. Aortic coarctation is especially frequent, and may occur in 25 to 40 per cent of cases;[1,93] in these patients aortic regurgitation is likely to be noted, being due either to hypertension or to the development of superimposed bacterial endocarditis. Indeed, the appearance of the latter complication in patients with coarctation of the aorta is associated with the presence of congenital bicuspid aortic valves in a high proportion of cases, 70.6 per cent in one series.[110] In coarctation associated with aortic rupture, bicuspid aortic valve was present in more than 50 per cent, and in cerebral hemorrhage accompanying coarctation in 32 per cent, in Abbott's series; both figures attest further to the frequency of association of the two anomalies.

Bacterial endocarditis occurs frequently in patients with congenital bicuspid aortic valves. The anomaly may be suspected when this infection occurs on the aortic valve in patients without rheumatic histories or prior clinical evidence of aortic valve disease, though in some such cases bacterial endocarditis has undoubtedly become engrafted on anatomically normal valves, rather then on congenitally malformed ones.

VENTRICULAR SEPTAL DEFECT

The association of aortic regurgitation with ventricular spetal defect is not uncommon; Plauth's group[106] found it in 6.6 per cent of their patients with isolated ventricular septal defect. In these patients aortic regurgitation is not present at birth, but generally appears during the first years of life.[106]

It is usually progressive in severity and associated with advancing symptoms of congestive heart failure.

In most cases the aortic valve lesion consists of prolapse of one or more aortic leaflets, the right coronary leaflet being most commonly affected, the noncoronary cusp next most often, both of these occasionally, and the left coronary cusp rarely. The size of the ventricular septal defect appears to be of less importance than its location in relation to the aortic valve; in these patients the defect is usually situated immediately beneath the aortic leaflets.[106] Secondary changes in the aortic cusps may be seen, including fibrous thickening, retraction, rolling, eversion, aneurysmal dilation, or, occasionally, superimposed bacterial endocarditis.

Historically it can often be established that the murmur heard first was systolic in time, and that the murmur of aortic regurgitation appeared later, usually before age 10 years. Fatigue, exertional light-headedness, and dyspnea are the commonest symptoms when the patient is first seen.

On examination the patients are not infrequently underdeveloped, especially those with large left-to-right shunts, or in whom aortic regurgitation appeared early.[106] Peripheral signs of aortic incompetence are often present. The left ventricular impulse is prominent, and a right ventricular heave may be found in those with substantial right ventricular systolic hypertension.

A systolic thrill may be noted, and a pansystolic murmur of ventricular septal defect is heard; the latter is often intense, and is best heard along the lower left sternal border. In the series reported by Plauth and his colleagues the aortic diastolic murmur was heard in both the right and left second intercostal spaces and radiated down the left sternal border. It was often intense and sometimes accompanied by a thrill. In 3 of their 15 patients a systolic ejection murmur accompanied by a thrill was found in the right second interspace and radiated along the carotid arteries.

The murmurs in this clinical setting are sometimes confused with the continuous murmur of patent ductus arteriosus; careful auscultation along the upper right and lower left sternal borders generally permits separation of the two murmurs in these patients. In addition, Harvey and Perloff[65] have pointed out that in aortic regurgitation with ventricular septal defect the "continuous" murmur does not envelop the second sound as is seen classically in patent ductus; the systolic component tends to be maximal in midsystole rather than in late systole and early diastole, and the murmur may be heard lower along the left sternal border than in patent ductus.

Aortography provides evidence of aortic valve incompetence and frequently of a left-to-right shunt. The deformed and redundant aortic leaflets may sometimes be seen, and occasionally associated dilation of the sinuses of Valsalva may be visualized[106] (Fig. 11).

Cardiac catheterization is required for definitive differentiation of the various malformations which may produce continuous or to-and-fro mur-

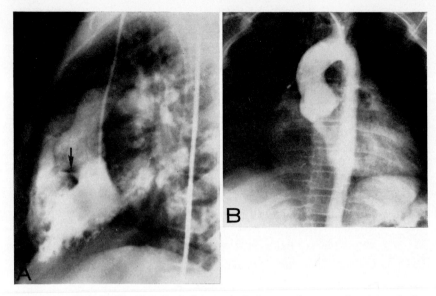

Fig. 11. (N.Y.H. No. 848611). Left ventriculogram and retrograde supravalvular aortogram. Male, age 10. Aortic regurgitation with ventricular septal defect. *A.* Lateral view. Systole. There is left to right shunting. At least one component of the defect is seen (arrow) just inferior to the right coronary sinus. *B.* Posteroanterior view. Diastole. A puff of regurgitant dye is seen in the left ventricle. On the full angiocardiographic study the aortic valve appeared to be tricuspid. There was deformity of the right coronary sinus with regurgitation of contrast material predominantly through this sinus and the noncoronary sinus.

murs. Scott and his group[121] have considered the differential diagnostic problems raised by this group of patients in some detail.

COARCTATION OF THE AORTA

Diastolic murmurs are not a feature of uncomplicated coarctation of the aorta.[110] When present they are associated with aortic valvular deformity or malformation, including congenital bicuspid aortic valve, bacterial endocarditis or associated rheumatic heart disease, or with patency of the ductus arteriosus.

As noted above, the commonest associated congenital lesion is bicuspid aortic valve, occurring in 42 per cent in Reifenstein's series.[110] As in other situations, some instances of acquired bicuspid aortic valve may be seen with coarctation; these seem to be chiefly old inflammatory changes, often rheumatic in origin. In addition, congenital bicuspid valves may be affected by inflammatory lesions which are superimposed. In all, Reifenstein found only 30 per cent of congenital bicuspid aortic valves in patients with coarctation to be unaffected by either bacterial endocarditis or by old inflammatory disease which he interpreted as rheumatic in origin.

Coarctation of the aorta occurs far more frequently in males than in females. Men with the anomaly are likely to be large, well developed, and heavily muscled.[130] The classical signs include especially a disproportion between the blood pressure readings obtained in the upper and lower extremities, usually but not invariably accompanied by small or absent pedal pulses. The systolic ejection murmur produced by the coarctation itself is usually loudest high in the left interscapular space, but may be widely heard over the precordium and in the left supraclavicular fossa. Continuous humming murmurs with systolic accentuation may be heard over areas rich in collateral vessels, especially the upper back; sometimes these murmurs are heard only in systole. Venous hums in the neck may occur with increased frequency in coarctation,[93] and not infrequently the left radial pulse is smaller than the right owing to impingement on the left subclavian ostium by the coarctation. An aortic early systolic click is a frequent finding.

Aortic diastolic murmurs occur in 10 to 35 per cent of cases, and the incidence and severity of aortic regurgitation increase with age. McKusick has concluded that dilation of the aortic root due to hypertension, in combination with a congenital bicuspid valve with or without secondary atherosclerotic change, probably accounts for most of these murmurs, and that aneurysm of a sinus of Valsalva is responsible for a few additional cases[93] (Fig. 12).

It is of importance, as McKusick has also emphasized, that in the presence of severe aortic regurgitation the signs of coarctation may be sub-

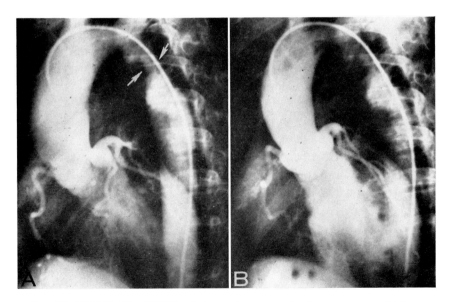

FIG. 12. (N.Y.H. No. 920539). Retrograde supravalvular aortogram. Male, age 19. Aortic regurgitation with coarctation of the aorta. A. Systole. Arrows indicate the coarctation. There is dilation of the ascending aorta. B. Diastole. There is moderate aortic regurgitation. The full angiocardiographic series showed a deep, eccentric, noncoronary sinus of Valsalva and abnormal motion of the valve cusps during systole. There was a partial doming effect and streaming posteriorly, suggesting the presence of a bicuspid valve.

merged; the femoral pulses may feel normally full if it is not noted that they lack the collapsing quality present in the upper extremities.[93]

The association of aortic regurgitation with coarctation should always raise the question of superimposed bacterial endocarditis, and appropriate studies to explore this possibility should be conducted.

SUBAORTIC STENOSIS

It is not clear that subaortic stenosis is invariably a congenital lesion, but, since it appears to occur with some frequency on this basis, it is considered here.

Experience with aortic diastolic murmurs in this condition has varied widely. They appear to be more common in the discrete form of the disease, in which a fibrous or fibromuscular band or diaphragm below the aortic valve obstructs left ventricular outflow.[4,14,49] In patients with the diffuse form, characterized by a hypertrophic, subvalvular muscle mass, aortic regurgitation is considerably less common. Thus, it was found in only 1 of the 64 cases studied by Braunwald and his group.[15]

Nagle[100] has reported a case of bacterial endocarditis occurring on a normal aortic valve in a patient with subaortic stenosis of the hypertrophic type; aortic regurgitation appeared. We[4] have noted a similar sequence in a patient with the discrete form of the disease, as have Brachfeld and Gorlin.[14] Thus, when the combination of subaortic stenosis and aortic regurgitation is noted, especially in association with fever, superimposed bacterial endocarditis should be considered.

Patients with subaortic stenosis are subject to episodes of syncope and to angina pectoris, dizziness, dyspnea, and sudden death. Symptoms may not appear until middle life, though early disability also occurs. Familial occurrence of the disease has been noted.

On examination cardiac enlargement is usually present. A double apical impulse, consisting of a presystolic expansion followed by the usual systolic outward thrust, was found in 45 of Braunwald's 64 patients with the hypertrophic variety of the disease.[15] A systolic thrill is noted in about half the cases, and is prominent along the lower left sternal border or at the apex. Third and fourth heart sounds are commonly heard, particularly the latter. Paradoxical splitting of the second sound may be present. A systolic murmur is a constant feature, and is usually loudest along the mid- or lower left sternal border or, less often, at the apex. Neck transmission is not prominent. The murmur may vary surprisingly in intensity from time to time; it tends to be of the late ejection type, and is somewhat more holosystolic at the apex.[15] It is higher-pitched and less rasping than the murmur of valvular aortic stenosis. Rarely it may be musical. Brisk carotid pulses and a prominent a wave in the jugular venous pulse are helpful ancillary findings.

The definitive diagnosis of subaortic stenosis and the distinction between the diffuse and discrete varieties depend on the findings on cardiac catheterization and angiocardiography.

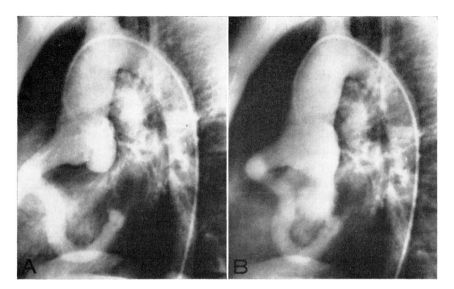

FIG. 13. (N.Y.H. No. 827437). Retrograde thoracic aortogram and selective right coronary arteriogram. Male, age 23. Huge fistula between right coronary artery and right ventricle. *A*. Systole. *B*. Diastole. Slight aortic regurgitation.

CORONARY ARTERIOVENOUS FISTULA

This congenital lesion is uncommon, but in recent years has received increasing attention, since it can now be identified by angiogram.[101],[126] The malformation is compatible with survival into adult life. It may produce continuous murmurs the location of which on the precordium is dependent on the anatomic site of the fistula. Congestive heart failure and various arrhythmias may be features of the clinical course.

While aortic regurgitation has not been a feature of the cases thus far reported, one patient* with angiocardiographic evidence of mild aortic regurgitation has been seen at The New York Hospital–Cornell Medical Center. In this case a huge fistula between the right coronary artery and the right ventricle was associated with deformity of the right sinus of Valsalva and slight regurgitation of dye through the aortic valve (Fig. 13). The patient was a 23-year-old man. A harsh, ejection-type systolic murmur was present in the left second interspace parasternally, and was faintly transmitted to the neck. A soft, blowing diastolic murmur was heard in the same region, and was transmitted down the right and left sternal borders. A murmur had been noted since birth but there had been no cyanosis or exercise limitation.

QUADRICUSPID AORTIC VALVE

This anomaly has been reported only nine times. Aortic regurgitation was described in two of these cases, [104],[112] and was responsible for congestive heart failure in both instances. The patients were 61 and 35 years old,

* Described here through the kindness of Dr. Israel Steinberg.

respectively, when their valvular lesions brought them to clinical attention. Both had had known murmurs since early life. In both cases it was demonstrated at operation that the four aortic cusps failed to approximate properly in diastole, accounting for the valvular incompetence. In one patient preoperative aortic root angiograms clearly showed the four cusps of the aortic valve. Corpora Arantii were found at the midpoints of the free edges of all four cusps in both cases, and were interpreted as reflecting abnormal embryogenesis with resultant formation of a true four-cusped valve rather than a pseudoquadricuspid valve due to old inflammatory disease.[104]

Atherosclerotic Aortic Regurgitation

Atheroma is a frequently invoked though rarely demonstrated cause of aortic regurgitation, though there are some instances of calcific disease of the aortic valve which may be due to atheromatous change in the valve itself and may, in some cases, be associated with evidence of aortic regurgitation. Mild aortic valve incompetence appearing in the elderly is likely to be ascribed to atherosclerosis, largely because of the advanced age of the patient, the frequent presence of demonstrable atheromatous disease elsewhere, and the lack of firm evidence of an alternative basis for the valve dysfunction. Supporting pathologic studies in such cases, however, are infrequent. Fenichel[41] reported 17 cases of aortic regurgitation which he ascribed to arteriosclerosis, but autopsy findings were described in only one, and in this case the anatomic diagnosis was calcific aortic stenosis and insufficiency; an arteriosclerotic origin was presumed.

Bedford and Caird,[7] in their review of valvular disease of the heart in old age, found most aortic incompetence in this group to be associated with aortic dilation due to loss of elastic fibers in the media. Further, they found atheromatous change involving the valve itself to be an unimportant cause of aortic regurgitation. Our own experience supports this view strongly; in the New York Hospital autopsy experience[4] of 258 cases only 1 was found in which atheromatous nodules or plaques involved the aortic cusps in such a way as to permit interference with cusp closure. In addition to this mechanism, atheroma may, on rare occasions, contribute to cusp rupture, leading to severe aortic valve incompetence, or may be associated with marked dilation of the aortic root with the production of relative aortic regurgitation, but, as Harvey and Bordley have commented, "Generally when this diagnosis is entertained it proves to be erroneous, since the condition is of such very rare occurrence." [62]

Aortic Regurgitation Due to Trauma and Cusp Rupture

Traumatic aortic regurgitation is usually due to severe blunt trauma to the chest, and is part of a group of cardiac injuries that may be produced in this manner. Others are myocardial contusion, pericardial effusion, cardiac rupture, and perforation of the interventricular septum; the latter two events may occur days after the trauma, as the bruised area undergoes softening. Varying degrees of atrioventricular block may follow cardiac trauma, as may various arrhythmias.

That such cardiac injury is not uncommon is reflected in one estimate that 38 per cent of patients sustaining chest injuries may show evidence of cardiac damage.[136] Other estimates have varied from 16 to 76 per cent, depending on the severity of the trauma. Although aortic valve rupture is uncommon, it is the commonest valvular lesion in patients surviving nonpenetrating cardiac injury. Most such patients are males in their middle years. More often than not no antecedent or associated heart disease is present. Usually only one cusp is involved, either by a tear in the body of the cusp itself or by separation of a commissure or of the point of attachment to the aortic ring. Severe anterior chest pain and syncope are common, usually immediately after the injury is sustained, but in some cases no acute symptoms are noted. Aortic regurgitation in these patients tends to be severe, with striking peripheral signs as well as a loud, often musical, diastolic murmur of which the patient himself, or those standing near him, may be aware. A harsh systolic murmur in the aortic region may also be present.

Penetrating cardiac injury may be associated with the development of aortic regurgitation, sometimes with long survival. The author has seen one case in which a murmur of aortic regurgitation appeared following an ice pick stab wound of the anterior chest, associated initially with acute cardiac tamponade. This patient developed tuberculous pericarditis within a few weeks, probably because of passage of the ice pick through a tuberculous mediastinal or pulmonary focus.

Rupture of the aortic valve in the absence of trauma is not infrequent. As Carroll[19] pointed out in his classical review, most such instances are due to bacterial endocarditis. Much less commonly syphilis is the underlying process. In addition, normal and diseased valves have been noted on occasion to rupture in association with muscular effort; the requisite exertion is ordinarily severe, but need not be, as exemplified in the patient of Cane and Kauntze,[18] who sustained aortic valve rupture while stooping to pick up a bottle of milk.

In the cases due to bacterial endocarditis any organism may be involved, though the pneumococcus, *Staphylococcus aureus*, and gonococcus are more likely to induce valve perforation or destruction quickly. Perforation of the belly of the cusp itself is the lesion immediately responsible for aortic regurgitation in about half the cases in which bacterial endocarditis is the underlying cause; ulceration of the cusp margin with rupture, or separation of one end of a cusp from its attachment to the aortic wall, is also seen.

Cusp rupture due to syphilis may be based not only on the fibrous changes in the leaflets themselves, but also on the associated aortic ring dilation, with failure of proper cusp apposition during valve closure, so that the the cusps fail to support each other in diastole and consequently sag and stretch.[19]

Occasional cases of cusp rupture have been ascribed to atheroma,[19] cusp fenestrations, and cystic medial necrosis of the aorta,[67] with or without the Marfan syndrome.[34] Valvular myxomatous transformation has also been implicated.[102] Normal valves have not infrequently been involved, however. As noted above, many of these cases occur in settings of muscular strain; the patients are usually males, frequently in occupations characterized by heavy labor. The lesion in the strain group is most often a vertical tear in the aortic intima near the base of the cusp, with consequent displacement or separation of the cusp attachment.[71] Usually only one cusp is affected, but sometimes two or even three are involved.

Pain in the chest is the commonest presenting symptom, and was noted in 92 per cent of Howard's series.[71] It is sudden and severe, precordial or epigastric, referred to the neck, arms, or back, and often accompanied by angor animi and syncope. Awareness of a roaring or other peculiar sensation in the chest is sometimes reported. Not infrequently it can be heard by those near the patient. Evidence of severe aortic regurgitation is usual. As in the traumatic group, the diastolic murmur is frequently musical; it has also been described as creaking, buzzing, piping, etc. An aortic systolic murmur, sometimes harsh or noisy, is common. Disappearance of the diastolic pressure as a diagnostic sign has been emphasized by Bean and Schmidt.[6]

Early and intractable congestive heart failure is common in aortic valve rupture; the outlook in these patients is grave.

Aortic Regurgitation Related to Aortic Valve Surgery

This new, iatrogenic type of aortic regurgitation has appeared in the past few years, and will be seen with increasing frequency in the future. Some idea of the dimensions of the population at risk may be gleaned from the fact that in mid-1967 Roberts and Morrow were able to state, "Since September, 1960, approximately 40,000 Starr-Edwards caged-ball prostheses have been furnished to surgeons by the Edwards Laboratories, and prosthetic valves of other design have also been employed with success." [111] The increasingly widespread use of valve prostheses, together with the steadily increasing number of long-term survivors of valve replacement, in whom many of these instances of aortic regurgitation occur, mean that this syndrome will be more commonly recognized as time passes.

Aortic valvulotomy may be followed by the appearance of the murmur of aortic regurgitation; this was not infrequent in the early cases. The degree of regurgitation varied, but was usually not severe. The murmur itself is usually soft, and heard at the usual location to the left of the upper sternum.

Following placement of aortic valve prostheses, early appearance of aortic regurgitation may be due to leaks around the suture line at the periphery of the prosthesis. Mechanical interference with proper functioning of the prosthesis may also be responsible; if the aortic prosthesis used is too large for the ascending aorta the aortic wall may protrude into the cage, preventing proper seating of the ball; on occasion the aortic wall is infolded during closure of the aortotomy, with similar results. Ball movement and seating may also be interfered with by protruding nodules of calcium or by the metallic struts of a simultaneously place mitral prosthesis.[111]

Bacterial endocarditis is an additional cause of early aortic regurgitation after prosthesis placement; *Staphylococcus aureus* is the commonest offender, but other organisms, including diphtheroids, have also been incriminated.[76] In most such instances aortic regurgitation has become apparent several weeks postoperatively, though premonitory persistent early fever may be seen. In some patients operative procedures such as dental extraction and skin grafts have preceded the septicemia; in others contamination of the cardiopulmonary bypass equipment may have been responsible; in still others infection may have been introduced at the time of operation.[76] In these cases vegetations have been found around the circumference of the annulus where the valve was placed, with extension of the infection into the surrounding myocardium and epicardium; in some instances the atrioventricular node has been involved in the inflammatory process with the production of high-grade atrioventricular block.[111] Partial or total detachment of the prosthesis from the infected annulus may occur with resultant abnormal movement of the prosthesis, which may be identified fluoroscopically or on long-exposure chest x-rays.[129] Bacterial endocarditis in this setting produces a severe degree of aortic regurgitation, and should be suspected when this appears days or weeks after insertion of a prosthesis, especially in the presence of fever, leukocytosis, or other collateral evidence of infection.

The late appearance of aortic regurgitation in patients with aortic valve prostheses has been noted in the past 2 years in a number of instances. On rare occasions this may reflect fistulae around the prosthetic valve ring, allowing regurgitation of blood from the aorta, alongside the prosthesis, into the left ventricle (Fig. 14).[111] More often, however, degeneration of the prosthetic ball (ball variance) has been responsible. This has been characterized by loss of the normal, glistening white appearance of the Silastic ball, with discoloration, swelling, appearance of grooves or fissures, sometimes with contained thrombus material, and occasionally shrinkage or fragmentation. Although not all the observed changes in these balls have been of hemodynamic significance, several patients have been seen in whom swelling of the ball resulted in impaired movement within the cage and fixation of the swollen ball against the metal struts, resulting in aortic regurgitation.[80,88,111] In these patients muffling or disappearance of one or both of the characteristic clicking sounds produced by the movement of the ball in the cage may be a valuable clue to the diagnosis. Peripheral embolization has been seen in association with this syndrome and has apparently been due to thrombus formation in fissures on the surface of the ball.[80] In occasional cases successful replacement of such a swollen, impacted ball has been possible.

Rarely the prosthetic ball may become dislodged from the cage. This

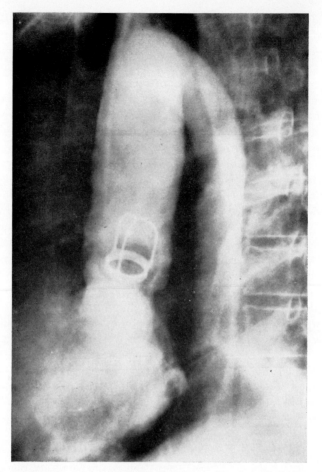

Fig. 14. (N.Y.H. No. 763473). Retrograde thoracic aortogram. Male, age 60. Aortic regurgitation 2 months following placement of a Starr-Edwards prosthesis for calcific disease of the aortic valve. The ball is well seated in the base of the cage in diastole, but there is gross reflux of dye into the left ventricle. At autopsy there were three small fistulae between the aorta and the left ventricle, at the periphery of the base of the prosthesis. No evidence of infection.

catastrophe may be suspected in patients who have undergone prosthetic aortic valve replacement and who develop sudden chest or abdominal pain, rhythm disturbances, shock, syncope, and evidence of free aortic regurgitation with absence of the usual opening and closing prosthetic clicks. Since the ball usually embolizes to the aortic bifurcation, leg pulses may be absent.[111]

In recent years all silicone rubber balls produced for these prostheses have been barium-impregnated, and are therefore relatively radiopaque; the diagnosis of ball variance with serial high-resolution films and cine-radiography should be facilitated by this change.[74]

Other Causes

RHEUMATOID DISEASE

The association of aortic regurgitation with rheumatoid disease, especially spondylitis, has been documented a number of times, chiefly in the past 15 to 20 years, during which time the rheumatoid state has become more clearly recognized as a systemic disease.[5,23,32]

Rheumatoid heart disease may occur with granulomatous lesions of the heart histologically similar to rheumatoid subcutaneous nodules, and with a curious form of aortitis with involvement of the aortic valve and clinical evidence of aortic regurgitation, often severe. The valve ring may be dilated, with resultant stretching of the cusps and commissural separation. Sometimes fibrous adhesions are found bridging the commissures. The valve cusps show fibrous thickening, rolling of the free margins, and retraction, sometimes with focal calcification. The aortitis is characterized by plaque-like intimal lesions placed in relation to the valve commissures, and extending into the sinuses of Valsalva and cusps. The lesions may extend up the ascending aorta for short distances. The coronary ostia may be distorted. Histologically there are perivascular accumulations of round cells, focal destruction of medial muscle and elastic fibers, subendothelial proliferation of connective tissue, and marked fibromuscular thickening of the vasa vasorum, sometimes with obliteration of the lumina.[23]

Clinical rheumatoid heart disease tends to occur in the more severe cases of rheumatoid arthritis, especially those with spondylitis;[32] most cases show evidence of involvement of peripheral joints in addition to spinal disease.[23] Males predominate; the average age at onset of the arthritis in Clark's series was 26 years, while the average age at onset of the heart disease in those in whom the dates of onset were known was 37 years. Average age at death in the same series was 45 years. Ninety-one per cent had spondylitis and 82 to 86 per cent presented evidence of involvement of hips, shoulders, or other peripheral joints. Subcutaneous nodules were not noted in this study.[23]

The aortic regurgitation may appear under observation, particularly during exacerbations of the disease, or may be present when the arthritic patient first comes under observation. Associated angina pectoris is not infrequent and is an ominous prognostic sign; all in Clark's series who developed it died within 4 years.

Congestive heart failure may not appear for years, but once decompensation begins its course tends to be relatively intractable. In Clark's group 7 of 10 patients died within 4 years of the appearance of heart failure.

Other clinical features include the occasional appearance of pericardial friction rubs, the Austin Flint murmur, and aortic systolic and apical systolic murmurs, the latter perhaps occasionally due to the similar but less severe changes that may occur in the mitral valve. Heart block of varying degrees of severity may occur, and may reflect granulomatous involvement of the conduction tissues.[125] Psoriasis occurs in about 18 per cent, and uveitis is also not infrequent at some point in the course. Constrictive pericarditis has been reported.

DISSEMINATED LUPUS ERYTHEMATOSUS

Involvement of the heart is common in disseminated lupus, though it rarely dominates the clinical course. In the series reported by Harvey et al.[63] 55 per cent experienced cardiac involvement at some time in the course of the disease. Most cardiac lupus consists of pericarditis, with or without effusion, but valvular lesions, chiefly nonbacterial verrucous endocarditis (Libman-Sacks), also occur frequently. These lesions generally involve the valves on the right and left sides of the heart with equal frequency. Murmurs, chiefly systolic, are common in patients with disseminated lupus and may, in some cases, be due to turbulence or valve dysfunction related to verrucous endocarditis; however, such factors as fever and anemia are often present and no doubt contribute importantly to the frequency with which such murmurs are heard. Diastolic murmurs thought to arise at the aortic valve are occasionally encountered; in the series of Brigden et al.,[17] 6 patients with such murmurs were found in a group of 60 studied; 2 of these came to autopsy, and in 1 of these "valvulitis" of the aortic valve was found.

Bernhard and his associates[9] have reported three instances of severe, rapidly progressive aortic regurgitation due to cusp thinning and perforation in patients with disseminated lupus. Death due to congestive heart failure occurred in each case. The basis for the valve lesion was unclear, but was not attributed by the authors to bacterial endocarditis. One patient had coexistent cystic medial necrosis of the aorta with aortic dissection. This is the only report associating disseminated lupus with aortic regurgitation of major severity. The relation of these cusp perforations to the fenestrations that may be seen under other circumstances (see below) is problematical.

In general, valvular dysfunction due to disseminated lupus is rarely significant hemodynamically, but valvular pathology due to the disease may be suspected when murmurs are encountered in patients with florid clinical evidence of the disorder.

Of additional importance is the fact that patients with disseminated lupus are prone to the development of superimposed infections, and that bacterial endocarditis is occasionally seen. Thus, the discovery of evidence of aortic regurgitation or of other murmurs in a patient with lupus requires investigation from this point of view.

OSTEOGENESIS IMPERFECTA

Aortic regurgitation of greater or lesser severity has been noted in patients with osteogenesis imperfecta, but the anatomic basis for this is obscure.[94] The major feature of the disease is multiple fractures, often after minor trauma, resulting in severe skeletal deformity. Blue sclerae are common, and deafness of the conduction type is not infrequent. A curious aspect of the disorder is the resemblance of some of these patients to those with the Marfan syndrome; thus, kyphoscoliosis, pectus excavatum, and pigeon breast may be seen, as may arachnodactyly.

CUSP FENESTRATIONS

Small fenestrations in the cusps of both the aortic and the pulmonary valves are common findings at autopsy, occurring in 72 per cent of hearts examined for this purpose in one study.[53] In other studies an even higher incidence has been found. Typically the fenestrations take the form of one or more tiny, often slitlike holes in one or more cusps, and are usually situated near the free edge; they are more numerous near the commissures. Aortic regurgitation is rarely associated with cusp fenestrations, since the lesions are usually located above the line of closure of the valve. Occasionally, either because of the presence of an unusually large fenestration or because of the coalescence of several smaller ones with extension below the line of closure, aortic regurgitation may occur; in some instances it may be severe and associated with peripheral signs and intractable heart failure, which may be fatal in a few months to 2 or 3 years.[20, 53] The diastolic murmur in these cases has not been unusual. In other instances cusp rupture may occur, with the production of a musical diastolic murmur and aggravation of congestive heart failure.[90]

The cause of cusp fenestrations is unclear. A process similar to cystic medial necrosis has been noted in the affected cusps in one case.[20] A congenital tissue defect has been mentioned as a possible basis by Friedman and Hathaway,[53] while acquired valvular disease may have played a role in the patient described by Matthews and Darvill.[90]

In general the incidence of fenestrations of the semilunar cusps increases with age, though they may be found in fetal hearts or in the first decade in 65 per cent.[53] Men are more likely to be affected, and hypertensives are slightly more likely to demonstrate them than normotensives. Under conditions leading to dilation of the valve ring it has been suggested that diastolic murmurs may be heard more often,[53] but in this situation their relation to the cusp fenestrations is problematical.

THE MUCOPOLYSACCHARIDOSES: THE MORQUIO SYNDROME; SCHEIE'S SYNDROME; THE HURLER SYNDROME

Among the mucopolysaccharidoses a number of cardiac lesions may be seen. The valvular lesions consist of increase in intercellular stroma with hyaline or mucoid changes, and fibrous thickening which may be nodular.[94]

The Morquio syndrome, also known as the Morquio-Ullrich syndrome, mucopolysaccharidosis IV, or keratosulfaturia, is characterized by marked dwarfism with knock knees, enlarged wrists, and misshapen hands. Barrel chest, pigeon breast deformity, and short neck are common. The characteristic facial deformity is marked by broad mouth, prominent maxillae, widely spaced teeth, and a short nose. Diffuse corneal opacification is common. Mentality may be normal or subnormal, and neurologic abnormalities including paraplegia may occur.[95] Most of these patients die before age 20. Aortic regurgitation is not infrequent, and is not unusual in its physical signs. It is generally present by the time these patients reach their teens.

In Scheie's syndrome, or mucopolysaccharidosis V, increased amounts of chondroitin sulfate B are excreted in the urine. In general the intellect is spared, and stature is normal or near normal. Broad-mouthed facies may be noted, as well as stiff joints, claw hands, increased body hair, and atypical retinitis pigmentosa. There is striking corneal clouding, especially peripherally. The carpal tunnel syndrome is frequently found. Most patients with Scheie's syndrome have aortic regurgitation.[95]

In the Hurler syndrome (mucopolysaccharidosis I) aortic regurgitation is seen less frequently, but occasionally occurs. Most of these patients are retarded mentally; dwarfing, corneal clouding, stiff joints, hepatosplenomegaly, and so-called gargoyle facies are additional features. Excess chondroitin sulfate B and heparitin sulfate are found in the urine. As in other mucopolysaccharidoses, involvement of the mitral or pulmonary valves may coexist, as may heart disease secondary to intimal thickening of the coronary arteries.[95]

REITER'S SYNDROME

The lack of a specific diagnostic test which may be applied to confirm the clinical diagnosis of Reiter's syndrome makes for some difficulty in classifying uncommon manifestations thought to represent expressions of the disease. Thus, some patients reported as exhibiting valvular heart disease due to Reiter's syndrome have had prior illnesses thought to be acute rheumatic fever[114] or acute gonococcal urethritis and polyarthritis.[33] Nevertheless, clinical evidence of acute pericarditis and myocarditis has been noted during the acute stages of illnesses thought to be Reiter's syndrome, and varying degrees of heart block have also been reported, as have nonspecific T-wave changes in the electrocardiogram. Various murmurs, including that of aortic regurgitation, have also been noted.[138] Autopsy examinations, however, are rare; in one[33] the aortic valve showed thickened and rolled edges without fusion or separation of the commissures; the aortic media showed patchy fibrosis and vascularization, while the adventitia was scarred and contained foci of perivascular round cell infiltration and endarteritic narrowing of the vasa vasorum. The similarity of these lesions to those found in rheumatoid spondylitis and scleroderma is to be noted. The specificity of the cardiac lesions in this patient is uncertain, however, as the mitral valve showed thickening, the chordae tendineae were shortened and scarred, and the mural endocardium of the left atrium showed opacification and thickening; these findings are suggestive of rheumatic heart disease.

In another autopsied case[114] similar lesions of the aortic valve were found, as well as aortic lesions of the type described above; the latter were confined to the ascending aorta. The other heart valves were normal.

In the reported cases of aortic regurgitation thought to be due to Reiter's syndrome recurrent episodes of urethritis and polyarthritis, often spread over a period of years, have been common. Evident polyarthritis, often chronic, has been a feature, and keratodermia blennorrhagica has been observed. In one series[33] iritis occurred in three out of four cases. The degree of aortic regurgitation has varied, but occasionally it has been severe. Current or prior evidence of conjunctivitis is often minimal. Radiologic examinations may reveal evidence of spondylitis, calcaneal spurs, and increased density of the sacroiliac articulations.

The diagnostic difficulties encountered in distinguishing such cases from some instances of rheumatoid disease and rheumatic heart disease may be substantial. It seems likely that on occasion Reiter's syndrome may be associated with lesions of the aortic valve and proximal aorta, but the frequency of this association appears to be very low; thus, Csonka's group found 3 such cases in 215 patients thought to have Reiter's syndrome.[33]

PROGRESSIVE SYSTEMIC SCLEROSIS (SCLERODERMA)

Cardiac involvement is not infrequent in progressive systemic sclerosis, and clinical evidence of heart disease may, on occasion, antedate cutaneous changes by 2 years or more. Heart failure is common, and usually reflects extensive myocardial fibrosis or cor pulmonale due to involvement of the lungs by the underlying disease. Pericarditis, sometimes with effusion, may also be seen. Heart murmurs are not infrequent, but clinically important aortic regurgitation is uncommon. Roth and Kissane[116] have described a young woman with progressive systemic sclerosis of 3 years' duration, who died in congestive heart failure, having presented murmurs suggesting aortic stenosis and regurgitation. The aortic cusps were thickened, rolled, and adherent; the proximal aorta showed fibrous thickening, loss of medial elastic tissue, and inflammatory infiltration. The aortic leaflets showed mucoid degeneration and capillary invasion. Such aortic lesions have been regarded by Marquis[89] as common to a number of diseases, as noted previously.

A somewhat similar patient, reported by Sabour and Mahallawy,[118] was thought to have significant mitral as well as aortic valve disease due to scleroderma, but autopsy was not performed.

PSEUDOXANTHOMA ELASTICUM

Lesions of the endocardium[94] and mitral valve[25] have been attributed to pseudoxanthoma elasticum. Coffman and Sommers[25] have described two cases with diastolic murmurs compatible with aortic valve origin, but the valve was normal at postmortem examination in one, and the other was not autopsied. In general valvular heart disease has not been a prominent feature of the disorder. Clinically it is dominated by cutaneous coarsening, grooving, and laxity; by angioid streaks in the optic fundi with or without accompanying hemorrhages and chorioretinitis; and by evidence of arterial disease which may be marked by diminution or absence of peripheral pulses, premature arterial calcification, evidences of coronary artery narrowing or occlusion, and hemorrhage from a variety of sites, notably the gastrointestinal tract, but also from the genitourinary tract, from the nose, and into the joints or subarachnoid space. The disease is inherited as an autosomal recessive trait.

VALVULAR MYXOMATOUS TRANSFORMATION

On rare occasions aortic regurgitation may result from cusp deformity or rupture associated with a peculiar histologic lesion. This is characterized by loss of the normal valve architecture with replacement by a myxoid, mucopolysaccharide-containing material as well as fibroblastic proliferation. Evidence of inflammation is lacking. Cystic medial necrosis of the aorta or major arteries has been a common accompaniment of this valvular lesion, and may result in aortic root dilation with aggravation of aortic incompetence.

This valvular abnormality has been observed in frank instances of the Marfan syndrome, and may affect the mitral or tricuspid valve as well as the aortic. In a number of patients such valvular lesions have been present without associated findings sufficient to permit definitive diagnosis of the Marfan syndrome; such individuals have often been tall and thin, with high palatal arches, scoliosis, pectus carinatum or excavatum, joint hypermobility, or other isolated findings suggesting this condition. Others have presented no such findings, and have been indistinguishable in habitus from normal individuals. The weight of clinical evidence has led to the impression that this valvular lesion frequently represents a *forme fruste* of the Marfan syndrome, though on occasion it may have some other basis.[108]

COGAN'S SYNDROME

A pecular nonsyphilitic interstitial keratitis associated with nerve deafness and vestibular symptoms was described by Cogan in 1945.[26] Since then a small number of additional cases have been reported; aortic regurgitation has been a feature of some of these.[27, 38, 56] The disorder tends to affect young adults, and usually presents abruptly with tinnitus, vertigo, and fulminating deafness. Lacrimation, visual blurring, granular corneal infiltrates, and foci of episcleritis may appear before, during, or at varying intervals following the vestibuloauditory symptoms. Peripheral neuropathy may be a feature. Histologic evidence of necrotizing angiitis has occasionally been noted.

Eisenstein and Taubenhaus[38] have estimated that about a third of the reported cases have had cardiovascular manifestations. In those with aortic regurgitation the valvular lesion has appeared months to years after the onset of the disease.[27, 56] On occasion the aortic diastolic murmur has been musical in quality; in one such case a perforation had occurred in the base of an aneurysmal outpouching of a cusp.[38] Congestive heart failure is not infrequently seen; it may prove fatal in days or may run a fluctuating course for a year or two. Acute aortitis,[27] fibrinoid changes in the valve cusps,[38] coexistent bacterial endocarditis,[38] and changes consistent with acute vasculitis in branches of coronary arteries[38] have all been reported. One of Gelfand's two cases[56] had a ruptured aortic cusp; the other demonstrated prolapse of all three cusps associated with aortitis which involved the coronary ostia.

DIAGNOSTIC APPROACH

It is important for the physician to develop a systematic method of approach in aortic regurgitation so that all the possible categories of potential causes may be considered in relation to the individual case. As a beginning, the possible bases for aortic regurgitation may be divided into common and uncommon causes, as follows:

Common Causes	Uncommon Causes
Rheumatic heart disease	Syphilis
Bacterial endocarditis	Congenital lesions
Calcific disease	Aortic dilation and distortion
Aortic dilation of old age	Postsurgical
	Traumatic
	Atherosclerotic
	Other

The causes listed as common accounted for more than 85 per cent of autopsied cases seen at The New York Hospital–Cornell Medical Center in the past decade; rheumatic heart disease was responsible for over 76 per cent of cases in this study in the same period.[4]

The statistical advantage derived from dividing the causes in this way is enhanced if the presence of coexistent aortic stenosis can be established with confidence; this may be difficult unless stenosis predominates hemodynamically, but the clear presence of aortic stenosis virtually excludes the rare causes of aortic regurgitation except for calcified congenital bicuspid valve and, in a sense, hypertrophic subaortic stenosis; it makes rheumatic heart disease or calcific disease of the aortic valve overwhelmingly the likeliest basis for the aortic regurgitation.

The general bedside evaluation of the patient with aortic regurgitation is helped by noting the age at which the lesion was first discovered. A history of murmurs in early childhood suggests a congenital cause; appearance of the diastolic murmur during the teens or twenties is most characteristic of rheumatic heart disease; syphilitic aortic regurgitation is most likely to be noted first in the thirties or forties, and the aortic incompetence of calcific disease after age 50. Senile aortic dilation tends to be noted after age 60. When the disorder appears at any age in relatively rapid fashion, over a period of days or weeks, bacterial endocarditis, aortic dissection, and cusp rupture should be considered, particularly if the regurgitation is severe.

Not infrequently aortic regurgitation of greater or lesser severity appears virtually under observation in middle-aged or elderly people in the absence of evidence of aortic stenosis; it may be noted to have developed between annual examinations, with or without associated symptoms suggesting the underlying cause. In the author's experience a variety of bases have been observed, including hypertension, aortic dissection, sinus of Valsalva aneurysm, bicuspid aortic valve, and bacterial endocarditis. Rheumatic heart disease has not been noted in these patients, and is a very rare cause of aortic regurgitation appearing after age 40.

Mild aortic regurgitation in patients of advanced age tends to be due to disease of the aorta rather than the valve cusps. In the prospective study by Bleich et al.[12] of 290 patients 65 years of age or older in a city hospital, 12 per cent had a soft diastolic murmur considered typical of aortic regurgitation, in the absence of pulse pressure widening; in this population serologic evidence of syphilis was found in 72 per cent of those with aortic incompetence; in the bulk of the remainder a clear cause could not be decided upon on clinical grounds; in these it was thought that dilation of the aortic ring and ascending aorta due to advanced age and accentuated by aortic disease was the probable basis. The experience of Bedford and Caird,[7] as noted above, was consonant with this, in that, in patients over age 65, aortic regurgitation was more often due to aortic ring dilation associated with loss of medial elastica than to any other cause.

The history, as obtained at the bedside, may be helpful, especially if developed systematically. Frank episodes of acute rheumatic fever or of clear-cut chorea are certainly important and may be elicited in two-thirds to three-fourths of cases of severe rheumatic aortic regurgitation; such a history is likely to be meaningful provided that the diagnosis at the time was based on adequate clinical and laboratory evidence and can be considered reasonably firm. Careful review of the recalled details of such illnesses with the patient or near relatives may be helpful. On the other hand, histories of less discrete manifestations, such as "growing pains," unexplained childhood fevers, and recurrent epistaxis, must be interpreted with caution, and are best not relied on heavily. In addition, it must be borne in mind that some patients with histories of rheumatic fever have aortic regurgitation on another basis; thus, even a clear-cut positive history should not interrupt sequential diagnostic thought.

In patients who give a history of bacterial endocarditis, and who later present with aortic regurgitation, the possibility of underlying rheumatic or, less often, syphilitic or congenital disease must be considered; as noted previously, such a history may be considered suggestive, to some extent, of the presence of rheumatic disease of the aortic valve.

It has been suggested in the past that severe angina pectoris in association with aortic regurgitation is most likely to reflect a syphilitic etiology with involvement of the coronary ostia. More recent observations indicate that angina is as common in rheumatic as in syphilitic aortic incompetence, occurring in about 50 per cent of those with severe degrees of regurgitation; it is not uncommon in severe aortic regurgitation due to any cause.[66]

Other historical features to be sought bear on evidence of syphilitic infection or antisyphilitic therapy. As noted above, once congestive failure appears, prolonged remissions with appropriate therapy are somewhat more characteristic of rheumatic than of syphilitic and some other types of aortic regurgitation. A relatively rapid downhill course after heart failure occurs is seen in aortic valve perforation or tear, rheumatoid heart disease, the Marfan syndrome, and traumatic incompetence, as well as in some postsurgical cases, as described previously. Thus, evaluation of the course of congestive heart failure may provide helpful initial diagnostic information.

A history of prior occurrence of episodes of chest pain compatible with aortic dissection may occasionally be developed at the bedside. In one patient of mine such an episode occurred 1 year before she was seen with newly acquired aortic root widening and sinus of Valsalva aneurysm with aortic regurgitation (Fig. 10).

A history of hypertension may suggest coarctation of the aorta, Takayasu's arteritis, or other less specific associations; the diastolic level should be sought in the history, though most patients are aware only of the systolic reading.

In addition to specific clinical details of the other potential causes of aortic regurgitation, evidence of familial disease should be sought, especially with reference to rheumatic fever, various aspects of the Marfan syndrome, the Ehlers-Danlos syndrome, and the mucopolysaccharidoses.

The physical examination must be comprehensive if maximal information relative to aortic regurgitation is to be developed. General aspects of the patient's habitus may suggest arachnodactyly, rheumatoid disease, or the mucopolysaccharidoses. Evidence of late syphilis may be noted, especially on examination of the eyes, the nasal septum, the liver, and the central nervous system. Search for the various manifestations of bacterial endocarditis should be especially careful in patients with recent appearance or worsening of aortic regurgitation; in those with prolonged endocarditis, general weakness, weight loss, and aberrant behavior may be prominent, and purpura, especially over the lower extremities, may be noted. The latter sign may occur with increased frequency in bacterial endocarditis involving the aortic valve, as opposed to the mitral.

Evidence of cartilaginous destruction in the external ear or nose suggests relapsing polychondritis; rheumatoid-type deformities are also seen in this condition and in disseminated lupus, as well as in rheumatoid arthritis per se.

Subluxation of the lens of the eye points strongly to the Marfan syndrome. It may be difficult to diagnose at the bedside, and may require slit lamp examination for confirmation. The combination of thick-lensed eyeglasses and aortic regurgitation raises the Marfan syndrome as a possibility, as does a high, arched palate. Blue sclerotics suggest this disorder or osteogenesis imperfecta.

The various features of disseminated lupus erythematosus which may be noted on examination need not be reviewed here, but for mention of this disorder as a cause of splenomegaly, joint pain, periungual erythema, pericarditis, pleural effusion, and purpura; association of these with aortic regurgitation should suggest this diagnostic possibility for consideration. If high-grade aortic incompetence is encountered in a patient with disseminated lupus the possibility of superimposed bacterial endocarditis should be entertained.

The cardiac examination may permit the diagnosis of rheumatic heart disease if the presence of coexistent mitral stenosis can be established. The importance of the presence of aortic stenosis has been noted previously. A musical quality of the aortic diastolic murmur is usually due to cusp eversion, which is most often seen in syphilitic disease of the aortic valve, but occasionally occurs in rheumatic heart disease, idiopathic cystic medial necrosis of the aorta, the Marfan syndrome, or acute rheumatic fever; a musical murmur may also be heard in some instances of cusp rupture, spontaneous or traumatic, or in bacterial endocarditis.

Transmission of the aortic diastolic murmur down the right sternal border in preference to the left is exceedingly uncommon in rheumatic aortic regurgitation, and suggests relatively uncommon causes of aortic incompetence, often associated with dilation and rightward displacement of the aortic root; these include aortic dissection, proximal aortic aneurysm, syphilis, cystic medial necrosis, and sinus of Valsalva aneurysm. Aortic valvular lesions may occasionally produce this transmission pattern, among them bacterial endocarditis, syphilis, trauma, and interventricular septal defect with aortic regurgitation.

The physical findings in congenital heart disease associated with aortic regurgitation have been reviewed above, as have those seen in patients with aortic valve surgery followed by aortic incompetence.

Laboratory examinations are sometimes of real help diagnostically, but must be selected and interpreted with care. Anemia in patients with aortic regurgitation is usually unrelated to the process at the aortic valve, but may be seen with disseminated lupus erythematosus, rheumatoid disease, and hemolysis related to aortic valve disease with or without prostheses.[40, 140] In patients with bacterial endocarditis anemia may be accompanied by leukocytosis and positive blood cultures. Blood cultures in patients suspected of having bacterial endocarditis should be inoculated with at least 10 ml of blood and should be held at least 3 weeks before being discarded as sterile. In addition to other media, thioglycolate broth should be routinely inoculated to aid in the recovery of anaerobic organisms. When three blood cultures are obtained over a 24- to 48-hour period and handled in this manner, the infecting organism is recovered in the overwhelming majority of cases unless antimicrobial therapy has already been administered.[139]

Serologic tests for syphilis and rheumatoid arthritis are useful adjuncts in the examination of patients with aortic regurgitation. As noted above, the fluorescent treponemal antibody absorption test is probably the most effective serologic test for syphilis now in use. In rheumatoid disease flocculation tests using latex particles, sheep erythrocytes, or bentonite particles are positive in two-thirds to three-fourths of cases. The tests involving inhibition techniques are probably positive in a higher proportion of cases.

Other laboratory procedures that may occasionally prove useful include the various serologic tests for disseminated lupus erthematosus, and demonstration of increased urinary excretion of specific mucopolysaccharides in the mucopolysaccharidoses. In addition, metachromatic staining of cultured white cells derived from the peripheral blood and stained with toluidine blue O may be demonstrated in the latter group of conditions.[46]

Electrocardiograms may on occasion be helpful diagnostically in aortic regurgitation. Generally speaking, evidence of left ventricular hypertrophy is common, though when valvular incompetence is mild or of brief duration there may be no electrocardiographic abnormalities. In the presence of a low-pitched apical diastolic murmur in a patient with aortic regurgitation, electrocardiographic evidence of right ventricular hypertrophy and right axis deviation point to organic mitral stenosis as opposed to the Austin Flint murmur, and hence to a rheumatic basis for the aortic valve lesion. Electrocardiographic evidence of right ventricular hypertrophy associated with clinical signs of free aortic regurgitation is also seen in the presence of cardioaortic fistulae involving the right heart, as with rupture of a sinus of Valsalva aneurysm into the right atrium or right ventricle.

Roentgenographic studies in aortic regurgitation are revealing of left ventricular enlargement in all cases of more than mild degree. Lateral and caudal shifting of the apex results in the typical boot-shaped configuration of the heart on posteroanterior films. Lateral films may reveal considerable increase in the posterior extent of the left ventricle, and should always be taken so that cardiac size is not underestimated.[120] Calcification of the ascending aorta or sinuses of Valsalva may be noted, and is strongly suggestive of syphilitic aortitis.

Aortic valve calcification is relatively uncommon unless a significant element of aortic stenosis is present. Schlant has estimated that it is seen in about 20 per cent of cases of pure aortic regurgitation,[120] but others[57] have found it to be rare unless there is substantial aortic stenosis.

Fluoroscopic study usually reveals increased left ventricular pulsations with relatively large systolic and diastolic excursions, and the appearance of a "rocking" heart, but is rarely of differential diagnostic usefulness. The presence of differential pulsations or disproportionate dilation of the ascending aorta makes the diagnosis of free rheumatic aortic regurgitation unlikely; under these circumstances there is usually an important element of aortic stenosis or aortic wall disease, the latter usually due to syphilis or the changes associated with the Marfan syndrome.[120]

The application of angiocardiographic techniques for diagnostic purposes to the patient with aortic regurgitation should be considered under three sets of circumstances: 1) when the diagnosis of aortic regurgitation is entertained, but cannot otherwise be made with confidence; 2) when the presence of coexistent disease of other valves or associated congenital lesions is suspected; and 3) when a rare cause of aortic regurgitation is suspected. It should be noted that aneurysm of the sinuses of Valsalva, aortic root dilation, and aortic dissection often produce little or no change suggesting their presence in posteroanterior and lateral plain films of the chest, and hence require vascular contrast studies for definition (Fig. 10). Stenosis or occlusion of the great vessels coming off the aortic arch in Takayasu's arteritis may also be visualized, as may the saccular aortic aneurysms associated with this disease or with syphilis. Of the congenital lesions sometimes associated with aortic regurgitation bicuspid aortic valve, ventricular septal defect, and aortic coarctation may be demonstrated, and subaortic stenosis may be suspected or established. Aortic incompetence following aortic valve surgery may also be characterized. On rare occasions a regurgitant jet lesion due to cusp perforation may be seen.

The use of cardiac catherization techniques, with or without associated dye dilution or other indicator studies, is not commonly required in the diagnostic study of patients with aortic regurgitation, but may be indicated when rare underlying causes are suspected, particularly one of the sometimes-associated congenital lesions, or in the presence of suspected coexistent disease of other heart valves which cannot be established otherwise.

Braunwald and Morrow[16] have shown that aortic regurgitation may be diagnosed and quantitated roughly by oximetric measurements at the ear lobe following intraaortic injection of indicator dye (indigo carmine) at various levels in the aorta through a catheter passed retrogradely via a peripheral artery. Frank and his co-workers[52] have suggested that upstream sampling during continuous infusion of indicator into the aortic root is more useful in quantifying aortic regurgitation. Neither technique is required with any frequency for general diagnostic use.

CONCLUSION

It will be seen from the foregoing that recent clinical observations have broadened substantially the diagnostic problem presented by the patient with aortic regurgitation. A few rules of thumb are helpful. Thus, it is well to remember that roughly three-quarters of cases are due to rheumatic heart disease; that the presence of clear-cut concomitant aortic stenosis virtually excludes rare causes and means almost always that the patient has rheumatic heart disease or calcific disease of the aortic valve; that aortic regurgitation appearing for the first time after age 40 is almost never due to rheumatic heart disease; that preferential transmission of the diastolic murmur down the right sternal border suggests an uncommon cause. Such correlations, however, must be supported by a broad clinical approach, a comprehensive consideration of all the facts available in relation to the individual patient, a considerable body of clinical information concerning a large number of disease states, and a willingness to consider all the etiologic possibilities in relation to the patient at hand.

REFERENCES

1. Abbott, M. E. On the relative incidence and clinical significance of a congenitally bicuspid aortic valve. With five illustrative cases. In *Contributions to The Medical Sciences in Honor of Dr. Emmanuel Libman by his Pupils, Friends and Colleagues*. International Press, New York, 1932.
2. Atwood, W. G., Miller, J. L., Stout, G. W., and Norins, L. C. The TPI and FTA-ABS tests in treated late syphilis. J.A.M.A. **203**:549, 1968.
3. Austen, W. G., and Blennerhassett, J. B. Giant-cell aortitis causing an aneurysm of the ascending aorta and aortic regurgitation. N. Engl. J. Med. **272**:80, 1965.
4. Barondess, J. A., and Sande, M. Some changing aspects of aortic regurgitation: An autopsy study. Trans. Amer. Clin. Climatol. Ass. **80**:23, 1968.
5. Bauer, W., and Clark, W. S. Systemic manifestations of rheumatoid arthritis. Trans. Ass. Amer. Physicians **61**:339, 1948.
6. Bean, W. B., and Schmidt, M. C. Rupture of the aortic valve. Disappearing diastolic pressure as a diagnostic sign. J.A.M.A. **153**:214, 1953.
7. Bedford, P. D., and Caird, F. I. *Valvular Disease of the Heart in Old Age*. J. & A. Churchill, Ltd., London, 1960.
8. Beighton, P. Ehlers-Danlos syndrome. Proc. Roy. Soc. Med. **61**:987, 1968.
9. Bernhard, G. C., Lange, R. L., and Hensley, G. T. Aortic disease with valvular insufficiency as the principal manifestation of systemic lupus erythematosus. Ann. Intern. Med. **71**:81, 1969.
10. Besterman, E. M. M. The use of phenylephrine to aid auscultation of early rheumatic diastolic murmurs. Brit. Med. J. **2**:205, 1951.
11. Bland, E. F., and Wheeler, E. O. Severe aortic regurgitation in young people. N. Engl. J. Med. **256**:667, 1957.
12. Bleich, A., Lewis, J., and Marcus, F. I. Aortic regurgitation in the elderly. Amer. Heart J. **71**:627, 1966.
13. Bousvaros, G. A., and Deuchar, D. C. The murmur of pulmonary regurgitation which is not associated with pulmonary hypertension. Lancet **2**:962, 1961.
14. Brachfeld, N., and Gorlin, R. Subaortic stenosis: a revised concept of the disease. Medicine **38**:415, 1959.
15. Braunwald, E., Lambrew, C. T., Rockoff, S. D., Ross, J., Jr., and Morrow, A. G. Idiopathic hypertrophic subaortic stenosis: a description of the disease based upon an analysis of 64 patients. Circulation **29**:30 (Suppl. IV): 1964.
16. Braunwald, E., and Morrow, A. G. A method for the detection and estimation of aortic regurgitant flow in man. Circulation **17**:505, 1958.
17. Brigden, W., Bywaters, E. G. L., Lessof, M. H., and Ross, I. P. The heart in systemic lupus erythematosus. Brit. Heart J. **22**:1, 1960.
18. Cane, C., and Kauntze, R. Acute aortic valve regurgitation. Guy's Hosp. Rep. **105**:197, 1956.
19. Carroll, D. Non-traumatic aortic valve rupture. Bull. Johns Hpokins Hosp. **89**:309, 1951.
20. Case Records of the Massachusetts General Hospital. N. Engl. J. Med. **245**:941 1951.
21. Case Records of the Massachusetts General Hospital. N. Engl. J. Med. **280**:208 1969.
22. Cecil, R. C., Parker, C. P., Jr., and Porter, W. B. Bacterial endocarditis. Report of a case in which a true musical diastolic murmur appeared and disappeared. Amer. Heart J. **36**:934, 1948.
23. Clark, W. S., Kulka, P., and Bauer, W. Rheumatoid arthritis with aortic regurgitation. Amer. J. Med. **22**:580, 1957.

24. Cobbs, B. W., Jr. In *The Heart*, Hurst, J. W., and Logue, R. B., Eds. McGraw-Hill Book Co., Inc., New York, 1966.
25. Coffman, J. D., and Sommers, S. C. Familial pseudoxanthoma elasticum and valvular heart disease. Circulation 19:242, 1959.
26. Cogan, D. G. Syndrome of nonsyphilitic interstitial keratitis with vestibulo-auditory symptoms. Arch. Ophthalmol. 33:144, 1945.
27. Cogan, D. G., and Dickersin, G. R. Nonsyphilitic interstitial keratitis with vestibuloauditory symptoms. A case with fatal aortitis. Arch. Ophthalmol. 71:172, 1964.
28. Cohen, P., Stout, G., and Ende, N. Serologic reactivity in consecutive patients admitted to a general hospital. Arch. Intern. Med. 124:364, 1969.
29. Cole, R., and Cecil, A. B. The axillary diastolic murmur in aortic insufficiency. Bull. Johns Hopkins Hosp. 19:353, 1908.
30. Corrigan, D. J. On permanent patency of the mouth of the aorta, or inadequacy of the aortic valves. Edinburgh Med. Surg. J. 37:225, 1832.
31. Cowper, W. Of ossifications or petrifications in the coats of arteries, particularly in the valve of the great artery. Phil. Trans. Roy. Soc. Lond. 24:970, 1705.
32. Cruickshank, B. Heart lesions in rheumatoid disease. J. Pathol. Bacteriol. 76:223, 1958.
33. Csonka, G. W., Lichfield, J. W., Oates, J. K., and Willcox, R. R. Cardiac lesions in Reiter's disease. Brit. Med. J. 1:243, 1961.
34. Dimond, E. G., Larsen, W. E., Johnson, W. B., and Kittle, C. F. Post-traumatic aortic insufficiency occurring in Marfan's syndrome with attempted repair with a plastic valve. N. Engl. J. Med. 256:8, 1957.
35. Dock, W., and Zoneraich, S. A diastolic murmur arising in a stenosed coronary artery. Amer. J. Med. 42:617, 1967.
36. Dolan, D. L., Lemmon, G. B., Jr., and Teitelbaum, S. L. Relapsing polychondritis. Analytical literature review and studies on pathogenesis. Amer. J. Med. 41:285, 1966.
37. Dry, T. J., and Willius, F. A. Interpretation of the electrocardiographic findings in calcareous stenosis of the aortic valve. Ann. Intern. Med. 13:143, 1939.
38. Eisenstein, B., and Taubenhaus, M. Nonsyphilitic interstitial keratitis and bilateral deafness (Cogan's syndrome) associated with cardiovascular disease. N. Engl. J. Med. 258:1074, 1958.
39. Erb, B. D., and Tullis, I. F. Dissecting aneurysm of the aorta. The clinical features of thirty autopsied cases. Circulation 22:315, 1960.
40. Eyster, E., Mayer, K., and McKenzie, S. Traumatic hemolysis with iron deficiency anemia in patients with aortic valve lesions. Ann. Intern. Med. 68:995, 1968.
41. Fenichel, N. M. Arteriosclerotic aortic insufficiency. Amer. Heart J. 40:117, 1950.
42. Fleming, P. R. The mechanism of the pulsus bisferiens. Brit. Heart J. 19:519, 1957.
43. Flint, A. On cardiac murmurs. Amer. J. Med. Sci. 44:29, 1862.
44. Flint, A. The occurrence of the mitral direct or presystolic murmur without mitral lesions. Lancet 1:131, 1883.
45. Flint, A. The mitral cardiac murmurs. Amer. J. Med. Sci. 91:27, 1886.
46. Foley, K. M., Danes, B. S., and Bearn, A. G. White blood cell cultures in genetic studies on the human mucopolysaccharidoses. Science 164:424, 1969.
47. Folts, J. D.. Young, W. P., and Rowe, G. G. A study of Duroziez's murmur of aortic insufficiency in man utilizing an electromagnetic flowmeter. Circulation 38:426, 1968.
48. Fowler, N. O. *Examination of the Heart*. Part Two: *Inspection and Palpation of Venous and Arterial Pulses*. American Heart Association, New York, 1965.
49. Fowler, N. O. *Cardiac Diagnosis*. Hoeber Medical Division, Harper and Row, New York, 1968.
50. Fowler, N. O., Hamburger, M. H., and Bove, K. E. Aortic valve perforation. Amer. J. Med. 42:539, 1967.
51. Fowler, N. O., Noble, W. J., Giarratano, S. J., and Mannix, E. P. The clinical examination of pulmonary hypertension accompanying mitral stenosis. Amer. Heart J. 49:237, 1955.

52. Frank, M. J., Casanegra, P., Nadimi, M., Migliori, A. J., and Levinson, G. Measurement of aortic regurgitation by upstream sampling with continuous infusion of indicator. Circulation 33:545, 1966.
53. Friedman, B., and Hathaway, B. M. Fenestration of the semilunar cusps, and "functional" aortic and pulmonic valve insufficiency. Amer. J. Med. 24:549 1958.
54. Garvin, C. F. Functional aortic insufficiency. Ann. Intern. Med. 13:1799, 1940.
55. Gelfand, D., and Bellet, S. The musical murmur of aortic insufficiency; clinical manifestations, based on a study of 18 cases. Amer. J. Med. Sci. 221:644, 1951.
56. Gelfand, M. Personal communication.
57. Glancy, D. L., Freed, T. A., O'Brien, K. P., and Epstein, S. E. Calcium in the aortic valve. Roentgenologic and hemodynamic correlations in 148 patients. Ann. Intern. Med. 71:245, 1969.
58. Gorlin, R., and Goodale, W. T. Changing blood pressure in aortic insufficiency; its clinical significance. N. Engl. J. Med. 255:77, 1956.
59. Gorlin, R., Klein, M. D., and Sullivan, J. M. Prospective correlative study of ventricular aneurysm. Mechanistic concept and clinical recognition. Amer. J. Med. 42:512, 1967.
60. Gouley, B. A., and Sickel, E. M. Aortic regurgitation caused by dilatation of the aortic orifice and associated with a characteristic valvular lesion. Amer. Heart J. 26:24, 1943.
61. Hamman, L. The diagnostic implications of aortic insufficiency. Cincinnati J. Med 25:95, 1944.
62. Harvey, A. M., and Bordley, J. Differential Diagnosis. The Interpretation of Clinical Evidence. W. B. Saunders Co., Philadelphia, 1955.
63. Harvey, A. M., Shulman, L. E., Tumulty, P. A., Conley, C. L., and Schoenrich, E. H. Systemic lupus erythematosus: review of the literature and clinical analysis of 138 cases. Medicine 33:291, 1954.
64. Harvey, W. P., Corrado, M. A., and Perloff, J. K. "Right-sided" murmurs of aortic insufficiency. (Diastolic murmurs better heard to the right of the sternum rather than the left.) Amer. J. Med. Sci. 245:533, 1963.
65. Harvey, W. P., and Perloff, J. K. Some recent advances in clinical auscultation of the heart. Progr. Cardiovasc. Dis. 2:97, 1959.
66. Harvey, W. P., Segal, J. P., and Hufnagel, C. A. Unusual clinical features associated with severe aortic insufficiency. Ann. Intern. Med. 47:27, 1957.
67. Hays, F. B., and Boggan, W. H. Rupture of aortic valve cusp attachment due to cystic medionecrosis of the aorta: a case report with necropsy findings. Ann. Intern. Med. 43:1107, 1955.
68. Herson, R. N., and Symons, M. Ruptured congenital aneurysm of the posterior sinus of Valsalva. Brit. Heart J. 8:125, 1946.
69. Hirst, A. E., Jr., Johns, V. J., Jr., and Kime, S. W., Jr. Dissecting aneurysm of the aorta; a review of 505 cases. Medicine 37:217, 1958.
70. Hodgkin, T. On retroversion of the valves of the aorta. London Med. Gaz. 3:433, 1829.
71. Howard, C. P. Aortic insufficiency due to rupture by strain of a normal aortic valve. Can. Med. Ass. J. 19:12, 1928.
72. Hudson, R. E. B. Cardiovascular Pathology. The Williams & Wilkins Co., Baltimore, 1965.
73. Hultgren, H. N. Calcific disease of the aortic valve. Arch. Pathol. 45:694, 1948.
74. Hylen, J. C., Judkins, M. P.. Herr, R. H., and Starr, A. Radiographic diagnosis of aortic-ball variance. J.A.M.A. 207:1120, 1969.
75. Jackman, J., and Lubert, M. The significance of calcification in the ascending aorta as observed roentgenologically. Amer. J. Roentgenol. 53:432, 1945.
76. Johnson, W. D., Cobbs, C. G., Arditi, L. I., and Kaye, D. Diphtheroid endocarditis after insertion of a prosthetic heart valve. J.A.M.A. 203:919, 1968.
77. Jones, A. M., and Langley, F. A. Aortic sinus aneurysms. Brit. Heart J. 11:325, 1949.
78. Kiger, R. G. Differentiation of Austin Flint and mitral stenosis murmurs by amyl nitrite. (Abstr.) Clin. Res. 11:24, 1963.
79. Koletsky, S. Congenital bicuspid aortic valves. Arch. Intern. Med. 67:157, 1941.

80. Laforet, E. G. Death due to swelling of ball component of aortic ball-valve prosthesis. N. Engl. J. Med. 276:1025, 1967.
81. Leatham, A. Auscultation of the heart. Lancet 2:703, 1958.
82. Leatham, A. Auscultation of the heart. Lancet 2:757, 1958.
83. Leonard, J. J., and Kroetz, F. W. *Examination of the Heart*. Part Four: *Auscultation*. American Heart Association, New York, 1966.
84. Lillehei, C. W., Bobb, J. R. R., and Visscher, M. B. Occurrence of endocarditis with valvular deformities in dogs with arteriovenous fistulae. Proc. Soc. Exp. Biol. Med. 75:9, 1950.
85. Logue, R. B. Dissecting aneurysm of the aorta. Amer. J. Med. Sci. 206:54, 1943.
86. Logue, R. B. Diagnostic clues on inspection of the patient presenting cardiovascular disease. Mod. Concepts Cardiovasc. Dis. 36:37, 1967.
87. Logue, R. B., and Sikes, C. A new sign in dissecting aneurysm of aorta. Pulsation of a sternoclavicular joint. J.A.M.A. 148:1209, 1952.
88. Magovern, G. J., Kent, E. M., and Cushing, W. B. Sutureless mitral valve replacement. Ann. Thorac. Surg. 2:474, 1966.
89. Marquis, Y., Richardson, J. B., Ritchie, A. C., and Wigle, E. D. Idiopathic medial aortopathy and arteriopathy. Amer. J. Med. 44:939, 1968.
90. Matthews, R. J., and Darvill, F. T., Jr. Fenestrations of the aortic valve cusps as a cause of aortic insufficiency and spontaneous aortic valve cusp rupture. Ann. Intern. Med. 44:993, 1956.
91. McDermott, W., Tompsett, R. R., and Webster, B. Syphilitic aortic insufficiency: the asymptomatic phase. Amer. J. Med. Sci. 203:202, 1942.
92. McGuire, J., Scott, R. C., and Gall, E. A. Chronic aortitis of undetermined cause with severe and fatal aortic insufficiency. Amer. J. Med. Sci. 235:394, 1958.
93. McKusick, V. A. *Cardiovascular Sound*. The Williams & Wilkins Co., Baltimore, 1958.
94. McKusick, V. A. *Heritable Disorders of Connective Tissue*, 3rd ed. The C. V. Mosby Co., St. Louis, 1966.
95. McKusick, V. A., Kaplan, D., Wise, D., Hanley, W. B., Suddarth, S. B., Sevick, M. E., and Maumenee, A. E. The genetic mucopolysaccharidoses. Medicine 44:445, 1965.
96. McKusick, V. A., Logue, R. B., and Bahnson, H. T. Association of aortic valvular disease and cystic medial necrosis of the ascending aorta. Circulation 46:188, 1957.
97. Meadows, W. R., VanPraagh, S., Indreika, M., and Sharp, J. T. Premature mitral valve closure. A hemodynamic explanation for absence of the first sound in aortic insufficiency. Circulation 28:251, 1963.
98. Meehan, J. J., Pastor, B. H., and Torre, A. V. Dissecting aneurysm of the aorta secondary to tuberculous aortitis. Circulation 16:615, 1957.
99. Morgan, W. L., and Bland, E. F. Bacterial endocarditis in the antibiotic era with special reference to the later complications. Circulation 19:753, 1959.
100. Nagle, J. P. Idiopathic hypertrophic subaortic stenosis and bacterial endocarditis. J.A.M.A. 200:643, 1967.
101. Neufeld, H. N., Lester, R. G., Adams, P., Anderson, R. C., Lillehei, C. W., and Edwards, J. E. Congenital communication of a coronary artery with a cardiac chamber or the pulmonary trunk ("coronary artery fistula"). Circulation 24:171, 1961.
102. O'Brien, K. P., Hitchcock, G. C., Barratt-Boyes, B. G., and Lowe, J. B. Spontaneous aortic cusp rupture associated with valvular myxomatous transformation. Circulation 37:273, 1968.
103. Pearson, C. M., Kroening, R., Verity, M. A., and Getzen, J. H. Aortic insufficiency and aortic aneurysm in relapsing polychondritis. Trans. Ass. Amer. Physicians 80:71, 1967.
104. Peretz, D. I., Changfoot, G. H., and Gourlay, R. H. Four-cusped aortic valve with significant hemodynamic abnormality. Amer. J. Cardiol. 23:291, 1969.
105. Phillips, J. H., Jr., and Burch, G. E. Selected clues in cardiac auscultation. (Editorial.) Amer. Heart J. 63:1, 1962.
106. Plauth, W. H., Jr., Braunwald, E., Rockoff, S. D., Mason, D. T., and Morrow, A. G. Ventricular septal defect and aortic regurgitation. Clinical, hemodynamic and surgical considerations. Amer. J. Med. 39:552, 1965.

107. Ray, C. T. In *The Heart*, Hurst, J. W., and Logue, R. B., Eds., p. 902. McGraw-Hill Book Co., Inc., New York, 1966.
108. Read, R. C., Thal, A. P., and Wendt, V. E. Symptomatic valvular myxomatous transformation (the floppy valve syndrome). Circulation 32:897, 1965.
109. Rees, J. R., Epstein, E. J., Criley, M., and Ross, R. S. Hemodynamic effects of severe aortic regurgitation. Brit. Heart J. 26:412, 1964.
110. Reifenstein, G. H., Levine, S. A., and Gross, R. E. Coarctation of the aorta. A review of 104 autopsied cases of the "adult type," 2 years of age or older. Amer. Heart J. 33:146, 1947.
111. Roberts, W. C., and Morrow, A. G. Anatomic studies of hearts containing caged-ball prosthetic valves. Johns Hopkins Med. J. 121:271, 1967.
112. Robicsek, F., Sanger, P. W., Daugherty, H. K., and Montgomery, C. C. Congenital quadricuspid aortic valve with displacement of the left coronary orifice. Amer. J. Cardiol. 23:288, 1969.
113. Robinson, M. J., and Ruedy, J. Sequelae of bacterial endocarditis. Amer. J. Med. 32:922, 1962.
114. Rodnan, G. P., Benedek, T. G., Shaver, J. A., and Fennel, R. H. Reiter's syndrome and aortic insufficiency. J.A.M.A. 189:889, 1964.
115. Ross, R. S., and McKusick, V. A. Aortic arch syndrome. Diminished or absent pulses in arteries arising from the arch of the aorta. Arch. Intern. Med. 92:701, 1953.
116. Roth, L. M., and Kissane, J. M. Panaortitis and aortic valvulitis in progressive systemic sclerosis (scleroderma). Amer. J. Clin. Pathol. 41:287, 1964.
117. Runco, V., Molnar, W., Meckstroth, C. V., and Ryan, J. M. The Graham Steell murmur versus aortic regurgitation in rheumatic heart disease. Results of aortic valvulography. Amer. J. Med. 31:71, 1961.
118. Sabour, M. S., and Mahallawy, M. N. Mitral and aortic valve disease in a patient with scleroderma. Brit. J. Dermatol. 78:15, 1966.
119. Scherf, D., and Brooks, A. M. The murmurs of cardiac aneurysm. Amer. J. Med. Sci. 218:389, 1949.
120. Schlant, R. C. In *The Heart*, Hurst, J. W., and Logue, R. B., Eds. McGraw-Hill Book Co., Inc., New York, 1966.
121. Scott, R. C., McGuire, J., Kaplan, S., Fowler, N. O., Green, R. S., Gordon, L. Z., Shabetai, R., and Davolos, D. D. The syndrome of ventricular septal defect with aortic insufficiency. Amer. J. Cardiol. 2:530, 1958.
122. Segal, J. P., Harvey, W. P., and Corrado, M. A. The Austin Flint murmur: its differentiation from the murmur of rheumatic mitral stenosis. Circulation 18:1025, 1958.
123. Segal, J., Harvey, W. P., and Hufnagel, C. A clinical study of one hundred cases of severe aortic insufficiency. Amer. J. Med. 21:200, 1956.
124. Self, J., Hammarsten, J. F., Lyne, B., and Peterson, D. A. Relapsing polychondritis. Arch. Intern. Med. 120:109, 1967.
125. Sobin, L. H., and Hagstrom, J. W. C. Lesions of cardiac conduction tissue in rheumatoid aortitis, J.A.M.A. 180:1, 1962.
126. Steinberg, I., Baldwin, J. S., and Dotter, C. T. Coronary arteriovenous fistula. Circulation 17:372, 1958.
127. Steinberg, I., and Finby, N. Clinical manifestations of the unperforated aortic sinus aneurysm. Circulation 14:115, 1956.
128. Stembridge, V. A., Hejtmancik, M. R., and Herrmann, G. R. Unusual musical murmurs of anterior cusp aortic regurgitation. Amer. Heart J. 48:163, 1954.
129. Stinson, E. B., Castellino, R. A., and Shumway, N. E. Radiologic signs in endocarditis following prosthetic valve replacement. J. Thorac. Cardiovasc. Surg. 56:554, 1968.
130. Taussig, H. B. *Congenital Malformations of the Heart*, 2nd ed. Harvard University Press, Cambridge, Mass., for The Commonwealth Fund, 1960.
131. Thayer, W. S. Observations on the frequency and diagnosis of the Flint murmur in aortic insufficiency. Amer. J. Med. Sci. 122:538, 1901.
132. Thorner, M. C., Carter, R. A., and Griffith, G. C. Calcification as a diagnostic sign of syphilitic aortitis. Amer. Heart J. 38:641, 1949.
133. Tucker, D. H., Miller, D. E., and Jacoby, W. J. Ehlers-Danlos syndrome with a

sinus of Valsalva aneurysm and aortic insufficiency simulating rheumatic heart disease. Amer. J. Med. 35:715, 1963.
134. Vakil, R. J. Ventricular aneurysms of the heart. Preliminary report on some new clinical signs. Amer. Heart J. 49:934, 1955.
135. Vinijchaikul, K. Primary arteritis of the aorta and its main branches (Takayasu's arteriopathy). Amer. J. Med. 43:15, 1967.
136. Watson, J. H., and Bartholmae, W. M. Cardiac injury due to nonpenetrating chest trauma. Ann. Intern. Med. 52:871, 1960.
137. Webster, B., Rich, C., Jr., Densen, P. M., Moore, J. E., Nicol, C. S., and Padget, P. Studies in cardiovascular syphilis. III. The natural history of syphilitic aortic insufficiency. Amer. Heart J. 46:117, 1953.
138. Weinberger, H. W., Ropes, M. W., Kulka, J. P., and Bauer, W. Reiter's syndrome, clinical and pathological observations. Medicine 41:35, 1962.
139. Werner, A. S., Cobbs, C. G., Kaye, D., and Hook, E. W. Studies on the bacteremia of bacterial endocarditis. J.A.M.A. 202:199, 1967.
140. Westring, D. W. Aortic valve disease and hemolytic anemia. Ann. Intern. Med. 65:203, 1966.
141. Wigle, E. D., and Labrosse, C. J. Sudden, severe aortic insufficiency. Circulation 32:708, 1965.

Primary Myocardial Disease

JAMES S. FORRESTER, HARVEY G. KEMP, JR. and RICHARD GORLIN

Among the diseases which have a major cardiac component there is probably none more consistently frustrating to the internist and cardiologist than the loosely amalgamated group known as primary myocardial disease. Although a careful physician can be confident of the presence of primary myocardial disease on clinical grounds in many cases, the ultimate establishment of the diagnosis may require a complicated and extensive work-up, including such sophisticated techniques as coronary arteriography and ventriculography. Furthermore, treatment is rarely curative, and etiology in the majority of cases remains unknown. Nonetheless, an accurate diagnosis is of considerable benefit to the patient, for it saves him the psychological and monetary expense of repeated diagnostic evaluation, as well as offering a rational basis for such therapy as is available. The recent development of cardiac transplantation raises further problems, as yet completely unanswered, particularly the incidence and severity of rejection phenomena in this group of disorders as opposed to other cardiac diseases.

Most cardiologists feel that the diagnosis of primary myocardial disease must be made by exclusion. While this is true for the majority of disorders so classified, the thrust of this view is essentially negative. It is the purpose of this chapter to outline the authors' approach to the problem of primary myocardial disease with emphasis on those factors in the history and physical and laboratory examinations which are most helpful in establishing a precise diagnosis.

DEFINITION AND CLASSIFICATION

The definition of primary myocardial disease is partly clinical and partly anatomic, so that no single characteristic is common to all cases. Primary myocardial disease encompasses a broad spectrum of myocardial disorders, usually associated with cardiomegaly and congestive heart failure. Individuals who have neither of these signs but have heart disease manifested by some combination of arrhythmias, embolic episodes, gallop

JAMES S. FORRESTER, M.D. Scientific Director, Myocardial Infarction Research Unit, Cedars of Lebanon Hospital, and Assistant Professor of Medicine, UCLA School of Medicine, Los Angeles, California. HARVEY G. KEMP, JR., M.D. Director, Division of Cardiology, St. Luke's Hospital Center, and Assistant Clinical Professor of Medicine, College of Physicians and Surgeons, Columbia University, New York, New York. RICHARD GORLIN, M.D. Chief, Cardiovascular Division, Peter Bent Brigham Hospital, and Associate Professor of Medicine, Harvard Medical School, Boston, Massachusetts.

sounds, or hemodynamic abnormality are also generally included. Anatomically, diffuse involvement of the myocardium is generally present.

Because of the vague nature of the defining characteristics and the use of other terms to signify this category of disease, considerable confusion has arisen. For purposes of this discussion, the terms cardiomyopathy, myocardiopathy, myocardosis, idiopathic cardiomegaly, and, in the older literature, chronic myocarditis, will be considered synonymous with primary myocardial disease. Further difficulties in classification arise from the lack of unanimity among authorities regarding the inclusion of myocarditis in the primary myocardial disease group. The myocarditis patient is usually acutely ill, and can generally be distinguished clinically from one with chronic primary myocardial disease. Therefore, acute myocarditis will be excluded from this classification, although there will be an unknown number of individuals who progress from acute myocarditis to the chronic form, and become indistinguishable from those with primary myocardial disease. The difficulty in classification becomes apparent when one realizes that no recent classifications are the same.[9, 10, 13, 19] Because it is useful to have an outline for teaching purposes as well as a diagnostic framework at the bedside, the authors employ the classification shown in Table 5. Not included in this classification is a diverse collection of specific disorders that occasionally may resemble primary myocardial disease. These include metastatic invasion of the heart, trichinosis, Chagas' disease, thyroid and other endocrine diseases with heart involvement, and beriberi.

TABLE 5

Primary Myocardial Disease

Unknown etiology
  1. Idiopathic cardiomyopathy
  2. Familial cardiomyopathy
  3. Endomyocardial fibrosis
  4. Endocardial fibroelastosis
  5. Postpartum heart disease
Specific etiology
  1. Alcoholic cardiomyopathy
  2. Collagen vascular disease
      a. Lupus erythematosus
      b. Scleroderma
      c. Polyarteritis nodosa and other angiitides
  3. Neuromuscular
      a. Friedreich's ataxia
      b. Progressive muscular dystrophy
      c. Myotonia dystrophica
  4. Infiltrative
      a. Sarcoidosis
      b. Amyloidosis
      c. Hemochromatosis
      d. Glycogen storage disease
      e. Mucopolysaccharidosis (gargoylism, Hurler's disease)

CLINICAL PRESENTATION

Although the noncardiac manifestations of the systemic diseases associated with primary myocardial disease may serve to distinguish one from the other, the cardiovascular manifestations are monotonously similar.[13] The two most common symptoms of cardiomyopathy are congestive heart failure and arrhythmia. Less common, but also frequent, are chest pain and syncope. In Harvey's series of over 200 patients with primary myocardial disease seen at Georgetown University Hospital, approximately two-thirds had congestive heart failure, one-third had arrhythmia, and one-fourth had chest pain.

The pain of primary myocardial disease is occasionally helpful in pointing toward a diagnosis. When it is dull, deep, unrelated to specific precipitating factors such as exertion, or prolonged in duration and unrelieved by nitroglycerin, one may be aided in ruling out other disorders, notably angina pectoris. Frequently, however, the pain may be pleuritic, or may in every way resemble angina pectoris, and in such cases an erroneous diagnosis is common.

Case 1:

A 50-year-old white man with a 20-year history of heavy alcohol consumption was referred for evaluation of undiagnosed chest pain. A year prior to admission he had an episode of severe substernal pain. Upon arrival at the hospital he had several episodes of ventricular fibrillation from which he was successfully resuscitated. From that time on he had frequent attacks of prolonged, nonradiating, substernal pain without clear-cut precipitating cause, occasionally relieved by nitroglycerin, and diagnosed as coronary insufficiency. Physical examination revealed atrial fibrillation and elevated neck veins; the heart was enlarged to percussion and there was a laterally displaced apical impulse. The first heart sound was loud, the second heart sound was split, and a third heart sound was audible. No murmur was heard. The remainder of the physical examination was not remarkable; stigmata of alcoholism were not present. The electrocardiogram revealed left bundle branch block. Chest x-ray revealed enlargement of the left ventricle, right ventricle, and right atrium as well as pulmonary congestion. The diagnosis prior to cardiac catheterization was coronary artery disease with treated congestive heart failure. Left cineventriculography revealed a large, markedly hypokinetic left ventricle. Stroke index was 18 cc/beat/m² ($n = 45$), and left ventricular end diastolic pressure was 18 mm Hg ($n = 10$ or less). Selective coronary arteriography revealed normal left and right coronary vessels. There were no valvular gradients, and mitral insufficiency was not detected by ventriculography.

This patient serves to illustrate the confusion in separating coronary artery disease from primary myocardial disease. Anginal pain and recurrent severe electrical instability suggest coronary atherosclerosis. The presence of atrial fibrillation and left bundle branch block are both suggestive of primary myocardial disease, as will be discussed later. In addition, the presence of congestive heart failure in the absence of a large aneurysm or prolonged severe history of coronary heart disease speaks against the latter diagnosis. This patient, however, presents a case in which definitive diagnosis required coronary arteriography.

Both right and left heart failure may occur, and symptoms of circulatory failure, such as ease of fatigue and generalized weakness, are common. Congestive heart failure secondary to primary myocardial disease usually presents with chronic failure of gradual onset, but initial presentation as acute pulmonary edema has been reported and should not, therefore, rule out the diagnosis. The congestive failure is frequently refractory to therapy, and this single observation should lead one to consider the diagnosis of primary myocardial disease. Another therapeutic difficulty characteristic of primary myocardial disease is increased sensitivity to digitalis, as manifested by arrhythmia.

Frequently the patient complains of palpitations, reflecting the high incidence of arrhythmia in this disease. Virtually every form of arrhythmia occurs, but premature ventricular and atrial beats are most common. Atrial fibrillation is also common, particularly in alcoholic myocardial disease. Less frequently one encounters atrial flutter, paroxysmal atrial tachycardia, or ventricular tachycardia. It is not surprising, therefore, that syncope and sudden death occur in an unusually high percentage of patients with primary myocardial disease.

Embolic complications, although not common in primary myocardial disease, are far more frequent than in most other cardiac disorders. One particular type of cardiomyopathy, seldom seen in the United States, has a strikingly high incidence of embolic disease; endomyocardial fibrosis, the most common heart disease in many parts of Africa, is associated with a 40 per cent incidence of embolic disease in reported series. The majority of emboli are cardiac in origin. Pulmonary emboli arise from the right atrium, whereas systemic emboli more commonly arise from the left ventricle, although the left atrium may occasionally also contain thrombi. The patient with primary myocardial disease, right atrial thrombi, and pulmonary emboli may present with features of pulmonary hypertension, and confusion with congenital heart disease may result if the emboli go unrecognized.[13] Primary myocardial disease should become a prime diagnostic consideration when a systemic embolic episode occurs and an adequate alternative explanation for its etiology does not exist.

PHYSICAL EXAMINATION

The physical examination, like the history, may reveal some very helpful clues to the correct diagnosis, but on occasion prominent physical signs may lead to an incorrect diagnosis, such as valvular heart disease.

The most frequent physical finding encountered in the cardiomyopathies is the gallop sound. The majority of patients have either an audible third heart sound (ventricular filling gallop) or fourth heart sound (atrial systole gallop). The third heart sound is more common, although fourth heart sounds have been reported in as many as half the patients with cardio-myopathy.[13] It seems likely that both gallop sounds reflect the decreased compliance of a fibrotic or infiltrated myocardium being distended by rapid filling. In the presence of moderate tachycardia and consequent decreased diastolic filling period, third and fourth heart sounds become superimposed, resulting in the loud summation gallop, which is quite common. Increasing the rate of ventricular filling by exercise will often make a previously unde-tected gallop sound audible. Congestive heart failure without an audible gal-lop is infrequent in primary myocardial disease. In the Georgetown experi-ence 140 patients had congestive heart failure secondary to cardiomyopathy; a gallop was heard in every patient. Even in the absence of congestive heart failure gallops are frequently heard; in the individual without congestive heart failure the third and fourth heart sounds may provide an early clue to the presence of myocardial disease. A word of caution must also be given regarding the gallop sounds. In the unusual case third and fourth heart sounds are prominent and occur quite close together in time, these low-pitched sounds can simulate a diastolic rumble and suggest mitral stenosis (Fig. 15). The consequences of this coincidence can be profound, particularly if other symptoms and signs, such as embolic phenomena or left atrial enlargement, are also present.

Case 2:

A 40-year-old state trooper was referred for evaluation of mitral valvular disease. He had no history of rheumatic fever and had drunk heavily for 10 years, but had ceased totally 10 years previously. He had had atrial fibrillation for the past 3 years. Three months prior to admission he had the sudden onset of global aphasia which subsequently cleared completely. A diagnosis of cerebral embolus was made, and treatment with anticoagu-

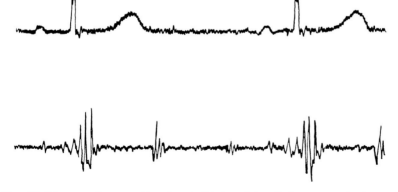

FIG. 15. Phonocardiogram. Prominent third and fourth heart sounds in an in-dividual with primary myocardial disease. In the presence of tachycardia the close proximity of these sounds may simulate a diastolic murmur.

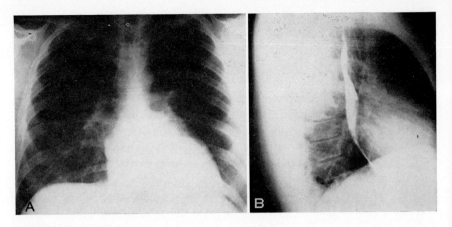

FIG. 16. Posteroanterior (A) and left lateral (B) chest x-rays. Note moderate enlargement of the left atrium as well as the left ventricle. Redistribution of pulmonary vascularity to the upper lobes is not present.

lants was begun. In the period before cardiac catheterization a number of physicians examined the patient. He was described as having atrial fibrillation, no left or right ventricular heaves, an increased first sound, a normally split second sound, a grade 2 mid-diastolic rumble, and an opening snap. A high-pitched systolic murmur was described by several observers; some physicians thought the opening snap was actually a third heart sound. The liver was palpable 2 cm below the costal margin and was not tender. Chest x-ray revealed biventricular enlargement. The left atrium was moderately enlarged, but the pulmonary artery segment appeared normal (Fig. 16). Precatheterization diagnosis was "pure" mitral stenosis, mild to moderate in degree. Phonocardiography demonstrated a third heart sound, but neither the systolic nor diastolic murmur was adequately demonstrated. Hemodynamic data revealed an elevated left ventricular end diastolic pressure (25 mm Hg), slightly diminished cardiac index (2.4 l/min/m^2), and no transvalvular gradient at rest or during isoproterenol stress. The pulmonary artery pressure was 36/20 mm Hg; the pulmonary capillary wedge pressure was 26 mm Hg. Selective coronary arteriography demonstrated normal vessels. Subsequent rectal mucosal biopsy for amyloid, as well as muscle biopsy, serum protein electrophoresis, serum iron and iron-binding capacity, and pulmonary angiogram for left atrial myxoma were all normal. While anticoagulation was being resumed following cardiac catheterization the patient experienced the sudden onset of a right homonymous hemianopsia, which subsequently cleared. He was discharged on anticoagulants with a diagnosis of primary myocardial disease, possibly a late sequel of alcohol usage. He serves to illustrate the occasional pitfalls inherent in auscultation, particularly when the history is supportive. The diagnostic rumble heard by most observers is unexplained, but does occasionally occur in primary myocardial disease. In addition, a sound has been recorded in primary myocardial disease with the same timing as an opening snap, but its mechanism is poorly understood.[13]

Murmurs are frequent in cardiomyopathy of all types, particularly those with congestive heart failure. The most frequent murmur encountered is a holosystolic murmur at the apex, consistent with mitral insufficiency. Since this murmur often diminishes or disappears with digitalis and diuretic therapy, it has been ascribed to dilation of the mitral valve annulus which recedes with decrease in cardiac size. In some cases papillary muscle dysfunction also plays a significant role. Particularly in those cases in which endomyocardial fibrosis is prominent, the papillary muscle may be bound down and the mitral valve held open.[27]

Diastolic mitral murmurs have been heard by many observers, although they are uncommon. Even though the murmur is frequently of higher pitch than the murmur of mitral stenosis, and is often confined to mid-diastole, confusion with mitral stenosis does occur. Pulmonic flow murmurs are also quite common, but seldom if ever are mistaken for the murmur of pulmonic stenosis, probably because the second sound and chest x-ray are not characteristic. The murmur of tricuspid insufficiency may also be heard in those individuals with severe congestive heart failure.

The nature of the second heart sound is of considerable interest. Generally it is loud and closely split, reflecting the pulmonary hypertension secondary to congestive heart failure or, less commonly, that due to pulmonary emboli. Many patients with primary myocardial disease have conduction defects, however, and widely and persistently split sounds may be heard in those with right bundle branch block; a paradoxically split second sound may be noted in the presence of left bundle branch block. In many patients both the first and second heart sounds are diminished in intensity, and confusion with pericardial effusion may occur, particularly when marked cardiomegaly coexists.

A frequently overlooked physical finding is the appearance of the facies. In several of the cardiomyopathies the facies alone will suggest the diagnosis, although this feature is often noted only retrospectively. Myotonia dystrophica is one such disorder, and gargoylism another. It is not uncommon for the physician to overlook the typical facies because several healthy members of the family have the same unusual appearance as the patient. The alcoholic facies is also suggestive.

Many patients with the unusual cardiomyopathies exhibit cutaneous manifestations. The alcoholic exhibits plethora or telangiectasia in an overwhelming percentage of cases. Hemochromatosis often gives rise to melanotic grayish pigmentation. Collagen vascular diseases abound in cutaneous manifestations, and many such patients have skin lesions that suggest the diagnosis. Sarcoid produces a great variety of cutaneous manifestations, most commonly nodules on the shoulder or face, amenable to a rapid biopsy diagnosis. Amyloidosis also has a characteristic cutaneous lesion, located especially on the face and at mucocutaneous junctions. Biopsy of the lesions or of the rectal mucosa will usually establish the diagnosis if amyloidosis is present. Because secondary cardiomyopathies are uncommon and not always easily recognized, there is often a considerable delay between the onset of symptoms and correct diagnosis. In such cases careful attention to these areas of the physical examination should aid in correct diagnosis.

DIAGNOSTIC STUDIES

The electrocardiogram is rarely normal in primary myocardial disease. Nonspecific ST- and T-wave abnormalities are the most frequent, followed closely by premature ventricular contractions. All types of arrhythmias are found, atrial fibrillation being particularly common. Of special note is the high incidence of Wolff-Parkinson-White syndrome in patients with familial cardiomyopathy. Bundle branch block has been more frequent in our experience than is generally reported, and is considerably less common in angiographically documented coronary heart disease than is generally stated.[12]

Several features of the ECG, while not diagnostic, are often helpful. P-wave abnormalities suggestive of biatrial enlargement are common, even when no apparent cause of atrial hypertrophy is present. One often encounters prominent P waves, greater than 2.5 mm in lead II, and biphasic P waves in the right precordial leads with prolonged intrinsicoid deflection and broad negative phase. Left ventricular hypertrophy or the ECG pattern of loss of septal Q wave, often attributed to septal fibrosis, is also frequently seen.[24] Evans[7] has described T-wave changes found frequently in alcoholic cardiomyopathy which he feels are suggestive, although not diagnostic, of this condition. Four abnormalities are described: the spinous, cloven, dimpled, and narrowly inverted T waves. Our experience has been that the overlap with other disorders is sufficiently great to make these interesting abnormalities of only limited usefulness.

A source of confusion in establishing the diagnosis of cardiomyopathy may be the presence of an ECG pattern of anterolateral infarction. Although a difference of opinion exists regarding the nature of the lesion associated with this finding, in some cases there is no anatomic correlation with the Q-wave abnormality.[30] About one-quarter of the patients in the authors' series have electrocardiograms suggestive of old myocardial infarctions (Fig. 17). Low voltage is found in a significant number of patients with cardiomyopathy, and may be misinterpreted as added evidence for pericardial effusion if there is also a large heart silhouette and distant heart sounds are noted.

The chest x-ray usually reveals cardiomegaly, although the magnitude of this need not be great. Cardiomegaly is by no means essential to the diagnosis, especially in individuals seen early in the course of the disease, or in patients manifesting arrhythmia. The authors have seen several young patients who presented initially with arrhythmias of unknown etiology associated with normal heart size, who have progressed to the classical clinical picture of idiopathic cardiomyopathy.

Hemodynamic studies have not been rewarding in establishing the

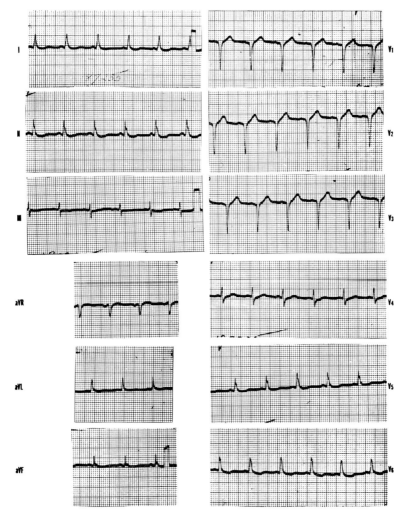

Fig. 17. ECG. Short PR interval (0.12 second). Loss of R-wave V₁₋₃ suggests old anteroseptal myocardial infarction.

diagnosis of cardiomyopathy.[33] The cardiac catheterization data are usually more helpful from the negative standpoint, in ruling out valvular and congenital heart disease. Cardiac output is generally reduced. The fibrotic or infiltrated myocardium results in the following functional abnormalities: decreased compliance (increased stiffness), diminished contractile state, and compensatory left ventricular dilation. In addition, altered intra-ventricular conduction and excitation may adversely affect synchrony of left ventricular contraction.

Restricted filling of the heart, indicated on the ventricular pressure curve by an early diastolic dip followed by a high diastolic plateau, is occasionally seen in cardiomyopathy. This phenomenon has been ascribed to the inabil-

ity of the ventricle to expand with inflow of blood from the atrium, so that
a high intraventricular pressure is achieved early in the rapid filling phase
of diastole. On a histologic basis this is secondary to fibrotic or hypertrophied myocardium, which results in a stiffer ventricle, an obliterated
cavity, or both. In our experience this finding is supportive of a diagnosis
of cardiomyopathy, but is also seen in constrictive pericarditis.

DIFFERENTIAL DIAGNOSIS

Coronary Heart Disease

Among patients with primary myocardial disesae, coronary heart disease
is probably the most commonly considered alternative diagnosis, for there
may be considerable overlap in both signs and symptoms. A typical problem
in differentiation might be that of a patient with a large heart, congestive
heart failure, ischemic type chest pain, ventricular gallop, and abnormal
ECG, possibly an anterolateral infarction pattern. Differential diagnosis
may be facilitated in younger patients by recalling that individuals with
premature onset coronary heart disease (before the age of 50) have several
characteristics that may distinguish them. Thus, there is a strong family
predilection. In addition, more than 90 per cent of these patients have a
demonstrably abnormal intravenous glucose tolerance test, abnormal serum
cholesterol or triglyceride concentrations, or an abnormal lipoprotein pattern on serum electrophoresis.[14] A smaller percentage are frankly diabetic.

A number of clinical points may be helpful in separating the primary
myocardial disease group from those with coronary heart disease. When
chest pain is dull, prolonged, unrelated to exertion, and unrelieved by
nitroglycerin, primary myocardial disease is suggested. Typical or atypical
angina pectoris, on the other hand, may occur in primary myocardial disease
and frequently leads to a misdiagnosis of coronary heart disease. The most
difficult clinical problems arise in the patient with congestive heart failure
and signs, symptoms, or historical features suggesting coronary heart
disease. It is unusual to see congestive heart failure in coronary heart disease
until a large amount of the myocardium has been damaged by myocardial
infarction. Thus, the heart is usually not greatly enlarged in coronary heart
disease unless the patient has extensive three vessel disease or an aneurysm
is present. It is our impression that, among these patients, the majority of
those who present with congestive heart failure, but without an electrocardiogram specific for coronary heart disease, have primary myocardial
disease and not coronary heart disease. In this group, however, coronary
angiography is essential to the diagnosis, since coronary heart disease
occasionally presents in a manner suggesting primary myocardial disease.

Case 3:

A 52-year-old white man complained of increasing shortness of breath
over a 6-month period; his symptoms began after a brief febrile illness
characterized by swelling of the lips and periorbital region, unaffected by

antihistamines, but rapidly relieved by a brief course of corticosteroids. He had had no prior cardiorespiratory complaints, but had a 3-year history of intermittent claudication. Physical examination revealed bilateral basilar rales, no cardiac enlargement, a prominent fourth heart sound, and hepatosplenomegaly. Laboratory data were within normal limits; ECG revealed sinus tachycardia, nonspecific ST-T-wave changes, and frequent premature ventricular beats. At the time of cardiac catheterization he was found to have elevated left ventricular end diastolic and right heart pressures and no valvular gradients. Selective coronary cineangiography revealed complete occlusion of the right coronary artery and severe disease in both the left anterior descending and left circumflex vessels. Medical therapy for congestive heart failure was begun, but he expired suddenly at home 2 weeks later. An autopsy was not performed.

This case history of coronary heart disease is unusual in our experience for several reasons. The patient presented with symptoms of congestive heart failure, but had no previous history of myocardial infarction. In addition, the heart was not grossly enlarged, which is the rule in coronary heart disease, but unusual in coronary heart disease with moderately severe congestive heart failure. Further, the absence of Q waves on the ECG is uncommon in the individual with congestive heart failure and coronary heart disease. On the other hand, the history of intermittent claudication weighed heavily in favor of the diagnosis of heart failure due to this cause.

The response of congestive heart failure to treatment is often helpful, in that the patient with primary myocardial disease is often refractory to therapy, and, even with successful treatment, may exhibit a persistent gallop.

Several physical findings may be helpful in distinguishing coronary heart disease from primary myocardial disease. Signs of arterial disease elsewhere in the body, while not definitive, are reasonably reliable, increasingly so with the severity of the findings. Any of the many physical findings suggesting diabetes favors coronary heart disease (or, rarely, hemochromatosis). The presence of xanthoma tendinosum or tuberosum usually indicates a familial lipid disorder, and strongly favors coronary heart disease. Paradoxical splitting of the second sound has been described in coronary heart disease.[34] The phenomenon is often transient, and occurs more commonly during acute ischemia. While the mechanism is not clear, it may reflect mechanical prolongation of systole or elevation of pulmonary artery pressure. Since both these phenomena occur with primary myocardial disease, the sign cannot be considered diagnostic of coronary artery disease in this setting. The gallop sound is probably more frequent in primary myocardial disease than in coronary heart disease, but the incidence of gallop in the latter is sufficiently great to minimize its usefulness in differential diagnosis.

Electrocardiography and other studies may be of help. The presence of 0.04-second Q waves clearly favors coronary heart disease. Discrete bundle branch block and intraventricular conduction defects, except those of the peri-infarction type, are not as common in coronary heart disease as once suspected, and should at least raise the question of etiologies other than coronary heart disease in those individuals who have bundle branch block. Among the patients referred to us for evaluation of suspected coronary heart disease with bundle branch block, about 50 per cent have been found to have primary myocardial disease. Exercise electrocardiography is probably more frequently productive of ST depression in coronary artery disease than in primary myocardial disease, but the authors have seen a strongly positive test in one individual with documented primary myocardial disease.

Apex cardiography is useful in detecting areas of anterior or apical paradoxical pulsation or localized akinesis, and this has been correlated by cinematographic techniques with abnormal ventricular motion.[22] Since both localized asynergy and paradoxical pulsation are seen much more often in the heart of the patient with coronary artery disease than in the patient with cardiomyopathy, this study may be of value when ventriculography cannot be performed. The cardiomyopathic ventricle is generally hypokinetic without localized abnormalities.

With all the above clinical data to distinguish these two groups, there will remain a number of individuals in whom a definite diagnosis cannot be made. In this group selective coronary arteriography, cineventriculography, and hemodynamic studies should be considered, particularly in the young, symptomatic individual in whom precise diagnosis is required, if only to render prognostication more accurate.

Rheumatic Heart Disease

Primary myocardial disease may simulate rheumatic heart disease, since both may occur in children and young adults. The most common problem involves interpretation of the systolic murmur of mitral insufficiency. In addition, primary myocardial disease may closely resemble mitral stenosis in some cases, either because of simulation of a murmur by merged third and fourth heart sounds or because of the actual presence of a diastolic murmur. To compound the problem further, an enlarged left atrium, as determined by chest x-ray, is not uncommon in primary myocardial disease, and Kerley's B lines are seen in both conditions.[9]

The presence of valvular calcification virtually rules out cardiomyopathy as the sole diagnosis. The great majority of individuals with valvular calcification have rheumatic heart disease, but healed subacute bacterial endocarditis and calcified mitral or aortic annulus must also be included in the differential diagnosis. The diagnostic accuracy of this finding is greatly enhanced by the use of image intensification fluoroscopy; yet this simple procedure is often not employed. When mitral insufficiency is present, the character of ventricular contraction becomes quite important. A vigorously contracting heart favors rheumatic heart disease; a hypokinetic ventricle favors primary myocardial disease.

Behavior of the murmur of mitral insufficiency with therapy is helpful,

for the murmur of primary myocardial disease often decreases as the atrioventricular annulus becomes less dilated or papillary muscle alignment
changes with decreasing left ventricular size. In contrast, a structural
valvular murmur may increase with compensation of function. It has been
suggested that the temporal relationship of the onset of the murmur to the
onset of symptoms of congestive heart failure might serve to distinguish
insufficiency due to structural valvular disease from that caused by annular
dilation, a murmur beginning with the onset of failure favoring primary
myocardial disease. The unreliability of timing each of these events makes
it difficult to put this observation to good clinical use.

Hypertensive Cardiovascular Disease

Hypertensive cardiovascular disease occasionally enters the differential
diagnosis when a patient presents with congestive heart failure, a large
heart, and evidence of left ventricular hypertrophy on electrocardiography.
In large series about 15 per cent of patients with primary myocardial disease are found to have increased blood pressure, a figure not dissimilar
from the incidence in the general population. The pressure elevation in
primary myocardial disease, however, is confined to those patients in whom
congestive heart failure supervenes. Severe diastolic hypertension rarely
occurs; the diastolic pressure usually ranges from 90 to 110 mm Hg. Hypertensive changes are not seen in the fundi. The pulse pressure is typically
narrow and the elevated diastolic pressure usually falls to normal levels
with treatment of the congestive heart failure. The disparity between the
duration and magnitude of elevated systemic pressure and the severity of
the congestive heart failure make it clear in most cases that hypertensive
cardiovascular disease is unlikely.

Pericardial Disease

Pericardial disease must be considered. The similarity between the two
disorders may be striking in a patient found to have congestive failure,
a large, bottle-shaped heart with diminished pulsations on fluoroscopy,
diminished heart sounds with a gallop, a pericardial knock which may be
interpreted on auscultation as a gallop, pulsus paradoxus, a Kussmaul
sign (inspiratory increase in jugular venous pressure), and low voltage on
the electrocardiogram. Prior to the extensive use of more sophisticated
radiologic techniques pericardial aspirations were occasionally attempted
to help make this distinction. In all but the most clear-cut or emergent of
such cases it is probably wise to employ right atrial dye injection in the
posteroanterior projection, intravenous carbon dioxide injection with the
patient in left lateral decubitus position, echo cardiography, or radioisotope scanning to determine the distance between the inner wall of the
right atrium and the outer border of the cardiac silhouette prior to the
decision to perform needle aspiration. Several clinical observations may
be helpful prior to the use of these techniques. In cases in which the maximum cardiac impulse is displaced considerably to the left and downward

primary myocardial disease is more likely, particularly if the impulse is strong. Further, the murmur of mitral insufficiency or tricuspid insufficiency is more commonly heard in primary myocardial disease. The ECG in pericardial disease usually shows only nonspecific ST-T-wave changes, whereas in primary myocardial disease it may have any of the many abnormalities described earlier. While the early diastolic dip in the ventricular pressure curve characteristic of restrictive pericardial disease is perhaps less common in primary myocardial disease, it occurs often enough to prohibit placing much emphasis on the finding. The same may be said for the "pressure plateau," wherein right heart pressures (right atrial mean, right ventricular diastolic, and pulmonary diastolic) are similar to left heart pressures (pulmonary capillary wedge, left atrial mean). This has been said to be more characteristic of pericardial disease than cardiomyopathy. In the latter, pulmonary capillary wedge pressure is said to exceed right ventricular diastolic and right atrial mean by more than 10 mm Hg. When one is able to obtain these data, dye studies should also be possible, and in our opinion these greatly outweigh the pressure data in diagnostic significance.

Primary Pulmonary Hypertension

Primary pulmonary hypertension may present with right heart failure of unknown etiology, usually in young women. Early in the course of the disease differentiation may not be difficult, for electrocardiography, chest x-ray, cardiac catheterization data, and clinical findings will point to cor pulmonale. When the patient with idiopathic pulmonary hypertension is seen late in the course of the disease, however, the two disorders may not be readily separable.

Congenital Heart Disease

In the young patient congenital heart disease will often be considered, owing to the presence of an enlarged heart and murmurs in the absence of historical or other evidence of rheumatic heart disease. The murmur of cardiomyopathic mitral insufficiency may be confused with that of a ventricular septal defect. Fortunately, cardiomyopathy mimics no specific congenital lesion exactly, and the extensive use of cardioangiography and pressure recordings make a definite diagnosis possible in most cases.

CLINICAL FORMS OF PRIMARY MYOCARDIAL DISEASE OF
UNKNOWN ETIOLOGY

Familial Cardiomyopathy

This is present by definition when the disease clusters in a family. There are several large families in which an autosomal dominant pattern of inheritance has occurred, but recessive patterns of inheritance may also be seen. It is important to note that earlier reports probably included cases now recognized as idiopathic hypertrophic subaortic stenosis. Left ventricular hypertrophy is almost invariable in familial cardiomyopathy, and an inordinate number of patients with the disease have the Wolff-Parkinson-White syndrome. One type of familial cardiomyopathy, recessively inherited, is also characterized by deafness, prolongation of the QT interval, recurrent syncope, and sudden death.[20] This disorder, however, is not characterized by cardiomegaly or symptoms of congestive heart failure. Careful histologic studies have revealed abnormalities of the small vessels of the heart, particularly the nutrient vessels of the sinoatrial and atrioventricular nodes, consisting primarily of thickening of the tunica media.[21] Abnormalities of small coronary arteries have been described in a few other unusual cardiac disorders, including Friedreich's ataxia, primary pulmonary hypertension, progressive muscular dystrophy, familial cardiomyopathy, and others. It is possible that such changes in the small coronary arteries and arterioles will be found to be characteristic of many of those disorders presently classified as primary myocardial disease.

Endomyocardial Fibrosis

This is a common form of heart disease in Africa, accounting for 10 to 15 per cent of patients with heart disease seen in several East and South African hospitals. A large number of predisposing factors, such as protein deficiency, parasitism, malaria, dysentery, climate, and season, have been suggested, but the etiology of this remarkable disorder is unknown. Pathologically the endocardium is found to be thickened by dense fibrosis. This fibrous material extends into the myocardium in such a way that the ventricular cavity tends to be obliterated. Often it also extends to involve the atrioventricular valves, holding them fixed, and creating severe mitral or tricuspid insufficiency. Calcification of the ventricular wall may occur, and mural thrombosis is almost invariable. Pulmonary and systemic emboli, therefore, are very common, occurring in as many as 40 per cent of the cases. Although long-term survivals are reported, many patients succumb in early adulthood to congestive heart failure, thromboembolic disease, or bacterial endocarditis. Specific lesions outside the heart are not encountered.

Endocardial Fibroelastosis

The similarity of the terms endomyocardial fibrosis and endocardial fibroelastosis makes confusion common. It is simplest if one recalls the pathology of each. The African disorder is characterized by dense proliferation of fibrous tissue that covers the endocardium and invades the myocardium; hence endomyocardial fibrosis. Endocardial fibroelastosis is characterized by proliferation of both fibrous and elastic tissue, and is largely confined to the endocardium. Endocardial fibroelastosis differs from the African disease in many other respects. It is seen primarily in children, often in association with other congenital heart lesions, such as coarctation of the aorta, aortic stenosis, and pulmonic stenosis; in such cases a separate diagnosis may not be made. The pathologic changes of fibroelastosis are, however, encountered in the absence of other cardiac abnormalities. Since 90 per cent of children so afflicted die before age 2 of congestive heart failure, it is seldom that an internist or adult cardiologist will see such a patient.

Postpartum Heart Disease

Postpartum heart disease maintains a tenuous position in the classification of cardiomyopathies. A few patients have been described who fulfill the following restrictive criteria: no evidence of previous heart disease, left ventricular failure occurring 1 to 20 weeks post partum, and no other apparent etiology.[31] Whether this group represents a separate etiology is uncertain. It is wisest to be vigorous in excluding other specific etiologies, particularly multiple pulmonary emboli.

CARDIOMYOPATHIES OF SPECIFIC ETIOLOGY

Alcoholic Cardiomyopathy

The secondary cardiomyopathies are usually accompanied by stigmata of the underlying disease, though these signs may not be prominent early in the course of the disease. Those with considerable experience in the treatment of alcoholics, for example, will often be able to suspect the presence of alcoholism even in the absence of a positive history. Alcoholic cardiomyopathy is one of the most interesting of the secondary cardiomyopathies. That idiopathic congestive heart failure occurs more frequently in alcoholics than in the normal population is generally accepted. Changes in myocardial metabolism in chronic alcoholics at rest and in both animal and human subjects during alcohol infusion are well documented.[8] Chronic ingestion of alcohol by laboratory animals has been shown to produce histologic changes in the myocardium similar to those seen in the human cardiomyopathy, and to impair the contractile state.

Electron microscopic changes in the myocardium of patients with alcoholic cardiomyopathy have been described.[16] Many of the changes are similar to those seen with myocardial ischemia: thus, swelling of the sarcoplasmic reticulum, lipid accumulation, myofibrillar damage, and mitochondrial swelling are seen. In addition, changes ascribed to a degenerative process are noted, including intramitochondrial inclusions, dense, parallel cristae, lysosome-like bodies, increased lipofuscin granules, and extensive fragmentation of the sarcoplasmic reticulum. The presence of virus-like particles has been debated and is at present unsettled.

The etiology of alcoholic cardiomyopathy remains obscure, although there is no lack of theories. Direct toxic damage by alcohol, induced metabolic abnormalities, the presence of toxic trace elements such as cobalt, associated but not necessarily related disorders, such as nutritional or vitamin deficiency, and diminished resistance to infection have all been suggested. Whether one factor predominates in the majority of cases is not known.

Clinically the patient presents with cardiomegaly, congestive heart failure, and arrhythmia. Atrial fibrillation is particularly common, and alcoholic heart disease should be suspected in any instance of "idiopathic" atrial fibrillation. There are no findings specific to the cardiac evaluation that allow one to distinguish this disorder from other cardiomyopathies. Therefore, it is essential to question all cardiomyopathy suspects in detail and with persistence regarding the use of alcohol. The quantity and duration of alcohol ingestion necessary to produce clinical cardiomyopathy is unknown and obviously varies with other factors, but Evans' estimate of 1 pint daily for 10 years may serve as a rough clinical guide.[6] There may be a delay in onset of symptoms for some years after discontinuing alcohol. The physical examination almost always alerts the examiner to the possibility of alcoholism. Plethoric facies, nervous oral movements such as pursing or lip smacking, telangiectasia on the face, chest, and back, mild tremor of the hands, and thenar and quadriceps wasting may appear somewhat earlier in the course of alcoholism than other chronic stigmata of this condition, and should be looked for carefully in those cases in which the etiology of the heart disease is not apparent.

Systemic Lupus Erythematosus

Cardiac involvement in collagen vascular disorders is quite common. In systemic lupus erythematosus (SLE) clinical evidence of heart disease is reported in more than half the cases,[15] and histologic evidence is present in nearly all cases. The pericardium and endocardium are more frequently and more strikingly involved than the myocardium. Pericarditis is the commonest manifestation. The incidence of systemic hypertension is much higher in cardiomyopathies secondary to collagen vascular disease than in other types. Persistence of hypertension after resolution of congestive heart failure is uncommon in other cardiomyopathies and very frequent in collagen vascular disease. Although the misdiagnosis of idiopathic cardiomyopathy will rarely be made in a patient actually afflicted with SLE, the examination of the blood for LE cells and antinuclear antibody is essential to the work-up of idiopathic cardiomyopathy.

Scleroderma

Scleroderma involves the heart in a somewhat smaller percentage of cases[25] than does SLE. Clinical evidence of cardiac disease is seen in about one-third of the cases. Scleroderma may afflict the heart either through primary myocardial involvement or through mechanical loading secondary to either systemic or pulmonary hypertension. Although patchy fibrosis occurs, with frequent dilation and development of heart block, the most frequent clinical cardiac manifestation is cor pulmonale. Other evidence of scleroderma is usually obvious.

Polyarteritis Nodosa

Of the collagen vascular disease group, the most severe involvement of the heart occurs in polyarteritis nodosa. In contrast to SLE, half the patients with polyarteritis die of congestive heart failure, and an even greater percentage have clinical signs of heart failure during the clinical course.[17] Vascular lesions predominate histologically, and small focal areas of myocardial infarction are seen in association with necrotizing angiitis of both the large epicardial and small intramural coronary vessels.

Heart failure frequently occurs in the absence of pericarditis, gross myocardial infarction, or systemic hypertension, all of which occasionally accompany polyarteritis.

Case 4:

A 58-year-old white man was admitted with a 2-year history of gradually increasing weakness and dyspnea on exertion, and a chronic nonproductive cough. He had suffered two syncopal episodes during this time, without clear-cut precipitating cause. In the 6 months prior to admission he experienced substernal heaviness and choking, brought on by exertion and relieved by rest. There was a strong family history of heart disease. Abnormalities on physical examination were confined to the heart. There was mild cardiomegaly, an aortic systolic ejection murmur without transmission, and a bifid left ventricular impulse. ECG showed evidence of a probable old anteroseptal myocardial infarction. An unexplained eosinophilia of 20 per cent was found. Other laboratory data, including LE preparations and urinary 17-keto- and 17-hydroxysteroids, were normal. The precatheterization diagnosis was coronary heart disease. Coronary arteriography revealed diffuse narrowing of the left anterior descending artery; there were normal ventricular pressures and an abnormal cardiac output. One year later the patient was readmitted, having sustained a 25-pound weight loss and increasingly severe chest pain in the interim. He was found to have an elevated blood urea nitrogen, and 3+ proteinuria; the hematocrit was 29 per cent and there was 50 per cent eosinophilia in the peripheral blood. In the ensuing 3 weeks uremia developed rapidly, and he expired with uremic encephalopathy. Postmortem examination revealed polyarteritis nodosa involving the heart, kidneys, spleen, and skin. There were multiple infarctions of both ventricles of 4 to 8 weeks' duration, as well as right ventricular mural thrombosis and multiple emboli.

Neuromuscular Disorders

Cardiomyopathy has been described in three neuromuscular disorders: myotonic dystrophy, progressive muscular dystrophy, and Friedreich's ataxia. From a differential diagnostic standpoint, only myotonic dystrophy is likely to be confused with idiopathic cardiomyopathy. This is largely because myotonic dystrophy is rare, and most physicians fail to recognize the typical facies. In some cases cardiac involvement precedes other manifestations,[18] and in such situations idiopathic cardiomyopathy would probably be erroneously diagnosed if a positive family history were not obtained. The disease is familial, being inherited as an autosomal dominant trait. There is characteristic atrophy of the muscles of the face, thighs, and forearms, and of the sternocleidomastoids. The resultant picture is one of an individual with droopy lids and slack jaw, with head thrust forward, and often with a stiff, uncertain gait. In addition, cataracts and premature balding are characteristic. The male patient is frequently impotent and has testicular atrophy. ECG abnormalities are far more frequent than are symptoms of heart disease.[26]

Myocardial involvement has been reported to occur in as many as 85 per cent of patients with progressive muscular dystrophy,[1] varying with the type of dystrophy. As with myotonic dystrophy, cardiac rhythm and conduction abnormalities predominate. In addition, thromboembolic complications and sudden death have been reported. Friedreich's ataxia, like muscular dystrophy, is not likely to enter the differential diagnosis of cardiomyopathy of unknown etiology, even though cardiac signs and symptoms are identical with those of other cardiomyopathies. Evidence of cardiac abnormality has been reported in about one-half the cases, and ECG abnormalities in 90 per cent of cases.[3]

Sarcoidosis

This condition often produces signs of congestive heart failure, usually late in the course of the disease. As in scleroderma, the majority of these individuals have pulmonary hypertension and cor pulmonale as a result of pulmonary sarcoid and pulmonary fibrosis. Direct myocardial involvement by sarcoid occurs in about 20 per cent of the cases, either as isolated or multiple granulomata, or as diffuse interstitial fibrosis.[28] Arrhythmias, intraventricular conduction defects, incomplete or complete atrioventricular block, Adams-Stokes syndrome, and sudden death characterize direct sarcoid involvement of the myocardium. In those individuals with myocardial involvement there is almost always involvement elsewhere in the body, so that a misdiagnosis of idiopathic cardiomyopathy is not likely to occur.

Cardiac Amyloidosis

Cardiac amyloidosis may be of several types, and debate continues concerning the validity of classification. Distinction has been made between secondary amyloid, which usually does not involve the heart, and primary amyloid, which involves predominantly the heart, tongue, lungs, blood vessels, and rectum. The overlap in distribution is considerable. When amyloid does affect the heart there is seldom a predisposing cause; involvement generally begins after the age of 40, and the patient commonly presents with congestive heart failure. It is usual for the diagnosis to be overlooked until late in the course. Eliot and his associates[5] have pointed out the high incidence of left axis deviation and intraventricular conduction abnormalities in this disease. Tissue biopsy is of considerable value in establishing the diagnosis, and is often included in the routine work-up of idiopathic cardiomyopathy. Biopsy of the rectal mucosa is positive in up to 80 per cent of individuals with amyloidosis,[11] and is associated with a low risk when properly performed. We have avoided liver biopsy because of the reported risk of intractable bleeding secondary to hepatic rupture after biopsy.

There is another form of amyloidosis which is seldom recognized ante mortem. Also termed senile amyloidosis, this form occurs in the elderly, usually in individuals over 80 years of age, and is confined to the heart. Buerger and Braunstein[4] reported finding cardiac amyloidosis in 24 per cent of autopsied patients over the age of 90. In most of these patients the finding was incidental and not associated with cardiac symptoms. In 20 per cent of those with senile cardiac amyloidosis the involvement may have contributed to congestive heart failure. The difficulties in distinguishing senile cardiac amyloidosis from coronary artery disease in the elderly is apparent, and tests required to confirm the diagnosis are probably not indicated in this age group.

Hemochromatosis

Hemochromatosis is most commonly diagnosed on the basis of diabetes, liver disease, gray-brown skin pigmentation, and testicular atrophy. The majority of patients, however, will also be found to have iron pigment deposition in the myocardium,[29] although clinical symptomatology does not necessarily follow. In those patients in whom pigment deposition is extensive and accompanied by fibrosis, cardiomyopathy may occur, although the disordered myocardial function may reflect alterations in intracellular metabolism as well. As with other infiltrative cardiomyopathies, the presentation of cardiac disease with reduced compliance is seen. This particular disorder, therefore, may simulate constrictive pericarditis, with elevated venous pressure, hepatomegaly, and cardiac catheterization data revealing an early diastolic dip and late diastolic plateau.[32] Although such cases are probably rare, hemochromatosis may involve the heart without producing skin pigmentation or diabetes. Serum iron and iron-binding capacity together with biopsy of the skin or liver should establish the diagnosis. Since this disease, unlike many of the other cardiomyopathies, is potentially amenable to specific therapy, one should obtain the serum iron and iron-binding capacity in any case of primary myocardial disease with clinical features that suggest the diagnosis of hemochromatosis.

Case 5:

A 36-year-old white male physician was evaluated for progressive heart failure. Fifteen years previously he had noted the onset of diminished sex drive. He had been married for 16 years, had no children and, on sterility evaluation 3 years previously had been found to have small testes and no spermatogenesis by testicular biopsy. One year previously he experienced the onset of diabetes mellitus requiring the use of 45 units of insulin daily. He had noted a slight increase in pigmentation at the ankles and belt line. An extensive endocrine evaluation led to the diagnosis of panhypopituitarism. In the 3 months prior to admission he gradually developed signs and symptoms of congestive heart failure, which were markedly accentuated just prior to admission, when he developed an influenza-like syndrome, along with other members of his family. On admission he had bilateral rales, bilateral pleural effusions, and a 2-cm enlargement in heart size as compared to previous examinations. There was a prominent third heart sound and tachycardia of 120 beats/minute. No murmur was heard. Laboratory data revealed a hematocrit of 54 per cent, serum glutamic-oxalacetic transaminase of 72 units/ml, lactic dehydrogenase of 136 units/ml, serum iron of 180 μg/100 ml, and iron-binding capacity of 210 μg/100 ml. The patient experienced sudden respiratory arrest 3 days later and expired. Viral studies done ante mortem for Coxsackie and adenovirus were all negative. Microscopic examination revealed severe hemochromatosis of the heart, pancreas, thyroid, and kidneys. Virtually all other organs were also involved. The changes in the heart consisted of severe degeneration, without evidence of active inflammation.

This unfortunate individual illustrates how the diagnosis of a chronic disease can be missed over a period of years. Although the correct diagnosis was made before death, it was too late to reverse the course of the disease.

Glycogen Storage Disease

This condition produces an infiltrative type of cardiomyopathy, but since the disease appears in infancy and almost invariably leads to death in the first year of life, it is involved in a diagnostic category different from the adult cardiomyopathies. Lingual enlargement, failure to thrive, cardiac failure without murmurs or cyanosis, and muscle flaccidity and atrophy usually lead to consideration of the diagnosis, which is confirmed by muscle biopsy.

Mucopolysaccharidosis (Gargoylism, Hurler's Syndrome)

This is not a difficult disease to recognize in its classical presentation. The individual has a distinctive facies. Stature is short, often with dorsal kyphosis, short neck, disproportionately short legs, and stubby fingers. A host of other abnormalities accompany these skeletal changes. Mental retardation, hepatosplenomegaly, corneal opacities, characteristic granulation of the polymorphonuclear cells (Alder's anomaly), and bone marrow mucopolysaccharide inclusions are also seen. The heart is involved in a majority of cases.[23] Many cases of mucopolysaccharidosis fail to achieve such classic proportions, however, and since survival into middle age is not uncommon, the diagnosis is probably often overlooked. Cardiomegaly is usual. Congestive heart failure may reflect myocardial damage by mucopolysaccharide deposition, or thickening of the mitral or aortic valves by the same material, with resultant valvular dysfunction. Diagnosis is largely clinical at the present time; the disorder should be suspected in undiagnosed heart failure if any of the aforementioned skeletal abnormalities are also present. Chondroitin sulfate, heparitin sulfate, or acid mucopolysaccharide is usually increased in concentration in the urine (See Chapter 2).[2]

CONCLUSION

Primary myocardial disease remains one of the great unresolved areas of cardiology. Since diagnosis is presently based primarily on clinical presentation rather than etiology, one may expect increasing clarity of classification as etiology is better defined. The major benefit of early diagnosis at present is not so much cure, but rather ability to establish a prognosis and to bring a halt to costly and often fruitless, repetitive medical tests and examinations. It is important in each case to rule out the rarer secondary cardiomyopathies because several, including hemochromatosis, sarcoid, collagen vascular disease, and alcoholism, are treated in a somewhat specific manner. The major diagnostic errors will occur in the area of overlap in signs and symptoms with coronary artery disease. Careful evaluation of the history, physical examination, and routine laboratory data will lead to a correct diagnosis in most cases, and will also point the way to appropriate diagnostic procedures, such as coronary arteriography, when these are indicated.

These studies were supported by United States Public Health Service Grants HE 05679 and HE 11306 and by a grant from Women's Aid for Research, Boston, Massachusetts.

REFERENCES

1. Berenbaum, A. A., and Horowitz, W. Heart involvement in progressive muscular dystrophy. Amer. Heart J. **51**:622, 1956.
2. Berenson, G. S., and Geer, J. C. Heart disease in the Hurler and Marfan syndromes. Arch. Internal Med. **111**:58, 1963.
3. Boyer, S. H., Chisholm, A. W., and McKusick, V. A. Cardiac aspects of Friedreich's ataxia. Circulation **25**:493, 1962.
4. Buerger. L., and Braunstein, H. Senile cardiac amyloidosis. Amer. J. Med. **28**: 357, 1960.
5. Eliot, R. S., McGee, H. J.. and Blount, S. G. Cardiac amyloidosis. Circulation **23**:613, 1961.
6. Evans, W. Alcoholic cardiomyopathy. Amer. Heart J. **61**:556, 1961.
7. Evans, W. Alcoholic cardiomyopathy. Progr. Cardiovasc. Dis. **7**:151, 1964.
8. Ferrans, V. J. Alcoholic cardiomyopathy. Amer. J. Med. Sci. **252**:89, 1966.
9. Fowler, N. O. Classification and differential diagnosis of the myocardiopathies. Progr. Cardiovasc. Dis. **7**:1, 1964.
10. Friedberg, C. K. *Diseases of the Heart*, 3rd ed., p. 992. W. B. Saunders Co., Philadelphia, 1966.
11. Gafni, J., and Sohar, E. Rectal biopsy for the diagnosis of amyloidosis. Amer. J. Med. Sci. **240**:332, 1960.
12. Haft, J., Herman, M. V., and Gorlin, R. Coronary arteriographic and left ventricular motion studies in left bundle branch block. Amer. J. Cardiol. **23**:117, 1969.
13. Harvey, W. P., Segal, J. P., and Gurel, T. The clinical spectrum of primary myocardial disease. Progr. Cardiovasc. Dis. **7**:17, 1964.
14. Heinle, R. A., Levy, R., Fredrickson, D. S., and Gorlin, R. Lipid and carbohydrate abnormalities in angiographically documented coronary artery disease. Amer. J. Cardiol. **24**:178, 1969.
15. Hejtmancik, M. R., Wright, J. C., Quint, R., and Jennings, F. L. The cardiovascular manifestations of systemic lupus erythematosus. Amer. Heart J. **68**:119, 1964.
16. Hibbs, R. G., Ferrans, V. J., Black, W. C., Weilbaecher, D. G., Walsh, J. J., and Burch, G. E. Alcoholic cardiomyopathy. Amer. Heart J. **96**:766, 1965.

17. Holsinger, D. R., Osmundson, P. J., and Edwards, J. E. The heart in periarteritis nodosa. Circulation 25:610, 1962.
18. Holt, J. M., and Lambert, E. H. N. Heart disease as the presenting feature in myotonia atrophica. Brit. Heart J. 26:433, 1964.
19. Hurst, J. W., and Logue, R. B. *The Heart Arteries and Veins*. Blakiston Division, McGraw-Hill Book Company, New York, 1966.
20. James, T. N. Congenital deafness and cardiac arrhythmias. Amer. J. Cardiol. 19: 627, 1967.
21. James, T. N. Pathology of small coronary arteries. Amer. J. Cardiol. 20:679, 1967.
22. Lane, F. J., Carroll, J. M., Levine, H. J., and Gorlin, R. The apexcardiogram in myocardial asynergy. Circulation 37:890, 1968.
23. Lindsay, S., Reilly, W. A., Gotham, T., and Skahen, R. Gargoylism: study of pathologic lesions and clinical review of 12 cases. Amer. J. Dis. Child. 76:239, 1948.
24. Marriott, H. J. L. Electrocardiographic abnormalities, conduction disorders and arrhythmias in primary myocardial disease. Progr. Cardiovasc. Dis. 7:99, 1964.
25. Oram, S., and Stokes, W. The heart in scleroderma. Brit. Heart J. 23:243, 1961.
26. Orndahl, G., Thulesinus, O., Enestrom, S., and Dehlin, O. The heart in myotonic disease. Acta Med. Scand. 176:479, 1964.
27. Parry, E. H. O. Endomyocardial fibrosis. In *Cardiomyopathies*, Ciba Foundation Symposium, G. E. W. Wolstenholme and C. M. O'Connor, Eds. Little, Brown and Co., Boston, 1964.
28. Porter, G. H. Sarcoid heart disease. N. Engl. J. Med. 263:1350, 1960.
29. Swan, W. G. A., and Dewar, H. A. The heart in hemochromatosis. Brit. Heart J. 14:117, 1952.
30. Tavel, M. E., and Fisch, C. Abnormal Q waves simulating myocardial infarction in diffuse myocardial diseases. Amer. Heart J. 68:534, 1964.
31. Walsh, J. J., Burch, G. E., Black, W. C., Ferrans, V. J., and Hibbs, R. G. Idiopathic myocardiopathy of the puerperium. Circulation 32:19, 1965.
32. Wasserman, A. J., Richardson, D. W., Baird, C. L., and Wyso, E. M. Cardiac hemochromatosis simulating constrictive pericarditis. Amer. J. Med. 32:316, 1962.
33. Yu, P. N., Cohen, J., Schreiner, B. F., and Murphy, G. W. Hemodynamic alterations in primary myocardial disease. Progr. Cardiovasc. Dis. 7:125, 1964.
34. Yurchak, P. M., and Gorlin, R. Paradoxical splitting of the second sound in coronary artery disease. N. Engl. J. Med. 269:741, 1963.

Systemic Arterial Hypertension

MORTON H. MAXWELL

Systemic arterial hypertension is a common, potentially life-limiting disorder. Studies in recent years have lengthened the list of known causes which are susceptible to surgical cure and have thus added substantial diagnostic responsibilities to the management of the hypertensive patient. Furthermore, since prolonged duration of arterial hypertension, regardless of its cause, may result in irreversible damage to multiple organ systems, the physician is obligated not only to make as precise an etiologic diagnosis as possible, but to do so as soon after the patient comes under his care as he reasonably can.

Systemic arterial hypertension may be arbitrarily defined as a diastolic blood pressure of 90 mm Hg or higher on repeated examinations in a subject with normal salt intake, regardless of age or sex. Although some consider arterial hypertension to represent simply the upper end of the normal blood pressure distribution[51] rather than a distinct disease,[52] there is conclusive evidence to indicate progressive increase in mortality and morbidity from vascular lesions of the central nervous system, heart, and kidneys with increments in blood pressure above 140/90 mm Hg.[1, 60] This relationship is present at all ages and correlates with both systolic and diastolic pressure.[33] Conversely, individuals with lower than "normal" diastolic pressures seem to have longer life expectancies and fewer cardiovascular complications than those with "normal" pressures.[19, 23] While mean blood pressure in populations tends to rise with age, this increase is *largely systolic*, and is due primarily to decreased elasticity of the aortic wall. Patients with diastolic hypertension in later life may therefore be considered to be hypertensive within the above definition.

Because the incidence of vascular complications in hypertension is related to the duration as well as the degree of elevation of the diastolic pressure, and because potentially curable forms of secondary hypertension, such as that due to renal artery stenosis, may become more resistant to corrective surgical therapy with prolonged duration, it is important to diagnose and, if indicated, treat hypertension at the earliest possible time. Not all patients with hypertension need necessarily be treated, however. Thus, the knowledge that a woman over 65 years of age with a diastolic pressure of 100 mm Hg may have a normal life expectancy is insufficient.

MORTON H. MAXWELL, M.D. Chief, Nephrology and Hypertension Service, Cedars-Sinai Medical Center, and Clinical Professor of Medicine, UCLA Medical Center, Los Angeles, California

Her life expectancy may indeed be normal if she has essential hypertension without evidence of secondary vascular damage, in which case treatment would not be mandatory; if the hypertension is secondary to early, progressive bilateral renal artery stenosis, however, her life expectancy is decidedly not normal, and it is imperative to make an accurate diagnosis at the earliest possible time. The decision regarding therapy must be individualized and reached only after consideration of all available clinical and laboratory information.

The definition of systemic arterial hypertension as a diastolic pressure of 90 mm Hg or greater eliminates from our usual diagnostic approach those patients with purely systolic hypertension. This may result from loss of elasticity of the aorta with age or may be due to a variety of other conditions, including thyrotoxicosis, anemia, heart block, arteriovenous fistulae, or the hyperkinetic heart syndrome. Systolic hypertension does not generally have the same serious prognostic implications as diastolic hypertension, and its treatment is that of the underlying condition.

The work-up of the patient with systemic arterial hypertension is aimed at establishing an etiologic diagnosis (Table 6) and ascertaining the severity of the hypertensive process (Table 7). These two factors dictate subsequent management.

HISTORY

There are very few clinical symptoms which can be attributed to arterial hypertension itself.[1] Perhaps the only symptom which is caused directly by the elevated blood pressure is headache. When this occurs, it is typically pounding and occipital in location, tends to be present upon awakening in the morning, and wears off during the day. True hypertensive headaches occur in fewer than 25 per cent of patients, and are unusual unless the diastolic blood pressure is greater than 110 mm Hg. There is no convincing evidence that dizziness or vertigo, seen in approximately 30 per cent of patients,[1] is caused by the high blood pressure per se. Likewise, the relationship of hypertension to epistaxis is unclear.

When symptoms are present in essential hypertension they are almost always attributable to secondary target organ damage, e.g., congestive heart failure, coronary artery disease, central nervous system vascular disease, or renal involvement, and indicate moderate to severe arterial hypertension. The two most common symptoms are dyspnea on exertion and tachycardia, both resulting from left-sided congestive heart failure. A careful history must be taken for evidence of encephalopathy or cerebrovascular accidents, such as changes in sensorium, seizures, transient weakness or paralysis of a limb, hemianopsia, or episodes of syncope. Angina pectoris may indicate associated coronary artery disease. The first symptom of renal involvement is often nocturia. Only with advanced renal failure do patients complain of pruritus, nausea, and vomiting.

Since arterial hypertension tends to occur as a familial disorder, a careful family history should be obtained. A positive family history of diabetes

TABLE 6

Causes of Secondary Hypertension

Renal
  Glomerulonephritis
  Pyelonephritis
  Congenital disorders
  Collagen diseases
  Diabetes mellitus
  Obstructive uropathy*
  Hypersensitivity angiitis
  Renal tumors
  Gouty nephropathy
Central nervous system
  Brain tumor*
  Increased intracranial pressure from any cause
  Bulbar poliomyelitis; Guillain-Barré syndrome
Adrenal
  Cushing's syndrome*
  Primary aldosteronism*
  Pheochromocytoma*
  Adrenogenital syndromes*
Vascular
  Coarctation of the aorta*
  Renal artery stenosis*
Miscellaneous
  Eclampsia*
  Polycythemia*
  Psychogenic*
  Drug-induced (oral contraceptives, licorice)*

* Potentially curable.

TABLE 7

*Hypertension Severity Index**

Degree	Diastolic pressure	Optic fundi	Left ventricular hypertrophy	Renal damage
	mm Hg	*grade*		
Mild	<100	0–I	None	None
Moderate	100–120	0–II	None, or left ventricular "strain" pattern	Few or no abnormalities
Severe	>120	III–IV	Yes	Yes

  * Worsened by Negro race; male sex; young age; encephalopathy, congestive heart failure, myocardial infarction, or angina pectoris (past or present); decreased glomerular filtration rate (creatinine clearance); and lack of lability of diastolic pressure.

mellitus, polycystic kidney disease, or pheochromocytoma may also be helpful, since these disorders have a familial occurrence and are frequently associated with secondary hypertension.

Certain symptoms or groups of symptoms may suggest or be pathognomonic of particular disorders causing secondary diastolic hypertension. Thus, transient "attacks" of any type are suggestive of adrenal tumors. Although 50 per cent of patients with *pheochromocytoma* have persistent diastolic hypertension, and are either asymptomatic or cannot be distinguished clinically from patients with essential hypertension, the other 50 per cent have attacks of paroxysmal hypertension from intermittently secreting tumors. The three most common symptoms during these attacks are headaches, excessive perspiration, and palpitations. Commonly associated manifestations are pallor, nervousness, tremulousness, weakness, nausea, chest and abdominal pain, dyspnea, flushing, and dizziness. Paroxysms are frequently spontaneous, but may be precipitated by physical exertion, abdominal palpation, and emotional upset. In full-blown *primary aldosteronism* the associated symptoms are typical of severe potassium deficiency: polyuria and nocturia, and attacks of severe muscle weakness or even muscle paralysis, particularly prominent in the proximal portions of all four extremities. *Cushing's syndrome*, even when not apparent from the appearance of the patient, is often manifested by severe personality changes and even by euphoria. Since all forms of *parenchymal kidney disease* may cause secondary hypertension, symptoms of these disorders must be elicited: nocturia, pallor, edema, dysuria, frequency of urination, flank pain, gross hematuria, pruritus, nausea, and vomiting. Rarely, a *brain tumor* may cause diastolic hypertension; the neurologic symptoms and subsequent examination usually make this diagnosis evident.

Although essential hypertension remains a diagnosis of exclusion and may, in fact, represent a heterogeneous group of disorders, we are in accord with others[8] that it is a distinct clinical entity with a characteristic natural history. Onset is rare in the first two decades of life or after the age of 50, the average age of onset being 32 years, and the average duration without treatment 20 years.[50] During the latter part of its natural history there is slowly progressive involvement of target organs (heart, brain, kidney), singly or in combination, with resulting symptomatology. Malignant hypertension is uncommon, occurring in fewer than 5 per cent of patients with essential hypertension.[27]

A history which is "inappropriate" for essential hypertension suggests secondary causes of high blood pressure, such as adrenal tumors, renovascular hypertension, or coarctation of the aorta.[35] In our experience the following inappropriate historical items have led most frequently to the diagnosis of secondary hypertension:

1. The onset of hypertension in a patient younger than 20 or older than 50 years of age, especially with a negative family history of hypertension.

2. The abrupt onset of severe hypertension, with or without preceding mild hypertension.

3. Malignant hypertension.

4. Inappropriate symptoms, particularly "attacks" (see above).

PHYSICAL EXAMINATION

Blood Pressure Determination

It is impossible to place enough emphasis on proper techniques for measuring blood pressure. Despite the fact that subsequent tests and therapy are based upon the results of this procedure, it is often performed casually and improperly.

In our clinic the blood pressure is recorded by a nurse after the patient has disrobed and has been resting quietly in a supine position in a semidarkened room for at least 15 minutes. The nurse has a minimal amount of conversation with the patient during this period, and does not suggest the level of pressure by words or by facial expression. The blood pressure is recorded rapidly five times, permitting the cuff to deflate completely and the mercury manometer to rest at zero for 15 seconds between readings. The patient then assumes the upright position and stands quietly for at least 2 minutes. Five successive blood pressure readings are then obtained in the upright position. This same procedure is repeated by the nurse at the termination of the physical examination, when the physician has left the examining room, but before the patient has dressed.

Although the resting blood pressure is not as reproducible or perhaps as significant as true basal blood pressure (taken after a full night's sleep and before arising from bed), it is preferable to the usual casual reading.[59] Having a nurse or a technician take the readings, rather than the physician, helps to reduce emotional responses to the physician's presence and to standardize the procedure. Repeated determinations tend to reduce the patient's emotional response to the procedure. When the physician considers the five recorded pressures, he utilizes the average figure if they are all reasonably close to each other. If one or two readings are disparate, particularly the first recorded pressures, he may choose to discard them and to average the other three or four. If there is extreme lability of blood pressures the physician will then take repeated readings himself.

Pressures recorded in the supine and upright positions sometimes suggest a particular circulatory abnormality or cause of secondary hypertension. The normal homeostatic adjustment to the upright position results in a slight decrease in systolic pressure and a slight increase in diastolic pressure with little change in mean arterial pressure. Orthostatic hypotension may occur in pheochromocytoma, in primary aldosteronism, or with generalized arteriosclerotic vascular disease. Furthermore, the recording of pressures in the supine and upright positions establishes a pattern of control measurements with reference to which the effects of subsequent antihypertensive drug therapy can be judged. This is particularly important when ganglionic blocking agents or sympatholytic drugs are used.

It is advisable to measure blood pressure in both arms and in the legs on the initial examination. If it is taken in only one arm and is elevated, hypertension will be diagnosed, but possible arterial disease or stenosis of the other subclavian artery may be overlooked. Conversely, if one measures it in the arm to which circulation is compromised one may find a normal or low pressure and miss the diagnosis of hypertension altogether. Determination of the blood pressure in the legs is important in excluding the possibility of coarctation of the aorta. This may be easily done by utilizing the palpatory method to estimate systolic blood pressure in comparison to that in the arm. The ordinary blood pressure cuff is applied to the calf of the leg and the systolic pressure is estimated by palpating the posterior tibial artery. The systolic pressure in the lower extremities is usually 10 to 30 mm Hg higher than that in the upper extremity when measured indirectly.

The following technical aspects of blood pressure recording deserve emphasis:

1. The size of the cuff must be appropriate to the arm girth, and the cuff must fit snugly around the upper arm before inflation.

2. Prior to actual blood pressure measurement the cuff must be inflated high enough to obliterate the radial pulse. This is to establish the true systolic pressure in case of an auscultatory gap.

3. The optimal position for placement of the diaphragm of the stethoscope on the arm is located by prior palpation for maximal pulsation of the brachial artery.

4. In both the supine and upright positions the patient's arm is elevated above the heart level during inflation of the cuff. This helps to eliminate venous filling, which may cause muffling of the Korotkoff sounds.

5. As the cuff pressure is slowly lowered, the sudden appearance of sharp clicking sounds indicates the systolic pressure (Korotkoff, phase 1). The disappearance of sound (Korotkoff, phase 5) is usually taken as the diastolic blood pressure,[57] although in an occasional patient the muffling of sounds (Korotkoff, phase 4) correlates better with diastolic pressure as measured by direct techniques.

General Examination

The physical examination in hypertensive patients provides evidence of the degree of hypertension and also the extent of end organ damage. In addition, there may be findings which suggest the presence of specific causes of secondary hypertension. Information obtained in the history and physical examination will also aid in directing the laboratory and radiologic evaluation of the patient, and in making decisions concerning the urgency of medical treatment and the need for hospitalization for specific diagnostic investigations.

In assessing the severity of the hypertensive process by physical examination, in addition to the actual level of the blood pressure particular note should be made of the optic fundi, the heart, and the lungs. Numerous studies have confirmed the validity of utilizing the state of the optic fundi to estimate the severity of the hypertensive process.[3, 16, 25] During the first examination, to ensure complete observation, the pupils may be dilated with a mydriatic agent. The fundi are then graded in accordance with the Keith-Wagener-Barker classification[25] as follows:

Normal.

Grade I—arteriolar constriction, either generalized or focal.

Grade II—venous notching, arterial-venous crossing defects.

Grade III—hemorrhages and/or exudates.

Grade IV—papilledema.

Constriction of the retinal arterioles indicates a reversible state of spasm. The severity of both generalized and focal arteriolar narrowing is closely correlated with the severity of diastolic hypertension.[3] This fact may be helpful in the initial study of patients with labile hypertension and spuriously high diastolic levels at the first examination; thus, those with little or no arteriolar narrowing often prove to have much lower blood pressures on subsequent examinations or when they are hospitalized.[16] It should be recognized that arteriovenous nicking and increased light reflex signify thickening of the arteriolar wall due to arteriolar sclerosis, and are more closely related to the duration of hypertension than to its severity. These findings, therefore, argue against recent onset of hypertension. In contrast to arteriolar constriction, which abates when blood pressure is reduced by appropriate therapy, sclerosis is an organic change in the wall of the arteriole which regresses little, if any, when blood pressure is reduced.[20, 28] Retinal hemorrhages in hypertensive patients are characteristically flame-shaped and most numerous adjacent to the optic discs. Retinal exudates secondary to hypertension are usually described as "cotton wool" or soft exudates, and signify increased permeability of capillaries and local ischemia, probably as a result of vascular damage from severe hypertension.[20] At times exudates may appear to be "hard" and sharply circumscribed. These punctate, more deeply placed exudates, particularly in malignant hypertension, may assume a radial configuration like spokes of a wheel, with the macula at the center, a configuration known as a "macular star." Both types of exudate regularly regress and ultimately disappear when blood pressure is reduced.[16] Papilledema is the hallmark of malignant hypertension, but may also be a sign of increased intracranial pressure of any cause, such as brain tumor or intracerebral hemorrhage. These latter possibilities must be carefully excluded when papilledema is seen in the absence of retinal hemorrhages and exudates. The mechanism of the papilledema secondary to diastolic hypertension is not clear, since not all patients with malignant hypertension have increased intracranial pressure.[27]

In addition to being a reliable index of the severity of diastolic hypertension, there is a direct relation between ophthalmoscopic grading, as described above, and the prevalence of certain complications of hypertension, e.g., electrocardiographic changes, cardiomegaly, proteinuria, and azotemia.[3] There is also a direct relation between severity of ophthalmoscopic grouping and mortality of untreated hypertensive patients.[16, 25] For any specific level of diastolic blood pressure the prognosis worsens from the lower to the higher ophthalmoscopic group.

Careful examination of the heart and lungs is important to ascertain the presence of left ventricular enlargement, congestive heart failure, or associated cardiac valvular lesions. Left ventricular enlargement results in a forceful apical impulse, often displaced laterally and caudally. Occasionally the apical impulse is reduplicated and associated with an S_4 gallop. In the presence of left ventricular failure an S_3 gallop may be heard, and pulmonary congestion may be indicated by moist, inspiratory basal rales. Systolic murmurs, if present, may reflect associated aortic valve disease, relative mitral regurgitation due to left ventricular failure with cardiac dilation, or turbulence created by muscular hypertrophy of the aortic outflow tract. A decrescendo diastolic murmur along the left or right sternal border may reflect relative aortic regurgitation due to dilation of the aortic root. Such murmurs, unless they are due to intrinsic valvular disease, are rarely heard when the diastolic pressure is less than 110 to 120 mm Hg, and often disappear when blood pressure is lowered by therapy.

A careful neurologic examination must be performed. Asymmetry of deep tendon reflexes, cranial nerve deficits, or localized motor or sensory defects may indicate previous, unsuspected cerebrovascular accidents or primary intracranial disease.

The presence of abdominal bruits suggests the possibility of renal artery stenosis.[22] In listening for such bruits one must press the bell part of the stethoscope deeply into the epigastrium in the midline, and then into both hypochondria beneath the lower rib margins. The bruit of renal artery stenosis is usually high-pitched and systolic, although it may be continuous. Occasionally it may be transmitted to the femoral arteries or flanks. It is almost impossible to cause a factitious bruit by pressure of the stethoscope in any of these areas, except in an occasional very thin individual with a lax abdominal wall. It must be remembered, however, that abdominal bruits may arise in vessels other than the renal arteries, particularly in older individuals with diffuse arteriosclerotic disease. Hence, the presence of a bruit should not be accepted as unequivocal evidence of renal artery stenosis without confirmatory arteriography.

Hypertensive patients do not present a characteristic appearance, nor do they necessarily have more evidence of vasomotor instability, such as sweating, than do other patients.

Findings on the physical examination which may suggest specific causes of secondary hypertension include the following:

1. Orthostatic hypotension (pheochromocytoma, primary aldosteronism).

2. Sudden rise in blood pressure with or without other symptoms suggesting catecholamine excess during or immediately after firm, bimanual palpation of the abdomen (pheochromocytoma).

3. "Moon" facies, hirsutism, "buffalo" hump, truncal obesity, plethoric appearance, and cutaneous striae (Cushing's syndrome).

4. Pallor of the mucous membranes, urochrome pigmentation of the skin, periorbital or pedal edema, and pericardial or pleural friction rubs (chronic parenchymal renal disease with uremia).

5. Retinal microaneurysms, sometimes accompanied by hemorrhages and exudates (diabetes mellitus).

6. Papilledema, usually with accompanying neurologic signs, in the presence of mild or moderate hypertension (brain tumor). This constellation may occasionally occur in malignant hypertension, when the hypertension is of acute onset (acute glomerulonephritis, eclampsia).

7. Irregular, firm abdominal masses in one or both hypochondria (polycystic kidney disease).

8. Delayed, weak, or absent pulsations of the femoral arteries with relative hypotension in the lower extremities (coarctation of the aorta).

9. Raynaud's phenomenon of the fingers or toes, skin rashes, joint swelling, and pleural or pericardial friction rubs in the absence of uremia (collagen diseases).

10. Chronic arthritis associated with tophaceous deposits in multiple joints and bursae and in the helices of the ears (gouty nephropathy).

DIAGNOSTIC EVALUATION

In our clinic, following the history and physical examination, patients are divided into three groups on the basis of the severity of the hypertensive process. The extent and pace of work-up are dictated by the group within which the patient falls.

Group 1: Borderline or Questionable Systemic Arterial Hypertension

This group consists of patients whose diastolic pressure readings on the first examination are less than 100 mm Hg and whose optic fundi are normal. It also includes those with purely systolic hypertension. These patients undergo a minimal laboratory work-up (Table 8), and blood pressure readings are repeated on several occasions in the clinic. If persistent diastolic hypertension is documented they are considered as being in group 2.

Group 2: Mild or Moderate Hypertension

These are patients who have diastolic pressures of 100 to 120 mm Hg, whose ocular fundi are Keith-Wagener-Barker grade II or less, and in whom there is no prior history or current evidence of hypertensive encephalopathy, cerebrovascular accidents, or left-sided congestive heart failure. Also included are those with minimal current hypertension but unequivocal diastolic hypertension in the past. These patients are seen as outpatients and undergo an appropriate laboratory work-up (Table 8) over a period of 1 to 3 weeks. During this time the blood pressure is determined repeatedly in order to ascertain its lability and to establish control readings for assessing the effectiveness of later antihypertensive therapy.

Patients in this group who have symptoms, signs, or laboratory evidence suggesting a cause of secondary hypertension such as coarctation of the aorta, renovascular disease, pheochromocytoma, primary aldosteronism,

TABLE 8

Laboratory Examinations in Systemic Arterial Hypertension

Test	Significance	Remarks
Urine		
Urinalysis	Sediment normal in mild hypertension, but hematuria and proteinuria may occur in severe hypertension. Abnormal sediment may suggest primary parenchymal renal disease (e.g., leukocyte casts in chronic pyelonephritis or erythrocytes with casts in glomerulonephritis or collagen disease)	Sediment examination must be performed on a *fresh* urine specimen, since formed elements may disintegrate, particularly in alkaline urine
Maximum specific gravity	Urinary concentrating defect may indicate primary renal disease, renal damage due to hypertension, or primary aldosteronism (due to potassium deficiency)	Discard morning urine after 12 hr of dehydration, and measure specific gravity on following specimen. Value $\geq$ 1.020 is "normal"
Quantitative protein excretion	Normal in mild hypertension and usually $<$ 1.0 g/24 hr even in severe hypertension with renal damage Protein excretion $>$1.0 g/24 hr suggests parenchymal renal disease	
Quantitative urine culture	Positive culture (100,000 organisms/cu mm) suggests active pyelonephritis	Asymptomatic chronic pyelonephritis is a common cause of hypertension, and may occur in the presence of a normal urinary sediment.
Phenolsulfonphthalein excretion (PSP test)	Detects renal function decrease, especially in pyelonephritis or other disorders with primarily tubular damage Roughly equated with renal plasma flow	$>$20% PSP excretion in 15 min considered "normal"
Creatinine clearance	Reflects glomerular filtration rate	Calculated from 24-hr urinary excretion of creatinine and serum creatinine
Catecholamines	Elevated in pheochromocytoma	Vanillylmandelic acid is the most reliable. May be normal during periods of normotension with intermittently secreting tumors. False negatives of VMA in patients taking monoamine oxidase inhibitors.

TABLE 8—*Continued*

Test	Significance	Remarks
Catecholamines— *continued*		False positives of metanephrine and normetanephrine in patients taking methyldopa, bronchodilators, and monoamine oxidase inhibitors
Aldosterone	Elevation suggests primary aldosteronism	Elevation may be secondary to severe hypertension alone, or to sodium depletion
17-Keto- and 17-hydroxysteroids	Elevated in Cushing's syndrome	
Blood		
Creatinine (or blood urea nitrogen)	Elevation reflects decreased renal function	
Potassium	Decreased in primary or secondary aldosteronism	No diuretics for 7 days before test
CO_2	Decreased in acidosis due to renal failure. Increased in alkalosis accompanying primary or secondary aldosteronism	No diuretics for 7 days before test
Uric acid	Elevation suggests gout or renal failure	Uric acid also mildly increased in a significant proportion of patients with essential hypertension without renal failure or clinical gout, and in patients taking thiazide diuretics
Glucose tolerance test	Abnormality may indicate diabetes mellitus or may be associated with pheochromocytoma, primary aldosteronism, or Cushing's disease	
Peripheral plasma renin activity	Low and suppressed in primary aldosteronism. Exaggerated with salt depletion in significant renal artery stenosis	Influenced by state of sodium balance and intake of certain drugs (oral contraceptives, hydralazine, etc.)
Miscellaneous		
Electrocardiogram	Evidence of left ventricular hypertrophy or "strain" may precede clinical cardiac enlargement. May reveal old myocardial infarction. May suggest hypo- or hyperkalemia	Useful in estimating "severity" of hypertension
Chest x-ray	Evidence of left ventricular hypertrophy and/or pulmonary congestion	Useful in estimating "severity" of hypertension

TABLE 8—*Continued*

Test	Significance	Remarks
Chest x-ray—*continued*	Notching of ribs may be seen in coarctation of aorta	
Rapid-sequence intravenous pyelogram	May be pathognomonic of renal disease (polycystic kidney disease, pyelonephritis) or suggest renal artery stenosis (disparity in size or function of kidneys) or adrenal tumor (displacement of kidney)	
Radioisotope renogram	Detects disparity in kidney size and function (renovascular hypertension, pyelonephritis)	Useful only if intravenous pyelogram cannot be done (sensitivity to iodides) or is unsatisfactory
Individual kidney function tests (so-called "split function tests")	May reveal typical pattern of "ischemia" in significant renal artery stenosis May distinguish unilateral pyelonephritis from renal artery stenosis in the presence of a small kidney	Requires catheters in both ureters
Arteriography	Detects coarctation of the aorta and renal artery stenosis May be useful in the diagnosis of renal and adrenal tumors	

or Cushing's disease are usually hospitalized for their diagnostic studies because of the necessity for arteriography and/or complex biochemical determinations which can be most reliably performed under metabolically controlled conditions. If hospitalization is not feasible, these studies, with the exception of arteriography and tests of function of the two kidneys individually, can be performed on an outpatient basis.

Group 3: Severe or Malignant Hypertension and Hypertensive Encephalopathy

Included in this category are patients who have resting diastolic blood pressures of 120 mm Hg or more and/or grade III or IV retinopathy. Left-sided congestive heart failure or central nervous system manifestations are common. These patients, who may be in danger of suffering a catastrophic vascular accident, are hospitalized and kept under observation while the characteristics of their blood pressure elevations are ascertained and necessary diagnostic tests performed with minimum delay prior to the institution of antihypertensive therapy. Also included in this group are patients with hypertensive encephalopathy manifested by mental obtundity, coma, and/or convulsions. Such patients present true medical emergencies and should receive prompt, effective antihypertensive therapy. Diagnostic evaluation can be initiated on admission, but complex procedures should be delayed until the acute hypertensive crisis is brought under control.

Our system for classifying the severity of hypertension appears in Table 7. In our opinion the best single indication of the severity of the hypertensive process is the state of the optic fundi (see above). Thus, any patient with grade III or IV fundi is considered to have severe or malignant hypertension, even if the diastolic pressure is less than 120 mm Hg. The diastolic blood pressure is probably the second most important criterion of severity, though marked lability on sequential examinations makes it a less reliable guide. When lability of blood pressure is demonstrated, our estimate of severity is revised downward. As can be noted, the severity classification is based almost entirely upon the history and the physical examination. The only laboratory procedures which are utilized are the electrocardiogram and simple estimates of renal function. Factors which worsen the prognosis are very carefully weighed in the evaluation (footnote to Table 7). Thus, hypertension is automatically considered to be "worse" in a Negro, in a male, and in a young individual. It is good clinical practice, if one is to err in his original estimate, to err in overestimating rather than underestimating the severity of the disease. This ensures a rapid and comprehensive work-up and treatment at the earliest possible time.

Every reasonable effort should be made to ascertain causes of hypertension amenable to specific curative therapy before a patient is labeled with the diagnosis of essential hypertension and hence committed to a lifetime of antihypertensive drug therapy. During the last decade the application of increasingly sophisticated techniques has resulted in the diagnosis of surgically treatable causes of hypertension, such as primary aldosteronism and renal artery stenosis, in significant numbers of patients who formerly would have been thought to have essential hypertension. It is probable that, with the wider application of tests presently available and the development of new ones, further definition of the population of "essential" hypertensives will be possible.

Laboratory examinations useful in the evaluation of the hypertensive patient are described in Tables 8 and 9. All patients with definitely elevated diastolic pressures should undergo certain screening procedures designed to supplement impressions gained from the history and physical examination with regard to the etiology and pathophysiologic severity of the hypertensive process. These might reasonably include a complete blood count, urinalysis, serum creatinine, serum potassium and CO_2, urinary catecholamines or vanillylmandelic acid (VMA), rapid-sequence intravenous pyelogram, electrocardiogram, chest x-ray, and peripheral plasma renin (low sodium intake, upright position).

Additional laboratory examinations, to establish the diagnosis of a specific cause of secondary hypertension suggested by the history, physical

TABLE 9

Laboratory Diagnosis of the Main Causes of Secondary Hypertension

I. Parenchymal renal disease
  A. Urinalysis
  B. Serum creatinine or blood urea nitrogen
  C. Phenolsulfonphthalein excretion
  D. Intravenous pyelogram
  E. Quantitative urine culture
  F. Urinary maximum specific gravity
  G. Serum calcium, phosphorus, and alkaline phosphatase activity
  H. Lupus erythematosus preparation; antinuclear antibodies; serum complement
  I. Renal clearances
  J. Renal biopsy
II. Cushing's syndrome
  A. Urinary 17-keto- and 17-hydroxysteroids
  B. Glucose tolerance test
  C. Serum potassium
  D. Plasma cortisol
  E. Adrenal stimulation (ACTH) and suppression (dexamethasone)
III. Primary aldosteronism
  A. Serum electrolyte concentrations
  B. Aldosterone excretion or secretion rate (normal salt intake)
  C. Peripheral plasma renin activity (normal and low salt intake)
  D. Glucose tolerance test
  E. Urinary maximum specific gravity
  F. Blood volume
  G. Urinary and salivary sodium-to-potassium ratios
  H. Adrenal vein aldosterone levels and venography
IV. Pheochromocytoma
  A. Urinary catecholamines and vanillylmandelic acid (VMA)
  B. Intravenous pyelogram
  C. Pharmacologic tests (histamine, phentolamine, glucagon,[32] tyramine[11])
V. Coarctation of the aorta
  A. Chest x-ray
  B. Aortogram
VI. Renal artery stenosis
  A. Rapid-sequence intravenous pyelogram
  B. Radioisotope renogram
  C. Renal arteriogram
  D. Bilateral renal venous renin activity
  E. Individual kidney function tests

examination, and screening procedures, should then be selectively chosen and performed.

When doubt exists, it is best to err on the side of doing an extra procedure, even if the indications for this procedure appear to be minimal. There is no valid evidence that essential hypertension of any degree ever resolves spontaneously, and the incidence of vascular complications in secondary as well as essential hypertension is related to the duration and the severity of the elevation of the diastolic arterial pressure. In addition, potentially curable forms of secondary hypertension, such as renal arterial hypertension, may become more resistant to corrective therapy with prolonged duration. It is imperative, therefore, to discover these potentially curable forms of hypertension at a relatively early stage, while they are still amenable to appropriate therapy.

CLINICAL FEATURES OF THE VARIOUS CAUSES OF SECONDARY HYPERTENSION

Hypertension Due to Renal Parenchymal Disease

Renal parenchymal diseases of diverse etiologies may be associated with systemic arterial hypertension.[10, 49] The mechanism of this renal hypertension has not been clarified, but it has been variously ascribed to increased secretion of a pressor substance (possibly renin), failure to destroy a circulating extrarenal pressor substance, failure to secrete a vasodilator substance (vasodepressor lipid), production of a substance which causes increased reactivity of blood vessels, and increased sensitivity to extracellular fluid volume expansion.[36]

It is rare for hypertension to occur with diffuse parenchymal renal disease until at least a moderate degree of renal functional impairment is present. Usually proteinuria and a persistently abnormal urinary sediment are evident. Renal disease can therefore, with rare exceptions, be eliminated as the cause of systemic arterial hypertension by a careful urinalysis and simple renal function tests, including a phenolsulfonphthalein excretion test (PSP) and serum creatinine. Long-standing benign essential hypertension may cause glomerulosclerosis and renal functional impairment. Proteinuria, if present, is mild, however, and the urinary sediment is normal except with severe or malignant hypertension, in which marked proteinuria and hematuria may be noted.

Measurements of peripheral plasma renin activity in patients with hypertension associated with parenchymal kidney disease have thus far been unrewarding.[29] Although acute glomerulonephritis may occur at any age, 80 per cent of the cases occur between the ages of 5 and 10 years. Renal function tests generally reveal a reduction in glomerular filtration rate with essentially normal tubular function, manifested by a reduced creatinine clearance (or elevated serum creatinine level) and normal concentrating ability. Nonstreptococcal glomerulonephritis may be differentiated from the poststreptococcal variety by the failure of serum antistreptococcal antibody titers to rise on serial determinations. Unlike the diastolic hypertension associated with chronic forms of parenchymal kidney disease, in which hemodynamic measurements reveal increased peripheral resistance with a relatively normal cardiac output, the hypertension associated with acute glomerulonephritis is secondary to markedly increased cardiac output with some increase in total peripheral resistance.[36] The majority of cases of acute glomerulonephritis heal spontaneously within several months, with return of the blood pressure to normal. The prevalence of hypertension in latent, inactive glomerulonephritis is variable; generally, persistence of diastolic hypertension following the acute episode signifies chronic active disease. This type of active glomerulitis, at any stage of the disease, may be recognized by the presence of red blood cell casts in the urine. The diagnosis of chronic glomerulonephritis may be evident from a history of preceding acute glomerulonephritis, or at times may be made presumptively in a patient with renal failure, diastolic hypertension, and a renal sediment demonstrating hyaline and granular casts and red blood cells. A familial history of renal failure occurring only in the males of the kindred, and associated with nerve deafness, suggests the possibility of hereditary nephritis.

Chronic glomerulonephritis must be differentiated by history and appropriate laboratory examinations from other forms of chronic renal parenchymal disease, including pyelonephritis, polycystic kidneys, disseminated lupus erythematosus, glomerulosclerosis (Kimmelstiel-Wilson disease), nephrocalcinosis, renal amyloidosis, and gouty nephropathy. Intravenous urography can be performed unless nitrogen retention is severe, and may reveal changes diagnostic or suggestive of chronic pyelonephritis or polycystic kidneys. Quantitative urine cultures of greater than 10^5 organisms/ml may indicate active renal infection. Occasionally pyelonephritis may be unilateral, with an atrophic kidney, and rare instances of cure of hypertension by unilateral nephrectomy have been reported.

Polycystic disease of the kidneys is a genetic disorder inherited as an autosomal dominant trait; it may result in death from uremia in infancy or may be essentially asymptomatic well into adult life. The diagnosis should be suspected if there is a family history of renal disease and a clinical history of abdominal pain, hematuria, and hypertension. Bilateral abdominal masses are usually palpable, and findings on intravenous urography are characteristic. Associated defects include hepatic cysts, which may cause hepatomegaly, and aneurysms of the intracranial arteries, which may rupture into the brain or subarachnoid space.

Other causes of chronic renal disease may usually be diagnosed from their symptom complexes and by specific laboratory findings. Occasionally renal biopsy may be of value. Percutaneous renal biopsy is a relatively safe procedure in expert hands, provided that the blood pressure is well controlled. Open renal biopsy may be employed if it is considered essential to have a pathologic diagnosis and the risk of percutaneous biopsy seems excessive.

Obstructive uropathy, unilateral or bilateral, due to bladder neck obstruction or ureteral obstruction from congenital defects, calculi, blood clots, tumor or retroperitoneal fibrosis, may also cause hypertension, and, if bilateral, chronic, and severe, may result in chronic renal failure as well. To prevent the latter consequence, early diagnosis and therapeutic intervention are essential. The lesion may be clinically silent or may be characterized by difficulty in micturition or by active cystitis or pyelonephritis with fever, chills, flank or abdominal pain, dysuria, frequency, and urgency. The diagnosis is established by intravenous or retrograde urography.

Renal tumors may be associated with hypertension. In the child this is most commonly an embryonal nephroma (Wilms' tumor), and, in the adult, renal cell carcinoma. Clinical findings include fever, weight loss, abdominal or flank pain, anorexia, nausea, and vomiting. An abdominal mass may be palpable, and urinalysis characteristically reveals microscopic hematuria. Renal cell carcinoma is prone to metastasize early to lung and bone, and may present initially with symptoms referable to these organs. Polycythemia, a leukemoid reaction, and markedly elevated erythrocyte sedimentation rate may be seen with this tumor. The diagnosis is confirmed by intravenous urography and/or renal arteriography. Nephrectomy usually results in return of blood pressure to normal.

Hypertension Secondary to Central Nervous System Disease

Hypertension may result from increased intracranial pressure of any cause. Thus, intracerebral hemorrhage is frequently associated with an elevated blood pressure; a slow heart rate in an obtunded or comatose patient should suggest this possibility. Brain tumor should be suspected in patients with papilledema and only mild or moderate hypertension. Usually a careful neurologic examination, together with study of the cerebrospinal fluid, skull x-rays, carotid and/or vertebral arteriography, and scanning procedures, will serve to establish these diagnoses. Bulbar poliomyelitis and the Guillain-Barré syndrome with respiratory failure may also cause hypertension. Whether this is due to brain stem or diencephalic involvement or to the necessity for artificial respiration in these patients is unclear. Usually the hypertension disappears as the clinical state of the patient improves.

Cushing's Syndrome

Cushing's syndrome is due to oversecretion of adrenal cortical hormones. The adrenal lesion may be an adenoma, carcinoma, or bilateral hyperplasia. The possible primary role of the anterior pituitary, particularly in the latter instance, is not clear, although anterior lobe tumors may be found in some cases. Rarely, excessive stimulation by ACTH-like substances secreted by a variety of malignancies, most notably oat cell carcinoma of the lung, has been described. Iatrogenic Cushing's syndrome occurs in patients taking large doses of glucocorticoids as therapy for other diseases. The syndrome, if due to intrinsic adrenal cortical disease, is approximately 3 times as common in women as in men. The diagnosis is usually evident from the history and characteristic findings on physical examination.

Hypertension develops in nearly 85 per cent of patients, but is rarely severe. Several cases of malignant hypertension have, however, been documented. Overt diabetes mellitus occurs in 10 to 15 per cent of patients, and generalized osteoporosis with or without pathologic fractures is common. Surgical removal of the adrenal neoplasm, or subtotal or total adrenalectomy in the case of bilateral hyperplasia of the adrenal cortex, relieves the clinical features of Cushing's syndrome and results in return to normotension in the large majority. In a few patients, especially those with pre-existing severe hypertension, blood pressures may remain elevated postoperatively. Presumably secondary mechanisms have become operative in these patients.

The clinical diagnosis can be verified by the finding of elevated urinary 17-hydroxysteroids and/or 17 ketosteroids and elevation of plasma cortisol levels with loss of their normal diurnal variation. The response of urinary steroid levels to exogenous ACTH and dexamethasone is also sometimes helpful. Additional common laboratory findings including polycythemia, hypokalemia, and a diabetic type of glucose tolerance test.

Primary Aldosteronism

Aldosterone, the most important mineralocorticoid secreted by the adrenal cortex, has its major site of action in the distal tubule, where it facilitates the reabsorption of sodium in exchange for potassium and hydrogen ions.[30] Since aldosterone does not directly cause peripheral vasoconstriction, and since some forms of secondary aldosteronism, such as cirrhosis with ascites and the nephrotic syndrome, are not associated with hypertension, the mechanism of elevation of blood pressure by excessive secretion from an aldosteronoma of the adrenal gland is unclear.[13]

Primary aldosteronism occurs in middle life and is twice as frequent in women as in men. The hypertension associated with it is almost invariably mild or moderate, though rare cases with malignant hypertension have been described. The signs and symptoms occur only in advanced cases, and can all be ascribed to severe, long-standing potassium deficiency.[4] Many patients have no symptoms at all and no signs other than mild systemic arterial hypertension. In the full-blown syndrome polyuria and nocturia, accompanied by polydipsia, result from defective urine-concentrating ability. Severe potassium depletion also leads to muscle weakness and, occasionally, paralysis.[4, 5, 7] Fifty per cent of patients exhibit abnormal glucose tolerance tests similar to those found in maturity onset diabetes. Usually these revert to normal when the hypokalemia is corrected.

Depletion of potassium and hydrogen ions leads to hypokalemic, hypochloremic alkalosis, which is responsible for the paresthesias and tetany seen in some patients. Serum sodium concentration is normal or increased, in contrast to secondary aldosteronism, in which it is normal or decreased. Severe kaliopenic nephropathy leads to demonstrable vasopressin-resistant isosthenuria.

Increased aldosterone excretion with normal excretion of glucocorticoids is characteristic of the disorder. Plasma renin activity is reduced or unmeasurable, and, contrary to results in normal individuals, fails to increase with upright posture and salt depletion. The combination of normal or increased aldosterone excretion during normal salt intake, along with low plasma renin activity after 5 days of sodium restriction and 2 hours in the upright position, is pathognomonic of primary aldosteronism.[5, 7]

An additional screening test which may be of value if properly performed is the determination of the salivary sodium-to-potassium ratio.[31] The mean salivary sodium-to-potassium ratio found in normal subjects is approximately 1.4, with a range of 0.6 to 3.0. A ratio of less than 0.25 is distinctly abnormal, and suggests increased aldosterone secretion.

Aldosterone excretion may occasionally be normal or only slightly elevated in patients with primary aldosteronism. In these cases the diagnosis can be made by demonstrating autonomy of aldosterone production, as judged by alterations in sodium and potassium balance during baseline studies and during stimulation and suppression tests (Table 10).[54, 56] To do this the patient is first placed on a normal intake of sodium and potassium to determine whether he excretes an excess of potassium in his urine in relation to the amount ingested. He is then kept on a normal potassium intake, but sodium intake is restricted to 10 mEq/day for 5 days. In primary aldosteronism this results in retention of potassium by the kidneys, because of diminished delivery of sodium to the distal exchange site. The serum potassium value returns toward normal. The salt intake is then increased to 200 mEq of sodium per day for 5 days. The increased delivery of filtered sodium to the distal tubule results in increased exchange of sodium for potassium, the rapid development of negative potassium balance, and a decline in the serum potassium value. In a normal individual these changes in sodium intake produce, respectively, compensatory increase and decrease in aldosterone secretion, tending to minimize alterations in potassium excretion. In primary aldosteronism sodium loading fails to suppress aldosterone secretion as it does in a normal patient or in one with secondary aldosteronism. Plasma renin activity remains low throughout these changes in sodium and potassium balance.

The differentiation between primary aldosteronism and secondary aldosteronism due to severe hypertension of other etiology may be difficult.

TABLE 10

Response to Alterations in Sodium and Potassium Intake in Primary Aldosteronism.

Diet		Urine Excretion		Serum		Plasma Renin	Aldosterone Secretion
Na+	K+	Na+	K+	Na+	K+		
mEq/day							
100	60	Normal	Normal or increased	Normal or increased	Normal or decreased	0	Increased
10	60	Decreased	Decreased	Unchanged	Increased	0	Increased
200	60	Increased	Increased	Unchanged	Decreased	0	Increased

See the text for details. Minor criteria include the following: salivary sodium-to-potassium ratio <0.25; increased blood volume; increased exchangeable sodium (Na_e) and decreased exchangeable potassium (K_e); abnormal glucose tolerance curve; and abnormal circulatory reflexes (postural hypotension).

As stated above, however, both malignant and accelerated hypertension are distinctly rare in primary aldosteronism. Furthermore, in secondary aldosteronism, the increased secretion of aldosterone is associated with increased renin secretion from a kidney presumably rendered ischemic by intrarenal vasoconstriction and/or organic damage to intrarenal vasculature.[9] In primary aldosteronism, therefore, one finds the unique combination of increased urinary aldosterone excretion and low plasma renin activity, in contrast to secondary aldosteronism, in which both these values are elevated.

When confronted with a patient with hypertension and hypokalemia one must consider, in addition to primary and secondary aldosteronism, hypokalemia of other etiologies. Hypokalemia may occur secondary to renal losses (e.g., renal tubular acidosis, Fanconi syndrome, damage induced by outdated tetracyclines) or gastrointestinal losses (chronic vomiting or diarrhea, villous adenoma). Commonest of all is hypokalemia due to thiazide derivatives used in the treatment of hypertension or congestive heart failure.

Ancillary findings which are sometimes helpful in the differential diagnosis of primary aldosteronism include increased blood volume and total exchangeable sodium (Na_e) and decreased total exchangeable potassium (K_e).[58] These findings, typical of continued, autonomous, high aldosterone secretion, may also be seen in Cushing's syndrome, but are not found in aldosteronism secondary to severe hypertension or in hypokalemia caused by potassium depletion from diuretic drugs, potassium-wasting renal disease, or gastrointestinal potassium losses.

Slaton and Biglieri[58] have described the depression of circulatory reflexes, as indicated by a loss of the post-Valsalva hypertensive "overshoot" and bradycardia, in hypertension associated with primary as opposed to secondary aldosteronism. The probable mechanism is a decrease in baroreceptor sensitivity due to the chronic volume expansion in primary aldosteronism.

Administration of large amounts of spironolactone (300 mg/day) generally reduces the blood pressure to normal and results in complete reversal of the biochemical derangement seen in primary aldosteronism.[61] Spironolactone therapy in secondary aldosteronism may correct the biochemical disorders, but never ameliorates the hypertension. The administration of spironolactone, therefore, may be used as a diagnostic test. It must be remembered, however, that it often takes from 6 to 8 weeks of continuous therapy before these results are seen.

A form of hypertension which may be associated with hypokalemic alkalosis and suppressed plasma renin activity is that seen following the excessive prolonged ingestion of licorice. Glycyrrhizinic acid, contained in the licorice, has a potent sodium-retaining effect. The dietary history and the findings of a low level of aldosterone secretion or excretion distinguish this syndrome from primary aldosteronism.[6]

A rare form of hypertension associated with suppressed aldosterone secretion and plasma renin activity is that associated with a deficiency of adrenal cortical 17α-hydroxylase.[2] These patients have hypertension associated with hypokalemia, presumably because of the non-aldosterone-related hypermineralocorticoidism secondary to increased ACTH production and an increased secretion of desoxycorticosterone and corticosterone, relatively weak mineralocorticoids.

Two other rare syndromes which may be confused with adult primary aldosteronism and are manifested by hypertension and hypokalemia are "juvenile" aldosteronism, a disease of children in which increased aldosterone secretion is found with malignant hypertension and bilateral adrenal hyperplasia,[21] and "familial pseudoaldosteronism," in which there are renal potassium wasting, sodium retention, and low aldosterone secretion.[34]

Primary aldosteronism should be considered whenever a patient has mild or moderate hypertension and unexplained hypokalemia. Whether, as suggested by Conn et al.,[7] primary aldosteronism with normal serum potassium values is common and may comprise as much as 20 per cent of the "essential" hypertensive population is not known. If this thesis is confirmed, it will become mandatory to measure urinary aldosterone excretion and peripheral venous plasma renin activity in all patients with systemic arterial hypertension.

Adrenogenital Syndromes

These are rare genetic disorders due to deficiency of one of the enzymes involved in synthesis of steroid hormones by the adrenal glands and gonads. The defect results in decreased secretion of cortisol, interruption of the negative feedback mechanism which normally governs the adrenal cortex, increased secretion of ACTH by the anterior pituitary, and overproduction of those steroid hormones which lie proximal, in the biosynthetic pathways, to the enzymatic block.

The diagnosis should be suspected in an infant or child who, on physical examination, has evidence of precocious virilization characterized by enlargement of the clitoris or penis, accelerated growth and bone maturation, adult musculature of male configuration, and male secondary sex characteristics, including early development of sexual hair, deepening of the voice, and acne. Overproduction of androgens by the adrenal gland is responsible for all these findings. In other patients the enzyme defect occurs at a point at which synthesis of androgens and estrogens is interrupted, and results in the clinical picture of continued sexual infantilism at the time of puberty, often associated with hyperpigmentation of palmar creases and mucous membranes and over pressure points.

Hypertension develops if the enzyme defect leads to the overproduction of hormones with mineralocorticoid properties. This occurs with 11β-hydroxylase and with 17α-hydroxylase deficiencies, but not with the most common form of adrenogenital syndrome, in which 21-hydroxylation is defective. The 11β-hydroxylase defect causes overproduction of both androgens and the mineralocorticoid, 11β-desoxycorticosterone. Patients show precocious virilization and hypertension and can be diagnosed by finding increased urinary 17-ketosteroids, tetrahydro-11β-desoxycorticosterone, and tetrahydro-11β-desoxycortisol. In 17α-hydroxylase deficiency, on the other hand, secretion of androgens and estrogens is diminished and that of 11β-desoxycorticosterone is increased. These patients remain sexually infantile at puberty, but are hypertensive. Study of urinary steroids reveals elevated pregnanediol, tetrahydro 11β-desoxycorticosterone, and corticosterone. In both defects, because of the abnormally high secretion rates of mineralocorticoids, there is hypokalemic alkalosis and suppression of aldosterone and renin secretion.

In all forms of the adrenogenital syndrome adequate replacement with cortisol restores operation of the normal feedback suppression of ACTH secretion and hence removes the excessive stimulus for the secretion of androgens and/or mineralocorticoids. Regression of the physiologic effects of these hormones follows, and both the hypertension and hypokalemic alkalosis subside. If complete suppression cannot be produced, the possibility that virilization may be due to an ovarian or testicular tumor must be considered.

Pheochromocytoma

When typical paroxysms of hypertension and symptoms characteristic of intermittent catecholamine release occur, little difficulty is encountered in making this diagnosis. Approximately 50 per cent of patients, however, display sustained hypersecretion of catecholamines and manifest persistent hypertension, with or without hypermetabolism and hyperglycemia. In these individuals, differentiation from essential hypertension may be difficult. Adverse reactions to abdominal palpation, anesthesia, surgical procedures, or other physiologic stresses may serve to stimulate suspicion, and marked postural hypotension may also be a helpful clinical clue. Recent studies[12] suggest that the orthostatic hypotension is due to functional autonomic blockade in most subjects, with the possibility that hypovolemia is a factor in a few others. Though a lean body habitus is characteristic, overweight patients have been described. Patients with pronounced symptomatic paroxysms usually have tumors which secrete significant quantities of epinephrine, whereas those with predominantly norepinephrine-producing tumors may manifest only hypertension, postural hypotension, and excessive sweating, with little or no evidence of hypermetabolism.

Other physical findings which raise the suspicion that pheochromocytoma may exist are *café au lait* spots, generalized hyperpigmentation, and cutaneous neurofibromatosis. Patients with von Hippel-Lindau disease, characterized by cerebellar and retinal hemangioblastomas, also have a high incidence of pheochromocytoma. Retinal hemangioblastomas must be differentiated from the papilledema, hemorrhages, and exudates seen in malignant hypertension of any etiology. In recent years the familial and nonfamilial association of amyloid-producing medullary thyroid carcinoma, pheochromocytoma, and hyperparathyroidism has stirred considerable interest.

Chemical and pharmacologic tests used in the diagnosis of pheochromocytoma are shown in Tables 11 and 12. Because of the ease and specificity of measurements of urinary catecholamines and their metabolites, the pharmacologic tests should generally be reserved for patients in whom the diagnosis is suspected, but in whom the chemical test results are negative or equivocal. An example of such a patient might be one with an intermittently secreting tumor who is normotensive at the time of testing. Measurement of urinary free catecholamines (epinephrine, norepinephrine), metanephrine and normetanephrine, or vanillylmandelic acid (VMA) are about equally sensitive and reliable if properly performed. Determination of VMA has the advantage of being relatively widely available and is the only method that can be used in a patient taking methyldopa for treatment of hypertension. Determination of metanephrine and normetanephrine is simpler to perform and is the most reproducible, but is falsely elevated in patients taking monoamine oxidase inhibitors, methyldopa, and sympathomimetic bronchodilators and nose drops. Determination of free catecholamines is similarly affected by the latter three agents and by certain foodstuffs, notably bananas. Bedside screening tests for VMA give false-positive reactions with a number of drugs and foodstuffs, and should be interpreted with caution. Plasma assay for catecholamines can be done, but is technically demanding and not generally available. Despite all precau-

TABLE 11

Normal Values of Chemical Tests in Diagnosis of Pheochromocytoma

Substance	24-hr Excretion	Excretion per mg creatinine
Plasma catecholamines..................	3.5 $\mu g/l$	
Urine		
Catecholamines.......................	150 μg	0.05 μg
Metanephrine + normetanephrine......	1.3 mg	2.1 μg
Vanillylmandelic acid.................	6.5 mg	9.5 μg

TABLE 12

Pharmacological Tests for Diagnosis of Pheochromocytoma

Provocative (blood pressure <170/110)
  Histamine: acetylcholine-like stimulation of adrenal chromaffin cells; initial hypotension (?)
  Tyramine: release of norepinephrine at nerve endings[11]*
  Glucagon: hypoglycemia releases adrenal catecholamines[32]*
Suppressive (blood pressure > 170/110)
  Phentolamine (Regitine): adrenergic block of circulating catecholamines
Useful in intermittent tumors, combined with blood or urine catecholamines

* Proposed new tests.

tions, false-positive and false-negative results occur with all tests.[26] Rarely, exploratory surgery may be necessary to establish the diagnosis.

Preoperative attempts to localize the tumor(s) are sometimes helpful. Tumors in the adrenal area can often be demonstrated by laminography or intravenous pyelography, and those in the thorax may be seen on chest x-ray in the paravertebral areas. Presacral or perirenal insufflation of carbon dioxide, adrenal arteriography, and venous catheterization for selective sampling of plasma catecholamines are additional techniques which have been employed. Results with these tests, used singly or in combination, have been disappointing, however, in reliably demonstrating the tumor(s). Since some are not without hazard in the brittle patient with pheochromocytoma, and since exploration of both adrenal glands and the entire abdomen is necessary in all patients because of the possibility of multiple tumors, most investigators do not insist on preoperative localization of the tumor.[17, 18]

Preoperative examinations should include, in addition to the above specific tests for pheochromocytoma, an evaluation of the patient's metabolic status and of his thyroid and parathyroid function, including radioactive scanning of suspicious glands, in light of the possible association with thyroid disease and hyperparathyroidism noted above.

Coarctation of the Aorta

This congenital anomaly is an important cause of hypertension in infancy and childhood, but occasionally may go undiagnosed until adult life. It occurs in males 3 to 4 times as commonly as in females. The hypertension associated with it may be predominantly systolic. Rarely, if ever, is malignant hypertension produced. When the anomaly is diagnosed in infancy, coarctation commonly presents with the picture of severe congestive heart failure, and is often associated with other congenital cardiac defects, including patent ductus arteriosus, ventricular septal defect, and valvular and subvalvular aortic stenosis. In these patients the coarctation is usually preductal in location. When coarctation is asymptomatic in infancy and goes undiagnosed until childhood or adult life, it is generally located adjacent or distal to the ligamentum arteriosum and is infrequently associated with cardiac anomalies other than a bicuspid aortic valve, which was found in 42 per cent of Reifenstein's series,[53] and may occasionally produce significant valvular obstruction or insufficiency. Older patients may be asymptomatic or may present symptoms referable to the hypertension (headaches, epistaxis), to diminished blood supply to the lower extremities (easy fatigability, weakness, cramps, coldness), or to cardiac failure, especially if there is associated valvular or myocardial disease.

The diagnosis can usually be made on physical examination by finding elevated blood pressure in the arms with normal or diminished pressures in the legs and weak and delayed femoral artery pulsations. One must be careful to take the blood pressure in both arms, since occasionally the left subclavian artery is stenotic, and one may get the false impression of normotension if the blood pressure is measured only in the left arm. Ancillary physical findings are related to the development of collateral circulation around the aortic obstruction and to the presence of other cardiac lesions. Enlarged intercostal arteries, which produce characteristic "rib notching" on chest x-ray, may become palpable along the inferior rib margins posteriorly, between the scapulae. Flow through these or through the coarctation may produce a systolic or continuous murmur heard over the precordium and in the interscapular area. If the patient has a bicuspid aortic valve, a basal systolic ejection murmur with or without the other findings of significant aortic valve obstruction may be present. The murmur of aortic insufficiency is also occasionally heard, and may be due to a bicuspid aortic valve, to dilation of the ascending aorta and aortic valve ring, or to destruction or distortion of aortic valve leaflets by infective endocarditis (see the chapter on Aortic Regurgitation.)

A patent ductus arteriosus, commonly present in infants with coarctation, occurs rarely in older patients as well, and may be identified by its characteristic machinery murmur in the second and third left interspaces anteriorly. Differential cyanosis of the lower extremities occurs when there is right-to-left shunting of unoxygenated blood through a patent ductus, which, when the coarctation is preductal, may be largely responsible for supplying blood to the lower part of the body.

In infants the presence of severe congestive heart failure and associated cardiac anomalies may make the clinical diagnosis obscure, and cardiac catheterization with aortography is often necessary to verify the diagnosis. In older patients radiographic procedures provide valuable confirmatory evidence of the diagnosis. The chest x-ray characteristically reveals left ventricular enlargement and rib notching. On cardiac fluoroscopy vigorous pulsations of the ascending aorta and subclavian arteries are seen, and the classic "inverted three" sign is produced in the barium-filled esophagus by its indention by dilations of the aorta proximal and distal to the coarctation. Aortography is helpful in defining the anatomy prior to surgical correction.

Prompt diagnosis of coarctation of the aorta is important both in infants and in older patients because of the poor prognosis of the untreated patient and the excellent results of corrective surgery. Untreated patients run a considerable risk of rupture or dissection of the aorta, bacterial endocarditis or endarteritis and cerebral hemorrhage. Sixty-one per cent of Reifenstein's series[53] were dead at less than 40 years of age from one of these complications. The risk of surgery in uncomplicated cases is less than 5 per cent and almost always results in "cure" of the hypertension. In infants with associated cardiac lesions this risk is higher, as it also is in older patients with degenerative changes in the aortic wall and large collateral vessels.

Renovascular Hypertension

Hypertension due to renovascular disease may vary in severity from mild to malignant, may occur in any age group and in either sex, and may simulate either essential or other secondary types of hypertension.[38, 40, 62] No single clinical sign is specific. The diagnosis should be suspected when hypertension is inappropriate to the age of the patient or when an upper abdominal bruit is heard. Although abdominal bruits may result from atherosclerosis of the aorta or stenosis of other intra-abdominal arteries (splenic, superior mesenteric), they are present in less than five per cent of patients with primary (essential) hypertension versus 60 per cent of patients with renovascular hypertension. They are, as would be expected, more easily detectable in thin than in obese individuals. Since renovascular hypertension may represent as much as 15 per cent of the hypertensive population[43] and is potentially curable, vigorous efforts should be made to establish or exclude it as a diagnostic possibility.

Renal damage due to essential hypertension is bilateral and symmetric. Asymmetry in renal function demonstrated on the intravenous urogram or the radioactive renogram,[42] therefore, should raise the suspicion of unilateral renovascular disease. Rapid-sequence intravenous urography, performed both in the dehydrated state and under conditions of water or osmotic diuresis, is highly sensitive and specific in detecting unilateral renal ischemia. When multiple diagnostic criteria are considered, including disparity in kidney length (1.5 cm or greater is generally considered to be significant), delay in the early nephrogram and pyelocalyceal appearance time on the ischemic side, and asymmetry in pyelocalyceal concentration, positive results are obtained in 80 to 90 per cent of patients with demonstrated anatomic renal artery stenosis.[37, 39]

Selective renal arteriography demonstrates whether lesions are unilateral or bilateral, and by their location and appearance suggests whether they represent atherosclerotic plaques or fibromuscular hyperplasia.[44] It also permits a judgment, if surgery is contemplated, as to whether revascularization may be feasible or a nephrectomy will have to be performed. The arteriogram tells nothing, however, about the functional significance of anatomic lesions.[40] Since stenosis of a renal artery is occasionally seen in normotensive patients,[14] and may be an incidental finding in hypertensive patients, unrelated to their elevated arterial pressures, additional examinations must be done to establish its functional importance before surgical correction of such a stenotic segment is undertaken.

The most sensitive test available for the detection of functional stenosis is the level of renin activity measured in blood drawn from both renal veins, obtained by percutaneous catheterization via the femoral vein. Considerable evidence is accumulating that elevation of renin activity in the renal venous effluent is the best single indicator that renal artery stenosis is responsible for the hypertension and that cure may be expected from corrective surgery.[15, 45] In unilateral lesions, the ratio of ipsilateral (stenotic) to contralateral renal venous renin activity is considered to be more important than the actual level, a ratio of 2:1 or greater generally being considered positive. Peripheral venous renin activity is not nearly as reliable, and may be normal despite a high concentration in one renal vein.

Individual kidney function tests have also been used to help ascertain the functional significance of stenosis.[41] Characteristically renal plasma flow, glomerular filtration rate, and urine volume are diminished on the ischemic side and urine creatinine concentration is correspondingly increased. If strict criteria are used, false-positive results are few with this test, but misleading or false-negative results may be obtained in bilateral or segmental renal arterial lesions.

Other screening tests which have been employed include the radioisotope renogram and the angiotensin infusion test. The former is abnormal in most instances of functional renal artery stenosis, but is relatively nonspecific and has a high incidence of both false-positive and false-negative results. Hyporeactivity of the blood pressure to an intravenous infusion of angiotensin is present in many patients with renovascular hypertension, but overlapping occurs with patients with essential hypertension, and consistently positive tests in subjects with malignant hypertension impair the specificity of this test.

In summary, an abnormal rapid-sequence intravenous urogram should suffice to distinguish the large majority of patients with significant renal artery stenosis. Renal arteriography should be performed in these patients, and bilateral renal vein blood samples for measurement of renin activity should be obtained. Individual kidney function tests can then be performed in selected instances to verify the degree of impairment of the ischemic kidney, and, if nephrectomy is contemplated, to estimate the functional adequacy of the contralateral kidney. Percutaneous bilateral renal biopsies may be done, but are often misleading and can be dangerous in subjects with systemic hypertension. In general, renal biopsy should be performed in these patients only at the time of surgery.

When judicious use of the above tests is made, identification and cure of renovascular hypertension is achieved by nephrectomy or renal artery repair in 70 to 80 per cent of patients in most reported series.

Hypertensive Disease of Pregnancy

The onset, after the 24th week of pregnancy, of hypertension associated with the development of proteinuria and edema is termed pre-eclampsia. If seizures supervene the syndrome is referred to as eclampsia. On rare occasions the syndrome appears in the postpartum period. In the presence of a hydatidiform mole eclampsia may occur earlier than the 24th week. The cause of this hypertensive disease of pregnancy is unknown. Secretion of a humoral pressor substance has been postulated, but not proven.

Impending pre-eclampsia should be suspected in a patient who gains weight rapidly and develops edema during the third trimester. Early diagnosis and treatment with salt restriction and diuretics is important, and may prevent emergence of the full-blown syndrome. Patients with pre-existing hypertension are particularly prone to develop pre-eclampsia, and, prior to the days of effective antihypertensive therapy, did so in approximately 28 per cent of cases. Whether careful control of blood pressure during pregnancy will lower this incidence has not been established, but fragmentary evidence indicates that it will.

The clinical diagnosis of pre-eclampsia may be difficult, especially if the patient is seen for the first time during the third trimester. The presence of hypertension, proteinuria, and edema at this time may indicate pre-eclampsia or may be due to chronic pre-existing renal disease. The definitive diagnosis can be verified only by renal biopsy, which, in pre-eclampsia, reveals characteristic glomerular changes, with swelling of the cytoplasm of endothelial cells, protein deposits under the basement membrane, and an increase in the number of intercapillary cells. This is not recommended as a routine diagnostic procedure, however, especially since the therapy is essentially the same regardless of the pathologic diagnosis.

Post partum the blood pressure of a patient with pre-eclampsia usually returns to normal within days or weeks. If hypertension persists another etiology should be sought. Approximately 40 per cent of patients manifesting pre-eclampsia do, however, develop sustained hypertension later in life. The reason for this is unclear.

Drug-Induced Hypertension

When confronted with a patient with hypertension, the physician must always keep in mind the possibility that this may be the result of ingestion of excessive amounts of a pharmacologic agent or food substance.

Sympathomimetic amines, such as amphetamines, taken as stimulants or for weight reduction, and phenylephrine or ephedrine taken as nasal decongestants or bronchodilators, may produce elevation of blood pressure. Oral contraceptives have recently been reported to cause exacerbation of pre-existing hypertension and, occasionally, to produce hypertension *de novo*. The estrogen content of "the pill" seems to be responsible, but the mechanism of its action has not yet been fully defined. Licorice, taken in large amounts as candy or in treatment of peptic ulcer, may cause hypertension associated with evidence of sodium retention and hypokalemic alkalosis, as described above. The clinical picture is similar to that of primary hyperaldosteronism, but aldosterone excretion and plasma renin activity are both diminished.

A careful history will exclude ingestion of these or other substances as the cause of hypertension. In all cases blood pressure will return to normal when the offending agent is withdrawn.

CONCLUSION

Systemic arterial hypertension of any etiology is a sign of a disorder in circulatory homeostasis. It is therefore, by definition, "secondary." Continuing study of "essential" hypertension, as indicated in the foregoing discussion, is helping to define increasing numbers of specific and potentially remediable causes in this group of patients, thereby permitting definitive therapeutic efforts to be made.

"Essential hypertension" is a disorder or group of disorders of unknown etiology which cannot be cured, but can only be controlled with varying degrees of success. It must remain a diagnosis of exclusion, made only after all known causes of secondary hypertension have been ruled out with reasonable certainty. Every hypertensive patient should have the benefit of careful diagnostic thought and such tests as are appropriate in light of the clinical facts he presents.

REFERENCES

1. Bechgaard, P. The natural history of benign hypertension—one thousand hypertensive patients followed from 26 to 32 years. In *The Epidemiology of Hypertension*, Stamler, J., Stamler, R., and Pullman, T. N., Eds., p. 357. Grune and Stratton, New York, 1967.
2. Biglieri, E. G., Slaton, P. E., Schambelan, M., and Kronfield, S. J. Hypermineralocorticoidism. Amer. J. Med. 45:170, 1968.
3. Breslin, B. J., Gifford, R. W., Jr., Fairbairn, J. F., II, and Kearns, B. P. Prognostic importance of ophthalmoscopic findings in essential hypertension. J.A.M.A. 195:335, 1966.
4. Conn, J. W. Aldosteronism in man. J.A.M.A. 174:775, 871, 1963.
5. Conn, J. W., Knopf, R. F., and Nesbit, R. M. Clinical characteristics of primary aldosteronism from an analysis of 145 cases. Amer. J. Surg. 107:159, 1964.
6. Conn, J. W., Rovner, D. R., and Cohen, E. L. Licorice-induced pseudo-aldosteronism. J.A.M.A. 205:492, 1968.
7. Conn, J. W., Rovner, D. R., Cohen, E. L., and Nesbit, R. M. Normokalemic primary aldosteronism. J.A.M.A. 195:111, 1966.
8. Cort, J. H., Fenci, V., Hejl, Z., and Jirka, A., Eds. *The Pathogenesis of Essential Hypertension*. State Medical Publishing House, Prague, 1961.
9. Davis, J. O. Aldosteronism and hypertension. Progr. Cardiovasc. Dis. 8:129, 1965.
10. Earle, D. P. Hypertension in parenchymal renal disease. Progr. Cardiovasc. Dis. 8:195, 1965.
11. Engelman, K., and Sjoerdsma, A. A new test for pheochromocytoma. Pressor responsiveness to tyramine. J.A.M.A. 189:107, 1964.
12. Engelman, K., Zelio, R., Waldmann, T., Mason, D. T., and Sjoerdsma, A. Mechanism of orthostatic hypotension in pheochromocytoma. Circulation 38 (Suppl. 6):72, 1968.
13. Espiner, E. A., Tucci, J. R., Jagger, P. I., and Lauler, D. P. Independence of blood pressure and aldosterone secretion. N. Engl. J. Med. 276:784, 1967.
14. Eyler, W. R., Clark, M. D., Garman, J. E., Rain, R. L., and Meininger, D. E. Angiography of renal areas including comparative study of renal artery stenosis in patients with and without hypertension. Radiology 78:879, 1962.
15. Fitz, A. Renal venous renin determinations in the diagnosis of surgically correctable hypertension. Circulation 36:942, 1967.
16. Gifford, R. W., Jr. The importance of retinal findings in essential hypertension. Bull. N. Y. Acad. Med. 14:922, 1969.
17. Gifford, R. W., Kvale, W. F., Maher, F. T., Roth, G. M., and Priestley, J. T. Clinical features, diagnosis and treatment of pheochromocytoma: a review of 76 cases. Proc. Staff Meet. Mayo Clin. 39:281, 1964.
18. Greer, W. E. R., Robertson, C. W., and Smithwick, R. H. Pheochromocytoma. Diagnosis, operative experience and clinical results. Amer. J. Surg. 107:192 1964.
19. Gubner, R. S. Life expectancy of the young hypertensive. In *Hypertension, Recent Advances*, Brest, A. N., and Moyer, J. H., Eds., p. 18. Lea and Febiger, Philadelphia, 1961.
20. Hodge, J. V., and Dollery, C. T. Retinal soft exudates: a clinical study of colour and fluorescence photography. Quart. J. Med. 33:117, 1964.
21. Holten, C., and Petersen, V. P. Malignant hypertension with increased secretion of aldosterone and depletion of potassium. Lancet 2:918, 1956.
22. Julius, S., and Stewart, B. H. Diagnostic significance of abdominal murmurs. N. Engl. J. Med. 276:1175, 1967.

23. Kagan, A., Gordon, T., Kannel, W. B., and Dawber, T. R. Blood pressure and its relation to coronary heart disease in the Framingham study. In *Hypertension*, Vol. VII: *Drug Action, Epidemiology and Hemodynamics*, Shelton, F. R., Ed., American Heart Association, New York, 1959.
24. Kaplan, N. M., and Silah, J. G. The effect of angiotensin II on the blood pressure in humans with hypertensive disease. J. Clin. Invest. 43:659, 1964.
25. Keith, N. M., Wagener, H. P., and Barker, N. W. Some different types of essential hypertension; their cause and prognosis. Amer. J. Med. Sci. 197:332, 1939.
26. Kelleher, J., Walters, G., Robinson, R., and Smith, P. Chemical tests for pheochromocytoma. J. Clin. Pathol. 17:399, 1964.
27. Kincaid-Smith, P., McMichael, J., and Murphy, E. A. Clinical course and pathology of hypertension with papilloedema (malignant hypertension). Quart. J. Med. 27:117, 1958.
28. Kirkendall, W. N., and Armstrong, M. L. Effect of blood pressure reduction on vascular changes in the eye. II. Results after two years. In *Hypertension, Recent Advances*, Moyer, J. H., and Brest, A. N., Eds., p. 624. Lea and Febiger, Philadelphia, 1961.
29. Kleinknecht D. et Maxwell, M. H. (Avec la collaboration technique de Mmes F. Huck et M. Sevignac). Etude Statistique des Variations de l' Activité Rénine Plasmatique Résultats. Preliminaires. In *Actualités Néphrologiques de l'Hôpital Necker*, Paris 1970.
30. Laragh, J. H. The role of aldosterone in man. J.A.M.A. 174:203, 1960.
31. Lauler, D. P., Hickler, R. B., and Thorn, G. W. The salivary sodium-potassium ratio. A useful "screening" test for aldosteronism in hypertensive subjects. N. Engl. J. Med. 267:1136, 1962.
32. Lawrence, A. M. Glucagon provocative test for pheochromocytoma. Ann. Internal Med. 66:1091, 1967.
33. Lew, E. A. *Build and Blood Pressure Study*. Society of Actuaries, Chicago, 1959.
34. Liddle, G. W., Bledsoe, T., and Coipage, W. S., Jr. A familial renal disorder simulating primary aldosteronism, but with negligible aldosterone secretion. Trans. Ass. Amer. Physicians 76:199, 1963.
35. Maxwell, M. H. Diagnosis and treatment of renovascular hypertension. Kidney 1:No. 5, 1968.
36. Maxwell, M. H. Rein et hypertension artérielle. Le Presse Medicale 77: 943, 1969.
37. Maxwell, M. H., Gonick, H. C., Wiita, R., and Kaufman, J. J. Use of the rapid sequence intravenous pyelogram in the diagnosis of renovascular hypertension. N. Engl. J. Med. 270:213, 1964.
38. Maxwell, M. H., Kaufman, J. G., and Bleifer, K. H. Stenosing lesions of the renal arteries: clinical manifestations. Postgrad. Med. 40:247, 1966.
39. Maxwell, M. H., and Lupu, A. N. Excretory urogram in renal arterial hypertension. J. Urol., 100: 395, 1968.
40. Maxwell, M. H., Lupu, A. N., and Franklin, S. S. Clinical and physiological factors determining diagnosis and choice of treatment of renovascular hypertension. Circ. Res. 21 (Suppl. 2):201, 1967.
41. Maxwell, M. H., Lupu, A. N., and Kaufman, J. J. Individual kidney function tests in renal arterial hypertension. J. Urol., 100: 384, 1968.
42. Maxwell, M. H., Lupu, A. N., and Taplin, G. V. Radioisotope renogram in renal arterial hypertension. J. Urol., 100: 376, 1968.
43. Maxwell, M. H., and Prozan, G. B. Renovascular hypertension. Progr. Cardiovasc. Dis. 5:81, 1962.
44. McCormack, L. J., Dustan, H. P., Gifford, R. W., Meaney, T. F., Stewart, B. H., and Kiser, W. S. Pathology of renal artery disease. Postgrad. Med. 40:348, 1968.
45. Michelakis, A. M., Foster, J. H., Liddle, G. W., Rhamy, R. K., Kuchel, O., and Gordon, R. D. Measurement of renin in both renal veins. Its use in the diagnosis of renovascular hypertension. Arch. Internal Med. 120:444, 1967.
46. Oberman, A., Lane, N. E., Narlan, W. R., Graybiel, A., and Mitchell, R. E. Trends in systolic blood pressure in the thousand aviator cohort over a twenty-four-year period. Circulation 36:812, 1967.
47. Page, I. H., and McCubbin, J. W., Eds. *Renal Hypertension*. Year Book Medical Publishers, Chicago, 1968.

48. Paul, O., and Ostfeld, A. M. Epidemiology of hypertension. Progr. Cardiovasc.
    Dis. 8:106, 1965.
49. Peart, W. S. Hypertension and the kidney. Brit. Med. J. 2:1353, 1421, 1959.
50. Perera, G. A., Clark, E. G., Gearing, F. R., and Schweitzer, M. D. The family
    of hypertensive man. Amer. J. Med. Sci. 241:18, 1961.
51. Pickering, G. W. The Nature of Essential Hypertension. Grune and Stratton, New
    York, 1961.
52. Platt, R. Heredity in hypertension. Lancet 7:899, 1963.
53. Reifenstein, G. H., Levine, S. A., and Gross, R. E. Coarctation of the Aorta.
    Review of 104 Autopsied Cases of "Adult Type," 2 years of Age or Older. Am.
    Heart J. 33: 146, 1947.
54. Relman, A. S. Diagnosis of primary aldosteronism. Amer. J. Surg. 107:173, 1964.
55. Sheps, S. G., Tyce, G. M., Flock, E. V., and Maher, F. T. Current experience in
    the diagnosis of pheochromocytoma. Circulation 34:473, 1966.
56. Silen, W., Biglieri, E. G., Slaton, P., and Galante, M. Management of primary
    aldosteronism. Ann. Surg. 164:600, 1966.
57. Simpson, J. A., Jamieson, G., Dickhaus, D. W., and Grover, R. F. Effect of size
    of cuff bladder on accuracy of measurements of indirect blood pressure. Amer.
    Heart J. 70:208, 1965.
58. Slaton, P. E., and Biglieri, E. G. Hypertension and hyperaldosteronism of renal
    and adrenal origin. Amer. J. Med. 38:324, 1965.
59. Smirk, F. H. High Arterial Pressure. Blackwell Scientific Publications, Oxford,
    1957.
60. Sokolow, M., and Perloff, D. The prognosis of essential hypertension treated
    conservatively. Circulation 23:697, 1961.
61. Spark, R. F., and Melby, J. C. Aldosteronism in hypertension: spironolactone
    response test. Ann. Internal Med. 68:1162, 1968.
62. Wilson, L., Dustan, H. P., Page, J. H., and Poutasse, E. F. Diagnosis of renal
    arterial lesions. Arch. Internal Med. 112:168, 1963.
63. Wurtman, R. J. Catecholamines. Little, Brown and Co., Boston, 1966.

Episodic Unconsciousness

JOHN E. LEE, THOMAS KILLIP III, and FRED PLUM

An episode of unconsciousness is usually a frightening experience for both the observer and the victim. Many a patient with a potentially treatable condition first comes to the attention of a physician following a transient lapse of his normal state of awareness because the patient and his family have become thoroughly alarmed. Although loss of consciousness is the most dramatic expression of the underlying condition, not infrequently a period of faintness, giddiness, confusion, or momentary forgetfulness may occur without progression to complete lack of awareness. Uncovering the cause of the presenting symptoms may challenge the skills of the physician assuming responsibility for the patient's welfare.

DEFINITION

Episodic loss of consciousness extends in degree from dulled awareness to complete unresponsiveness, and in duration from fractions of seconds to minutes or even hours. Loss of consciousness implies an extensive disturbance of brain function (but not necessarily disease of the brain itself), and "episodic" implies that the disturbance is reversible and repetitive. The explanation for a single unwitnessed episode of unconsciousness is often elusive, but recurrent episodes require careful investigation, for their causes can produce permanent neurologic damage or death.

CONSCIOUSNESS AND UNCONSCIOUSNESS

Intact consciousness is the sum of the many motor, sensory, and psychologic functions mediated by the cerebral hemispheres. The hemispheres are maintained in a constant state of activity by a continuous physiologic interplay between their neurons and those of a highly specific neural activating system located in the reticular formation of the upper brain stem.

For a disorder to cause unconsciousness, therefore, it must meet certain anatomic and physiologic "requirements." The anatomic requirements are 1) involvement of the central gray matter core of the upper brain stem, which includes the diencephalon, midbrain, and pons, or 2) nearly complete

JOHN E. LEE, M.D. Clinical Associate Professor of Neurology, Cornell University Medical College, and Associate Attending Neurologist, New York Hospital, New York. THOMAS KILLIP III, M.D. Roland Harriman Professor of Medicine, Cornell University Medical College, and Attending Physician, New York Hospital, New York. FRED PLUM, M.D. Anne Parrish Titzell Professor and Chairman, Department of Neurology, Cornell University Medical College, New York, New York.

involvement of both cerebral hemispheres. A disorder affecting only one cerebral hemisphere does not usually interrupt consciousness, although it may seriously impair the patient's ability to communicate his awareness. For example, a patient with an internal carotid artery occlusion producing cerebral infarction may be hemiplegic, aphasic, and behaviorally blunted, but he remains conscious as long as only one cerebral hemisphere is affected.

A major factor that governs the ease with which an appropriately located disturbance causes unconsciousness is its speed of onset. The relative plasticity of the nervous system compensates for slowly developing injuries, but not for rapidly developing ones.

Although the anatomic bases for loss of consciousness are fairly clearly defined and are not commonly a diagnostic problem, the physiologic requirements are less precisely understood, but diagnostically more important. In general terms they include 1) deficiencies of brain metabolism, 2) disorders of intrinsic brain bioelectrical activity, and 3) mechanical disturbances within the cranium. The first of these categories is the most frequent clinical cause of episodic unconsciousness.

Brain metabolism fails and consciousness is impaired whenever the utilization of oxygen by neurons and glial cells falls below a critical level. The rate of oxygen consumption in a normally functioning brain is 3.3 cc/100 g of brain tissue per minute.[21, 29] Brain function is disturbed whenever cerebral respiration falls about 20 to 30 per cent below this value, and consciousness is usually lost when the rate falls below about 2.0 cc. Again, the rate at which the decline occurs is important, with more severe symptoms following rapid changes. Oxygen utilization by the brain can be decreased by an inadequate cerebral blood flow, by an inadequate oxygen supply, by an inadequate supply of glucose, or by "toxic" factors which obstruct the normal enzymatic processes of cerebral oxidative metabolism. By far the most important of these, and indeed the most common cause of transient unconsciousness, is an inadequate cerebral blood flow.[28]

Brain metabolism is rarely, if ever, impaired by a moderate decrease in cerebral blood flow, such as occurs in most patients with heart failure, because a greater volume of oxygen can be extracted from each unit of blood to maintain the oxygen supply of brain tissue. However, when cerebral blood flow decreases to less than 50 to 60 per cent of normal, the oxygen uptake begins to decline and brain function deteriorates.

Cerebral arterioles have the intrinsic ability to constrict or dilate in response to changes in intra-arterial pressure. The cerebral vessels constrict when systemic blood pressure rises and dilate when it falls, so as to maintain a constant level of cerebral blood flow in the face of a changing blood pressure. This cerebral autoregulation loses its capacity to maintain a normal cerebral blood flow when the mean arterial blood pressure falls to about 60 mm Hg or less.[21, 29] Below this level the cerebral blood flow decreases as the arterial blood pressure falls. In addition, there may be a transient failure or lack of autoregulation with a rapid fall of arterial blood pressure, so that cerebral blood flow may decrease linearly with the blood pressure in sudden hypotension. Extremely high blood pressure levels may be accompanied by such severe cerebral vasoconstriction that cerebral blood flow may be impaired under these circumstances as well.

Seizures are disturbances in cerebral electrical activity, and the physiologic "requirement" for unconsciousness to result from such a disorder is that the seizure involve the central reticular network of the brain stem. Some seizures begin as focal cortical phenomena, but these will not impair consciousness unless they spread into the deeper reticular system. If the seizure begins in the reticular system, however, it produces an immediate loss of consciousness, as in pure petit mal and grand mal epilepsy. This differentiation has important diagnostic and therapeutic implications which will be discussed later.

Transient intracranial effects of head trauma, either through damage to brain cells or by producing ischemia, impair brain function and produce unconsciousness. In concussion following blows to the head both these mechanisms are involved, and ischemia may result from the sudden increase in intracranial pressure. Whenever trauma or ischemia involves the brain stem unconsciousness is all the more likely to occur.

These, then, are the general principles determining whether, with any given illness, consciousness will be maintained or lost, Tables 13 and 14 outline the most common specific causes of transient unconsciousness. In subsequent sections each of these conditions is discussed in detail.

EVALUATION OF UNCONSCIOUSNESS

This chapter will discuss various causes of episodic unconsciousness; the case report below vividly illustrates the necessity for a careful diagnostic approach to the unconscious patient.

Case 1

An 18-year-old man was found lying in the street banging his head on the pavement. Speech was unintelligible. He was taken to a large city hospital, where a diagnosis of catatonic schizophrenia was made. Waxy flexibility of the limbs was demonstrated to a group of medical students. The patient's mother then arrived and told the physicians that her son was diabetic. Intravenous glucose promptly restored apparently normal mental function. Blood glucose obtained prior to therapy was 24 mg/100 ml.

With an inadequate history, a cursory examination, and no laboratory data, a wrong and potentially disastrous diagnosis was considered established. Certainly the history was incomplete, but perhaps careful inspection would have revealed evidence of insulin injection sites on the skin, and examination of the optic fundi might have shown microaneurysms. In attempting to evaluate episodic unconsciousness both the patient and the physician deserve the benefit of a careful history and physical examination, buttressed by appropriate laboratory tests.

TABLE 13

Classification of Episodic Unconsciousness Due to Abnormal Function of the Cardiovascular System

I. Low cardiac output due primarily to insufficient venous return
  A. Abnormal vasomotor function
    1. Simple faint (vasovagal syncope)
    2. Postural hypotension
    3. Primary autonomic insufficiency
      a. Idiopathic orthostatic hypotension
      b. Shy-Drager syndrome
      c. Disorders of central and peripheral nervous system
    4. Sympathectomy
      a. Surgical
      b. Pharmacologic
  B. Reduced blood volume
    1. Blood loss
    2. Low serum proteins
      a. Enteropathy
      b. Burns
    3. Dehydration
    4. Addison's disease
  C. Mechanical block
    1. Valsalva's maneuver
    2. Cough syncope
    3. Micturition syncope
    4. Pregnancy, third trimester
    5. Atrial myxoma
    6. Varicose veins
    7. Pericardial tamponade
II. Low cardiac output due to obstruction to ventricular outflow
    1. Aortic stenosis
    2. Hypertrophic subaortic stenosis
    3. Primary pulmonary hypertension
    4. Pulmonary embolism
III. Anoxia
    1. Cyanotic heart disease
IV. Arrhythmia
  A. Tachycardia
    1. Supraventricular
    2. Ventricular
    3. Multiple extrasystoles
  B. Bradycardia
    1. Sinus
    2. Post-tachycardia asystole (overdrive suppression)
    3. Ventricular asystole
  C. Heart block
    1. Type II: sudden asystole
    2. Morgagni–Adams-Stokes syndrome
  D. Vagal reflex and carotid sinus syndromes
  E. Ventricular fibrillation

TABLE 14

Classification of Episodic Unconsciousness Due to Abnormal Function of the Central Nervous System

I. Systemic disorders impairing cerebral metabolism
    A. Hypoxia
    B. Anemia
    C. Hypoglycemia
II. Cerebral arterial occlusion
    A. Basilar-vertebral artery insufficiency
    B. Carotid occlusion plus insufficiency
    C. Intracranial arterial spasm
        1. Subarachnoid hemorrhage
        2. Hypocapnia
        3. Hypertensive encephalopathy
        4. Basilar migraine
III. Primary neurologic disorders
    A. Epilepsy
        1. Generalized seizures
            a. Grand mal (generalized major motor seizure)
            b. Petit mal (generalized minor seizure)
            c. Drug withdrawal seizures
            d. Syncopal seizures
        2. Focal seizures
            a. Focal seizures becoming generalized
            b. Temporal lobe (psychomotor) seizures
    B. "Mechanical" disturbances of brain function
        1. Concussion
        2. Transient intracranial hypertension
        3. Developmental abnormalities
IV. Other episodes of unconsciousness
    A. Narcolepsy-cataplexy
    B. Post-traumatic syndrome
    C. Menière's disease
    D. Psychogenic unconsciousness
        1. Hysteria
        2. Malingering—compensation

Examination of the Unconscious Patient

Discussion of the differential diagnosis of coma is beyond the scope of the present chapter. It is essential to recognize and treat certain immediate threats to life in the unconscious patient. Answers to several questions should be immediately sought. Is the patient responsive? Is he breathing? Is the airway open? Does he have a heart beat? What is the heart rate? Is blood pressure being maintained? Has there been an injury?

Satisfactory answers to these queries can be obtained by a rapid and efficient examination of the patient that is limited to essentials and utilizes the techniques of inspection and palpation. It is far quicker, for example, to palpate a carotid or femoral artery to estimate heart rate and blood pressure than to spend precious time attempting to auscultate the heart or measure blood pressure with a cuff.

Examination of the unconscious patient might be organized according to the following general procedure: A brief glance will note the position of the patient, the attitude of the limbs and the head and neck. Does the victim respond to voice or touch? A major artery such as the carotid or femoral is quickly palpated to determine heart rate and pulse volume. Are the extremities warm or cold? Is skin color normal, or are the lips or nail beds cyanotic? Does extreme pallor suggest anemia? As important as a rapid survey of the cardiovascular system is an evaluation of respiration and patency of the airway. Any uncertainty about respiratory rate or volume can usually be resolved by placing a hand on the anterior neck and feeling for chest wall motion. Rapid search for injury should include palpation of the skull, torso, and extremities. A more thorough neurologic evaluation, including careful flexion of the neck, inspection of the eyes and pupils, and evaluation of deep tendon and plantar reflexes, is usually best performed after the physician is assured that the cardiovascular and respiratory systems are supporting the patient adequately.

The immediate threats to life are cardiac or respiratory arrest, bleeding, and severe injury. If these conditions appear to be absent in the initial survey a more leisurely evaluation can take place. Recognition of a life-threatening complication, on the other hand, should impel immediate emergency measures. It is well to remember that the brain can only survive 3 to 4 minutes after cessation of effective cerebral blood flow. Even this brief margin is reduced in older patients. The need for prompt recognition and effective therapy of cardiac or respiratory arrest is paramount.

DIAGNOSIS

Episodes of unconsciousness are frequently not witnessed. Even when trained or medically oriented observers are present, the excitement of the moment may engender inaccurate statements and as many versions of the event as there are observers, a vexing problem. As much information as possible should be obtained by carefully questioning the victim and available witnesses. Areas of important information include the presence or absence of a warning, the time of day when the attack occurred, activity, medicines, and possible predisposing conditions.

To help the physician focus his approach to the unconscious patient, Table 15 provides a guide according to age, the patient's activity at the time of the attack, and observations that are likely to be recalled by the patient or untrained witnesses.

In obtaining a history of an episode of unconsciousness, one must inquire in meticulous detail as to precisely what the circumstances were, what the patient felt, and what any observer saw. This should provide information sufficient at least to categorize the episode, for example, as systemic circulatory failure, a disorder of brain metabolism, cerebrovascular disease, or epilepsy.

TABLE 15

Guide to Diagnosis of Causes of Episodic Unconsciousness

Age	
Childhood:	Epilepsy, cyanotic heart disease, hypoglycemia, hypocapnia-Valsalva, basilar migraine
Young adults:	Simple faint, epilepsy, hypoglycemia, drug withdrawal, postural hypotension, blood loss, pregnancy, hysteria
Middle and old age:	Aortic stenosis, heart block, arrhythmia, pulmonary emboli, postural hypotension (extracellular fluid loss, autonomic insufficiency), cerebral arterial disease, cough and micturition syncope
Activity at onset	
Exertion:	Aortic stenosis, arrhythmia, dehydration and postural hypotension
Emotional stress:	Simple faint, hysteria, arrhythmia

Observations at time of episode
  Initial symptoms
    Weakness, light-headedness: low cardiac output, hypoglycemia
    Unusual pattern of psychological or visceral symptoms: psychomotor epilepsy
    Vertigo, weakness, visual blurring: basilar artery insufficiency
    Palpitations or angina: arrhythmia
  Physical abnormalities
    Pallor: low cardiac output
    Cyanosis: anoxia, inadequate ventilation, intracardiac shunt
    Bradycardia: heart block, simple syncope, pulmonary embolus
    Convulsive movements: epilepsy, severe syncope from any cause, cerebrovascular insufficiency, hypoxia, hypoglycemia
    Postictal confusion: epilepsy, cerebrovascular insufficiency, hypoglycemia

Warning of Impending Attack

Cardiac faints usually are not preceded by an aura. Some patients with Stokes-Adams syndrome, however, describe a loss of vision, a gray film, or the sensation of color in the visual field, especially blue or purple, before losing consciousness. Following the episode the victim may feel a hot or warm flush over his body. This latter sensation presumably reflects the intense vasodilation that follows momentary loss of peripheral blood flow. The mechanism probably is similar to the vasodilation which follows release of arterial occlusion. The increased blood flow is related to the local accumulation and subsequent washout of metabolic products with vasodilator properties.

Although most episodes of unconsciousness due to cardiac abnormality are sudden, in some patients the onset is more gradual. This may be the case in patients with arrhythmia. The patient may be aware of tachycardia, irregular heart beat, or skipped beats preceding unconsciousness.

Age and Sex

The probability that a certain diagnosis will be established is often influenced by the age and sex of the patient. Simple fainting, postural hypotension, and orthostatic hypotension are most common in young women. Primary pulmonary hypertension is a disease found predominantly in women, and periodic unconsciousness may be a troublesome symptom in the second and third decades. Syncope is a well-recognized complication of aortic stensosis. This condition usually is manifest after the age of 50, and occurs predominantly in men, though severe congenital aortic stenosis may occur in infants and children. Unconsciousness caused by intermittent heart block or in established complete heart block, the Stokes-Adams syndrome, has its highest incidence in the sixth and seventh decades, and occurs with equal frequency in both sexes.

Family History

A number of cardiovascular conditions which predispose to episodic unconsciousness may be familial. Such entities include the Wolff-Parkinson-White syndrome, supraventricular tachycardia with short PR interval and normal QRS, and complex congenital malformations, including supravalvular aortic stenosis, hypertrophic subaortic stenosis, heart block , and the tetralogy of Fallot. Several families have been described in which a prolonged QT interval, apparently a heritable defect, is associated with recurrent bouts of ventricular fibrillation. This condition has been described in association with congenital deafness, a combination also observed in the Dalmatian coachhound. The list is by no means exhaustive, but valuable clues or unusual constellations of familial disorders may be uncovered by a carefully detailed family history.

Medications

A variety of medications utilized in the treatment of hypertension may be associated with severe postural hypotension (Table 16). Reserpine,

TABLE 16

Drugs with Postural Hypotension as a Prominent Side Effect. Drug-induced hypotension can be a side effect of any of the agents listed below, but is more likely if the dose is poorly controlled, if the drugs are used in combination, if they are used parenterally, or if the patient is hypovolemic or has arterial disease or impaired vascular reflexes.

Phenothiazines
  Promazine (Sparine)
  Chlorpromazine (Thorazine)
  Thioridazine (Mellaril)
Imipramine (Tofranil)
Antiadrenergic agents
  Bretylium
  Guanethidine (Ismelin)
  Methyldopa (Aldomet)
  Reserpine
  Propranolol (Inderal)
Ganglionic blocking agents
  Hexamethonium
Bethanechol (Urecholine)
Nitrites and nitrate vasodilators

hexamethonium, and ganglionic blockers such as guanethidine inhibit the normal vasoconstriction which occurs with the assumption of the upright position. Syncope in a patient taking digitalis should raise a suspicion of digitalis-induced arrhythmia or heart block. The β-blocking agent propranolol may induce bradycardia and faintness with exertion or with change in posture. Postural hypotension and light-headedness may complicate the use of a variety of antidepressant medications. Serious reactions, including severe hypotension with unconsciousness, may occur with drugs which inhibit monoamine oxidase. Severe reactions are triggered when certain foods, such as cheese, containing high concentrations of catecholamines, especially tyramine, are ingested.

Activity and Symptoms at Onset

One of the most important questions a physician should seek to answer concerns the activities of the patient preceding the episode of unconsciousness. A change in position, especially from lying or sitting to standing, points to a postural mechanism. Preceding palpitations or ischemic cardiac pain suggest a cardiac arrhythmia. Patients with aortic stenosis or hypertrophic cardiac disease characteristically faint during or immediately following exertion. A left atrial myxoma or a mitral ball valve thrombus may obstruct ventricular inflow when the patient leans over, as to tie a shoelace. Fainting when the patient is on the toilet suggests that a Valsalva maneuver or excessive "vagotonia" producing bradycardia may have been causative. Syncope during a stressful situation in an anxious patient suggests a vasovagal faint.

Physical Examination

Especial care should be taken in relation to detection of cardiovascular and neurologic abnormalities. One should observe the pulse rate and rhythm, the response of the blood pressure to standing and to vagal stimulation, and any evidence of venous stasis. Focal neurologic signs in a patient suspected of having a seizure disorder suggest intracranial disease, and require further study. Conversely, the absence of neurologic abnormality on careful examination is usually reliable evidence that the patient does not have a structural defect of the nervous system. Pupils which react poorly to light, defective sweating, and postural hypotension suggest autonomic insufficiency. Excessive tremulousness may indicate that the patient is undergoing drug or alcohol withdrawal.

The best way, of course, for a physician to determine the cause of an episode of unconsciousness is to witness the attack and make the appropriate observations at the time. Since he rarely has this opportunity, he must usually rely on the recollections of the patient and of nonprofessional observers and on his own examination of the patient after the event has passed. In many cases, such as simple vasodepressor fainting or epilepsy, this information is reliable and sufficient. But if one has only the patient's history to go on, diagnosis of the more complex causes of episodic uncon-sciousness can be exceedingly difficult.

CAUSES OF EPISODIC UNCONSCIOUSNESS

Abnormal Cardiovascular Function

Insufficient Venous Return

The venous network of the body plays a crucial role in the maintenance of cardiac output and hence systemic blood pressure.[26] More than 80 per cent of the total blood volume is contained in the venous bed. An adequate venous flow into the right heart is dependent upon sufficient blood volume, normal sympathetic reflex control of venous tone, a venous capacity appro-priate for the available blood volume, and an unobstructed return pathway to the heart. Table 6 lists a variety of causes of unconsciousness which result from inadequate venous return.

Any mechanism which interferes with venous return may lead to a reduction in cardiac output. When venous return and cardiac output are reduced, adequate blood pressure is maintained by peripheral vasocon-striction. Should this adjustment fail or be overcome, as for example in the febrile patient with low blood volume, or if the venous insufficiency is sudden, as with change in position, systemic arterial pressure will fall and unconsciousness may ensue.

SIMPLE FAINTING OR VASOVAGAL SYNCOPE

This is the most common form of episodic unconsciousness. Fainting accompanies many varieties of physiologic and psychologic stress.[11] Al-though it is more commonly a response to pain, actual physical injury, loss of blood, or peripheral vasodilation, syncope may follow even apparently trivial emotional or physical stress. Its psychologic setting is often one of pain or fear that cannot be avoided or counteracted by appropriate action. In his extensive studies on fainting, Engel has concluded that "careful psychological study of many instances of vasodepressor syncope consist-ently reveals the faint to be preceded by some combination of anxiety of an actual or threatened injury and at the same time some restriction or inhibition of action."[11] He points out that this reaction is more common as a neurotic trait in men than in women because of masculine concern with physical strength and courage. A faint rarely occurs without some warning, such as weakness, tremor, nausea, sweating, yawning, light-headedness, or giddiness. The warning symptoms are generated largely by increased circulating catecholamines; presyncopal urinary levels of epinephrine and norepinephrine have been found to be higher in "fainters" than in "non-fainters."[6] The pulse rate increases with these initial symptoms and then slows considerably as the systolic blood pressure reaches the critical level of 55 to 60 mm Hg and the patient loses consciousness. Whereas tachy-cardia usually accompanies low blood pressure, a cardinal sign of the simple faint is bradycardia.[10, 30] During and sometimes for a period after unconsciousness, the pulse rate may be as slow as 50 to 60/minute. Because the cutaneous blood flow is decreased, the skin is pale and cold, and increased sympathetic activity induces sweating.

Vasodepressor syncope has a duration measured in seconds to minutes, and recovery is usually prompt when the subject reclines and an adequate cerebral blood flow is restored. If the subject is unable to fall (as in a telephone booth or when tied into a wheelchair) inadequate cerebral blood flow will continue, and cerebral ischemia may lead to seizures or even to permanent neuronal damage. Syncope is frequently accompanied by a few tonic convulsive movements, especially if the hypotension is profound or accompanied by an additional cause of reduced cerebral circulation, such as arteriosclerosis.

Simple fainting is the result of complex interactions, largely under reflex control, among venous capacity, heart rate, and resistance in the arterial circuit.[34] In susceptible individuals, especially when they are anxious or frightened, autonomic discharge markedly reduces venous tone, slows the heart rate and causes arterial dilation. The change in venous tone increases capacity and pools blood in the large veins. Venous return, and hence cardiac output, fall. Both bradycardia and decreased arterial resistance contribute to the decrease in blood pressure. Cerebral blood flow cannot be maintained and the victim loses consciousness. This process can be so profound as to cause syncope even when the subject is reclining.[10, 30]

The following case report is a typical example of several stressful factors leading to an episode of vasovagal syncope.

Case 2

A 19-year-old secretary agreed to donate blood to the Red Cross bloodmobile. Her appointment was in the evening, and she had a large dinner before appearing. A vein in the antecubital fossa was punctured and 400 ml of blood were collected. During the procedure the young woman began to hyperventilate, broke into a sweat, turned pale, and lost consciousness. Her pulse rate was 40. Systolic blood pressure by palpation was 55 mm Hg. After some 15 seconds she had a convulsion. The withdrawn blood was rapidly reinfused, 1.0 mg of atropine was administered, and the foot of the bed was elevated. Heart rate and blood pressure rose and the patient regained consciousness after about 6 minutes. Following recovery the patient described a feeling of considerable apprehension and anxiety during the venepuncture.

An unaccustomed procedure, anxiety, and postprandial visceral pooling of blood provided the setting in which a simple faint or vasovagal syncope occurred. Pallor, sweating, low blood pressure, slow pulse, and the response to atropine and increased venous return established the diagnosis. The occurrence of convulsions is not helpful in differential diagnosis, since seizures may occur 15 to 20 seconds after cessation of effective cerebral blood flow, no matter what the mechanism. Thus, convulsions do not necessarily indicate a primary neurogenic cause of loss of consciousness.

POSTURAL HYPOTENSION

This occurs when peripheral vasomotor mechanisms fail in response to the erect posture. When man stands upright a complex series of reactions, largely reflex in origin, take place.[2, 23] Arterial blood pressure is maintained by increases in peripheral resistance, venous tone, and heart rate. As normal human subjects are passively raised from supine to 65° in tilt table experiments, the mean cerebral arterial pressure falls 34 percent and the cerebral blood flow decreases by 21 per cent. With the assumption of the vertical position venous pressure in the thorax falls, venous return is reduced, and cardiac stoke volume decreases, but cardiac output or minute volume is maintained by an increase in heart rate. There may be a slight fall in arterial pressure. The largely passive reduction in venous return is counteracted by an increase in autonomic nerve discharge which leads to venoconstriction and improved venous return. These changes are accompanied by increases in plasma norepinephrine and urinary catecholamines and have been attributed to increased sympathetic activity and release of transmitter substance from the nerve endings.

In this complex interaction, it is small wonder that malfunction may occur on sudden standing. All of us, at one time or another, have experienced a momentary feeling of faintness upon standing quickly after prolonged sitting or lying. Postural syncope is most often associated with prolonged motionless standing, with standing after prolonged recumbency because of illness or debility, with pregnancy, and with malfunction of the sympathetic nervous system. Fainting while standing in parades or dull meetings is a common experience. Excessive heat, hunger, dehydration, and anxiety add to the risk. Deliberate leg muscle contraction, even shuffling the feet, is an effective preventive measure. The symptoms of postural syncope are with few exceptions those of vasodepression, and consciousness is quickly regained when the patient becomes horizontal.

Postural adaptive mechanisms can fail at least partially after as little as a week of bed rest, especially in the elderly or in those with painful, debilitating, or frightening illnesses.[1] Leg exercises while in bed, early ambulation, and the awareness of the possibility of postural hypotension help to prevent syncope. Elderly or immobile patients risk syncope when sitting in a chair for long periods.

Idiopathic Orthostatic Hypotension. In some individuals the normal compensating reflex responses for maintaining blood pressure with assumption of the upright position appear to be deficient.[2] The normal increase in blood norepinephrine level on standing does not occur. This lack presumably reflects an inadequacy of the primary reflex adjustments. Venous tone does not increase and systemic arterial vasoconstriction is limited. Such individuals may suffer from debilitating orthostatic hypotension, and are said to have the idiopathic variety. This condition is thought to be a primary disorder of the autonomic nervous system, and may include defective sweating and sexual impotence. In addition, some patients have a gradual progressive involvement of corticobulbar and corticospinal tracts, the basal ganglia, and the cerebellar system. Some have a parkinsonian appearance. This condition is known as the Shy-Drager syndrome. The most frequent early symptoms of this uncommon disorder are dizziness and faintness with intermittent postural loss of consciousness. Orthostatic hypotension can be easily elicited on a tilt table. After lying supine for several minutes, the subject, strapped to the tilt table, is swung erect. Within a short time blood pressure falls, the pulse rate fails to rise, and the subject may faint. Treatment is designed to increase blood volume and compensate for reduced venous tone by filling the capacious venous bed. The salt-retaining steroid fluorohydrocortisone, in adequate dosage, is the most useful available drug.

Autonomic Insufficiency. Postural hypotension may be the most prominent symptom of a generalized neurogenic autonomic insufficiency which accompanies a variety of neurologic disorders.[8, 15] The most common conditions causing this state are the peripheral neuropathies, such as those associated with diabetes, the Guillain-Barré syndrome, alcoholism, malnutrition, porphyria, and tabes dorsalis. Disorders of the central nervous system can also be associated with autonomic insufficiency, and include Wernicke's disease (thiamine deficiency), structural lesions of the medulla oblongata, and idiopathic orthostatic hypotension, already described. In addition to the loss of postural vasomotor reflexes, the patient with autonomic insufficiency usually has decreased sweating, gastrointestinal hypomotility, and sexual impotence. The normal increase in blood norepinephrine level on standing does not occur. Characteristic of syncope due to autonomic insufficiency is the absence of the usual warning symptoms. These patients may not experience the weakness, nausea, giddiness, and sweating preceding the usual vasovagal attack, and for this reason are in greater danger of injury from falling.

A number of physiologic and pharmacologic tests help to establish the presence or absence of autonomic insufficiency. Postural hypotension in these patients is often unaccompanied by tachycardia. Also, there is an abnormal blood pressure response to the Valsalva maneuver: in the normal subject the raised intrathoracic pressure during the Valsalva maneuver interferes with the venous return to the heart, and arterial blood pressure falls, then rises slightly as reflex vasoconstriction occurs. When intrathoracic pressure is released the arterial pressure overshoots its resting level because of persisting vasoconstriction. In the patient with impaired vascular reflexes raised intrathoracic pressure evokes a steady fall in arterial blood pressure; on release there is a gradual return to the resting level instead of an overshoot. Patients with defective neurovascular control also may show abnormal responses to administered nitroglycerine and norepinephrine as detailed by Birchfield.[4]

Sympathectomy. Insufficient venous return plays a dominant role in the syncope or postural hypotension which may be troublesome following sympathectomy. Orthostatic hypotension may also complicate the use of certain drugs, such as the ganglionic blockers used in the management of hypertension, some tranquilizers and antidepressants, and the antiadrenergic agents (see Table 16). In both surgical and "pharmacologic" sympathectomy the normal autonomic reflex responses to assumption of the upright position are inhibited. The importance of venous return in the maintenance of arterial pressure can be demonstrated experimentally by placing the postsympathectomy or drug-treated patient in water to his chin. Postural hypotension is eliminated by this maneuver, which is unfortunately not very practical, because the external hydrostatic pressure improves venous return, thus overcoming the expansion of the venous bed with upright position. An antigravity suit has similar effects.

DECREASED BLOOD VOLUME

A number of conditions associated with decreased blood volume may predispose to unconsciousness. Included are anemia, acute blood loss, low serum proteins and thus low plasma volume, dehydration, and Addison's disease. Recurrent syncope or orthostatic hypotension may be the first sign of deficient blood volume. In the patient with a suspected or potential blood volume deficit an inordinate tachycardia when sitting up in bed may be an important clue alerting the physician to the impending difficulty.

The likelihood of postural hypotension and syncope with blood loss depends on how much blood is lost and how fast, on how frightened the patient is, and on the state of the cardiovascular system. In professional donors, who presumably have no fear of venepuncture or bleeding, syncope occurs only when as much as 15 to 20 per cent of the blood volume is removed within 6 to 13 minutes.[9] Syncope associated with less profound traumatic or pathologic hemorrhage is as much the product of pain and fear as of blood loss. Slow and occult bleeding is usually well compensated for, and leads to syncope only when the additional stresses of prolonged standing or exertion are added.

Any condition causing vasodilation will reinforce pre-existing postural hypotension. Thus, if the stage is set, fainting is more likely to occur in a warm room or if the patient has fever.

MECHANICAL BLOCK

Various forms of mechanical block can inhibit venous return to the right heart. Among these are the Valsalva maneuver, vigorous coughing, and forceful micturition. Syncope may result from increased intrathoracic pressure, impeding venous inflow to the chest. The simple childhood trick of hyperventilation followed by thoracic compression against a closed glottis (the Valsalva maneuver) will lead to unconsciousness. Sometimes the ritual is reinforced by having a partner squeeze the subject's chest manually.[19] The hyperventilation lowers arterial CO_2 pressure causing systemic vasodilation and cerebral vasoconstriction. The Valsalva maneuver abruptly reduces cardiac output, and the youngster who has been standing loses consciousness.

According to experimental studies the loss of consciousness with the Valsalva maneuver is caused by systemic hypotension, with the possible addition of increased intracranial pressure. A high intrathoracic pressure inhibits venous return to the heart, which results in decreased cardiac output and systemic hypotension. This phenomenon was nicely demonstrated by two patients we studied during the Valsalva maneuver with continuous monitoring of arterial, venous, and cerebrospinal fluid pressures: syncope occurred only when the arteriovenous pressure difference (net perfusion pressure) fell below 40 mm Hg. Syncope is produced more readily when the Valsalva maneuver is preceded by a short period of hyperventilation (which itself reduces the cerebral blood flow). In one study recumbent subjects lost consciousness when the mean arterial blood pressure fell to an average level of 51 mm Hg. associated with an arterial blood PCO_2 of 26 mm Hg or less.[19] With greater degrees of hypocapnia less hypotension was required to induce syncope. The rapidity with which syncope appears during the Valsalva maneuver has suggested to some workers that the abrupt accompanying rise in intracranial pressure compresses brain cells and capillaries and produces additional ischemic and concussive effects. However, the peak of the rise in cerebrospinal fluid pressure during the Valsalva maneuver does not consistently correlate with the onset of syncope.

Cough Syncope. The same mechanisms that operate during the Valsalva maneuver account for cough syncope.[24] During a cough intrathoracic pressure may rise to 300 mm Hg or more. Cough syncope usually occurs in overweight men with chronic lung disease following vigorous coughing or laughter, but it has been described in women and occasionally in children. The patient, who is otherwise asymptomatic, has a bout of violent coughing, suddenly loses consciousness, and falls, only to regain both his senses and his feet within a few seconds.

Micturition Syncope. This condition is uncommon. It occurs in men, and is usually nocturnal. The patient arises from sleep to urinate and suddenly loses consciousness as he stands at the toilet either before, during, or after voiding. The causative factors are several. Sudden rising from sleep induces postural hypotension; the Valsalva sequence reduces cerebral blood flow; there is a vasovagal hypotensive response to sudden relief of a distended bladder. Alcohol ingestion during the evening makes bladder distension and peripheral vasodilation more likely to occur.

Other Causes. Two less common forms of episodic unconsciousness may be due to mechanical obstruction of venous return. During the third trimester of pregnancy the distended uterus may compress the inferior vena cava when the subject is supine, and thus cause faintness. Change of position is usually sufficient to alleviate symptoms. In atrial myxoma a ball valve tumor in the left atrium prolapses through the mitral valve and may cause prolonged unconsciousness.

Obstructed Aortic Outflow

AORTIC STENOSIS

Syncope is a common presenting complaint in severe aortic stenosis.[25] It is usually an indication of a high degree of obstruction and implies a poor prognosis. Development of syncope in the patient with aortic stenosis should mandate a careful evaluation of the severity of the lesion, since sudden death is a distinct hazard. The possibility that surgical intervention may be necessary should be carefully considered, as illustrated in the following case.

Case 3

A 53-year-old man had had a heart murmur for many years. He had served in the Pacific theater during World War II and was an active individual who enjoyed sports. He considered himself in good health. While hurrying up an inclined ramp at a racetrack in order to place a bet, he suddenly fell, unconscious. He recovered fully in about 5 minutes. Thoroughly frightened, he sought medical advice. He had never had angina pectoris or symptoms suggesting heart failure. Physical examination revealed signs of aortic stenosis. Cardiac catherization revealed a 100 mm Hg peak systolic gradient across the aortic valve. Valve area was calculated to be 0.6 cm^2 (normal, 3 to 4 cm^2). The aortic valve was subsequently removed during an operative procedure, and a ball valve prosthesis was inserted. Recovery was uneventful. Syncope has not recurred postoperatively.

The unconsciousness of aortic stenosis usually occurs during or following exercise. Presumably it reflects the inability of the left ventricle to overcome the fixed aortic obstruction. During exertion the anticipated increase in cardiac output fails to occur, yet the peripheral arterial bed dilates. Perfusion pressure drops and cerebral blood flow decreases abruptly. In some patients syncope has been related to bouts of ventricular arrhythmia, including recurrent but self-limited ventricular fibrillation. In many instances the arrhythmia is probably a reflection of changes in coronary blood flow and myocardial metabolism associated with ventricular hypertrophy.

The recognition of aortic stenosis should not be difficult, provided that the patient is subjected to a systematic and careful physical examination. Although most patients with significant aortic stenosis have a palpable slurred upstroke or anacrotic notch in the carotid pulse, significant obstruction may be present without the classic pulsus parvus and tardus. Indeed, systemic arterial hypertension may coexist with severe aortic stenosis.

The hallmark of aortic stenosis is a coarse, harsh, "ejection-type" or "diamond-shaped" murmur, which may be heard to the left or right of the sternum in the second or third intercostal space. Almost every patient with significant aortic stenosis has a systolic thrill accompanying the murmur. The thrill may be overlooked unless assiduously sought for by having the patient lean forward or even get on his hands and knees. It is important to search for a thrill, since its presence is confirmatory evidence of aortic stenosis.

In some patients, especially older patients with barrel chests and displacement of the upper sternum anteriorly, the murmur of aortic stenosis has a honking or musical quality and is heard best at the apex. The thrill may also be most prominent in the so-called mitral area. Not infrequently a diagnosis of mitral regurgitation is erroneously entertained. It is important to be alert to this confusing clinical picture, since the physiologic implications of the two lesions are quite different. Although mitral regurgitation may cause important disability because of left ventricular failure, it is usually a well-tolerated lesion with a slow devolutionary phase. Aortic stenosis, on the other hand, may be clinically silent for many years, only to precipitate episodic unconsciousness, heart failure, or sudden death.

The aortic valve is invariably heavily calcified in individuals over 35 years of age with aortic stenosis. This fact has two important clinical implications. First, valve calcification should be searched for to confirm the diagnosis in patients suspected of having aortic stenosis. Second, failure to find calcification should raise questions about the accuracy of the clinical assessment. Valve calcification may be recognized on a well-exposed lateral chest film. A more sensitive technique is fluoroscopy with an image intensifier.

HYPERTROPHIC SUBAORTIC STENOSIS

Syncope is a well-known complication of idiopathic left ventricular hypertrophy or the so-called idiopathic hypertrophic subaortic stenosis syndrome.[5] In this condition left ventricular muscle mass is markedly increased. The velocity of myocardial contraction is increased and is associated with a characteristic bifid form of the aortic pressure pulse. In some patients there is evidence of subaortic stenosis due to hypertrophied muscle. Although it is tempting to relate the syncope to spasm of the outflow tract, and hence increased subaortic obstruction, a left ventricular-aortic systolic pressure gradient has not been demonstrated in a number of cases. It is probable that the episodic unconsciousness in this condition is related to a complex series of factors, including further impairment of cardiac performance with exercise, a drop in stroke volume, and a marked rise in left ventricular end diastolic pressure. Mechanisms similar to those described for calcific aortic stenosis may also be operative, so that, in the face of reduced stroke volume, arrhythmia or excessive vasodilation may develop during exercise.

Hypertrophic heart disease has been diagnosed as a clinical entity only in the past decade. It is now apparent that the condition, although uncommon, is by no means rare. It is frequently overlooked or misdiagnosed as mitral valve regurgitation or valvular aortic stenosis. The condition may be familial, and sudden death has been reported. Incision into the hypertrophied ventricular septum in the left ventricular outflow tract has been undertaken for treatment of severe cases associated with signs of infundibular aortic stenosis, but the natural history of the disease is so variable that considerable uncertainty now exists as to the value of this form of therapy. Reducing the velocity of ventricular contraction by means of β-adrenergic blockade with propranolol has been reported to be beneficial.

Bouts of unconsciousness are characteristic of two other cardiac conditions, namely pulmonary arterial hypertension without shunt and tetralogy of Fallot.

PULMONARY HYPERTENSION

In pulmonary hypertension, either idiopathic or secondary to often unrecognized pulmonary emboli, the pressure in the pulmonary artery may be at systemic levels or higher. Since cardiac output is low and relatively fixed in these conditions, syncope may have causes similar to those described for aortic stenosis. Bouts of acute right ventricular failure have also been postulated as an explanation for the recurrent syncope in these conditions. In primary pulmonary hypertension signs of right heart overload predominate. Usually there is a systolic parasternal heave, a loud pulmonic second sound, and occasionally a diastolic murmur of pulmonic regurgitation. The electrocardiogram shows right ventricular hypertrophy.

TETRALOGY OF FALLOT

In the tetralogy of Fallot a large ventricular septal defect combines with severe infundibular pulmonic stenosis to produce a right-to-left intracardiac shunt and cyanosis. Pulmonary blood flow and hence systemic oxygenation depend on the bronchial collateral circulation and the varying flow through the obstructed right ventricular outflow tract. Infundibular spasm or hypertrophy may reduce pulmonary blood flow, increase the right-to-left shunt, and hence worsen the systemic anoxia. If systemic blood pressure should fall, as during excitement, emotion, or exercise, a large amount of the blood in the right ventricle may follow the path of least resistance and be shunted through the defect to the systemic circulation. In either of the above situations arterial hypoxia may be profound and syncope may ensue.

PULMONARY EMBOLISM

The initial symptom of pulmonary embolism may be sudden loss of consciousness. Massive embolization with obstruction of the main stem or both branches of the pulmonary artery rapidly leads to systemic circulatory collapse, but this requires occlusion of 60 to 80 per cent of the pulmonary arterial bed.[14] We have observed several patients who suddenly lost consciousness with pulmonary embolization that was otherwise clinically silent. In these cases apnea, bradycardia, hypotension, and unconsciousness followed pulmonary embolization that neither obstructed the main pulmonary arteries nor caused massive infarction. This is not a commonly recognized clinical pattern, but it is not rare and should be considered whenever a patient has any degree of respiratory distress with unexplained loss of consciousness. The following two case reports illustrate this important point.

Case 4

A 64-year-old Hungarian architect was waiting at the airport on his way home when he suddenly fainted. He regained consciousness shortly and was brought to the Cornell Neurological Division of Bellevue Hospital because of a presumed stroke. The examination showed no focal neurologic signs, but he was intellectually somewhat slow. He was moderately hypotensive and tachypneic, and it was thought that he had suffered a myocardial infarct. The electrocardiogram, however, showed only minor ischemic changes. Over the next 2 days he had three more episodes of unconsciousness, each one leaving him a little more obtunded. Repeated electrocardiograms recorded slight right axis deviation; a tracing recorded during an episode of unconsciousness showed no change in cardiac rhythm. Auscultation of the chest revealed clear breath sounds, and a single chest x-ray was unremarkable. On the third day he died suddenly. At autopsy multiple emboli occluded the smaller branches of the pulmonary arteries. There was no myocardial infarction or gross brain lesion.

Case 5

A 55-year-old woman with severe polyneuropathy was being examined on ward rounds. She suddenly stopped talking, developed a fixed stare, had clonic movements in the left arm, and was incontinent. This lasted no more than 15 seconds, and was followed by a minute of confusion, then full alertness. Her skin was gray and clammy, and she was diaphoretic. A radioactive lung scan showed several small peripheral areas of decreased pulmonary blood flow.

These events are not readily explained, but experimental studies suggest that multiple pulmonary emboli may produce circulatory and respiratory inhibition by stimulation of stretch receptors in small pulmonary vessels which induces a vagal reflex response.

Arrhythmia

Unconsciousness may occur when the heart is beating too fast or too slowly if an adequate cardiac output cannot be sustained. In a normal man heart rates as low as 30 beats/minute may be tolerated as long as the subject remains supine. Cardiac output is usually well maintained until a heart rate of greater than 180/minute is reached. However, patients with abnormal hearts, cerebral vascular disease, or other disorders, such as anemia or blood loss, may have disturbances of cerebral function at heart rates well within the limits tolerated by normal individuals.

SINUS BRADYCARDIA

Although extreme slowing of the ventricular rate is most commonly associated with heart block, it has been recognized recently that sinus bradycardia may be troublesome in elderly patients. Slowing of the heart due to sinus bradycardia implies abnormality of the cardiac pacemaker at two levels, usually the sinus node and the atrioventricular (A-V) node. Since the latter acts as escape pacemaker at rates between 40 and 50 beats/ minute, failure of an escape nodal rhythm to appear when the primary sinus rate falls below this range indicates that the A-V node is not functioning normally.

Persistent sinus bradycardia is thought to reflect a reduction in blood supply to the heart's prime pacemaker. The artery to the sinus node is a relatively long, easily identified vessel which arises from the proximal right coronary artery in 54 per cent and from the circumflex artery in 42 per cent of human hearts. The major blood supply to the A-V node comes from the A-V node artery. This short vessel arises from the crux of the heart posteriorly, where the circumflex vessel turns to become the posterior descending artery. Coronary arteriosclerosis may impair the blood supply to either the sinus or A-V node, and result in slow heart rates not necessarily accompanied by heart block. Disease of the smaller coronary arteries and fibrosis apparently unrelated to coronary arteriosclerosis may also be associated with bradycardia. Dramatic examples of the former condition have now been encountered in patients with transplanted hearts during rejection.

Sinus bradycardia may complicate acute myocardial infarction, especially within the first few hours after onset. It is likely that the arrhythmia reflects an acute disturbance in blood supply to the pacemaker tissues. Reflex factors and excessive "vagotonia" secondary to stimulation of receptors within the heart have been postulated, especially as complications of diaphragmatic or inferior infarctions. Firm proof of this thesis is lacking. Fortunately the sinus bradycardia complicating acute myocardial infarction responds readily to small doses of atropine, and usually persists but a few hours. Occasionally the arrhythmia is refractory and requires insertion of a pacemaker.

Case 6

A 67-year-old woman was admitted to the coronary care unit with crushing precordial pain that persisted for an hour. An electrocardiogram confirmed the diagnosis of acute myocardial infarction. One hour following admission the heart rate fell to 40 beats/minute. An electrocardiogram showed slow nodal rhythm. No P waves were identified. The patient became confused. Blood pressure was 90/60 mm Hg and the lungs were congested. Following atropine, 1.0 mg, the anticipated increase of heart rate failed to develop. A pacemaker electrode was inserted into the right atrium and the heart was paced at a rate of 90. Blood pressure rose, signs of heart failure cleared, and the patient became alert and oriented. Three weeks later a permanent pacemaker was inserted, since the sinus node remained apparently functionless.

OVERDRIVE SUPPRESSION

It is an electrophysiologic principle that rapid discharge of a subsidiary pacemaker may suppress the dominant pacemaker. Thus, following the abrupt cessation of a bout of atrial tachycardia, for example, asystole may persist for several seconds. This phenomenon, known as a postoverdrive suppression of the dominant pacemaker, is an uncommon cause of syncope. It apparently reflects an unusual sensitivity to a normal mechanism, since postoverdrive suppression can easily be demonstrated in laboratory preparations. This arrhythmia may be misdiagnosed as a form of heart block, which it is not. Once it is recognized that the fundamental problem is a normal, albeit exaggerated, physiologic response, treatment may be directed toward suppression of the bouts of tachycardia rather than avoidance of heart block. If the tachycardia cannot be prevented, implantation of a demand pacemaker may be required to overcome the periods of asystole.

Case 7

A 59-year-old secretary had the sudden onset of "blackouts" with convulsions. She was admitted to the hospital after experiencing six episodes of syncope in 1 day. Several had occurred when she was lying down. Physical examination revealed rapid atrial fibrillation. There were no murmurs and no neurologic abnormalities. Observations on a monitoring oscilloscope revealed episodes of sinus rhythm, followed by bouts of rapid atrial fibrillation. After some time the fibrillation would cease spontaneously, to be followed by long periods of asystole before sinus rhythm returned. When the asystolic period exceeded 6 seconds, the patient lost consciousness. A permanent pacemaker was required to overcome the asystolic intervals, since the paroxysmal atrial fibrillation could not be suppressed with digitalis or quinidine.

HEART BLOCK

In 1876 Stokes described episodes of unconsciousness in an elderly patient who had a slow heart rate. Based on the original description, the term Stokes-Adams syndrome should properly be applied only to syncope caused by ventricular asystole in the presence of established complete heart block. Generally, however, the term is applied to any attacks of unconsciousness associated with heart block. It is known that recurrent syncope in patients with established heart block may also be triggered by self-limited episodes of ventricular tachycardia or ventricular fibrillation. If the ventricular tachycardia is sufficiently rapid stroke volume may be so low that syncope ensues. Unconsciousness may also reflect postoverdrive suppression of the slower rates. Satisfactory treatment of permanent heart block or the Stokes-Adams syndrome usually requires insertion of a permanent artificial pacemaker.[20]

Episodic or intermittent heart block occurs in two modes. In the first form, termed Mobitz type I, the block is progressive, and the electrocardiogram shows a prolonged PR time with regularly dropped beats, the Wenckebach phenomenon. In the second type, or Mobitz type II, the block is sudden and is not preceded by less severe conduction difficulties. The patient with type II heart block will conduct normally under ordinary circumstances. Seemingly at random, and often quite abruptly, complete heart block with syncope will develop. The block may be rate-related, and is more likely to develop when the heart rate is increased. Recognition of this form of episodic unconsciousness in the elderly patient may be very difficult. The history may be vague. The physical examination is usually not helpful unless there is associated calcific aortic or mitral valve disease. Scrutiny of the electrocardiogram for diagnostic clues, such as left axis deviation or bundle branch block, or long-term monitoring of the heart rate and rhythm may be necessary to establish the diagnosis. In general, treatment requires the insertion of a permanent pacemaker into the ventricle.

Techniques have recently become available which permit recording of electrograms directly from the bundle of His in the intact human heart.[7] Data obtained with this technique suggest that type I block is associated with conduction defects in the A-V node and type II block is caused by lesions distal to the bundle of His, presumably bilateral bundle branch block.

The conducting system of the ventricles consists of the main bundle of His, which arises in the atrium at the atrioventricular node and penetrates the fibrous skeleton of the heart. The main bundle then divides into the left and right main branches. The left bundle branch further divides into two fascicles: a septal or anterior, and a parietal or posterior, trunk. Knowledge of the anatomy of the system is important, since it is now recognized that blockage of the right branch and one of the two rami of the left branch may give rise to a characteristic electrocardiographic pattern. Furthermore, many instances of complete heart block are probably caused by bilateral bundle branch block rather than blocks in the main bundle.[22] Often the electrocardiogram has shown conduction disturbances for many years prior to the development of complete block. Thus, the patient with blockage of two of the three main branches of the bundles is a candidate for sudden heart block and syncope should the remaining branch, the only one carrying impulses from atrium to ventricle, be damaged or cease to function. Recognition of an electrocardiogram suggesting involvement of the right bundle with a portion of the left in a patient with a history of episodic unconsciousness represents an important step in initiating proper therapy.

Case 8

A 59-year-old man suffered two "blackout" spells within a week. Both occurred without warning when he was walking in his apartment. He fell suddenly to the floor and was unconscious for several minutes. Physical examination was within normal limits. An electrocardiogram showed marked left axis deviation and right bundle branch block. Prolonged oscillographic monitoring eventually revealed an episode of complete heart block which lasted no more than a few seconds and did not cause unconsciousness. It was assumed that the "blackouts" represented intermittent bilateral bundle branch block, and a permanent pacemaker was inserted into the right ventricle.

TACHYCARDIA

Syncope may be caused by intermittent and self-limited episodes of ventricular tachycardia or ventricular fibrillation. Recurrent bouts of these arrhythmias with spontaneous recovery have been reported in persons with otherwise apparently "normal" hearts. Most often, however, such rhythms are associated with organic heart disease. Ventricular fibrillation and tachycardia are frequent and dangerous complications of acute myocardial infarction, and may cause clinical cardiac arrest. Unless resuscitative efforts are initiated promptly and effective circulation is maintained, brain death will quickly ensue.

VAGAL REFLEX BRADYCARDIA

Vagal reflex bradycardia or cardiac arrest can produce syncope in the absence of heart disease. The stimulus for this response can arise from a number of organs, the afferent innervation of which may be vagal, trigeminal, glossopharyngeal, or spinal. Presumably emotional reactions can also induce the response, although this is difficult to document. Probably this is a hyperactive vagal reflex in most cases, but Gastaut and Fischer-Williams[13] were able to produce at least transient cardiac arrest by ocular compression in 71 of 100 patients with a history of syncope, suggesting that many patients with recurrent syncope have some degree of autonomic instability and vagal overresponsiveness. Some patients respond to vagal stimulation with hypotension without bradycardia, and this too may induce syncope. Vagal reflex syncope can be produced by many different stimuli, including ocular compression, esophageal dilation, esophageal spasm from drinking carbonated beverages, and distension of the rectum or vagina. A common factor in these phenomena would seem to be visceral pain. Atropine is often effective in preventing vagal reflex syncope.

CAROTID SINUS SYNDROME

Carotid sinus syncope is just as rare as the other forms of vagal reflex syncope. The vasodepressor and cardioinhibitory reflexes evoked by massaging the carotid sinus were first described by Hering more than 100 years ago. Weiss and Baker[33] described two forms of carotid sinus syncope, one involving primarily bradycardia and a second due to systemic hypotension and vasodilation. The carotid sinus is a component of a neurogenic control system, mediated through the vagus, which regulates cardiac performance.[33] Stretch receptors located in the wall of the carotid artery, when stimulated by increased arterial pressure, initiate a withdrawal of sympathetic impulses to the peripheral circulatory tree, resulting in vasodilation and hypotension. The vagal discharge also slows the sinus node. In addition, varying degrees of heart block may be mediated by the vagal influence on the A-V node.

Individual sensitivity to carotid sinus stimulation varies. An occasional individual is extraordinarily responsive and develops bradycardia and unconsciousness with minimal stimulation of the sinus area. If and when loss of consciousness occurs, it is induced by pressure at the carotid bifurcation, which may be as mild as the squeeze of a tight collar or as vigorous as strong massage. The diagnosis is uncertain unless asystole and syncope can be reproduced by a degree of carotid sinus pressure that is consistent with the circumstances in which the patient has had previous symptoms. Any more vigorous compression runs the risk of decreasing carotid blood flow and does not prove the existence of carotid sinus syncope. In any patient who loses consciousness with carotid massage, but does not develop asystole, one must suspect that the other carotid is thrombosed and that the massage merely interrupts the remaining internal carotid artery circulation.

Systemic Disorders Impairing Cerebral Metabolism

Hypoxia

An otherwise healthy man requires a severe degree of hypoxia to cause a failure of brain metabolism and loss of consciousness. Under normal conditions the brain extracts 6.6 cc of O_2 from each 100 ml of blood circulating through it to maintain its metabolic rate. As the oxygen concentration of the inspired air decreases, cerebral vasodilation occurs and cerebral blood flow increases, so that a normal rate of oxygen delivery is maintained. In one study, for example, subjects breathing 8 per cent oxygen increased their cerebral blood flow by 36 per cent to maintain a normal rate of cerebral oxygen consumption.[32] Humans maintain consciousness until jugular venous blood PO_2 decreases to below 20 mm Hg (normal, 34 mm). At this level brain tissue PO_2 is about 4 mm Hg, and enzymatic reactions lose efficiency.[31] Given a normal hemoglobin concentration, these conditions correspond to an arterial PO_2 of about 35 mm Hg, an uncommon degree of hypoxia, but one that rapidly produces unconsciousness. On rapid decompression to an altitude of 38,000 feet ($PO_2 < 30$ mm Hg), subjects lose consciousness within 10 to 15 seconds.[12]

Anemia

The effects of anemia on neurologic function are variable, and depend on the degree of anemia, its chronicity, and the extent of associated vascular disease. Patients with chronic anemia can increase the cerebral blood flow 30 per cent or more to maintain adequate brain metabolism. Theoretically, it should be possible to maintain consciousness with a hemoglobin concentration of 3.5 g/100 ml, and we have studied a young woman with this degree of anemia who was alert and could conduct a reasonable conversation.

Despite this theoretical and occasional tolerance of profound anemia, less extreme conditions of anemia or hypoxia endanger brain function when other factors, such as hypotension or arterial stenosis, are added. Fainting and transient blindness are among the dangers of sudden bleeding, and hematocrit levels below 12 to 16 per cent subject the patient to grave risks of neurologic damage. We have cared for three patients with hematocrit levels between 12 and 20 per cent who developed cerebral infarction and died while awaiting completion of diagnostic studies of the anemia. Transfusion rarely, if ever, interferes with one's ability to diagnose the cause of anemia, and should never be withheld in older patients when the hematocrit falls below 20 per cent, and probably in any patient whose hematocrit falls below 15 per cent.

Hypoglycemia

Loss of consciousness from hypoglycemia usually occurs when the blood sugar falls to 20 to 30 mg/100 ml. At this level cerebral oxygen uptake decreases and the electroencephalogram contains diffuse slow wave activity.

The symptoms of hypoglycemia follow no uniform pattern, and there is no orderly course of neurologic events as cerebral glucose deprivation progresses. The physiologic principles of unconsciousness discussed earlier require that there be metabolic failure either diffusely through the cerebral cortex or within the brain stem activating system. Patients with hypoglycemia exhibit the clinical symptoms of either of these patterns. Some patients have changes primarily in mental function, with delirium, quiet confusion, or agitation. Others rapidly become comatose and have signs of multifocal brain stem dysfunction, such as decerebrate spasms, central neurogenic hyperventilation, and hypothermia; the pupillary light reflex usually remains intact, which helps to differentiate this metabolic brain stem disorder from a destructive one. Hypoglycemia sometimes presents as a focal neurologic disorder closely resembling a hemispheral stroke or as a generalized convulsion with postictal coma. It is important to recall this possibility when faced with a convulsing patient not known to be epileptic. Blood should be drawn for glucose determination and intravenous glucose injected immediately without waiting for the laboratory result.

Subsequent attacks of hypoglycemia need not take the same form as previous ones. With recurrent attacks a patient may experience a variety of these syndromes, and the focal neurologic signs may shift from side to side.

Recovery from hypoglycemia is usually prompt after glucose injection or ingestion, but is sometimes delayed. Normal brain function may not return immediately, even though blood sugar levels are restored, suggesting that glucose deprivation has caused temporary or permanent neuronal damage.

Any unconscious hypoglycemic patient runs a strong risk of permanent brain damage, a risk which accumulates with each recurrence. The gradual and subtle loss of intellect that follows repeated hypoglycemia further increases the likelihood of improper insulin regulation. Episodic unconsciousness in diabetics should alert the physician to this possibility and to the tragic potentials of recurrent hypoglycemia.

Cerebral Arterial Occlusion

Independently of systemic hypotension or failure of cardiac output, cerebral blood flow can be impaired by occlusion, constriction, or stenosis of the carotid, vertebral-basilar, or cerebral artery systems. It is unusual for local arterial obstruction to cause ischemia of the whole brain. Selective brain stem ischemia is a more common cause of episodic unconsciousness.

Basilar Artery Insufficiency

This produces transient attacks of brain stem ischemia.[3] Loss of consciousness is a prominent symptom. Episodes of unconsciousness may recur along with or independent of other focal brain stem symptoms, such as weakness, sensory loss, visual blurring, diplopia, and vertigo. Each episode may be different, and it is this variety of cranial nerve and shifting motor and sensory symptoms that leads to the diagnosis in patients with arteriosclerotic or hypertensive vascular disease. One pattern of basilar vertebral insufficiency is the drop attack, which results from ischemia of the long motor tracts but not of the reticular area supporting consciousness. The patient suddenly falls and may appear to have a "blackout," but gets up quickly and can usually recall that he did not lose consciousness. Recovery from transient brain stem ischemia can sometimes be rapid and complete, but is often slow, with confusion and dullness persisting for several hours.[35]

The precipitating cause of transient ischemic attacks cannot always be determined. Presumably there is a partial obstruction, such as an arteriosclerotic plaque within the artery involved, but some dynamic circulatory change must be added to produce the transient episode. Anemia, polycythemia, nicotine-induced vasoconstriction, transient drops in cardiac output, and changes in blood pressure are among the factors which have been implicated. Some transient ischemic attacks may be caused by small emboli breaking off from atheromatous plaques or from a thrombus formed on a plaque. The episodes can occur with the patient lying down as well as standing, an important difference from syncope. Head and neck position may be important. The vertebral artery, as it pursues its tortuous course through the cervical spine, runs a special risk of being compressed by osteoarthritic spurs. One of our patients, an elderly man, sat among the front rows of his church congregation close to the elevated pulpit, a position which represented a certain status in his community but also required considerable extension of his neck as he attended to the preacher. As a result he had repeated episodes of unconsciousness. Cerebral arteriography demonstrated that the vertebral arteries were being compressed by osteoarthritic spurs when the neck was extended.

Carotid Artery Insufficiency

Carotid artery insufficiency does not cause transient loss of consciousness unless there is so much obstruction to flow in other neck vessels that a decrease in flow through one carotid causes ischemia in both cerebral hemispheres or the upper brain stem.

Spasm of Cerebral Arteries

Spasm of cerebral arteries, often under unusual circumstances, may lead to temporary unconsciousness. Irritation or inflammation of the circle of

Willis can occur with bacterial meningitis or with the chemical meningitis of subarachnoid hemorrhage. This leads to arterial spasm and to diffuse brain ischemia. One of the effects of the hypocapnia of overbreathing is cerebral vasospasm and ischemia, even to the point of unconsciousness. Severe arterial hypertension produces cerebral vasospasm, and loss of consciousness sometimes accompanies the headache and other symptoms of hypertensive encephalopathy.

Basilar Migraine

Impairment of consciousness in basilar migraine has been described by Bickerstaff.[3] All the patients were adolescent girls with a family history of migraine. Loss of consciousness was never abrupt and never profound. It was often preceded by a dreamlike state, visual scotomata, ataxia, and vertigo and followed by severe headache. The neurologic symptoms of migraine are thought to result from transient spasm of intracranial arteries.

Subarachnoid Hemorrhage

Displacement or stretching of the arteries at the base of the brain or stimulation of the medial aspect of the temporal lobe readily produces changes in heart rate and blood pressure, and ECG signs of "myocardial ischemia" are common in patients with subarachnoid hemorrhage. The following case dramatically illustrates these relationships in a patient with recurrent loss of consciousness.

Case 9

A 44-year-old construction worker arrived at the New York Hospital emergency room at 11 a.m. complaining of having blacked out $\frac{1}{2}$ hour earlier. During the preceding year the patient had complained of occasional frontal-occipital headaches. Four months prior to admission he felt dizzy and lost consciousness briefly. Three days prior to admission he felt transiently weak and dizzy as if he would faint, but he had no pain. On the day of admission he felt "exceptionally well." At work he was climbing stairs and suddenly fell, unconscious. Within 2 minutes he was awake and complained of severe generalized headache. He arrived at the emergency room feeling well with a pulse of 76/minute and a blood pressure of 108/76 mm Hg. At 11:30 a.m. he complained of progressing headache and lost consciousness. An ECG recorded complete A-V dissociation with a nodal rhythm at a rate of 52/minute. At 12:05 p.m. he was awake with a blood pressure of 180/90 mm Hg. The ECG recorded normal sinus rhythm with ST elevation and T-wave inversion suggesting early myocardial infarction or ischemia. By 12:15 p.m. he lost consciousness again, with a blood pressure of 160/100 mm Hg. The ECG recorded normal sinus rhythm, changing in minutes to complete A-V dissociation with a rate of 50/minute, then to ventricular tachycardia, followed by supraventricular tachycardia as the blood pressure rose to 250/180 mm Hg. The cerebrospinal fluid was grossly bloody. He remained unconscious and died the next morning. Dissection of the brain at autopsy disclosed a saccular aneurysm of the right posterior communicating artery which had ruptured into the subarachnoid space and the adjacent medial temporal lobe. There were no abnormalities in the myocardium or the cardiac interventricular septum.

Primary Neurologic Disorders

Epilepsy[27]

A seizure, in order to produce unconsciousness, must be either generalized or confined to the upper brain stem (diencephalon). Focal cerebral seizures do not disturb consciousness unless they spread to become generalized. It is not difficult to recognize typical grand mal and petit mal seizures, nor should they be difficult to differentiate from syncope if the facts of the event are clear. Both are generalized seizures, originate in the upper brain stem, and show no focal components.

GRAND MAL SEIZURES

There is no stereotyped aura or introductory symptom to the generalized seizure. The primary event is sudden loss of consciousness. Grand mal (or generalized major motor) seizures are characterized by loss of consciousness along with loss of postural tone, followed by tonic then clonic convulsive movements. After the movement has ceased the patient only slowly regains full consciousness; he commonly is confused, complains of headache, and falls asleep.

PETIT MAL EPILEPSY

Petit mal epilepsy is a disease of children and never begins in adults, although it may persist into adult life from childhood. The clinical event is a sudden loss of consciousness that lasts a few seconds, without loss of postural tone. It may be accompanied by slight 3/second picking, chewing, or blinking movements. The child is usually unaware that anything has happened, but may be confused for a few seconds postictally. An electroencephalogram taken during a seizure and often between seizures shows regular 3/second spike wave activity. Petit mal attacks or the electroencephalographic abnormality can frequently be precipitated by 1 or 2 minutes of hyperventilation.

DRUG WITHDRAWAL SEIZURES

A generalized seizure occurring in a person without a history of previous seizures may be the initial sign of drug withdrawal. This is especially apt to occur in an alcoholic or hypnotic drug addict who is hospitalized for another illness, and thus abruptly deprived of his usual drug. Seizures are not a part of the opiate withdrawal syndrome. Alcohol withdrawal seizures, or "rum fits," occur within 48 hours after alcohol is stopped or reduced, often preceding the more easily recognized symptoms of delirium tremens. Complete abstinence is not required, a reduction in the usual level of intake being sufficient. Dependence on hypnotic drugs may develop with as little as three or four hypnotic doses daily, a level ingested chronically by many anxious or insomniac patients. The usual drugs involved are the barbiturates, meprobamate, glutethimide, and chloral hydrate; recently glutethimide has been particularly apt to be associated with withdrawal seizures. Isbell points out that when five or six hypnotic doses of any of these drugs are taken daily, 50 per cent of the patients convulse on withdrawal.[17] Withdrawal from either alcohol or hypnotics may be a life-threatening illness, and should be treated as a medical emergency with temporary resumption of hypnotic or sedative drugs, which can then be tapered off.

FOCAL SEIZURES

The focal seizure is one that begins as an electrical disturbance in a specific area of cerebral cortex rather than in the brain stem. It is important to recognize focal seizures and to distinguish them from generalized or "centrencephalic" seizures. A focal seizure always implies a structural brain lesion (tumor, infarct, scar), which requires a vigorous diagnostic search. The patient will lose consciousness only if the focal discharge spreads to produce a generalized seizure. Unfortunately, some focal seizures become generalized so rapidly that neither the patient nor an untrained observer notes the signs of focal onset. A careful history must be obtained, with special reference to any cortically localizable symptoms preceding unconsciousness—for example, twitching or tingling of a foot, a thumb, or a corner of the mouth. Postictal weakness of the face or an extremity is also evidence of focal origin of a seizure.

TEMPORAL LOBE OR PSYCHOMOTOR EPILEPSY

This is a focal seizure disorder which causes an alteration in consciousness or behavior, but does not initially cause complete loss of consciousness. The patient may be unaware of what he is doing, and term the event a "blackout." To an observer, however, he is awake but has lost some degree of contact with his environment. His actions may be repetitive or bizarre. He may become violent or wander until he is lost. More commonly, however, the event is less dramatic, and is announced by an aura, often a feeling of fullness in the chest or throat, a sense of something about to happen, a feeling of detachment or unreality, of drifting away. This is often a frightening experience. Distortions of visual or auditory perceptions and olfactory or gustatory hallucinations accompanying a lapse of awareness are strong evidence for temporal lobe epilepsy. Temporal lobe seizures, of course, are focal cerebral attacks and must be investigated as such.

The differentiation of syncope from epilepsy is often difficult. A description of the situation and the initial events of the attack is most valuable. Patients are often amnesic for the events preceding and during a seizure, but can recall in at least foggy detail the events preceding syncope. Both syncope and seizures often occur in a general setting of stress or fatigue, but an epileptic attack, unlike syncope, is rarely precipitated by a specific emotional or physiologic stress.

The recollection of warning symptoms of weakness, nausea, sweating, and light-headedness supports the diagnosis of syncope. The patient turns pale, his pulse becomes weak and slow, and he falls to the ground. Almost immediately he begins to recover, and his recovery is rapid, without lingering confusion. If he stands up quickly he may faint again. Warnings are unusual before generalized seizures, and the initial symptoms of psychomotor seizures tend to be some of the specific sensations already mentioned. During a seizure the patient is more likely to appear plethoric or cyanotic than pale. Recovery is delayed by a period of bewilderment and confusion. Neither the onset nor recovery from seizures is related to posture; epilepsy may continue or even begin with the patient horizontal. Incontinence, tongue biting, and glassy stares occur with severe syncope as well as with seizures and do not differentiate the two.

When syncope is associated with profound cerebral anoxia it can produce a seizure. This usually consists of only a tonic spasm or a few twitches, but readily progresses to a generalized convulsive seizure if the anoxia is prolonged. It should be remembered that anoxia was the means Robert Boyle used to produce the first experimental epilepsy.

At times it is impossible to distinguish on the basis of clinical evidence alone between syncope and seizures. Kershman[18] proposed the term "cerebral syncopal seizures" to include the patient with loss of consciousness who has an abnormal electroencephalogram and a history of vasomotor instability, nervousness, dizziness, and anxiety. Here lies the borderland between faints and fits.

The electroencephalogram is only occasionally useful in determining the cause of episodic unconsciousness. A normal EEG can be reassuring, but it does not rule out epilepsy or cerebrovascular disease when the history suggests one of these disorders. If, by rare chance, an EEG can be recorded during the episode of unconsciousness, syncope can be differentiated clearly from a seizure. As syncopal symptoms begin, the EEG shows bilaterally synchronous slow waves without spike discharges, and if unconsciousness persists, as in cardiac arrest, the EEG becomes flat. The EEG pattern usually returns to normal along with clinical recovery. Seizures are accompanied by high-voltage, sharp wave or spike activity, which is usually followed by diffuse slowing during the postictal period. During hysterical unresponsiveness the EEG will be normal or show excessive muscle tension artifact. The interictal record in a patient with epilepsy is often normal, but repeated records during light sleep and with hyperventilation increase the yield of abnormality. The discovery of paroxysmal abnormalities over the inferior frontal or temporal lobe areas helps to distinguish patients with psychomotor seizures from those with syncope or hysterical "fainting." However, patients with vasomotor instability and clinical syncope may have diffuse disturbances of the electroencephalographic rhythm.

Mechanical Disturbances of Brain Function

TRAUMA

Episodic unconsciousness can be caused by trauma to the brain even though there is no gross anatomic disruption of brain tissue. Cerebral concussion, by definition, is associated with no structural damage, but is a frequent cause of unconsciousness. The history of a blow to the head is usually obtained, but retrograde amnesia, another characteristic result of cerebral trauma, may obscure the patient's recall of the injury.

ACUTE CEREBRAL VENTRICULAR OBSTRUCTION

In this situation what might be considered an internal concussion occurs, with a transient severe increase in intraventricular pressure. Transient occlusion of the aqueduct of Sylvius can be caused by a posterior fossa tumor or by decompensation of a developmental abnormality of the aqueduct. These are uncommon events, and more typical than sudden loss of consciousness would be paroxysmal headaches or a gradual progression of mental dullness. A pedunculated tumor or cyst of the third ventricle can suddenly obstruct the foramina of Monro and produce acute dilation of the lateral ventricles. This may occur when the patient puts his head forward, and is associated with sudden headache and loss of consciousness which clears rapidly if the tumor falls back into its nonobstructing position.

DEVELOPMENTAL ABNORMALITIES

Certain developmental abnormalities of the posterior fossa make the lower brain stem more vulnerable to external trauma. Illingworth[16] reported a child who would suddenly lose consciousness when trying to reach something above her head, and another who had repeated episodes of unconsciousness from the age of 7 to 8 months onward whenever he was struck on the back of the head. Both children had abnormal fusion of the cervical vertebrae (Klippel-Feil syndrome), and it was presumed that the medulla oblongata was being compressed at the foramen magnum.

Other Episodes of Unconsciousness

Narcolepsy

Sleep is both clinically and physiologically different from unconsciousness. The recurrent somnolence of narcolepsy is not, strictly speaking, a form of episodic unconsciousness. The narcoleptic patient usually complains not of fainting, but of feeling abnormally sleepy, and he can be aroused easily. Its relationship to strong emotion, however, gives the narcoleptic syndrome a place in the differential diagnosis of episodic unconsciousness. Emotional excitement (great laughter, joy, or fear) may induce a sudden loss of postural tone known as cataplexy. Usually the patient with cataplexy has been laughing or is frightened or angry, when his legs suddenly give way and he falls to the ground without losing consciousness. He may appear to be fainting, but on careful questioning it is revealed that he has not actually lost consciousness.

Post-traumatic Syndrome

The post-traumatic syndrome which occurs in the weeks or months following a head injury often includes attacks of loss or near loss of consciousness. Patients report recurrent "blackouts," dizziness, or giddiness, and it is often difficult to define these events as either syncope or vertigo. Emotional instability, headache, poor concentration, depression, and lack of energy are other features of the syndrome. It may be attractive to ascribe all this to neurosis or to the wish for compensation, but many neurologists note the remarkable consistency of the symptoms, and suspect that the condition has a structural mechanism even though the pathophysiology is unclear. The symptoms often respond to reassurance and supportive care. Vague dizziness is a more common complaint than actual unconsciousness, but the latter does occur and may be difficult to distinguish from post-traumatic epilepsy. If the attacks persist, anticonvulsant drugs may be used as a diagnostic therapeutic trial, but always with the expressed expectation that the symptoms will eventually subside.

Ménière's Disease

Some patients lose consciousness with attacks of vertigo in Ménière's disease. The mechanism may be a vasodepressor response to the intense vertigo, but the association is not common and warrants careful consideration of brain stem disease, especially in older persons potentially susceptible to basilar artery insufficiency.

Hysterical Fainting

In order to achieve its goal of psychological gain, hysterical fainting must occur in a dramatic setting with an appropriate audience. The subject swoons without pallor or change in pulse rate, and either lies motionless or becomes involved in some form of thrashing about or more purposeful movement. Consciousness is not regained as soon as the patient becomes horizontal, as it is in most types of syncope. Among the diagnostic criteria of hysterical faints should be consistent abnormalities of previous behavior or personality. Hysteria is essentially a disorder of youth, and unless financial compensation is involved, "hysterical" symptoms almost never begin for the first time in patients over 20 to 25 years old. The diagnosis of hysterical fainting in the middle-aged or elderly is risky at best and, if made, should be based on only very firm evidence of previous hysterical symptoms and with the clear exclusion of organic disease. Caloric stimulation of the vestibular system during hysterical unconsciousness demonstrates nystagmus, with the fast phase away from the ear being stimulated. The test is performed by first ensuring that the ear drum is intact and that the external auditory canal is free of obstruction, then elevating the head 30° from horizontal and irrigating the canal with 30 cc of ice water. Tonic eye deviation without the rapid component of nystagmus indicates true cerebral depression. Absence of any ocular response to caloric stimulation usually indicates structural damage or profound metabolic depression of the brain stem.

CONCLUSION

This chapter has outlined the basic requirements for the maintenance of consciousness, described a variety of syndromes that can present with episodic loss of consciousness, and classified these syndromes into primarily cardiovascular and neurologic disorders. Such a classification is to some degree arbitrary, since unconsciousness is itself a neurologic disorder and implies a disturbance of brain function. The importance of searching for the basic cause of unconsciousness is to minimize the risk of its recurrence and consequent permanent brain injury, for the preservation of cerebral function is in large measure the ultimate goal of all medical diagnosis and treatment.

REFERENCES

1. Barroclough, M. A., and Sharpey-Schafer, E. P. Hypotension from absent circulatory reflexes: effects of alcohol, barbiturates, psychotherapeutic drugs and other mechanisms. Lancet 1:1121, 1963.
2. Bickelmann, A. G., Lippschutz, E. J., and Brunjes, C. F. Hemodynamics of orthostatic hypotension. Amer. J. Med. 30:26, 1961.
3. Bickerstaff, E. R. Impairment of consciousness in migraine. Lancet 2:1057, 1961.
4. Birchfield, R. I. Postural hypotension in Wernicke's disease. Amer. J. Med. 36: 404, 1964.
5. Braunwald, E., Lambrew, C. T., Rockoff, S. D., Ross, J., Jr., Morrow, A. G., and Pierce, G. E. Idiopathic hypertrophic subaortic stenosis. Circulation 30 (Suppl. IV): 63, 1964.
6. Chosy, J. J., and Graham, D. T. Catecholamines in vasovagal fainting. J. Psychosom. Res. 9:189, 1965.
7. Damato, A. N., Lau, S. H., Helfant, R., Stein, E., Patton, R. D., Scherlag, B. J., and Berkowitz, W. D. A study of heart block in man using His bundle recordings. Circulation 39:297, 1969.
8. Diamond, M. A., Murray, R. H., and Schmid, P. G. Idiopathic postural hypotension: physiologic observations and report of a new mode of therapy. J. Clin. Invest. 49:1341, 1970.
9. Ebert, R. V. Syncope. Circulation 27:1148, 1963.
10. Ebert, R. V., Stead, E. A., and Gibson, J. G. Response of normal subjects to acute blood loss. Arch. Internal Med. 68:578, 1941.
11. Engel, G. L. Fainting, p. 11. Charles C Thomas, Springfield, Ill., 1962.
12. Ernsting, J. Some effects of brief profound anoxia upon the central nervous system. In Selective Vulnerability of the Brain in Hypoxemia, Schade, J. P., and McMenemey, W. H., Ed., p. 41. F. A. Davis Co., Philadelphia, 1963.
13. Gastaut, H., and Fischer-Williams, M. Electroencephalographic study of syncope. Its differentiation from epilepsy. Lancet 2:1018, 1957.
14. Gorham, L. W. A study of pulmonary embolism. Arch. Internal. Med. 108:189, 1961.
15. Hohl, R. D., Frame, B., and Schatz, I. J. The Shy-Drager variant of idiopathic orthostatic hypotension. Amer. J. Med. 39:134, 1965.
16. Illingworth, R. S. Attacks of unconsciousness in association with fused cervical vertebrae. Arch. Dis. Child. 31:8, 1956.
17. Isbell, H. Drug dependence (addiction). In Cecil-Loeb Textbook of Medicine, Beeson, P. B., and McDermott, W., Eds., p. 1499. W. B. Saunders Co., Philadelphia, 1967.
18. Kershman, J. Syncope and seizures. J. Neurol. Neurosurg. Psychiat. 12:25, 1949.
19. Klein, L. J., Saltzman, H. A., Heyman, A., and Sieker, H. O. Syncope induced by

the Valsalva maneuver. A study of the effects of arterial blood gas tensions, glucose concentration and blood pressure. Amer. J. Med. 37:263, 1964.

20. Landegren, J., and Biorck, G. The clinical assessment and treatment of complete heart block and Adams-Stokes attacks. Medicine 42:171, 1963.

21. Lassen, N. A. Cerebral blood flow and oxygen consumption in man. Physiol. Rev. 39:183, 1959.

22. Lepeschkin, E.: Electrocardiographic diagnosis of bilateral bundle branch block in relation to heart block. Progr. Cardiovasc. Dis. 6:445, 1964.

23. Marshall, R. J., and Shepherd, J. T. *Cardiac Function in Health and Disease*, p. 409. W. B. Saunders Co., Philadelphia, 1968.

24. McIntosh, H. D., Estes, E. H., and Warren, J. V. The mechanisms of cough syncope. Amer. Heart J. 52:70, 1956.

25. Morrow, A. G., Roberts, W. C., Ross, J., Jr., Fisher, R. D., Behrendt, D. M., Mason, D. T., and Braunwald, E. Obstruction of left ventricular outflow. Ann. Internal Med. 69:1255, 1968.

26. Rushmer, R. F. *Cardiovascular Dynamics*, 3rd ed., p. 559. W. B. Saunders Co., Philadelphia, 1970.

27. Schmidt, R. P., and Wilder, B. J. *Epilepsy*. F. A. Davis Co., Philadelphia, 1968.

28. Schneider, M. Critical blood pressure in the cerebral circulation. In *Selective Vulnerability of the Brain in Hypoxemia*, Schade, J. P., and McMenemey, W. H., Eds., p. 7. F. A. Davis Co., Philadelphia, 1963.

29. Sokoloff, L. Metabolism of the central nervous system in vivo. In *Handbook of Physiology*. Sect. I: *Neurophysiology*, Filed, J., Magoun, H. W., and Hall, V. E., Eds., Vol. 3, Chap. 77. American Physiological Society, Washington, D. C., 1960.

30. Stead, E. A. Fainting. Amer J. Med. 13:387 1952

31. Thews, G. Implications to physiology and pathology of oxygen diffusion at the capillary level. In *Selective Vulnerability of the Brain in Hypoxemia*, Schade, J. P., and McMenemey, W. H., Eds., p. 27. F. A. Davis Co., Philadelphia, 1963.

32. Turner, J., Lambertsen, C. J., Owen, S. G., Wendel, H., and Chiodi, H. Effects of .08 and .8 atmospheres of inspired PO_2 upon cerebral hemodynamics at a "constant" alveolar PCO_2 of 43 mm Hg. Fed. Proc. 16:130, 1957.

33. Weiss, S., and Baker, J. P. The carotid sinus reflex in health and disease: its role in the causation of fainting and convulsions. Medicine 12:297, 1933.

34. Weissler, A. M., Warren, J. V., Estes, E. H., McIntosh, H. D., and Leonard, J. J. Vasodepressor syncope. Factors influencing cardiac output. Circulation 15:875, 1957.

35. Williams, D., and Wilson, T. G. The diagnosis of the major and minor syndromes of basilar insufficiency. Brain 85:741, 1962.

Chronic and Recurrent Diarrhea

THOMAS P. ALMY

Though the lower intestines are not essential to life, their malfunctioning in the form of protracted diarrhea leads some unfortunates to their deaths, and produces in others a formidable yet ignoble disability. Discriminating among the many possible causes for this phenomenon is a challenging task for the physician. They are indeed so numerous, and some so rare, that even the most mature clinician cannot depend on experience alone as a diagnostic guide. Though much remains to be learned about the mechanisms of diarrhea, the efforts of many able investigators in the last 20 years now permit an approach to the problem which is at least partly rational.

While the clinician at the bedside, prior to extensive laboratory procedures, often fails to make an exact etiologic diagnosis, he can frequently formulate in terms of pathophysiology the general bodily mechanism at work. This is a useful intermediate step, as it serves to direct the diagnostic studies toward a well-conceived goal. There follows an outline of recognized mechanisms, which the author has found can be carried in his head. A more formal clinicopathologic classification of diarrheas is offered in Table 10, for reference purposes. It is clear that there is no one-to-one relationship between mechanisms and pathologic entities—for example, a wide variety of diseases seem to produce diarrhea by allowing bacterial overgrowth in the small bowel; yet one or more of three mechanisms may be involved in the diarrhea of patients with a non-β-islet cell tumor of the pancreas.

DEFINITION

Everyone with a sixth-grade education knows what diarrhea is; yet it signifies different things to different patients. The physician's first task is to be sure what *his* patient means by this complaint. He may mean that his stools are overly large, loose, or excessively frequent; that he has a frequent urge to defecate, whatever the result; or that he cannot keep from soiling himself. In the diagnostic schema developed here, the short-lived diarrhea of acute infections will be excluded, except in explanation of mechanisms, and the special problems of infantile diarrhea will not be discussed.

THOMAS P. ALMY, M.D. Nathan Smith Professor and Chairman, Department of Medicine, Dartmouth Medical School, and Director of Medicine, Dartmouth-Hitchcock Affiliated Hospitals, Hanover, New Hampshire

MECHANISMS

Normal Fluid Exchanges; Normal Motility

The passage of 0.5 to 3 stools/day, with 24-hour output averaging about 150 g, is the composite result of a large number of processes, disturbance of which may give rise to diarrhea. The volume and the physical and chemical characteristics of ingested food and fluid, the quantity of digestive juices, their admixture with the ingesta, the absorption of nutrients, and the motility of the intestines all have an influence on stool size and frequency. The average stool consists of only about one-third unabsorbed food, the remainder being made up of cast-off intestinal epithelial cells, microbes, and partially dried secretions. The continued passage of stools in patients on a clear liquid diet, or even in short periods of fasting, is thus not surprising.

Although it has long been known that 8 to 9 liters of fluid enter the intestine daily in the bile and in gastric and pancreatic juice, and that this water is subtotally reabsorbed in the lower bowel,[7] only recently has the dynamic character of fluid and electrolyte exchanges at all levels of the intestine been recognized.[12] Using isolated *in vivo* loops of intestine and isotopically labeled water and electrolytes, various investigators have been able to show that normal traffic across the intestinal mucosa is two-way and rapid.[9, 10, 38] Even in areas where net absorption of water is most rapid, *influx* into the body fluids (insorption) is partially counterbalanced by *efflux* into the intestinal lumen (exsorption, or secretion). Similar opposing fluxes exist for the major electrolytes, the result of simple diffusion down gradients of concentration or electrical charge, facilitated diffusion, or energy-dependent active transport mechanisms such as the sodium pump. Though most of the luminal water and electrolyte is recovered in the small bowel, the process continues in the colon,[24] which shares with the renal tubules the role of conservation of body water and sodium, responding in similar fashion to aldosterone and to antidiuretic hormone. In addition, potassium and bicarbonate are actively secreted, in concentrations several times higher than those in extracellular fluid. Nevertheless, the total osmolality of luminal contents is maintained throughout at about the same level as in plasma.

Normal motility throughout the bowel may be summarized as the purposeful alternation of propulsive and nonpropulsive patterns. Specialized segments having relatively high levels of intraluminal pressure in the resting state (sphincter zones) are recognized at the pylorus, the ileocecal junction, and the anus, and a similar function is served by the sigmoid colon. Pressure at each of these points is controlled by local reflexes, rising when the bowel wall below the sphincter is tensed, and falling when contraction or distension occurs just above.[22] Thus, all segments of the gut except the stomach are normally protected from great distension, and time for digestion and absorption is assured. In the colon in particular, nonpropulsive motility, conducive to water absorption, predominates throughout the day except following meals, when "mass peristalsis" establishes an aboral gradient which fills the rectum and initiates the signal for defecation.

Mechanisms of Diarrhea

Diarrhea may be due to accumulation of excessive fluid volume within the gut, or to primary increase of propulsive motility.

Excessive Volume

Excessive volume, distending the gut wall at some point and initiating strong propulsive movement, is the common feature in most cases of diarrhea. Its mechanisms, however, are diverse.

EXCESSIVE WATER INTAKE

Excessive intake of water is never the sole cause, but is a controllable factor in many complex disorders.

ABRUPT ENTRY

Abrupt entry into any segment of gut of a large volume of fluid is a factor in many disorders. The tap water enema is a familiar model, and the dumping syndrome,[28] the effects of ileocolic anastomoses, and spontaneous enteroenteric fistulae are other examples.

MALABSORPTION

Malabsorption of various substances, including the products of digestion, leads to accumulation in the lumen of osmotically active solutes, and thence to exsorption of a larger volume of water. (A simple model of this is the saline cathartic or mannitol in high concentration, in which insorption is essentially zero.) The diarrhea of certain postgastrectomy patients is worsened by sugar; that of sprue is related to multiple unabsorbed nutrients; that of lactase deficiency is due in part to unabsorbed lactose.

SECRETION OF FLUID

Secretion, or excessive exsorption, of large volumes of fluid into the intestine is a predominant mechanism in only a few well-recognized states. The now-classic example is cholera, in which the vibrio's exotoxin clearly stimulates exsorption in the small bowel while maintaining normal rates of insorption.[6] Villous adenoma of the colon or rectum secretes a copious fluid,[14] but much larger volumes (up to 10 to 12 liters/day) are secreted by the bowel under the stimulus of certain non-β-islet cell tumors of the pancreas unassociated with gastric hypersecretion.[32] It is probable that the diarrhea of patients with lymphangiectasia of the intestine, as well as that in certain cases of congestive heart failure and cirrhosis of the liver, is due in part to exsorption resulting from high lymphatic or venous pressure in the mucosa.

Increased Propulsive Motility

This may be due to local reflex stimulation or to generalized neural or humoral stimulation of the intestine.

PARTIAL OBSTRUCTION

Partial obstruction (localized) of the lumen of small bowel or colon leads to strong contractions above and relaxation below the lesion. This may initiate a peristaltic rush, with resulting diarrhea.

INFLAMMATION

Inflammation and engorgement of the gut wall, resulting from specific or nonspecific infections (shigellosis, ulcerative colitis), cause higher pressures to arise from muscular contractions in the inflamed zone, and may thus establish an aboral gradient. Certain irritant cathartics may have similar effects.

CHEMICALS

Chemical agents which stimulate bowel movements may act systemically, as in the case of the emodin cathartics or serotonin, or locally, as do phenolphthalein, hydroxylated fatty acids (either as castor oil or as the products of bacterial degradation of ingested fat), and deconjugated bile acids.[17] The last is particularly significant in the diarrhea of the "blind loop syndrome."

AUTONOMIC STIMULATION

Patterns of autonomic stimulation, apparently integrated in the central nervous system as bodily accompaniments of emotional tension, appear to be the chief mechanism in the diarrhea of irritable colon[2] and the related dysfunction of the small bowel.

MODUS OPERANDI

The management of a patient with diarrhea may repuire many of the diagnostic and therapeutic facilities of a modern medical center, but the most important elements remain the thoroughness and resourcefulness of the internist or family physician. His most important acts will be taking the history, inspection of the stools, and formulation of key hypotheses which can be resolved sequentially by laboratory studies or therapeutic trials.

History

The history should permit early inferences regarding the *location* and general nature of the underlying process. A few accurate facts about the frequency, volume, and appearance of the stools, and a clear description of any accompanying pain, make it possible to distinguish between "large-stool diarrhea" and "small-stool diarrhea."

TABLE 17

An Etiologic Classification of Diarrhea

I. Intrinsic disease of the intestine
   A. Inflammatory
      1. Due to pathogenic bacteria and their toxins—cholera, shigellosis, *Salmonella* infections, staphylococcal food poisoning, intestinal tuberculosis, etc.
      2. Due to viral agents—ECHO, Coxsackie, lymphogranuloma venereum, etc.
      3. Due to pathogenic fungi—histoplasmosis, mucormycosis
      4. Due to protozoa—amebiasis, giardiasis, leishmaniasis
      5. Due to metazoan parasites—e.g., *Strongyloides*, *Schistosoma mansoni* or *japonicum*, *Trichuris trichiura*, *Trichinella spiralis*
      6. Nonspecific inflammatory disease, with altered immunological state and/or bacterial overgrowth
         a. Ulcerative colitis, Crohn's disease, diverticulitis, adult celiac disease, Whipple's disease
         b. Blind loop syndrome, tropical sprue, hypogammaglobulinemia
         c. Pseudomembranous enterocolitis, postantibiotic alterations in fecal flora
         d. Allergy to ingested foods or drugs; Henoch-Schoenlein purpura
   B. Neoplastic
      1. Benign tumors—adenoma, leiomyoma, lipoma; multiple polyposis of colon, Peutz-Jeghers syndrome
      2. Carcinoma, lymphoma, leiomyosarcoma, carcinoid
   C. Primary metabolic abnormality, such as lactase deficiency, cystinuria (celiac disease?)
   D. Congenital or acquired structural defects, such as diverticula of the jejunum
   E. Due to chemical agents
      1. Poisons and industrial toxins—parathion, other insecticides; mercury and arsenic; carbon tetrachloride, etc.
      2. Drugs—cathartics, colchicine, antimetabolites, sympathetic blocking agents, etc.
   F. Due to untoward effects of surgical procedures—gastrectomy, extensive resection of small bowel, ileocolostomy; blind loop formation; gastrojejunocolic fistula
II. Extrinsic disease affecting the intestine
   A. Neurogenic and adaptive disorders
      1. Psychophysiologic reaction—irritable colon; mucous colitis
      2. Tabes dorsalis; diabetic neuropathy; orthostatic hypotension
      3. Increased intracranial pressure
      4. Vagotomy
      5. Withdrawal of opiates
   B. Metabolic disorders and hormonal mechanisms
      1. Pancreatic insufficiency
      2. Non-β-islet cell adenomas of pancreas—Zollinger-Ellison syndrome, others
      3. Liver and biliary tract disease, with exclusion of bile from intestine or portal hypertension
      4. Malignant carcinoid syndrome
      5. Pellagra, porphyria
      6. Renal insufficiency
      7. Graves' disease, Addison's disease

TABLE 17—*Continued*

C. Vascular and "collagen" disorders
    1. Passive congestion of the viscera—portal vein or lymphatic obstruction, constrictive pericarditis
    2. Mesenteric arterial insufficiency
    3. Scleroderma, systemic lupus erythematosus, polyarteritis nodosa

---

"Large-Stool Diarrhea" and "Small-Stool Diarrhea." When the stools are consistently large, and movements occur not more often than 6 to 10 times daily, the underlying disorder is likely to involve the small intestine or the proximal colon. The reservoir area of the distal colon is reacting to exceptionally large volumes of fluid or to irritating intestinal contents, though its own irritability is normal. Such stools are likely to be watery, free of gross blood, and to contain undigested food particles. When pain is present it is most often cramplike, with borborygmi, and located in the periumbilical area or in the right lower quadrant (Fig. 18). These areas have been identified, by both clinical and experimental observations, as sites of pain reference from the mesenteric small intestine and the right colon.[1, 21]

In "small-stool diarrhea" some of the stools are actually smaller in volume than a normal deposition, and the frequency of defecation may at times greatly exceed six times per day. The patient may at times experience much urgency, even tenesmus, yet pass only 15 ml or so of feces, or only flatus, with a partial sense of relief. The stool is rarely liquid, but often mushy or jelly-like, dark in color, with visible mucus and rarely some blood or pus. Pain, when present, is usually aching or griping, located in the hypogastrium, the right or left lower quadrant, or the sacral region (Fig. 18), and relieved by an enema.[1, 21] All these features indicate impairment of the reservoir function of the distal colon by disease or disorder of that segment. Though this complex of symptoms best fits the designation "irritable colon," it is seen also in cancer, ulcerative colitis, and other diseases of the distal colon.

Other Characteristics of the Stool. These may be reported by the patient but must be confirmed by direct inspection, and may be valuable diagnostic clues. The watery green stool of enteric infection can often be distinguished by history from the pale tan, foamy, floating stool of steatorrhea. (It should be remembered, of course, that some nonfatty stools also float, because they hold within them pockets of gas.)

Diurnal Variations. Diurnal variations in the intensity of diarrhea may indicate the extent to which it is related to normal physiologic events. In many patients stool frequency is greatest in the morning before and after breakfast, and again after the evening meal, reflecting normal variations in colonic activity. In others the lack of these variations, particularly the awakening of the patient from sleep in order to defecate, indicates an overriding and continuous stimulus, such as an infection or a carcinoid tumor secreting serotonin. The urgent nocturnal diarrhea of diabetic

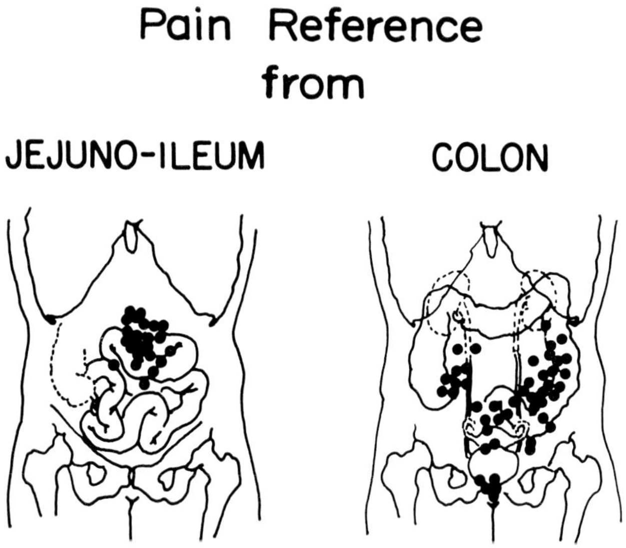

Pain Reference from

JEJUNO-ILEUM   COLON

Fig. 18. Comparison of sites of pain reference to the abdominal wall from the jejunoileum (*left*) and the colon (*right*). (Redrawn from data of Jones.[21])

neuropathy is characteristic,[29] but not wholly specific.[40] The persistence of voluminous stools for more than 12 hours after all oral intake has been stopped strongly suggests that the secretion of fluid into the gut is a dominant mechanism.

Loss of Weight. Weight loss is conspicuously absent in most cases of mild diarrhea, those that are truly intermittent, and those involving only a motility disturbance in the distal colon. When wasting has occurred in the presence of undiminished appetite, either hyperthyroidism or the malabsorption syndrome is strongly suggested. In others the association of weight loss with fever, anorexia, weakness, and other signs of a systemic illness bespeaks an infection or other inflammatory disease of the bowel. Patients with bowel cancer rarely lose weight until their appetites fail.

Associated Symptoms of Disease. Naturally, associated symptoms of disease elsewhere in the body often give valuable clues to the pathogenesis of diarrhea, as does a careful review of all medications being taken. Concurrent vomiting may reflect partial intestinal obstruction or may be a symptom of uremia. Chronic respiratory symptoms may suggest cystic fibrosis, scleroderma, or tuberculous enteritis. Joint pains may be a clue to inflammatory bowel disease, or may be due to gout which has been treated with colchicine, with resultant diarrhea. A sore mouth may be the result of treatment of leukemia with antimetabolites, which may also cause the loose stools.

Duration and Fluctuation in Severity. The duration and long-term fluctuations in severity of the symptoms should be carefully noted and correlated in time with other events in the patient's life, seeking circumstantial evidence for etiologic factors. The coincidence of diarrheal episodes with emotional conflicts occasioned by stressful experiences is at once the most common association and the most difficult to validate (see Tables 18 and 19). Patient, indirect inquiry, without the use of leading questions, is best, and the patient's subjective reactions to his experiences, often conveyed by nonverbal signals, are essential in evaluating their possible connection with his illness. Temporal correlations with operations and other illnesses may be relevant for physical or psychologic reasons. Exposure to specific illnesses through epidemics or family contacts, or exposure to unsanitary conditions through travel or confinement in poorly managed institutions, may indicate the possibility of specific infections. Relation of attacks to ingestion of specific foods or drugs should be carefully tested for consistency, and may indicate allergic mechanisms or mucosal enzyme de-

TABLE 18

Object Lesson: People with Parasites Have Problems. J. M., 47-year-old housewife.

Age	Life Situation	Symptoms
5–7	Mother died; "stepmother was mean to me"	Not recalled
17	Married without parents' blessing	Not recalled
18	1st pregnancy	*Constipation; vomiting,* headache, "asthma," "hay fever"
19–26	6 pregnancies, then first husband died	As above, plus occasional *diarrhea, abdominal pain*
37	Remarried; stepdaughters	Same
42	Eldest son killed	*Severe diarrhea;* onset same day
46	*Entamoeba histolytica* found in stools . . . treated . . . stools thereafter negative . . . symptoms continued	
47	Above history elicited . . . supportive psychotherapy, placebos . . . symptoms abated	

TABLE 19

Object Lesson: People with Problems Have Parasites. C. H., 21-year-old single woman, waitress.

Age	Life Situations	Symptoms
0–12	Parents fought	Not recalled
13	Ran away from home	Not recalled
16–19	Reform school	Not recalled
20–21	Mistress to ill-tempered bartender; feared she was becoming insane	Alternating diarrhea and constipation, periumbilical and right lower quadrant pain
	Entamoeba histolytica found in stools . . . treated; stools then negative	None

ficiencies. The occurrence of diarrhea on beginning a new job (or a new hobby) may lead to recognition of a causative toxic chemical.

Clinical Examination

Physical examination is of value chiefly for clues to associated diseases elsewhere in the body, and for assessment of the nutritional effects of the diarrheal disease. Such signs as exophthalmos, jaundice, uremic breath, pigmented mucous membranes, macroglossia, general lymphadenopathy, hydrarthrosis, and erythema nodosum may quickly suggest the underlying cause of diarrhea. The characteristic flushing of the patient with metastatic carcinoid tumor, the localized peripheral lymphedema of lymphangiectasia, or the Argyll Robertson pupil of diabetic neuropathy may lead promptly to a hypothesis which may prove correct.

Acute depletion of extracellular fluid and electrolytes may be evidenced by diminished skin turgor, muscle weakness, and postural changes in pulse and blood pressure. More chronic nutritional losses may be shown by muscle wasting, reduced thickness of skin folds, and edema; specific nutritional losses may be suggested by marked pallor, glossitis, and koilonychia (iron, folate, B_{12}), the Chvostek or Trousseau signs (calcium, vitamin D), and cutaneous or mucosal hemorrhages (usually vitamin K). Aphthous ulcers and clubbing of the fingers are not uncommon in sprue and ulcerative colitis. Fever, of course, is a key finding, though it is sometimes present in neoplastic lesions of the bowel, often absent in specific infections, and usually absent in ulcerative colitis.

The abdomen itself may reveal useful signs, including localized tenderness, masses, palpable viscera, visible and audible peristalsis, and ascites. The surgical experience of the patient is usually obvious from his scars. Gaseous distension, particularly that which is minimal in the morning and increases through the day, is consistent with partial intestinal obstruction, the malabsorption syndrome, or simple aerophagia.

The rectal and pelvic examination will permit bimanual palpation of diseased loops of small or large bowel. The perineum itself may reflect the duration and severity of the diarrhea, in general reddening and maceration of the perianal skin, and in relaxation of the anus, which is common in colitis. The presence of hemorrhoids may correlate with excessive straining due to rectal involvement in an inflammatory or neoplastic process. Anal fistulae are often early signs of regional enteritis, but may be seen in ulcerative colitis as well. Strictures due to cancer, colitis, or lymphogranuloma venereum are likely to be found 2 cm or more inside the anus, while those due to previous surgery begin at the anus itself. A rectal shelf or a "frozen pelvis" may provide the first clue to an advanced neoplastic process. A retroverted uterus and adnexal mass may lead to consideration of endometriosis with bowel involvement. But one of the greatest rewards of digital examination is the most mundane—a *fecal impaction* is a common cause of watery brown diarrhea!

TABLE 20

Diagnostic Clues from the Physical Examination

Finding	Possible Etiology of Diarrhea
Skin:	
Reddish-purple flush	Malignant carcinoid syndrome
Jaundice, excoriations	Exclusion of bile from duodenum, with steatorrhea
Induration and attachment over fingers, face	Systemic sclerosis (scleroderma)
Ecchymoses	Malabsorption, treatment with antimetabolites, or Henoch-Schönlein purpura
Erythema nodosum	Ulcerative colitis or regional enteritis
Pyoderma gangrenosum	Ulcerative colitis
Pigmentation (melanotic spots)	Addison's disease; Peutz-Jeghers syndrome
Telangiectasia (of abdomen)	Radiation enteritis
Head:	
Exophthalmos, lid lag	Graves' disease
Pigmented mucous membranes	Addison's disease
Macroglossia	Amyloidosis
Hypertrophied gums	Amyloidosis or treatment with antimetabolites
Aphthous stomatitis	Sprue; ulcerative colitis
Miosis, salivation	Poisoning with insecticide (anticholinesterase)
Tophi of ears	Colchicine treatment of gout
Neck and spine:	
Lymph node enlargement	Lymphoma; carcinoma of bowel; tuberculosis; Whipple's disease
Thyroid enlargement (or surgical scar)	Graves' disease; medullary carcinoma of thyroid
Ankylosis of neck or spine	Regional enteritis; ulcerative colitis
Chest:	
Rales; pneumothorax; pleural effusion	Tuberculosis
Hyperresonance; coarse rhonchi	Cystic fibrosis
Left pleural effusion	Chronic pancreatitis
Right pleural effusion	Amebiasis (with liver abscess)
Severe hypotension	Cholera, gastrointestinal hemorrhage, pseudomembranous enterocolitis, ganglionic blocking agents
Hypertension, pericarditis, endocarditis	Polyarteritis, other diffuse vascular disease
Abdomen and pelvic regions:	
Gaseous distension	Malabsorption, various causes
Ascites, hepatomegaly, splenomegaly	Cirrhosis, constrictive pericarditis, congestive heart failure, schistosomiasis
Firm, misshapen liver	Carcinoma (or carcinoid) of bowel, amebiasis
Surgical scars:	
Upper abdominal	Gastrectomy, vagectomy
Lower abdominal	Colonic or ileocolonic resection or bypass
McBurney or right lower rectus	Regional enteritis (!)
Inguinal adenopathy	Lymphoma: lymphogranuloma venereum
Anal abscess or fistula	Regional enteritis

TABLE 20—*Continued*

Finding	Possible Etiology of Diarrhea
Extremities and Neurological:	
Hydrarthrosis	Ulcerative colitis, regional enteritis, Whipple's disease
Podagra	Colchicine toxicity
Edema of one limb	Intestinal lymphangiectasis
Peripheral neuropathy	Diabetic diarrhea
Tetany (Chvostek's and Trousseau's signs)	Malabsorption syndrome
Pupils fixed to light	Diabetic diarrhea
Stroke, or ischemia of foot	Mesenteric arterial insufficiency

Laboratory Data

The Stool. The importance of the physician's immediate personal inspection of the stool should need no emphasis; yet in many well-run hospitals and clinics it is delayed or omitted—apparently for reasons of revulsion, of the scientific snobbery that accepts only precise biochemical evidence, and because of the sense of efficiency that comes from delegating batches of messy tests to a faceless laboratory technician, who reports via a computerized printout.

To the thinking clinician, however, the stool has much to tell. The diagnostic significance of its volume has already been mentioned. Its consistency fairly reflects the fluidity of the luminal contents at the uppermost level of the intestine involved by disease: hence the stool in *Salmonella* enteritis resembles ileostomy fluid, while a mushy stool gives assurance that the trouble lies chiefly in the distal colon. Homogenization of the stool is quite complete before the distal colon is reached; hence streaks or flecks of blood, mucus, or pus, on or separate from the stool itself, must have come from somewhere in the left colon, usually the sigmoid or rectum. The pale, foamy, greasy, foul stool of severe steatorrhea is readily recognized; for those who have not observed one its odor is best described as offensive and overpowering (Fig. 19). In lactase deficiency the fermentation of lactose may yield a definite aroma of sour milk; an ammoniacal smell bespeaks *Proteus* organisms: and no odor at all, an overgrowth of *Staphylococcus*. In acute diarrheas actual recording of the total weight or volume of the stools each 24 hours may be crucial, as in cholera; the pH may indicate fermentative production of organic acids, and direct measurement of losses of sodium and potassium may be a valuable guide to therapy.

Testing of the stool for occult blood should begin at the time of rectal examination, the specimen being obtained on filter paper from the soiled glove. Fresh stool specimens should then be smeared and examined microscopically for cellular content and for fat. Uniformly dispersed polymorphonuclear leukocytes in large numbers are seen mainly in ulcerative colitis. Amebae, other protozoa, and parasitic ova should be sought; for special

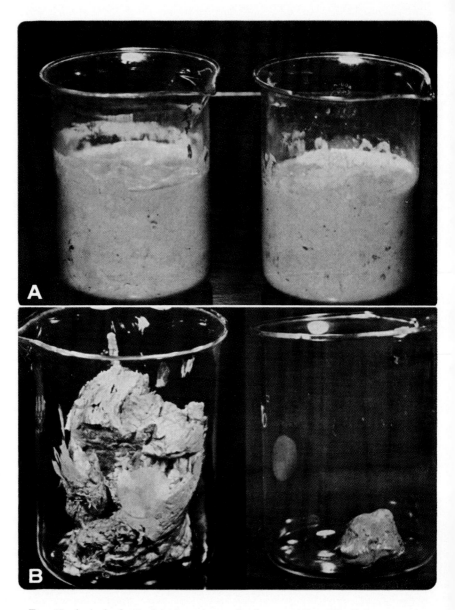

FIG. 19. *A*. A single stool (volume in two beakers, totaling 500 ml) from a patient with steatorrhea. *B*. Two subsequent stools from the same patient, during progressive clinical improvement. Note, however, that chemically proven *steatorrhea* (over 10 g of fat in stool per 24 hours) *was present throughout this period*—i.e., while certain gross characteristics of stool may indicate presence of steatorrhea, their absence does not exclude it.

methods applicable to different species standard texts should be consulted. Staining with Sudan III following acetic acid treatment may give an early indication that steatorrhea is indeed present.[15] Cultures should always be obtained from fresh specimens (or at sigmoidoscopy), and flecks of blood or mucus should be "fished"; otherwise true pathogens may be overgrown by saprophytic organisms. In many hospitals it may be necessary to request the laboratory to report the predominant organism even though it is not ordinarily pathogenic, and to culture specifically for fungi, or else the effects of antibiotics on fecal flora will be ignored. In numerous instances appropriately timed serologic tests for *Salmonella* or *Shigella* infections, the complement fixation test for amebiasis, or the tuberculin or Frei test may be indicated.

Sigmoidoscopy. In severe diarrhea early use of *sigmoidoscopy* may require a degree of bravery, but the information obtained may greatly expedite diagnosis. It should first be attempted without preliminary cleansing of the bowel; if the field is obscured with feces, excellent specimens can be obtained for culture and microscopic examinations for bacteria and amebae. A curette, a wire loop, or a bronchoscopist's specimen collector in the suction train can be used. Following preparation with an enema of tapwater, physiologic saline, or Travad (not longer than 1 hour before the examination), proctosigmoidoscopy then may reveal gross evidence of disease in the bowel.

The minimal criteria for ulcerative colitis deserve comment: In the rectum, discrete ulcers are usually *not* seen, but the whole mucosa is diffusely dull or velvety, lacking the usual sheen; hemorrhage, if not spontaneous, can be induced by simple swabbing with a cotton pledget—after a few seconds, petechiae appear. The finding of discrete areas of inflammation, with normal mucosa between, suggests Crohn's disease or sometimes amebiasis.

Mucosal Biopsy. Mucosal biopsy by small biting forceps or suction tubes may be rewarded, even in the absence of focal lesions, by the finding of diffuse inflammation characteristic of (not diagnostic of) ulcerative colitis,[16] or mucous inspissation indicating cystic fibrosis, or periarterial metachromatic changes diagnostic of amyloidosis. Excision of a tiny piece of the edge of a rectal valve and immediately pressing the specimen between glass slides in a drop of tap water for microscopic examination often affords rapid identification of the ova of schistosomes, especially *Schistosoma mansoni*.[23] Biopsies should be taken generally from a point 5 to 10 cm from the anal margin—above the anal canal with its nonspecific inflammation, and below the peritoneal reflection. The depth of insertion of the sigmoidoscope should always be recorded, in case later x-ray findings question the normality of the sigmoid or rectosigmoid region.

Laboratory Studies

It is assumed that the clinical laboratory will be wisely and selectively used to supply data bearing on any systemic disease (see Table 17) which might be related to the diarrhea. In relation to urinalysis, the output of

5-hydroxyindole-3-acetic acid, a metabolite of serotonin, is markedly elevated in the malignant carcinoid syndrome and moderately so in nontropical sprue. The output of indole-3-acetic acid is a fair nonspecific reflection of small intestinal bacterial overgrowth from whatever cause, but this test is not widely available.

Blood Analysis. Anemia in the presence of diarrhea may be of great diagnostic interest. Iron deficiency anemia is usually due to blood loss, sometimes to malabsorption, and almost never to dietary deficiency. Megaloblastic anemia provides important leads to the differential diagnosis of steatorrhea (see below). Leukocytosis and the appearance of immature polynuclear cells ("shift to the left") may give unexpected evidence of the magnitude of an inflammatory disease or infarction of the bowel, as these changes are often seen in the absence of fever. Elevation of the erythrocyte sedimentation rate may be the clearest indication, prior to x-ray examinations, that an inflammatory and not a psychophysiologic process is present. In any patient with severe diarrhea the serum electrolytes should be measured, and also the serum proteins, by the salting-out method or by electrophoresis. Though hypokalemia is common in ulcerative colitis, its association with diarrhea is a striking feature of a rare form of pancreatic adenoma.[32] The recognition of protein-losing enteropathy,[20] usually by otherwise unexplained reductions of serum albumin and γ-globulin, narrows the diagnostic range of diarrheal mechanisms.

Radiography. Because barium in the stools interferes with a number of the laboratory tests mentioned above, as well as for reasons of expense and radiation hazards, x-ray studies are often deferred until many of the other steps are completed. The diagnostic importance of the radiologic studies must in every instance be carefully weighed against the contribution they will make to the cumulative, lifetime exposure of the patient to ionizing radiation. It has been calculated that each abdominal x-ray procedure delivers from 0.6 to 2.5 rads to the skin, and the estimated exposure of the spinal bone marrow and the ovaries is a significant fraction of this. Fortunately neoplasms and other important findings from gastrointestinal x-rays occur predominantly in later life, and the principal caution which must be observed is avoidance of their uncritical use in young women, particularly in the second half of each menstrual cycle.

A plain film of the abdomen and x-rays of the spine can of course be obtained as soon as need for them is perceived. The high prevalence of significant disease in the colon, together with the risk of impaction of barium given by mouth when the colon is partially obstructed, dictates that a barium enema be performed prior to upper GI series. Efforts to produce an "ileal leak" are particularly important, if the colon itself appears normal. It is noteworthy that a gastrojejunocolic fistula can often be demonstrated by barium enema and not with a barium meal.

As lesions directly or indirectly related to the cause of diarrhea may be found at any level of the gastrointestinal tract, the GI series must be painstaking and complete. The esophageal motor disorder of scleroderma, revealed only by special films in the supine position, may be the initial lead to the cause of an obscure diarrhea. The exact location of a gastrojejunos-tomy, the filling of an afferent loop in a Billroth II anastomosis, unusually coarse gastric rugae, extrinsic pressure in the region of the pancreas or the liver, and evidence of excessive dilution of barium with intestinal fluid may be important clues. At times, when a local lesion in a single jejunal or ileal loop is suspected, it is wise in repeating the x-rays to administer barium via a long intestinal tube passed to or just above the suspected lesion ("small bowel enema").

The radiologic characteristics of typical neoplastic and inflammatory lesions of the small bowel need not be recited here. The finding of a so-called "deficiency pattern" (actually a coarsening of the feathery barium outline due to reduced number and increased breadth of the valvulae conniventes) is often presented as evidence for malabsorption, while it may occur in many other conditions which produce mucosal edema and/or hypomotility of the bowel. Paradoxically, stasis of barium in the small intestine is *most* relevant to the diagnosis of diarrhea, though its causes are legion (see remarks on the "blind loop" syndrome, below).

Recent advances in radiology, of course, extend our reach beyond mere delineation of the intestinal lumen. Selective abdominal arteriography may reveal a partial occlusion of a major vessel or a vascular tumor. Lymphangiography via lymph channels in the leg or foot may demonstrate enlarged periaortic nodes and suggest the presence of an abdominal lym-phoma.

Clinical Trials

Clinical trials of potent therapeutic agents are often justified in the absence of a clear etiologic diagnosis, but rarely as a "shot in the dark." The most abused form of clinical trial is probably the resort to antibiotics or sulfonamide drugs in the treatment of diarrheas due to viral agents, resistant bacteria, or nonspecific infections such as occur in ulcerative colitis. The risks of emergence of highly drug-resistant intestinal flora are rarely justified. In a variety of conditions associated with bacterial over-growth in blind loops or in the presence of small intestinal stasis, however, small amounts of tetracyclines given orally for 2 weeks often acutely re-lieve the diarrhea (see section on malabsorption). This is apparently due in part to the prevention of bacterial degradation of bile acids; the same result may be achieved by the oral administration of cholestyramine, which sequesters and renders chemically inert the bile acids deconjugated by bacterial action.

The diagnostic use of adrenal steroids in patients only suspected of having ulcerative colitis or other inflammatory bowel disease is fraught with difficulty. Patients with psychophysiologic disorders may be inconstantly benefited by the mood-elevating properties of these drugs. Tuberculosis of the intestine and certain other infections may be permitted to spread even while inflammation is suppressed and symptomatic benefit obtained. Again, the risks are great and the reliability of diagnostic conclusions is low.

An almost indispensable application of the clinical trial is the elimination diet. Elimination of gluten, lactose, and other foods for which terminal digestive pathways are defective may dramatically illuminate the diagnosis (see section on differential diagnosis). For years the elimination of all potential food allergens, and the gradual refeeding of suspected foods one at a time, has been known to provide the only reliable evidence of true gastrointestinal allergy, especially if the barium-filled intestine is observed fluoroscopically after the allergen is ingested unbeknownst to the patient.[19]

The ultimate elimination diet, of course, is total parenteral alimentation. As indicated previously, all diarrheas should thus be controlled unless the mechanism is one of primary hypermotility or excessive exsorption of fluid.

MALABSORPTION

Clinical recognition of features of the malabsorption syndrome imposes an obligation, first, to establish beyond reasonable doubt that a persistent defect of absorption truly exists, and, second, to discover the causative mechanism. This obligation has become especially stringent in recent years, as the techniques of differential diagnosis have been multiplied and truly effective means of therapy, in many instances quite specific for one of the possible causes, have been discovered.

Diagnosis

Diarrhea is, of course, an inconstant feature of the malabsorption syndrome. When present, it usually consists of bulky, pale, foul stools, which have already been described in this chapter, and are highly variable in frequency. The persistence of diarrhea when oral intake is suspended for 2 days or longer, however, or the alternation of diarrhea with periods of true constipation is virtually incompatible with this syndrome. On the other hand, progressive weight loss in the absence of severe anorexia, fever, or evident hypermetabolism strongly suggests malabsorption, and the appearance of any of a wide range of symptoms and signs of nutritional deficiency often points to this diagnosis.

Thus, the catabolism of proteins resulting from defective absorption and excessive enteric protein loss is reflected clinically in muscular wasting and weakness, edema, and hypoalbuminemia. (Vitamin E deficiency probably also contributes to the muscular weakness.) Excessive losses of calcium lead in some patients to hypocalcemia, with latent or manifest tetany, and in others to demineralization of bones with complaints leading to orthopedic consultations. Hemorrhages and bruises associated with reductions of plasma prothrombin and related clotting factors, easily correctible by parenteral injection of vitamin K, are the result of loss of this fat-soluble vitamin in the stool. Aphthous ulcers (*sprouw* is Dutch for aphthous ulcer), cheilosis, and sore tongue, though not specific for this syndrome, are commonly ascribed to losses of B vitamins. Anemia may be microcytic, due to malabsorption of iron and/or pyridoxine; or megaloblastic, due to deficiencies of folic acid or vitamin B_{12}.

Any two or three of the above manifestations, or any one of them in the presence of typical fatty stools, should lead to careful laboratory studies to establish or rule out the presence of malabsorption. The most broadly applicable screening tests are the microscopic study of the stools for fat (see above) and the serum carotene determination (under 50 μg/100 ml is presumptive evidence of steatorrhea). The xylose absorption test (the excretion of less than 5.0 g in the urine after a 25-g oral load) is widely used, but is negative in a considerable proportion of patients with significant malabsorption. The clinically available indices of absorption of isotopically labeled fats have not proven consistently reliable.

Although rare unquestioned examples of malabsorption without steatorrhea do exist, the best and most direct laboratory criterion is the quantitative chemical determination of total fat in the stools; a 3-day collection of all stools from a subject on a dietary fat intake in the range of 50 to 150 g/day should contain not more than 20 g of fat (approximately 7 g daily). Because the diagnosis of malabsorption is usually so important, it is recommended that, if a reasonable suspicion has been aroused by significant symptoms and signs, it should be considered as ruled out only by the demonstration by chemical methods of a normal amount of fat in the stools.[37, 41]

Differential Diagnosis

The considerable range of etiologic possibilities to be considered in the differential diagnosis of proven steatorrhea can be considerably narrowed by careful review of the history and physical findings, but the ultimate identification of a specific mechanism may require the sharpest tools of the modern morphologist, biochemist, or microbiologist. The writer has found it useful, as a routine bedside thought process, to consider in order the many steps in the digestion and absorption of the critical molecule, the long-chain triglyceride, any one of which may be impaired. These fall into three basic stages: intraluminal, intraepithelial, and lymphatic transport.

Intraluminal Stage. In the intraluminal stage (Fig. 20), preliminary emulsification is dependent upon the normal gastric reservoir and antral pumping of aliquots of chyme into the duodenum, where pancreatic lipase and conjugated bile salts together lead to partial degradation to mono- and diglycerides and the formation of a micellar solution of fat.[34] Thus a history of gastric surgery or pancreatitis, or the physical findings of jaundice or appropriate surgical scars, may promptly suggest the true etiology of malabsorption. The surgical history may reveal other clues of importance: the "blind loop" syndrome may result from a bowel anastomosis for regional enteritis or neoplastic disease, or from a long afferent loop in a gastrojejunostomy, in which stasis of bile-stained, infected contents is reflected clinically in episodes of postprandial bilious vomiting. Symptoms suggesting a marginal (gastrojejunal) ulcer may suggest an associated gastrocolic fistula, and symptoms of recurrent low-grade intestinal obstruction should always raise the possibility of stasis and bacterial overgrowth as a cause of steatorrhea. A similar mechanism might be thought

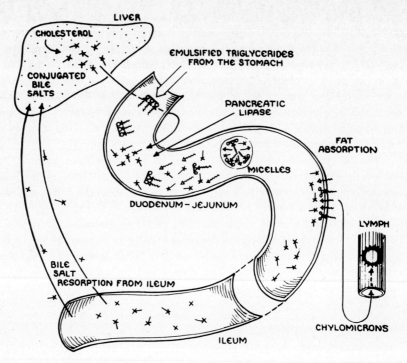

FIG. 20. Factors in intraluminal micelle formation, and the absorption of fats and bile salts. (Reprinted, with permission, from Senior, J. R., J. Lipid Res. 5:495, 1964.)

of in the presence of peripheral neuropathy (diabetes) or symptoms of scleroderma.

Intraepithelial Stage. The intraepithelial stage (Fig. 21) may be defective because of extensive surgical resection of the small bowel, or because of diffuse mucosal disease such as tropical or nontropical sprue. Actual *or prior* residence in the tropics or subtropics is a common clue to the former condition, and some areas (e.g., Puerto Rico, Haiti, Madras, and Viet Nam) have a particularly high prevalence. The insidious onset of nontropical sprue (adult celiac disease) may be signaled by any of the nutritional consequences of steatorrhea previously described. The only special clue is an intestinal or nutritional disorder of childhood, with onset usually within the first year of life and clearing before puberty. Characteristic diarrhea may have been absent, but abdominal distension, retardation of growth, anemia, and food intolerances may be recalled. A history of radiation therapy or the use of alkylating agents, antimetabolites, colchicine, neomycin, or triparanol may provisionally implicate one of these agents as a cause of epithelial injury.

Mesenteric Lymphatic Obstruction. The several causes of mesenteric lymphatic obstruction should be thought of in the general study of the patient. The extraintestinal manifestations of tuberculosis, lymphoma, and amyloidosis are familiar. It should be noted that intestinal amyloidosis

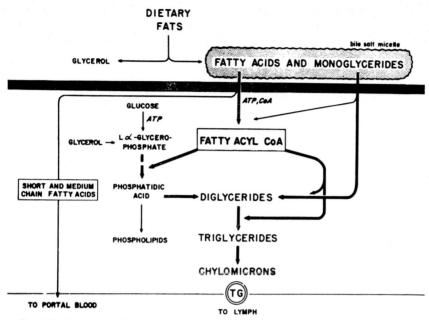

FIG. 21. Intraepithelial pathways for absorption of fatty acids and monoglycerides across intestinal mucosa, involving the resynthesis of triglycerides and the formation of lipoproteins (chylomicra) from long-chain fatty acids. Note that short- and medium-chain fatty acids are transported directly to portal blood, the basis for their use in nutritional supplements. (Reprinted, with permission, from Isselbacher, K., Fed. Proc. 24:16, 1965.)

corresponds more closely to the "primary" variety, in which hepatosplenomegaly is rare and the more obvious lesions may be found in the heart, skin, and tongue. Whipple's disease should be thought of when prolonged fever, abdominal pain, arthritis, and lymphadenopathy are observed. The presence of peripheral (often localized) lymphedema or of a chylous effusion may suggest lymphangiectasia of the intestine.

When none of the above clinical clues points to a provisional diagnosis the following sequence of laboratory procedures is recommended—they of course apply equally to the confirmation of suspicions already aroused:

1. *Complete gastrointestinal x-rays*—barium enema followed by GI series with small bowel films. The routine chest x-rays should be searched for evidence of tuberculosis or lymphoma.

2. *Suction biopsy of the jejunum*, just beyond the ligament of Treitz (Fig. 22). If a portion of the muscularis mucosae is included in the specimen, and if it is carefully embedded so that vertical sections can be taken through it, it may clearly show the villous atrophy and mild mononuclear infiltration characteristic of adult or childhood celiac disease.[33] The same may also be appreciated on examination of the fresh specimen under the dissecting microscope. Lesser mucosal atrophy and greater inflammation of the lamina propria are characteristic of tropical sprue and of stronglyloidiasis, and in patients with diffuse lymphoma the malignant cells are sometimes

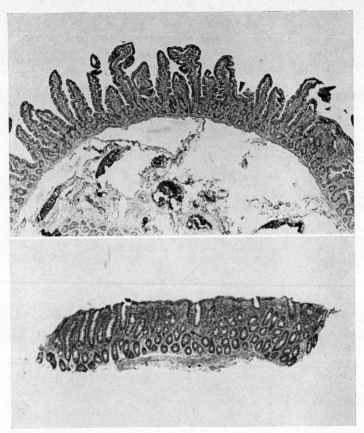

Fig. 22. *A*. Suction biopsy of normal jejunum. Note finger- and leaf-like villi, and height of villi much greater than depth of crypts. *B*. Suction biopsy of jejunum in untreated adult celiac disease (nontropical sprue). Note complete villous atrophy, much-elongated crypts.

seen. Stained with periodic acid–Schiff, the typical macrophages of Whipple's disease may be recognized. Stained with cresyl violet, a small blood vessel bearing an amyloid deposit may be found, but a deeper biopsy of the rectal mucosa is more likely to be positive. *Giardia lamblia* may be observed, clinging in large numbers to the surface of the villi. A biopsy in a child with abetalipoproteinemia, taken an hour after a feeding of corn oil, is likely to show the retention of excessive quantities of neutral fat in intraepithelial droplets, with little or no fat in the lamina propria (this rare entity could be earlier suspected from the findings of acanthocytic red cells on smear of peripheral blood and of an excessively low serum cholesterol concentration—under 60 mg/100 ml, and from the absence of β-lipoproteins on plasma electrophoresis.)

   3. A *modified Schilling test*—urinary excretion of orally administered C^{60}-labeled vitamin B_{12} *with intrinsic factor*, followed by the usual intramuscular "flushing" dose of "cold" B_{12}. Failure to absorb B_{12} under these conditions usually results either from massive steatorrhea (dilution in large volume

of luminal fluid) or, more significantly, from bacterial overgrowth and utilization of the vitamin at or above the ileal level. The latter hypothesis can be tested by repetition of the test after a trial of tetracycline (see below).

4. The *secretin-pancreozymin test* of pancreatic exocrine function, measuring the volume, pH, bicarbonate, and enzyme content of duodenal fluid before and after injection of these hormones. While the test must be carefully done and gastric juice quantitatively aspirated via a separate tube, the patient with pancreatogenous steatorrhea usually has a profound depression in pancreatic secretion, if not achylia.

5. *Miscellaneous studies.* In still-obscure cases, the diagnosis may be suggested by the finding of tubercle bacilli in the stools, or even an infiltrate characteristic of tuberculosis in the chest x-ray. Suspicion of mesenteric arterial insufficiency may require a selective angiogram for confirmation. Serum electrophoresis may reveal hypogammaglobulinemia as the cause of steatorrhea, and the possibility of hypothyroidism or hypoparathyroidism may be sufficient to indicate the need for protein-bound iodine levels or serum calcium and phosphorus determinations, respectively. An excessive output of 5-hydroxyindole-3-acetic acid in the urine (more than 300 mg/24 hours) will confirm suspicions of the malignant carcinoid syndrome, and excessive nocturnal gastric secretion (over 1 liter in 12 hours) will indicate that the steatorrhea may be due to the Zollinger-Ellison syndrome.

The final recourse in many differential diagnostic problems in steatorrhea is a trial of therapy. The effects on the patient can be measured by the abatement of diarrhea and other symptoms, by gain in weight, and at times by actual weighing of the stools, before the stool fat output is again chemically measured. The more rewarding stratagems are the following:

1. The *gluten-free diet.* With meticulous exclusion of all gluten-containing foods, clinical improvement may begin in a few days to several weeks or months after institution of this diet in patients with celiac disease, and rarely in other conditions (lymphoma, Whipple's disease).[5, 35] Earlier than this the modestly elevated (15 to 20 mg/24 hours) urinary 5-hydroxyindole-3-acetic acid excretion may be returned to normal. Histologic improvement in the intestinal mucosa follows in most but not all instances in months or years. Clinical, chemical, and eventually morphologic relapse follows return to gluten-containing diets.

2. *Broad-spectrum antibiotics*, if therapeutically effective, reinforce the suspicion of any of the causes of bacterial overgrowth (see Table 17) or of Whipple's disease, even in the absence of specific laboratory support. Reduction of a previously elevated level of urinary output of indole-3-acetic acid may presage clinical improvement in the former condition. The best procedure is to give 0.25 g of tetracycline orally four times daily for 14 to 21 days before considering the trial to be ineffective. Less often, neomycin or chloramphenicol is substituted.

3. *Pancreatic enzyme replacement* is usually strikingly effective within 2 to 3 weeks in relieving pancreatogenous steatorrhea, provided that an adequate amount of a potent preparation is used Thus, 4.0 g of U.S.P.

pancreatin three times a day before meals (36 standard tablets daily) is required; alternatively, 3.0 g of Viokase or 0.6 to 0.9 g of Cotazym is given with each meal.

4. When fever, weight loss, and continued diarrhea give clear clinical parameters to follow, a blind trial of streptomycin and isoniazid is occasionally justified, lest an obscure case of intestinal tuberculosis go unrecognized.

FERMENTATIVE DIARRHEAS

Although clinicians have long suspected that some cases of diarrhea are due to the bacterial fermentation of unabsorbed carbohydrates, only in the last 10 years has this phenomenon been clearly linked to specific deficiencies of intraepithelial disaccharidases in the small bowel.[13] Of these, the most common deficiency is that of lactase, although sucrase, isomaltase, and multiple maltase deficiencies have been found in successively smaller numbers of persons. Lactase deficiency is much more frequent in nonwhite populations.[4] Though the stools are often watery and profuse and sometimes smell like sour milk, these features may be absent and the diarrhea itself may be inconstantly related to ingestion of recognized milk or milk products. Temporary depression of intestinal lactase activity has been observed after acute viral or bacterial enteritis, hepatitis, and even "grippe," and patients with adult celiac disease and those who have had a gastrectomy may have a similar deficiency. Hence, on the one hand a history of milk intolerance in a patient with diarrhea should not be dismissed lightly, and on the other hand this mechanism should be considered as one of a number of factors causing diarrhea in various identifiable diseases.

Clinically a presumptive diagnosis of lactase deficiency can be made on the basis of a lactose tolerance test (50 g/m^2 of body surface, but not more than 100 g orally). If the maximal rise in blood glucose is not over 25 mg/100 ml, and if the patient has intestinal symptoms which are not reproduced by testing with an equal weight of a 1:1 mixture of glucose and galactose, one can be confident that lactase deficiency exists and could be confirmed, if desired, by measurement of enzyme activity in a small intestinal biopsy specimen. This conclusion can then be verified by clinical trial of a diet free of milk and milk products.

This form of milk intolerance may be contrasted with that often attributed to hypersensitivity to one or more of the proteins of cow's milk. Though it probably is a significant cause of diarrhea in infants, its importance in intestinal disorders of adults is by no means clear. The frequency and the titers of serum antibodies to these proteins are not consistently greater in these patients than in controls. The empirical trial of an elimination diet, avoiding therapeutic suggestion insofar as possible, seems the only practical recourse for the physician.

INFLAMMATORY BOWEL DISEASE

Inflammatory bowel disease is a term now acquiring increased currency; it connotes diffuse or multifocal involvement of the large and/or small intestine in an acute or chronic inflammatory process of undetermined etiology, and subsumes in particular the entities *idiopathic ulcerative colitis* and *Crohn's disease* (including regional enteritis and granulomatous colitis). Both diseases are highly destructive to the bowel and may chronically disable the patient. Hence, although the effectiveness of current medical therapy leaves much to be desired, their early recognition is at least of prognostic importance, and offers the best chance of minimizing damage to the intestine.

Though these are properly classified as diarrheal diseases, the diarrhea is often preceded or overshadowed by evidences of systemic illness. Fever, general malaise, anorexia, and weight loss may suggest a broad range of diagnostic possibilities; less often, but more characteristically, one sees one or more signs of a delayed hypersensitivity reaction or altered immune response—erythema nodosum, pyoderma gangrenosum, iritis, aphthous stomatitis, and arthritis. When involving the peripheral joints, the arthritis usually simulates early rheumatoid arthritis, yet is asymmetrical, affecting the larger and more proximal joints; it is associated with negative latex fixation reactions, and rarely leads to ankylosis. On the other hand, a true ankylosing spondylitis occurs with startling frequency in these diseases, and almost as commonly in women as in men.

The intestinal symptoms and signs vary with the location and the type of inflammatory process (see below), but this group of diseases can usually be distinguished from psychophysiologic reactions by fever, significant weight loss, greater tendency to diarrhea during hours of sleep, peripheral blood leukocytosis or elevated erythrocyte sedimentation rate, or the finding of abundant leukocytes in fresh thin smears of the stool. The differentiation from amebiasis, shigellosis, lymphogranuloma venereum, tuberculosis, and other specific infections must be made on culture of the pathogenic organisms, tissue pathology, or at times clinical trial of specific chemotherapeutic agents.

Ulcerative Colitis

Crohn's disease and ulcerative colitis differ from each other in important morphological features, which are reflected in differences in symptomatology, clinical course, and complications. *Ulcerative colitis* is a diffusely spreading, superficial inflammation of the colonic mucosa, usually appearing earliest in the rectum and sigmoid. Rectal bleeding is a common early symptom, in 50 per cent of cases preceding the diarrhea. The inflammation is acutely necrotizing, not proliferative; fibrosis, obstruction, and fistula formation are very rare, but acute perforation and peritonitis are seen in severe cases. The stools, often small but very frequent (up to 30 to 40/day), consist mainly of exudate. Tenesmus and griping in the lower abdomen are common, cramps uncommon; the disease is often entirely painless. The onset and recurrences of bloody diarrhea are often abrupt and are frequently associated with clear-cut episodes of stress and emotional conflict.

On examination the patient with ulcerative colitis of average severity often looks younger than the stated age, has little or no fever and negative abdominal findings, and may have some of the extraintestinal manifestations characteristic of both diseases. Hemorrhoids may be present (probably the result of straining), and sigmoidoscopy usually directly demonstrates the morbid process. The most significant features are 1) a diffusely edematous, velvety mucosa; 2) spontaneous oozing of blood from its surface, or bleeding easily induced by light trauma, as by a cotton swab (this property is called *friability*); 3) less commonly, sloughing of mucosa and polypoid islands of surviving hyperplastic mucosa (pseudopolyps) are seen. Biopsy of the mucosa characteristically reveals a marked infiltration of the lamina propria with lymphocytes, plasma cells, macrophages, polymorphonuclear leukocytes, and eosinophils. Rupture of this exudate into the epithelial crypts (crypt abscess) and sloughing of epithelium may be seen.[16]

It should be emphasized that most of the above features may be seen in a patient whose barium enema is negative. Perhaps because only the mucosa is likely to be involved early in the process, the colon x-rays are often misleading. At the same time, they provide the only valid clinical indication of the *minimal* upward limits of the disease process in the bowel, and serial examinations over time can indicate its spread or its abatement. In moder-

TABLE 21

Object Lesson: Colitis Is Not a "Wastebasket" Diagnosis. E. F., 54-year-old professional woman.

Age	Clinical Features	Diagnosis and Treatment
40	Onset alternating diarrhea and constipation; rectal bleeding on occasion. Proctoscopy: negative. Barium enema: loss of haustration, distal colon	Diagnosis: colitis. Rx: antibiotics
44	Symptoms continued, findings unchanged	Same
53	Rectal bleeding more severe. Proctoscopy, barium enema as before (no "spot" films)	Diagnosis: ulcerative colitis. Rx: adrenal corticoids
54	Symptoms same. Proctoscopy: normal mucosa; blood coming from above. Barium enema: on *"spot"* films a 4-cm polypoid tumor of sigmoid colon	Operation: sigmoid resection (no metastases found). Pathologic diagnosis: adenocarcinoma of colon, grade 2, Dukes 2. No evidence of ulcerative colitis
64	Well. No evidence of recurrent disease	None

Comment
1. Diagnosis of ulcerative colitis is usually evident on proctoscopy.
2. Radiologic criteria should be strictly observed.
3. "Spot" films are needed to rule out small neoplasms.
4. Carcinoma of the colon can cause *prolonged* diarrhea. In this case there are no clinical grounds for ascribing the prolonged bloody flux to any other cause.

ately ill patients the barium shadow of the colon is not grossly distorted, but in profile minute spicules of barium, filling the tiny ulcers, project outward from the luminal mass. Reduction or absence of haustration in the distal colon is of no significance by itself, as this segment in normal persons may have this appearance when filled with barium under pressure.

Except for sigmoidoscopy, mucosal biopsy, and barium enema, no other diagnostic measures in this disease have proved highly reliable in common use. If the above characteristics are present and specific pathogens are not found the diagnosis can be made with considerable (though not complete) confidence.

Crohn's Disease (Regional Enterocolitis)

This chronic, granulomatous, cicatrizing enteritis, the microscopic pathology of which resembles intestinal tuberculosis except for the absence of caseation necrosis, was first identified in the terminal ileum by Crohn and his associates.[11] Since then it has been recognized in every segment of the intestinal tract. The pathologic and clinical characteristics of such lesions in the small bowel are well known, are the subject of many excellent reviews,[25, 26] and will not be restated here. In the differential diagnosis of diarrhea, that of regional enteritis may be considered a clear example of "large-stool" diarrhea, and the disease, when extensive, must be considered among the causes of the malabsorption syndrome.

In recent years the occurrence of Crohn's disease in the large bowel, with or without involvement of the jejunoileum, has been increasingly recognized. At times indistinguishable from idiopathic ulcerative colitis, it usually differs from that disease in the following particulars:[30]

1. The inflammatory process is localized to one or more segments of the colon, with sharply demarcated areas bordered by normal bowel.

2. The earliest lesions are more often not in the rectum or sigmoid, but are located more proximally, even in the cecum.

3. The inflammation from the beginning involves the submucosa and even the serosa, thickening the bowel wall, narrowing its lumen, and leading to deep fissure-like ulcerations but less mucosal sloughing. Fistulae are common, and may extend to the skin or to other hollow viscera, but free perforation of the bowel is rare.

Clinically, rectal bleeding is less prominent and stool frequency not as great as in ulcerative colitis. The onset is less abrupt, the leukocytosis less severe. *Fistula in ano*, fever of unknown origin, or extracolonic manifestations more often precede diarrhea in the unfolding history. Rectovaginal fistula, pneumaturia, and other fistulous phenomena sometimes occur. Examination not infrequently reveals, in addition, firm, tender abdominal masses of thickened, inflamed bowel, mesentery, and other attached organs. If visible at proctosigmoidoscopy, the mucosal lesions are usually not grossly or microscopically distinguishable from ulcerative colitis, although in a minority of *deep* biopsies of the rectum the typical Langhans giant cell systems may be found. The barium enema is, by contrast, much more valuable, as the deep and irregular fissuring of the bowel as well as the segmental or proximal distribution of the lesions may be quite apparent.

Aside from the differentiation from ulcerative colitis, Crohn's disease of the colon must be distinguished from a number of other conditions leading to segmental thickening of the bowel wall and encroachment upon the lumen.

Tuberculous Enterocolitis. This involves the same lymphatic tissues in ileum and ascending colon,[18] and in the absence of a history of tuberculosis may be signaled by findings on the chest x-ray or by calcified mesenteric nodes on plain abdominal films. Symptomatically such cases may at first respond very favorably to adrenal corticoids, administered for a mistaken diagnosis of Crohn's disease. The use of isoniazid is occasionally justified in the absence of tissue diagnosis or recovery of tubercle bacilli.

Ischemic Colitis. This condition is being recognized with increasing frequency. In patients without intestinal infarction, but with extensive atherosclerosis of the mesenteric arteries, a stenotic, sharply demarcated segment of transverse and upper descending colon may be recognized on barium enema, sometimes with irregular indentions of the lumen on the antimesocolic border ("thumb printing").[31] Selective abdominal angiography then may show the sites of obstruction or narrowing in the superior and inferior mesenteric arteries and their branches.

Diverticulitis and Carcinoma. Extensive diverticulitis of the sigmoid or descending colon may at certain stages appear on x-ray very like granulomatous colitis, without visible diverticula. Even more rarely, a short segment of the colon affected by Crohn's disease may appear as an obstructing carcinoma. In these latter two instances the true diagnosis is usually first apparent at the operating table; the bowel resection would be required in any case, but a clear preoperative or intraoperative diagnosis is important in determining the desirable extent and character of the operation performed.

DIARRHEA DUE TO PSYCHOPHYSIOLOGIC DISTURBANCES (IRRITABLE COLON, MUCOUS COLITIS, ADAPTIVE COLITIS, ETC.)

Life stress and emotional tension are almost ubiquitous in human experience, and both careful clinical observation[8, 42] and laboratory studies have shown that colonic propulsive mechanisms are included among the body's reactions to emotional arousal.[2, 3, 8] As people with other diseases competent to cause diarrhea are not exempt from these psychophysiologic disorders of the bowel, the physician who would make an accurate diagnosis of diarrhea must learn to do two things: 1) identify these disorders from positive as well as negative evidence, and 2) judge the relative importance of "functional" and "organic" disorders in the total picture of illness.*

* The terms "functional" and "organic" are here used in their conventional, but inappropriate, sense. In reality, there is probably structural change in both groups, but in the "functional" group it resides elsewhere than in the bowel.[36]

The typical patient with mucous colitis exhibits alternating constipation and diarrhea for varying proportions of the time, with periodic griping pains in the lower abdomen only partially relieved by defecation or the passage of flatus. The stools are often small, and even when loose may consist of only 10 to 30 ml of material of mushy or jelly-like consistency; they often contain visible mucus and (not rarely) streaks or stains of blood, the latter mostly because of associated hemorrhoids. Other patients may consistently have larger, more watery stools and almost total freedom from pain. There may or may not be dyspepsia, recurrent headache, palpitation, excessive sweating, angioneurotic edema, and other signs of autonomic lability.[8, 42] On examination the sigmoid or cecum may be firmly contracted masses, tender on deep pressure. Sigmoidoscopy may show moderate to marked mucosal engorgement, excessive mucus secretion, and spasmodic occlusion of the lumen—but no more. If the mucosa bleeds easily on swabbing with cotton, ulcerative colitis should be suspected and a biopsy performed; alternatively, the inflammatory disease can be recognized by finding a profusion of polynuclear leukocytes in a smear of rectal mucus. The barium enema in some patients with mucous colitis may show extensive narrowing of the lumen, imitating the "string sign" of granulomatous disease, or may show many closely set, ringlike constrictions in the distal colon.[27] These findings are the more convincing if the bowel has *not* been prepared with castor oil or soapsuds enemas, as these agents can produce similar changes in normal persons.

These clinical features, characteristic of irritable colon, are not distinctive enough to permit that diagnosis to be made with confidence, and the study of the patient should include one or more cultures of the stool for bacterial pathogens, two or more examinations of the fresh stool for amebae and other parasites, as well as the search for neoplasms, diverticulitis, ulcerative colitis, and other diseases of the lower bowel by proctosigmoidoscopy and barium enema. Unless the syndrome of "small-stool" diarrhea is clearly present, it is wise to examine the small bowel as well by x-ray, and in some instances to seek evidence of malabsorption in the serum carotene level or the stained smear of the stool for fat. The relationship of diarrhea to ingestion of specific foods or drugs should be carefully reviewed; the most rewarding "find" of this sort in recent years has been the discovery of intestinal lactase deficiency in some adults with this syndrome.[39]

But irritable colon as a psychophysiologic reaction should not be a diagnosis of exclusion. The intermittent pattern of its symptoms is often correlated in time with the appearance and disappearance of periods of emotional arousal in the patient, resulting from understandably stressful life situations.[42] Such coincidences often strongly reinforce the diagnosis, and should regularly be sought; the closer they are in time, the smaller the likelihood that they are due to chance alone. To avoid prejudice in the mind of either the physician or the patient, it is best to obtain the social history separately from the account of bodily symptoms, record their chronology with care, and then match them on a "life chart" (see Table 18).

Signs of emotion, both verbal and nonverbal, in the taking of the history must be carefully noted and interpreted. The acquisition of such direct evidence of psychophysiologic responses does not ensure a correct diagnosis, but contributes greatly to it, and is often the cornerstone of truly effective treatment of the patient.

As previously mentioned, many patients with "organic" disease of the bowel also have a significant "functional" (psychophysiologic) disturbance. Hence, the discovery of one plausible explanation for diarrhea may leave another condition undiscovered. When the "organic" cause is discovered first, an underlying neurosis may be ignored which may perpetuate the diarrhea long after the supposed infection or tumor is successfully treated. When the emotional disturbance is striking, the search for a structural lesion in the bowel may not be sufficiently thorough. When both are clearly defined and carefully studied, more discriminating and effective management is possible.

CONCLUSION

It should be clear from the above that understanding of mechanisms of diarrhea has advanced rapidly in recent years. The application of the newer methods of cell biology to the biochemical events in the intestinal mucosa and the luminal contents has opened up new opportunities in treatment and hence new challenges to the diagnostician. The concept of food intolerance due to failure of an essential intramucosal enzymatic process in the terminal phase of digestion, and that of the intraluminal elaboration by bacteria of chemical compounds capable of producing diarrhea, will probably lead to the discovery of other related mechanisms in the near future. It cannot be hoped that this article will be an adequate guide to the subject 10 years hence. On the other hand, it is reasonable to believe that the general pathophysiologic approach to this clinical task will be increasingly useful as it becomes, with the accretion of new knowledge, even more complex.

REFERENCES

1. Almy, T. P. In *The Differential Diagnosis of Abdominal Pain*, S. M. Mellinkoff, Ed., p. 23. McGraw-Hill Book Co., Inc., New York, 1959.
2. Almy, T. P. Experimental studies on the "irritable colon." Amer. J. Med. 10:60, 1965.
3. Almy, T. P., Abbot, F. K., and Hinkle, L. E., Jr. Alterations in colonic function in man under stress. IV. Hypomotility of the sigmoid colon, and its relationship to the mechanism of functional diarrhea. Gastroenterology 15:95, 1950.
4, Bayless, T. M., and Rosensweig, N. S. Incidence and implications of lactase deficiency and milk intolerance in white and negro populations. Johns Hopkins Med. J. 121:54, 1967.
5. Benson, G. D., Kowlessar, O. D. and Sleisenger, M. H. Adult celiac disease with emphasis upon response to the gluten-free diet. Medicine 43:1, 1964.
6. Carpenter, C. C. J., Slack, R. B., Feeley, J. C. and Steenberg, R. W. Site and characteristics of electrolyte loss and effect of intraluminal glucose in experimental canine cholera. J. Clin. Invest. 47:1210, 1968.
7. Carter, C. W., Coxon, R. V., Parsons, D. S. and Thompson, R. H. S. 1945, cited by Fordtran, J. S., and Ingelfinger, F. J., in *Handbook of Physiology*. Vol. III: *The Alimentary Canal*, p. 1466. American Physiological Society, Washington, D. C., 1968.

8. Chaudhary, N. A., and Truelove, S. C. The irritable colon syndrome—a study of the clinical features, predisposing causes, and prognosis in 130 cases. Quart. J. Med. (N.S.) 31:307, 1962.
9. Code, C. F. Sorption of water and electrolyte in healthy persons: a brief review. Proceedings of the Cholera Research Symposium, University of Hawaii, p. 87. U. S. Government Printing Office, Washington, D. C., 1965.
10. Code, C. F. The semantics of the process of absorption. Perspect. Biol. Med. 3:560, 1969.
11. Crohn, B. B., and Yarnis, H. Regional Ileitis, 2nd ed. Grune and Stratton, New York, 1958.
12. Curran, P. F., and Solomon, A. K. Ion and water fluxes in the ileum of rats. J. Gen. Physiol. 41:143, 1957.
13. Dahlqvist, A., Hammond, J. B. and Crane, R. K. Intestinal lactase deficiency and lactose intolerance in adults. Gastroenterology 45:488, 1963; 54:807, 1968.
14. Davis, J. E., Seavey, P. W. and Sessions, J. T., Jr. Villous adenomas of rectum and sigmoid colon with severe fluid and electrolyte depletion. Ann. Surg. 155:806, 1962.
15. Drummey, G. D., Benson, J. A., Jr., and Jones, C. M. Microscopic examination of stool for steatorrhea. N. Engl. J. Med. 264:85, 1961.
16. Flick, A. L., Voegtlin, K. F. and Rubin, C. E. Clinical experience with suction biopsy of the rectal mucosa. Gastroenterology 42:691, 1962.
17. Hofmann, A. F. The syndrome of ileal disease and the broken enterohepatic circulation: cholerheic enterology. Gastroenterology 52:752, 1967
18. Howell, J. S. and Knapton, P. J. Ileocecal tuberculosis. Gut 5:524, 1964.
19. Ingelfinger, F. J. Medical progress—gastrointestinal allergy. N. Engl. J. Med. 241:303, 337, 1949.
20. Jeffries, G. H., et al. Protein-losing enteropathy. N. Engl. J. Med. 266:652, 1962.
21. Jones, C. M. Digestive Tract Pain. The Macmillan Co., New York, 1938.
22. Kelley, M. L., Jr. The ileocolonic junction: an inaccessible "sphincteric zone." Gastroenterology 53:811, 1967.
23. Latty, S. G., Jr., Hunter, G. W. III, Moon, A. P., Sullivan, B. H., Jr., Burke, J. C. and Sproat, H. F. Studies on Schistosomiasis. X. Comparison of stool examination, skin test, rectal biopsy, and liver biopsy for the detection of schistosomiasis mansoni. Gastroenterology 27:324, 1954.
24. Levitan, R., and Ingelfinger, F. J. Effect of d-aldosterone on salt and water absorption from the intact human colon. J. Clin. Invest. 44:801, 1965.
25. Lockhart-Mummery, H. E., and Morson, B. C. Crohn's disease (regional enteritis) of the large intestine and its distinction from ulcerative colitis. Gut 1:87, 1960.
26. Lockhart-Mummery, H. E., and Morson, B. C. Crohn's disease of the large intestine. Gut 5:493, 1964.
27. Lumsden, K., Chandhary, N. A. and Truelove, S. C. The irritable colon syndrome. Clin. Radiol. 14:54, 1963.
28. Machella, T. E. Mechanism of the post-gastrectomy dumping syndrome. Gastroenterology 14:237, 1950.
29. Malins, J. M., and French, J. M. Diabetic diarrhea. Quart. J. Med. (N.S.) 26:467, 1957.
30. Marshak, R. H., and Lindner, A. E. Ulcerative and granulomatous colitis. J. Mt. Sinai Hosp. 33:444, 1966.
31. Marston, A., Pheils, M. T., Thomas, M. L. and Morson, B. C. Ischemic colitis. Gut 7:1, 1966.
32. Matsumoto, K. K., et al. Watery diarrhea and hypokalemia associated with pancreatic islet cell adenoma. Gastroenterology 50:231, 1966.
33. Rubin, C. E., et al. Studies of celiac disease. I. The apparent identical and specific nature of the duodenal and jejunal lesion in celiac disease and idiopathic sprue. Gastroenterology 38:28, 1960.
34. Senior, J. R. Intestinal absorption of fats. J. Lipid Res. 5:495, 1964.
35. Sleisenger, M. H. Diseases of malabsorption. In Textbook of Medicine, Beeson, P. and McDermott, W., Ed. 12th ed. p. 880. W. B. Saunders Co., Philadelphia, 1967.

36. Stead, E. A., Jr. Meaning of human behavior to the physician of tomorrow. (Editorial.) Arch. Internal Med. 110:409, 1962.
37. Van de Kamer, J. H., et al. A rapid method for the determination of fat in feces. J. Biol. Chem. 177:347, 1949.
38. Visscher, M. B., et al. Sodium ion movement between the intestinal lumen and the blood. Amer. J. Physiol. 141:488, 1944.
39. Weser, E., et al. Lactase deficiency in patients with the "irritable colon" syndrome. N. Engl. J. Med. 273:1070, 1965.
40. Whalen, G. E., et al. Diabetic diarrhea. A clinical and pathophysiological study Gastroenterology 56:1021, 1969.
41. Whitby, L. G., and Lang, D. Experience with chromic oxide method of fecal marking in metabolic investigations on humans. J. Clin. Invest. 39:854, 1960.
42. White, B. V., Cobb, S., and Jones, C. M. Mucous colitis. Psychosom. Med. Monogr. No. 1, 1939. (See also Ann. Internal Med. 14:815, 1940.)

Weakness

DAVID GROB

Weakness is among the commonest complaints presented to the physician. It is one of the presenting symptoms in the majority of patients with acute or chronic illness of any etiology. Less often it is the sole or predominant complaint. This chapter will consider both local and general weakness from a diagnostic point of view.

THE MOTOR SYSTEM

Weakness may result from impairment of any part of the motor system which governs the function of voluntary muscle (Fig. 23). The stimulus for voluntary movement begins in the highest cerebral centers, including the frontal lobes, which initiate passage of the motor impulse from the motor cortex down the corticospinal (pyramidal) tract to the motor nuclei of the brain stem and anterior horn cells of the spinal cord, and thence to the motor nerves. The stimulus must then cross the neuromuscular junctions between the endings of the motor nerve and the muscle fibers, following which it initiates contraction of the muscle fibers. This path taken by the stimulus for voluntary movement has been termed the motor system. It is made up of the centers for volitional activity in the frontal cortex, the upper motor neuron (motor cortex and cortiscospinal tract), lower motor neuron (anterior horn cell and motor nerve), neuromuscular junction, and muscle fibers. Muscle tone and movement are also influenced by other efferent as well as afferent systems, including the second motor cortex and the extrapyramidal (basal gangliar, brain stem nuclear), cerebellar, labyrinthine, reticulospinal, vestibulospinal, and proprioceptive pathways.[38]

MANIFESTATIONS OF DYSFUNCTION OF THE MOTOR SYSTEM

It is evident that a great variety of diseases may affect one part or another of the motor system, resulting in skeletal muscle dysfunction and ensuing signs and symptoms (Table 22). The manifestations of muscle dysfunction are limited, and consist, in decreasing order of frequency, of weakness, atrophy, stiffness, spasm, pain, tenderness, and abnormal movements[36] (Table 23). Weakness occurs in almost all disorders of the motor system, and is usually the presenting complaint. It may be subjective or objective, localized or generalized, and of acute or gradual onset. It may be accompanied by fatigue, i.e., decreasing work output on repeated effort. Subjective fatigue, which is the patient's self-appraisal in terms of body feelings, and which usually is described as tiredness, must be distinguished

DAVID GROB, M.D. Director, Department of Medicine, Maimonides Medical Center, and Professor of Medicine, State University of New York, Downstate Medical Center, Brooklyn, New York

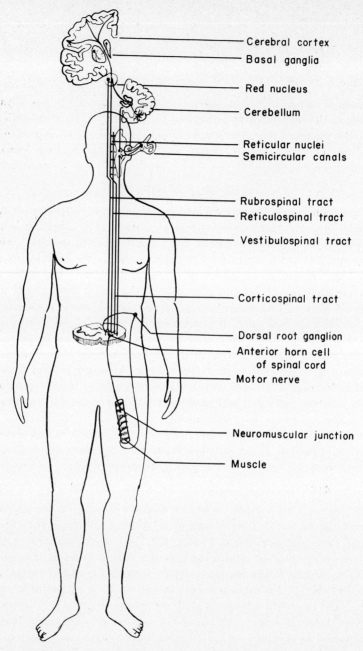

Cerebral cortex
Basal ganglia
Red nucleus
Cerebellum
Reticular nuclei
Semicircular canals
Rubrospinal tract
Reticulospinal tract
Vestibulospinal tract
Corticospinal tract
Dorsal root ganglion
Anterior horn cell
   of spinal cord
Motor nerve
Neuromuscular junction
Muscle

FIG. 23. The motor system. The stimulus for voluntary movement begins in the highest cerebral centers, which initiate passage of the motor impulse from the motor cortex down the corticospinal tract to the anterior horn cell of the spinal cord and thence down the motor nerve to the neuromuscular junction and to the muscle. Muscle tone and movement are also influenced by the effect of the cerebellar, extrapyramidal, and proprioceptive pathways on the anterior horn cells.

TABLE 22

Causes of Weakness

I. CENTRAL NERVOUS SYSTEM Emotional Upper motor neurone Extrapyramidal motor system Cerebellum	Vascular, infection, tumor, trauma, demyelinating, hereditary
II. LOWER MOTOR NEURON Anterior horn cells	Poliomyelitis, progressive muscular atrophy, syringomyelia, myelitis, tumor, disc, trauma
Nerves	Peripheral neuritis (*infections:* mononucleosis, polyneuritis, herpes zoster; *toxins:* diphtheria, lead, arsenic; *deficiency:* thiamine, nicotinic acid, B_{12}; *metabolic:* porphyria, amyloidosis; *vascular:* periarteritis) Tumor, disc, trauma
III. NEUROMUSCULAR JUNCTION Chemical agents	Depolarizing (acetylcholine, anticholinesterases, decamethonium, succinylcholine) Competitive (*d*-tubocurarine) Electrolyte concentration of plasma or muscle affecting neuromuscular junction, muscle, or nerve: low or high K^+, Ca^{++}, Na^+, Mg^{++}
Toxins	Botulinus, tetanus, venoms
Disease	Myasthenia gravis
IV. MUSCLE Infectious and debilitating diseases	Trichinosis, epidemic myalgia, neuromyasthenia, other
"Mesenchymal" tissue diseases	Dermatomyositis, myositis, scleroderma, lupus, periarteritis
Endocrine diseases	Hyper- or hypofunction of thyroid, adrenal cortex, anterior pituitary, parathyroid
Unknown cause	Muscular dystrophy, myotonic dystrophy, myoglobinuria

from objective fatigue, which can be measured. Weakness due to muscle dysfunction must be distinguished from limitation of motion due to joint, bursa, tendon, or bone pain, or to contracture.

EXAMINATION OF THE MOTOR SYSTEM

History

In addition to a general medical and family history of disease, note should be made of the patient's handedness (right or left). The examiner

TABLE 23
Manifestations of Dysfunction of the Motor System

Weakness	In almost all disorders
Wasting	In diseases of the lower motor neuron and of muscle
Stiffness or spasm	In diseases of the upper motor neuron and extrapyramidal system, poliomyelitis, tetany, tetanus, myalgia, scleroderma, muscle trauma, occasionally polymyositis
Pain	In poliomyelitis, spinal tumor, disc or osteoarthritis, some causes of peripheral neuritis, trichinosis, paroxysmal hemoglobinuria, epidemic myalgia, occasionally polymyositis
Abnormal movements	In some diseases of the extrapyramidal system, tetany, tetanus; fasciculations in progressive muscular atrophy and anticholinesterase poisoning

should obtain a careful description of the patient's complaint and symptoms, including time and nature of onset, distribution, progression, remissions, and variation. The patient's disabilities should be described. Inquiry should be made concerning visual impairment, ptosis, diplopia, hearing, balance, sensation to touch, pain, and temperature, and morning-evening variation in symptoms. Pain should be described, and localized if possible to muscle, joint, tendon, or bone. The marital and occupational history, variations in mood, and emotional and social aspects of the patient's complaint and disability should be recorded.

Physical Examination

A complete physical examination, with particular attention to the neuromuscular system, is mandatory in every patient who complains of weakness, whether generalized or localized. During examination the patient should be warm enough to prevent shivering, which may be mistaken for muscular fasciculations. The gait, posture, deformities, if any, and muscle bulk, tone, and strength should be observed. The range of active and passive movement at all joints and the power of each movement should be tested and graded. Joint disease, dislocation, or ankylosis may be revealed. Pain on motion should be noted, as it limits activity and may be mistaken for weakness.

The *distribution of weakness* should be delineated, to determine whether it is due to involvement of a specific muscle, of several muscles innervated by a peripheral nerve, nerve root, or segment of the spinal cord, of an entire extremity, or of a specific movement involving more than one muscle. The *degree of weakness* should be estimated as quantitatively as possible. Grip strength may be recorded by a hand dynamometer or ergometer. Flexors of the neck may be tested by timing the patient's ability to elevate his head while lying supine, and neck extensors may be similarly tested with the patient lying prone. Shoulder girdle muscles may be evaluated by noting the length of time the patient can elevate his arms when seated. Flexors of the thigh may be tested by determining the length of time the straight leg can be elevated from the supine position, and extensors tested from the prone position. Levators of the eyelids should be tested by measurement of the width of the palpebral fissures at rest, on maximal upward deviation, and after 1 minute of maximal upward deviation. The range of eye movement in each direction should be recorded (normal 45° laterally and medially, 40° up, and 60° down). Dysphagia may be evaluated by the use of the fluoroscope with barium swallow, and dysarthria by speech tests. The performance of any muscle should be recorded as a percentage of the normal value or in levels of 0 to 5.[20] This enables one to assess the effect of administration of pharmacologic agents for diagnostic tests, and the effects of placebo, suggestion, and therapy. It is important to keep in mind that clinical evaluation of muscle strength relies on the patient's effort, which needs encouragement to be maximal, and on the examiner's estimation of performance, and is therefore not entirely objective. A truly objective determination of muscle strength and fatiguability can be obtained by measuring the response of muscle to repetitive supramaximal nerve stimulation. While this is a valuable tool for research, it is rarely necessary for diagnosis.

Muscle *atrophy* is determined not only by inspection, but also by palpation, including comparison of muscles on opposite sides. At the same time muscle *tenderness* may be elicited. Muscle *tone* is evaluated by moving the extremity passively, first slowly through a complete range of motion, and then at varying speeds. *Coordination* is tested by the finger-nose-finger test, the heel-knee-toe test, standing with feet together and eyes open and then closed, gait, including tandem walking, and other voluntary activities. *Abnormal movements* should be observed, as should the effect on them of rest, voluntary activity, tension, fatigue, and, in some instances, sleep.

The *tendon reflexes* are elicited (jaw, biceps, triceps, supinator, quadriceps, and Achilles), and, if absent, the effect of reinforcement observed. The *superficial abdominal and cremasteric reflexes* are elicited. Rapid stretching of the tendons of the ankle, knees, and wrist is carried out to attempt to produce *clonus*. The *plantar reflex* is elicited by stroking the plantar surface of the foot as lightly as possible. The normal response, after the age of 1 or 2 years, is plantar flexion of the toes. A lesion of the upper motor neuron characteristically results in slow, tonic dorsiflexion of the toes, especially the great toe, and fanning of the toes (Babinski's sign).[77] Failure of the toes to move ventrally or dorsally in response to plantar stimulation may be significant, particularly if there is a difference between the two sides. Other forms of stimulation may also be tried: stroking the lateral aspect of the foot (Chaddock), or applying pressure to the tibia (Oppenheim), Achilles tendon (Schaeffer), or calf muscles (Gordon). The Babinski sign is the easiest to elicit, but occasionally it is worth trying two forms of stimulation simultaneously, particularly the Babinski and the Oppenheim or Gordon.[81]

Laboratory Studies

Serum

Enzymes Derived from Muscle. A number of enzymes leak into the plasma when membrane permeability is increased in certain diseases of muscle, particularly polymyositis, muscular dystrophy, paroxysmal myoglobinuria, and alcoholic myopathy (Table 24). These include glutamic and pyruvic transaminases (SGOT and SGPT), lactic dehydrogenase (LDH), aldolase, and creatine phosphokinase (CPK).[16] Since the transaminases are also present in liver, glutamic transaminase in heart, lactic dehydrogenase in liver, heart, lung, various neoplasms, and red blood cells, and aldolase in liver, heart, and red blood cells, it is not always possible to ascribe an increase in serum levels of these enzymes to disease of muscle. Creatine phosphokinase is absent from liver and red blood cells, and nearly absent from lung. The highest concentration of this enzyme is in skeletal muscle; the heart has $\frac{1}{3}$ this concentration, the brain $\frac{1}{6}$, and the uterus $\frac{1}{25}$. Since the mass of skeletal muscle is 50 times that of heart or brain, comprising 40 per cent of body weight, a moderate or marked increase in serum level of creatine phosphokinase can almost always be ascribed to disease of muscle. Minor elevations may also result from disease of the heart or brain, as well as from exercise, convulsions, lower motor neuron disease, menstruation, or pregnancy. Determination of

TABLE 24

Serum Enzymes Derived from Muscle and Other Tissues. Elevated in certain diseases of muscle (polymyositis, muscular dystrophy, paroxysmal myoglobinuria, alcoholic myopathy, clofibrate myopathy).

Enzyme	Concentration in Tissue
Glutamic-oxalacetic transaminase (GOT)	Liver > heart > skeletal muscle
Glutamic-pyruvic transaminase (GPT)	Liver > skeletal muscle
Lactic dehydrogenases	
LDH 1, 2	Heart > lung > erythrocytes > brain > kidney
LDH 3	Lung > thyroid > pancreas > nodes > adrenal > leukocytes
LDH 4, 5	Skeletal muscle > liver > lung > neoplasms
Aldolase	Liver > skeletal muscle > heart > erythrocytes > neoplasms
Creatine phosphokinase (CPK)	Skeletal muscle 18,000 $\times$ 10^{-4} unit/mg
	Heart 5,500 $\times$ 10^{-4} unit/mg
	Brain 3,000 $\times$ 10^{-4} unit/mg
	Uterus 700 $\times$ 10^{-4} unit/mg
	Gall bladder 500 $\times$ 10^{-4} unit/mg
	Adrenal 130 $\times$ 10^{-4} unit/mg
	Thyroid 113 $\times$ 10^{-4} unit/mg
	Lung 0.5 $\times$ 10^{-4} unit/mg

the serum level of creatine phosphokinase is the most useful chemical test for confirming the diagnosis of the diseases of muscle mentioned above, evaluating the activity of these diseases, and detecting preclinical stages and carriers of muscular dystrophy.

Potassium. Measurement of the serum level of potassium is important in the diagnosis of hypokalemia, hyperkalemia, and the periodic paralyses. Elevated serum levels are also encountered in paroxysmal myoglobinuria and alcoholic myopathy.

Glucose. The fasting and postprandial levels of glucose enable detection of diabetes and hypoglycemia.

Urine

Creatine. This compound is synthesized in the kidney, liver, and pancreas from glycine, arginine, and methionine. It is rapidly taken up from the serum by muscle fibers and converted reversibly into creatine phosphate, which is an important reserve of energy for muscular contraction. Creatinine, the anhydride of creatine, is formed from this compound and its phosphate in skeletal muscle and excreted in the urine in considerable and constant amounts (1 to 2 g/day). Normally little or no creatine is excreted in the urine: in adult males the upper limit of normal per day is 2 mg/kg, and in adult females and children 4 mg/kg, by the usual analytical techniques. In almost all disorders associated with muscle atrophy there is increased excretion of creatine in the urine, a proportionate decrease in excretion of creatinine, and usually an increased serum level of creatine. These changes are due in part to decreased uptake of creatine by the wasted muscles and decreased conversion to creatinine, but are not always proportional to the degree of atrophy. Creatinuria (mean figures in milligrams per kilogram per day) is most marked in some myopathies, such as muscular dystrophy[18] and polymyositis,[14] of moderate degree in neurogenic atrophy, such as progressive muscular atrophy and poliomyelitis,[9] of mild degree in disuse atrophy,[5] and absent in myasthenia gravis and other disorders not associated with muscular atrophy.[76] It is not clear why creatinuria is absent in myotonic dystrophy, and less marked in thyrotoxic myopathy than in uncomplicated hyperthyroidism. The determination of creatine in a 24-hour collection of urine is most helpful in the investigation of weakness of unknown origin not associated with obvious muscle atrophy, since increased creatinuria then provides evidence for loss of muscle bulk. It does not distinguish between neurogenic and myopathic disease, except that marked creatinuria suggests the latter.

Myoglobin. Myoglobinuria is most striking in paroxysmal myoglobinuria and alcoholic myopathy, and following crush injury of muscle. Minor degrees may occur in polymyositis or muscular dystrophy.

Electromyography

This technique is the study for diagnostic purposes of the electrical activity of skeletal muscle. The clinical examination indicates which muscles are to be studied. Recording electrodes are inserted in order to record electrical activity that occurs spontaneously or is evoked by voluntary muscle contraction or nerve stimulation. The information provided rarely supplies the diagnosis, but is often helpful in indicating the presence of a lesion of the lower motor neuron, neuromuscular junction, or muscle, and in localizing the lesion.[2]

Lower Motor Neuron Disease

Spontaneous electrical activity of muscle occurs following denervation resulting from a lesion anywhere in the lower motor neuron. Spontaneous discharges occur from muscle fibers and groups of fibers (*fibrillation potentials and positive sharp waves*) and from motor units and groups of motor units (*fasciculation potentials*). The latter may also be found in normal individuals, and hence are indicative of lower motor neuron disease only if accompanied by clinical evidence of such disease, particularly weakness and atrophy, or if they are of abnormal configuration, e.g., polyphasic or of increased amplitude or duration.

Voluntary muscle contraction results in no buildup of motor unit activity if denervation is complete. If incomplete, there is less buildup than normal on maximal effort (*incomplete interference pattern*), owing to reduction in the number of motor units. Even though there are fewer action potentials than normal, some may be of greater amplitude and longer duration than normal (*giant potentials*), as a result of reinnervation of denervated muscle fibers. There are also more *polyphasic potentials* (four or more phases) than the normal 2 to 4 per cent.

Muscle Disease

Voluntary muscle contraction results in normal buildup of motor unit activity (*complete interference pattern*), except in severe myopathy, since some activity is retained in all motor units. However, there are more *potentials of short duration and lower amplitude* and more *polyphasic potentials*, particularly of low amplitude, than normal.

Spontaneous electrical activity in the form of fibrillation potentials and high-frequency discharges may occur in some muscle diseases, probably owing to hyperirritability of muscle fibers. Such activity is most marked in the stiff man syndrome, myotonia congenita, myotonic dystrophy, and hyperkalemic periodic paralysis; long bursts of "myotonic" potentials, which oscillate in amplitude and frequency, may occur in these disorders, particularly after needle insertion, movement, or tapping of the muscle. Lesser degrees of spontaneous electrical activity may occur in polymyositis, muscular dystrophy, and hyperthyroidism, but fasciculations are very uncommon in muscle disease, in contrast to lower motor neuron disease.

Neuromuscular Junction Disease

Supramaximal stimulation of the nerve to the affected muscle of patients with myasthenia gravis results in progressive diminution (decrement) in the amplitude of the evoked action potentials. In patients with the Eaton-Lambert syndrome, usually associated with bronchogenic carcinoma, there is progressive increase (facilitation) in the evoked potentials, which are initially abnormally small.

Nerve Conduction Velocity

This measurement is useful for the detection of disease or injury of the peripheral nerves. *Motor nerve conduction* velocity is determined by stimulating a nerve at two points, recording the muscle action potential responses, and dividing the distance between the two points by the difference in time interval between nerve stimulation and each of the muscle responses. When stimulation of the nerve at two points is not feasible, measurement of prolongation of the latency between nerve stimulation and muscle response provides evidence of a lesion distal to the point of stimulation. *Sensory nerve conduction* is determined by stimulating the finger tip and recording the sensory potentials in the nerve at the wrist (orthodromic conduction), or by stimulating the nerve at the wrist and recording the sensory potential at the finger tip (antidromic conduction). A more precise procedure is to stimulate the finger tip and record the sensory potentials at two points along the nerve, and to divide the distance between the two points by the difference in time interval between nerve stimulation and each of the sensory potentials.

Slowing of motor nerve conduction occurs in motor peripheral neuropathy or injury, and of sensory nerve conduction in sensory peripheral neuropathy or injury. No change in motor nerve conduction rate occurs in diseases of the anterior horn cells or anterior roots, since, while some motor nerve fibers degenerate, the remaining fibers conduct at a normal rate. Likewise, no change in sensory nerve conduction occurs in spinal cord disease affecting sensory tracts or the posterior roots proximal to their ganglia.

Muscle Biopsy

This procedure is important in distinguishing between myopathic and neurogenic muscular atrophy, and in the diagnosis of many diseases of muscle, such as polymyositis, muscular dystrophy, paroxysmal myoglobinuria, trichinosis, and the rare myopathies.[28]

Nerve Biopsy

This procedure is employed far less often than muscle biopsy, and is less often helpful. Diagnosis of peripheral neuropathy can usually be made by clinical examination and measurement of nerve conduction velocity, but in the occasional instance when further confirmation is necessary, the sural or anterior tibial nerve may be biopsied to demonstrate histologic evidence of sensory (sural) or motor neuropathy of the lower extremity.[26] There are relatively few diseases in which the specific diagnosis can sometimes be made on the basis of nerve biopsy: periarteritis nodosa, amyloidosis, sarcoidosis, leprosy, and metachromatic leukodystrophy.

DIFFERENTIAL DIAGNOSIS OF WEAKNESS

In the initial approach to the patient with weakness it is helpful to localize the cause anatomically, if possible, and then to consider etiology. Anatomic localization is aided by considering the path taken by the motor stimulus down the motor system: frontal lobes → upper motor neuron (cerebral cortex and corticospinal tract) → lower motor neuron (anterior horn cells and motor nerves) → neuromuscular junction → muscle (Fig. 23).

Lesions of the upper motor neuron are recognized by characteristic changes: weakness with spasticity, increased tendon reflexes, clonus, and extensor plantar reflex, but no atrophy. Lesions of the lower motor neuron and most diseases of muscle produce weakness with atrophy, flaccidity, and decreased tendon reflexes. Other diseases of muscle or of neuromuscular transmission produce weakness without atrophy, usually without alteration in tendon reflexes. Some disorders of the motor system are associated with pain or with abnormal tone or movements.

The history and physical examination usually enable identification of the following settings in which weakness occurs:

I. Weakness with signs of upper motor neuron lesion
   Monoplegia, hemiplegia, paraplegia, quadriplegia
II. Weakness with atrophy
   Monoplegia, hemiplegia, paraplegia, or quadriplegia
      Acute onset
         Lower motor neuron
      Gradual onset
         Lower motor neuron
         Muscle
III. Weakness without atrophy or signs of upper motor neuron lesion
      Acute onset
         Neuromuscular junction
         Muscle
      Gradual onset
         Neuromuscular junction
         Muscle
IV. Weakness with pain
V. Weakness with abnormal tone or movements
VI. Subjective weakness

WEAKNESS WITH SIGNS OF UPPER MOTOR NEURON LESION

Injury to the upper motor neuron (motor cortex and corticospinal tract) may result from vascular disease (thrombosis, hemorrhage, or embolism of cerebral or spinal vessels), infection (encephalitis, meningitis, abscess, syphilis), disseminated sclerosis, pernicious anemia, amyotrophic lateral sclerosis, or brain or spinal cord tumor. An upper motor neuron lesion can usually be identified by its characteristic manifestations: weakness, spasticity, exaggerated tendon reflexes, clonus, extensor plantar reflex, and diminished abdominal and cremasteric reflexes. Muscle atrophy does *not* occur, or is slight, resulting from prolonged disuse rather than from disease.

If the lesion is in the motor cortex or in the corticospinal tract above the decussation of most fibers in the medulla, the side of the body opposite the lesion is affected, while if the lesion is in the spinal cord, the same side of the body is affected. After the initial period of paralysis, some movements gradually improve, in spite of the irreparable nature of destruction of central nervous system pathways. Groups of muscles, rather than individual muscles, are affected, and the proper relationship between synergists and antagonists is preserved. Movements are lost in approximate proportion to the unilaterality of their representation in the brain, and they are preserved or regained in proportion to the bilaterality of their representation. Therefore, the paralysis never involves all the muscles on one side of the body. Strictly unilateral movements, such as isolated movements of the extremities, are lost and never regained following a complete lesion of the corticospinal tract; movements which are sometimes bilateral and sometimes unilateral, such as those of the shoulders and hips, are regained to a large extent; and movements which are always bilateral, such as those of the pharynx, larynx, eyes, forehead, chest, abdomen, and spine, are never more than slightly affected, perhaps because they are represented almost equally in the two cerebral hemispheres. In the limbs the finer movements are impaired more than the grosser. Of the cranial musculature only the muscles of the lower face and tongue are involved to any significant degree. Movements of the upper part of the face are little affected.

Immediately after the occurrence of injury to the upper motor neuron the tone of the affected muscles is decreased ("spinal shock"), but after several days or weeks it becomes markedly increased; i.e., flaccidity is followed by spasticity. The abnormally increased muscle tone is attributed to removal of the inhibitory influence normally exerted by some of the fibers of the corticospinal and reticulospinal tracts on the reflex maintenance of tone by the anterior horn cells. The spasticity is usually greatest in the flexors of the arm and in the extensors of the leg, giving rise to the characteristic hemiplegic posture. The arm is adducted at the shoulder, semiflexed at the elbow, pronated at the forearm, and flexed at the wrist and fingers, while the leg is adducted, extended at the knee, and flexed and inverted at the ankle. The increased muscle tone and more synchronous discharge of the anterior horn cells in response to muscle stretch result in exaggeration of tendon reflexes and the appearance of ankle and patellar clonus. Upper motor neuron lesions also result in disappearance of the abdominal, cremasteric, and plantar reflexes. The last becomes extensor, as a result of release of the withdrawal reflex from inhibition by the corticospinal tract.

Injury transecting the spinal cord results in bilateral upper motor neuron lesions with paralysis which is at first flaccid but soon becomes spastic, as reflex activity returns to the distal cord and restores muscle tone. The tone of the flexor muscles of the legs is usually restored to a greater degree than that of the extensors, and function of the bladder is impaired.

Following an upper motor neuron lesion the *electromyogram* is normal, and the reaction of the muscle to stimulation by faradic current is normal; i.e., there is no reaction of degeneration. The *serum enzymes* are normal. The *muscle biopsy* is normal or shows minimal changes.

Monoplegia

Monoplegia refers to severe weakness or paralysis of all the muscles in one arm or leg. If muscle atrophy does not develop the most likely cause of monoplegia is an upper motor neuron lesion. The site of such a lesion is most likely the cerebral cortex or, less frequently, the thoracic or lumbar region of the spinal cord, since interruption of the corticospinal tract between these sites—i.e., the internal capsules, brain stem, or cervical cord—is much more likely to produce hemiplegia. A vascular lesion (thrombosis or embolism) is the commonest cause, but a tumor, abscess, or encephalitis may have the same effect. Multiple sclerosis or spinal cord tumor may, early in the course, cause weakness of one extremity, usually the leg. Monoplegia due to an upper motor neuron lesion is characteristically accompanied by spasticity, increased reflexes, extensor plantar reflex, and absent abdominal and cremasteric reflexes. However, during the first few days after onset of an upper motor neuron lesion, the period of "spinal shock," the muscles may be flaccid and the tendon reflexes normal or diminished.

Hemiplegia

Hemiplegia (weakness of an arm and leg on one side of the body) is the commonest distribution of severe weakness or paralysis. It almost always results from an upper motor neuron lesion. The commonest cause of hemiplegia is vascular disease of the cerebrum[3] or brain stem,[83] most often due to thrombosis superimposed on an arteriosclerotic plaque, and less often to intracranial hemorrhage; it may also reflect embolization from an auricular thrombus (especially in the presence of auricular fibrillation or mitral stenosis), from a mural thrombus following myocardial infarction, or from bacterial vegetations on the aortic or mitral valve (Table 25). The second commonest cause is trauma, resulting in contusion of the brain or subdural or epidural hemorrhage. Less common causes include primary or metastatic brain tumor, abscess, encephalitis, meningitis, disseminated sclerosis, tuberculosis, meningovascular syphilis, and encephalopathy associated with a distant neoplasm.[15] The site of the lesion can usually be deduced from the associated neurologic findings. A lesion of the cerebral cortex, corona radiata, or internal capsule produces weakness of the face, arm, and leg on the opposite side. A cortical lesion may also result in aphasia (if the lesion is on the dominant side), convulsions, cortical sensory loss (astereognosis, loss of two-point discrimination), or visual field defects. A lesion of the brain stem may cause paralysis of the muscles supplied by the oculomotor or facial nerve or of the tongue or palate on the same side as the lesion, owing to injury to anterior horn cells, as well as paralysis of

TABLE 25

Causes of Hemiplegia

Vascular	Arterial thrombosis (intracranial, extracranial); arterial embolus (from auricle, mural thrombus, bacterial endocarditis); arterial hemorrhage (hypertension, atheroma, aneurysm, thrombocytopenia, hypoprothrombinemia); venous or sinus thrombosis; infarction due to hypotension resulting from heart block, ventricular tachyarrhythmia, or other cause; hypertensive encephalopathy
Infection	Bacterial: meningitis, abscess
	Tuberculous: meningitis, tuberculoma
	Viral: encephalitis
	Fungal: cryptococcosis, moniliasis, aspergillosis, mucormycosis
	Syphilitic: meningovascular
Neoplasm	Primary, metastatic, tumor meningitis
Hypersensitivity	Polyarteritis, lupus erythematosus
Congenital	Aneurysm: berry, arteriovenous
Trauma	Laceration, subdural hematoma, birth injury
Toxic	Lead encephalopathy
Demyelination	Disseminated sclerosis, Schilder's disease

the arm and leg on the opposite side. A lesion of the corticospinal tract in the cervical spinal cord causes weakness of the arm and leg on the same side. This may result from disseminated sclerosis, syringomyelia, tumor, epidural abscess, cervical disc, spondylosis, or myelitis. Vascular disease of the spinal cord is uncommon, presumably owing to the collateral circulation network, but when thrombosis, hemorrhage, or arterial dissection does occur, the lesion is usually bilateral. Damage to the adjacent spinal tracts from any of these causes may result in loss of vibratory and position sense on the same side and of sense of pain and temperature on the opposite side (Brown-Séquard syndrome). Damage to adjacent anterior horn cells may cause a lower motor neuron lesion (weakness with wasting) at the level of the lesion.

Vascular Disease

Cerebral vascular disease is the commonest cause of paralysis of one or more extremities. It usually results in hemiplegia, less often monoplegia, and least often quadriplegia as a result of bilateral hemiplegia. Weakness due to cerebral vascular disease almost always results from a lesion of the corticospinal tract or motor cortex, and hence is accompanied by upper motor neuron signs, as previously described. On occasion it may be due to a lesion of the extrapyramidal motor system, or there may be loss of purposive movement without paralysis (apraxia).

Two-thirds of cerebral vascular accidents are due to *arterial thrombosis*, 20 per cent to *intracerebral hemorrhage*, 8 per cent to *subarachnoid hemorrhage*, and 5 per cent to *embolus*.[58] The onset of a cerebral vascular accident is usually sudden, with maximum intensity of weakness attained within minutes to hours after onset. However, at least 15 per cent of patients have premonitory manifestations for hours or days; these consist of headache, dizziness, drowsiness, mental disturbances, and focal neurologic signs, especially transient hemiparesis, aphasia, or paresthesia over half the body.[83] Headache is prominent at the onset of weakness in all patients with subarachnoid hemorrhage, 60 per cent of those with intracerebral hemorrhage, 25 per cent of those with cerebral embolus, and 6 per cent of those with thrombosis. Vomiting at onset occurs in half of patients with hemorrhage and in 10 per cent of those with embolus or thrombosis. Coma at onset occurs in half of those with hemorrhage and one-fourth of those with embolus or thrombosis, and convulsions (usually generalized, occasionally Jacksonian) at onset occur in 15, 9, and 7 per cent, respectively. Hence, the occurrence of headache, vomiting, coma, or convulsions at the onset of a cerebral vascular accident suggests that this is due to hemorrhage, but does not exclude embolus or thrombosis. Stiffness of the neck is usually, though not always, present after hemorrhage, and is only occasionally present after embolus or thrombosis, but cervical osteoarthritis, which is common in the elderly, may simulate this sign. Cheyne-Stokes or labored respiration, pupillary changes, conjugate deviation of the eyes, quadriplegia, and bilateral extensor plantar reflexes are also more common after hemorrhage.

The spinal fluid is grossly bloody in all patients with subarachnoid hemorrhage, in 85 per cent of those with intracranial hemorrhage (the remainder having encapsulated bleeding), and 15 per cent of those with cerebral embolus.[29] It is grossly clear in those with cerebral thrombosis, though there may be slight xanthochromia and red blood cells may be seen on microscopic examination. In patients with cerebral thrombosis the spinal fluid protein level is normal (below 45 mg/100 ml) in 69 per cent, slightly elevated (46 to 99 mg/100 ml) in 29 per cent, and more markedly elevated in only 2 per cent.

It is frequently difficult to distinguish between cerebral thrombosis and embolus. Cerebral embolus should be considered whenever there is sudden onset of paralysis in a patient with bacterial endocarditis, fever of undetermined origin with a cardiac murmur, or auricular fibrillation, mitral valve disease, or recent myocardial infarction.

Approximately one-fourth of patients with cerebral vascular accidents have extracranial thrombosis of the carotid, vertebral, or subclavian artery, which can be revealed by arteriographic studies. These must be undertaken before the hemiplegia is complete if arterial reconstruction is to have any value. The finding of a systolic bruit in the neck may provide supportive evidence of arterial stenosis.

Approximately 60 per cent of patients with subarachnoid hemorrhage bleed from a ruptured berry aneurysm, 30 per cent from a ruptured arteriosclerotic vessel, and 10 per cent from an arteriovenous aneurysm, tumor, or following trauma.[55] Since 75 per cent of berry aneurysms are in the anterior part of the circle of Willis, there may be premonitory signs of third, fourth, or sixth cranial nerve palsies, or visual changes due to pressure on the optic nerve, tract, or chiasm.[71] Following rupture there are signs of meningeal irritation (headache, stiff neck) and increased intracranial pressure (drowsiness, vomiting, coma, papilledema, and occasionally convulsions), focal signs (third, fourth, or sixth nerve palsies, hemiplegia, aphasia), and bloody spinal fluid. About 50 per cent of patients die (20 per cent during the first 2 days), and one-fourth to one-half of those who survive have one or more recurrences of bleeding, with the same mortality. Cerebral angiography usually identifies the berry aneurysm, and in 15 per cent of patients demonstrates multiple aneurysms.

Arteriovenous aneurysms produce recurrent episodes of subarachnoid hemorrhage in 50 per cent of patients with this lesion, but these episodes are less severe than in patients with berry aneurysm, and hemiplegia is less common. About 50 per cent of patients also have intermittent convulsions, usually focal and less often generalized, which may respond to anticonvulsant drugs.

Intracerebral hemorrhage usually results from rupture of an arteriosclerotic vessel, most often in a patient with arterial hypertension. Less often it may result from a tumor, berry aneurysm, or arteriovenous aneurysm, or may be due to thrombocytopenia or trauma. Focal neurologic signs, including hemiplegia, cranial nerve palsies, and coma, are more severe than following subarachnoid hemorrhage, and the mortality is even higher.

Brain Tumor

Four-fifths of brain tumors are primary and one-fifth are metastatic, particularly from the lung, breast, skin (especially melanoma), gastrointestinal tract, and kidney.[69] The manifestations of the tumor depend on its location, size, and invasiveness. Involvement of the pyramidal tract may cause hemiplegia; involvement of the motor cortex, monoplegia or hemiplegia; and involvement of the cranial nerves or their nuclei, signs of cranial nerve palsy. The development of slowly progressive hemiplegia or monoplegia, spreading from one part of the limb to another, is particularly suggestive of brain tumor, though in some patients the paralysis may set in rapidly. If increased intracranial pressure occurs there may be headache, vomiting, papilledema, visual impairment, and diplopia due to sixth nerve palsy. Focal or generalized convulsions, ataxia, incoordination, sensory changes, personality change, or impairment of consciousness may also occur. Examination of the spinal fluid protein and performance of an electroencephalogram, carotid and vertebral angiogram, radioisotope brain scan, and, if necessary, pneumoencephalogram or ventriculogram are helpful in diagnosis.

Occasionally a malignant tumor in almost any location may be associated with neurologic manifestations not attributable to metastases. The commonest is polyneuropathy. Less common are multifocal leukoencephalopathy involving the cerebral hemispheres, with hemiplegia, visual field impairment, and dementia. Myelopathy with paraplegia and segmental sensory loss, as well as cerebellar degeneration, may also occur.[15]

Syphilis

Manifestations of central nervous system involvement may appear at any time from a few weeks to 50 years after infection.[10] Approximately 3 per cent of patients develop acute meningitis or meningovascular syphilis a few weeks to 3 years following infection, with headache, stiff neck, and sometimes cranial nerve palsies, hemiplegia, or convulsions.[57] The serologic test for syphilis is positive in the blood in 75 per cent, and in the spinal fluid in 90 per cent, and protein and lymphocytes (100 to 2000/cu mm) are usually elevated in the spinal fluid.

If primary or secondary syphilis is untreated 9 per cent of patients develop tabes dorsalis, 5 per cent general paresis, and smaller numbers develop syphilitic meningitis or meningovascular syphilis, with manifestations as described above. Others may develop spinal spastic paraplegia, polyneuropathy, or syphilitic amyotrophy, resembling amyotrophic lateral sclerosis, usually 10 to 25 years after the infection.

General paresis is manifested by personality change or dementia in nearly all patients, and in half by paralytic attacks, often with hemiplegia. Other manifestations include slurred speech, tremor, or occasionally convulsions. Nearly all patients have pupillary abnormalities, chiefly miosis, and half have Argyll Robertson pupils. In 90 per cent the serologic test for syphilis is positive in the blood and spinal fluid, and spinal fluid protein and lymphocytes are increased. In *tabes* three-fourths of the patients complain of lancinating pains, half of ataxia, one-third of urinary incontinence or retention, and fewer of rectal incontinence, gastric or visceral "crisis" with pain, nausea, vomiting, or diarrhea, or visual impairment due to optic atrophy. Nearly all patients have pupillary abnormalities with miosis, and half have Argyll Robertson pupils. Half the patients have impairment of position sense, which is responsible for the ataxia and for a positive Romberg sign, half have impairment of vibratory sensation, and fewer have impairment of pain or touch. Nearly all patients have absent ankle jerks, and three-fourths have absent knee jerks. The serologic test for syphilis is variable in both blood and spinal fluid.

Paraplegia

Paralysis of both legs of acute onset is relatively infrequent, and is usually due to a lesion of the corticospinal tracts below the cervical cord. When paralysis occurs suddenly, in a matter of minutes, it is usually the result of traumatic or vascular necrosis of the spinal cord produced by fracture, dislocation of the spine, bleeding from a tumor or vascular malformation (hematomyelia from angioma or telangiectasis), or, less commonly, the result of a bleeding diathesis or hypertension. Other causes include occlusion of a spinal artery by a thrombosis on an arteriosclerotic plaque or by a dissecting aneurysm.[13, 68] When paralysis or weakness develops over hours or days, it may be the result of demyelinating disease (e.g., disseminated sclerosis), postinfectious or postvaccinal transverse myelitis, meningovascular syphilis, epidural abscess, Pott's disease, vertebral metastases, cord tumor, subacute combined degeneration, protruded cervical disc, spondylosis, syringomyelia, amyotrophic lateral sclerosis, or hereditary spastic paraplegia.[59] In each instance the upper motor neuron lesion is identified, after the initial period of spinal shock, by increased tendon reflexes and clonus in the legs and by extensor plantar reflexes. The muscles below the level of damage to the corticospinal tract are affected. If the adjacent spinothalamic tracts are damaged there will be loss of pain and temperature sensation below a particular level, and, if the posterior columns are damaged, loss of vibratory and position sense. In bilateral disease of the spinal cord the bladder and bowel sphincters may also be impaired. Lumbar puncture may show increased protein or cells in the spinal fluid and failure of spinal fluid pressure to rise on pressure over the jugular vein (positive Queckenstedt test).

Less frequently paraplegia developing over hours or days may be due to disease of the lower motor neuron, whether at the level of the anterior horn cells, cauda equina, or peripheral nerves. In this case the muscles are flaccid, tendon reflexes are diminished, fasciculations may occur, and atrophy develops within 2 to 3 weeks. Rarely, paraplegia developing over hours may be due to muscle disease, such as periodic paralysis or paroxysmal myoglobinuria, which are recognized by the transient nature of the weakness and by laboratory studies.

Spinal Cord Compression

When paraplegia occurs as a result of spinal cord compression it is vital to localize the lesion by myelography and relieve the compression by laminectomy before thrombosis of spinal vessels and complete or irreversible paraplegia occur. Causes of compression which produce sudden paraplegia include fracture or dislocation of the spine and epidural hematoma, while paraplegia may develop over hours or days as a result of epidural abscess, Pott's disease, vertebral metastases, cord tumor, ruptured cervical disc, or spondylosis.[6] The paraplegia is often preceded by evidence of compression of posterior nerve roots, resulting in pain, paresthesia, and sensory loss of segmental distribution, and of anterior nerve roots, resulting in lower motor neuron signs of weakness, diminished tendon reflexes, sometimes fasciculations, and eventually atrophy of segmental distribution. Damage to the corticospinal tracts results in paraplegia, with spasticity after the initial period of spinal shock has worn off, as well as increased tendon reflexes, clonus, extensor plantar reflexes, and urinary sphincter impairment. Damage to the spinothalamic tracts and posterior columns results in diminished sensation, with a sensory level near the lesion. The location of the lesion is indicated by the segmental distribution of root signs, by the sensory level, and sometimes by vertebral tenderness. Epidural abscess, which is more common in children, is suggested by the sudden development of pain in the back or legs and signs of cord compression in a patient who has, or is recovering from, a bacterial infection.[6]

Disseminated Sclerosis

This disease begins between the ages of 10 and 50 years, usually between 20 and 40 years. Its manifestations are due mainly to demyelination of the corticospinal tracts, cerebellum, spinocerebellar and spinothalamic tracts, posterior columns, and optic nerves.[47] Weakness of one or more extremities, usually the legs, of either acute or gradual onset, and due to upper motor neuron lesion, is the commonest presenting symptom, occurring in one-half the patients. Paresthesias, ataxia, or blurred vision are the initial symptoms in most of the others, and vertigo or urinary sphincter disturbance occur initially in a few. Weakness of one or more extremities is the commonest sign on examination (69 per cent), usually accompanied by spasticity and occurring mainly in the legs, with increased tendon reflexes and extensor plantar reflex in 89 per cent and absent abdominal reflexes in 70 per cent. The next most common signs are cerebellar: nystagmus in 68 per cent, intention tremor in 43 per cent, and ataxia and scanning speech in 20 per cent. Next in frequency are posterior column signs (diminished vibratory and postural sensation) in nearly one-half, temporal pallor of the optic discs in one-third, spinothalamic tract signs (decreased cutaneous sensation to pain and temperature) in one-fourth, and changes in affect in one-third, frequently with euphoria and occasionally with eventual mental deterioration. The diagnosis is difficult to make unless there is evidence of two or more spatially separated lesions and a history of spontaneous remission. The finding of an elevated γ-globulin concentration in the spinal fluid supports the diagnosis.

Subacute Combined Degeneration (Posterolateral Sclerosis)

This neurologic disorder is due to vitamin B_{12} deficiency, which results in degenerative, demyelinating lesions in the posterior and lateral (corticospinal) tracts, the peripheral nerves, and the brain. The commonest cause of vitamin B_{12} deficiency is pernicious anemia, a disease of late adult life, usually beginning in the fourth to sixth decade, and due to disappearance from the gastric secretions of intrinsic factor, necessary for absorption of vitamin B_{12}. Less common causes include dietary deficiency of vitamin B_{12} and decreased absorption of the vitamin due to total or partial[82] gastrectomy, intestinal malabsorption syndromes, intestinal blind loop or dilation proximal to a stricture, or fish tapeworm. Vitamin B_{12} deficiency of any cause results in macrocytic anemia, megaloblastic hyperplasia of the bone marrow, and soreness of the tongue. Patients with pernicious anemia also have gastric achlorhydria which is resistant to histamine administration, and an increased incidence of gastric carcinoma. In 80 per cent of patients with pernicious anemia, and in a smaller proportion of patients with other causes of vitamin B_{12} deficiency, neurologic symptoms gradually develop, and may appear at the same time as the anemia or later. Occasionally neurologic symptoms appear before the anemia, or in the absence of anemia, particularly in patients who have received folic acid, which produces a hematopoietic response but does not prevent the neurologic lesions of subacute combined degeneration.[9]

The initial complaints of subacute combined degeneration are usually due to sensory neuropathy, and consist of numbness, tingling, and occasionally pain in the distal portions of the extremities. Loss of sensitivity to pain, touch, and temperature may be present in minimal fashion. Posterior column damage results in loss of perception of vibration and position, particularly in the lower extremities. The proprioceptive loss causes sensory ataxia which is aggravated when the patient closes his eyes (positive Romberg sign). The motor symptoms begin as weakness in the lower extremities, followed by difficulty in walking and stiffness. If motor neuropathy is severe the weakness is flaccid, atrophy occurs, and tendon reflexes are diminished. If the lesion of the corticospinal tract predominates the weakness and gait are spastic, and tendon reflexes may be increased. The plantar reflex is usually extensor, and clonus may be present. In severely affected patients sphincter disturbances develop, and involve the bladder more often than the rectum. Lesions in the brain are believed to be responsible for the blurring of vision sometimes noted, and for mental disturbances, which are common and include irritability, confusion, amnesia, depression, and occasionally paranoia. The *spinal fluid* is usually normal, but may contain increased concentrations of protein.

Since signs of involvement of the posterior and lateral columns of the cord may also occur in multiple sclerosis, spinal cord tumor, spondylosis, arachnoiditis, and taboparesis, and since peripheral neuropathy of any cause may produce sensory ataxia and weakness, it is essential to demonstrate deficiency of vitamin B_{12} before initiating therapy. In the Schilling test, Co^{60}-labeled vitamin B_{12} is administered orally and absorption of vitamin B_{12} is determined by the urinary excretion, fecal elimination, or hepatic deposition of the cobalt. If urinary excretion is measured, a massive parenteral "flushing" dose of nonlabeled vitamin B_{12} is given prior to the labeled vitamin B_{12}. In normal subjects 62 to 82 per cent of ingested vitamin B_{12} is absorbed, and 7 to 10 per cent is excreted in the urine, while in patients with pernicious anemia only 5 to 15 per cent is absorbed and 1 per cent is excreted. Measurement of reduced plasma levels of vitamin B_{12} and observation of a reticulocyte response to parenteral administration of vitamin B_{12} are also of diagnostic value in previously untreated patients.

Quadriplegia

If the lesion affecting both corticospinal tracts is in or above the cervical cord weakness of all four extremities occurs. If the damage is in the lower segments of the cervical cord and the anterior horn cells are affected, as in syringomyelia or occlusion of the anterior spinal artery, the arms may show signs resulting from a lower motor neuron lesion, and the legs signs of an upper motor neuron lesion. If the damage is above this region of the cord all four extremities will show the signs of an upper motor neuron lesion. If the damage is above the cranial nerve nuclei concerned with swallowing pseudobulbar palsy will ensue. The commonest cause of quadriplegia is repeated cerebral vascular accidents or basilar artery insufficiency leading to bilateral hemiplegia.[83] Other causes are the same as those noted for paraplegia.

WEAKNESS WITH ATROPHY

Weakness with atrophy, flaccidity, and decreased tendon reflexes results from lesions of the lower motor neuron, and from most diseases of muscle (Table 22).

Disease of the Lower Motor Neuron

The anterior horn cells or cranial motor nerve nuclei and the motor fibers of the spinal or cranial nerves comprise the *lower motor neuron*, injury to which results in muscle weakness, atrophy, flaccidity, and decreased tendon reflexes. Destruction of either the cell body or axon fiber results in degeneration of the latter distal to the point of destruction. The muscle fibers which are thereby deprived of their motor nerve supply become paralyzed. The distribution of the palsied muscles depends on whether the lesion is in the anterior horn cells (or cranial nerve nuclei) or in the spinal roots or nerves, but in general distal muscles are more affected than proximal. All muscle reflexes, including tendon reflexes and reflexes responsible for the maintenance of muscle tone, are abolished after denervation, so that the muscle becomes flaccid. The contractile response of muscle to direct percussion is usually preserved. Within 3 weeks there begin spontaneous electrical discharges of single muscle fibers, or of groups of fibers constituting a fraction of a motor unit, giving rise to contractions called *fibrillations*. The resulting muscle movements are very fine, visible only in the tongue except in very thin individuals, and usually detected by electromyography. Within 3 months the denervated motor endplates and muscle fibers atrophy, resulting in about a 30 per cent reduction in muscle bulk, and then gradually disappear over a period of about 3 years. Slow degeneration of the anterior horn cells, as in progressive muscular atrophy or syringomyelia, or less often of the ventral roots, as in spondylosis or tumor, results in spontaneous discharges of single motor units or groups of motor units, which produce visible muscular twitchings termed *fasciculations*.

Weakness is the main manifestation of disease of the lower motor neuron, whether the lesion is in the anterior horn cells (or cranial nerve nuclei) or in their axons in the anterior roots or motor nerves. Sensory changes are absent when the lesion is localized to the anterior horn cells (as in progressive muscular atrophy) or anterior roots, and are usually present when the lesion is in the peripheral nerves, most of which consist of sensory as well as motor fibers. However, sensory changes may accompany an anterior horn cell lesion when there is simultaneous involvement of spinal sensory tracts, as in syringomyelia, and they may accompany anterior root disease when the posterior roots are also affected, as by a spinal cord tumor or intervertebral disc. Occasionally peripheral neuropathy may be purely motor. The coexistence of upper motor neuron signs below the level of a lower motor neuron lesion points to intraspinal disease.

LABORATORY STUDIES

The *electromyogram* is of great value in establishing the diagnosis of lower motor neuron disease and in differentiating this from disease of muscle. In lower motor neuron disease there occur in most patients spontaneous electrical discharges from muscle fibers and groups of fibers (fibrillation potentials and positive sharp waves) and from motor units and groups of motor units (fasciculation potentials). The latter are more frequent in diseases of the anterior horn cells than in diseases of the ventral roots, and least common in diseases of the peripheral nerves. They are more frequent in slowly progressive disease than in lesions of acute onset. During voluntary muscle contraction in patients with lower motor neuron disease the number of motor unit potentials is reduced; they are more likely to be discrete and of increased amplitude and duration ("giant potentials"), and there are more polyphasic potentials than are seen in normal subjects. Following complete degeneration of the motor nerve fibers the muscle continues to respond to galvanic (uninterrupted) stimulation, but no longer responds to faradic (interrupted) stimulation. This is known as the eaction of degeneration. The short duration of current flow in faradic

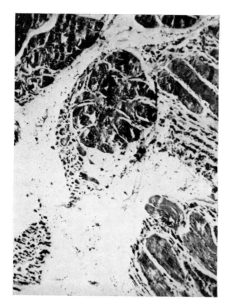 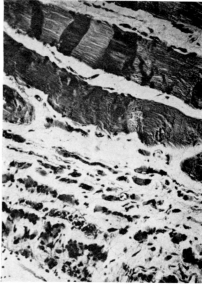

FIG. 24. Muscle atrophy of neurogenic origin, due to a lower motor neuron disease (progressive muscular atrophy). Note the grouped atrophy of muscle fibers in some fascicles, and normal fibers in adjacent fascicles. *Left,* cross-section; *right,* longitudinal section. ×130.

stimulation is capable of stimulating nerve, but not muscle, which has a longer chronaxie.

Motor and/or sensory *nerve conduction velocity* is usually below normal in diseases of the peripheral nerves, but is normal in diseases of the anterior horn cells or anterior roots.

The *serum level of enzymes derived from muscle* is normal or only slightly elevated. *Creatine excretion* in the urine is usually elevated in proportion to the extent of muscle wasting.

Muscle biopsy is of value in distinguishing between lower motor neuron disease and muscle disease.[4] In neurogenic disease atrophied fibers are more likely to be grouped, following the distribution of the destroyed motor units, with adjacent groups of normal fibers (Fig. 24), though in advanced disease the atrophy may become generalized. Atrophic fibers are more likely to be angular on cross-section, and target fibers, with darkly stained centers, may be identified. In myopathic disease muscle atrophy is more likely to be diffuse (Figs. 31 and 37).

Disease of Muscle

Some diseases of muscle result in weakness with atrophy, flaccidity, and decreased tendon reflexes. These include hyperthyroidism, hyperadreno-corticism, polymyositis, muscular dystrophy, myotonic dystrophy, and a number of rare myopathies. These diseases of muscle must be distinguished from diseases of the lower motor neuron which produce similar signs (Table 26). The distribution of weakness and wasting tends to be more proximal in diseases of muscle than in diseases of the lower motor neuron, and the

TABLE 26

Differentiation between Weakness Arising from Disease of Lower Motor Neuron (Neuropathy) and of Muscle (Myopathy). Similarities: weakness with wasting, flaccidity, and decreased tendon reflexes.

Differences	Neuropathy	Myopathy
Site of weakness	Distal	Proximal
Tendon reflexes	Decreased early	Decreased late
Muscle response to direct percussion	Present	Decreased (except in myotonia and hypothyroidism)
Sensory loss	May be present	Absent
Fasciculations	May be present	Absent
Complete paralysis	May occur	Rare (except in periodic paralysis)
Electromyogram: nerve conduction	May be delayed	Normal
Fibrillations and fasciculations	May be present	Rare
Biopsy: atrophy of muscle fibers	Grouped	Diffuse
Serum enzymes: aldolase, creatine phosphokinase, glutamic-oxalacetic transaminase, lactic dehydrogenase	Normal	Usually elevated

wasting and decrease in tendon reflexes tend to be less severe. The contractile response of muscle to direct percussion is usually reduced in diseases of muscle, except for myotonic dystrophy, hyperkalemic periodic paralysis, and hypothyroidism, while it is usually preserved in diseases of the lower motor neuron. Fascicular twitching does not occur in diseases of muscle, except rarely in hyperthyroidism; this finding usually indicates slowly progressive disease of the lower motor neuron. Sensory change does not occur in diseases of muscle, except rarely in polymyositis; this finding usually indicates disease of the peripheral nerves, posterior roots, spinal cord, or brain. If neither fascicular twitching nor sensory change is present, it may be difficult to distinguish between disease of muscle and of the lower motor neuron, and laboratory studies must be employed to localize the lesion.

LABORATORY STUDIES

The *electromyogram* in some diseases of muscle, particularly polymyositis and muscular dystrophy, shows more polyphasic motor unit potentials, usually of reduced amplitude, than are seen in normal subjects. These resemble to some extent the polyphasic potentials seen in patients with lower motor neuron disease, but are usually smaller and are much less likely to be accompanied by spontaneous electrical discharges. *Nerve conduction velocity* is normal.

The *serum levels of enzymes derived from muscle* are markedly elevated in muscular dystrophy and during the active stage of polymyositis. If the serum levels of these enzymes are elevated disease of muscle is indicated, but normal serum levels do not exclude inactive or chronic polymyositis or other diseases of muscle. *Creatine excretion* in the urine is usually elevated in proportion to the extent of muscle wasting.

Muscle biopsy is of great value in the diagnosis of some diseases of muscle, including polymyositis, muscular dystrophy, and the rare myopathies, and in distinguishing between myopathic and neurogenic disease. In myopathic disease muscle atrophy is more likely to be diffuse (Figs. 31 and 37), in contrast to the grouping of atrophic fibers in neurogenic disease. Atrophic fibers are more likely to be round in cross-section, and target fibers are rare. Muscle fibers may show evidence of degeneration, including swelling, hyalinization, basophilia, vacuolar degeneration, flocculation, fragmentation, and phagocytosis. In both neurogenic and myopathic atrophy there may be an increase in sarcolemmal nuclei, fat, and connective tissue, and infiltration with round cells, but these changes tend to be more marked in some myopathic diseases.

Monoplegia with Atrophy

Monoplegia is more frequently due to lesions of the lower motor neuron than of the upper motor neuron or of muscle. The lower motor neuron lesions, which may be in the anterior horn cells, spinal roots, or nerves, are recognized by the presence of muscular atrophy, flaccidity, decreased or absent tendon reflexes, and electromyographic changes.

Monoplegia with atrophy is relatively rare in the upper extremity. In infants the commonest cause is brachial plexus trauma, in children poliomyelitis, and in adults these causes or syringomyelia, early progressive muscular atrophy, spinal cord tumor or myelitis, protruded cervical intervertebral disc, spondylosis, or peripheral neuropathy, including that due to compression of the brachial plexus by cervical rib or scalenus muscles. Monoplegia with atrophy is more common in the lower extremity, and may result from any of these lesions affecting the thoracic or lumbar cord or its roots and nerves. Protruded intervertebral disc and mononeuropathy rarely paralyze all or even most of the muscles of a limb. While primary diseases of muscle, such as muscular dystrophy and polymyositis, may begin in one limb and produce weakness with atrophy, simulating diseases of the lower motor neuron, other limbs become involved soon after onset.

Hemiplegia with Atrophy

Hemiplegia is almost always due to an upper motor neuron lesion, in which case there is no associated atrophy, or only mild atrophy due to disuse, if the paralysis begins after skeletal growth has been completed. However, if the lesion occurred during infancy or childhood, the normal development of the muscles and skeletal system of the affected limbs is retarded, and these limbs, and even the trunk on one side, are small. When hemiplegia occurs as a result of spinal cord injury at any age, the anterior horn cells or ventral roots at the level of the corticospinal tract lesion may also be damaged, resulting in muscular atrophy at the level of the lesion, but not below it. Only rarely does a lower motor neuron disease, such as poliomyelitis, progressive muscular atrophy, or neuropathy, or a myopathy, such as facioscapulohumeral muscular dystrophy, produce weakness of an arm and leg on one side of the body. In these diseases atrophy occurs, and is usually visible within a few weeks after onset of weakness.

Paraplegia or Quadriplegia with Atrophy: Acute Onset

The association of weakness with atrophy, flaccidity, and diminished tendon reflexes enables one to localize the lesion to either the lower motor neuron or muscle. However, since atrophy may not be evident until 1 to 3 weeks after onset of a lesion at these sites, and since upper motor neuron lesions may cause weakness with flaccidity and diminished tendon reflexes during the initial period of spinal shock, localization of an acute lesion may be difficult. Limb weakness that develops very acutely, in a matter of minutes, is likely to be due to an upper motor neuron lesion, of the spinal cord in the case of paraplegia or quadriplegia, or of the cerebrum or brain stem in the case of hemiplegia. Limb weakness that develops over a period of hours or days is attributed to a lesion of the upper motor neuron if upper motor neuron signs appear, or to a lesion of the lower motor neuron, particularly peripheral neuropathy or poliomyelitis, if atrophy ensues. The occurrence of a sensory level or paralysis of bladder or bowel sphincters indicate a lesion in the cord. Distal sensory and motor loss, greater impairment of touch, vibration, and position sense than of pain and temperature, and sparing or only brief disturbance of sphincter function would point to a lesion of the peripheral nerves. Limb weakness, usually of all four extremities, develops rapidly, over minutes or hours, in a few diseases of muscle, such as periodic paralysis, paroxysmal myoglobinuria, and phosphorylase deficiency. However, muscular wasting does not ensue in these disorders, in contrast to lower motor neuron disorders, which result in atrophy within a few weeks.

In flaccid paralysis of acute onset occurring over hours or days poliomyelitis and polyneuritis must be considered, particularly if there is a preceding acute febrile illness. Poliomyelitis may usually be differentiated by the occurrence of meningeal signs, asymmetrical distribution of the paralysis and of the diminished tendon reflexes, pleocytosis in the spinal fluid, and absence of sensory impairment. Encephalitis may produce similar signs, but is less likely to produce weakness of the extremities. Polyneuritis is usually characterized by fairly symmetrical paralysis and diminished tendon reflexes, and by pain and paresthesias; other features include some sensory diminution (though this is not invariable), infrequency of ocular palsies, and, particularly in acute "infective" polyneuritis of unknown origin, increased protein without much pleocytosis in the spinal fluid.

Disease of Anterior Horn Cells

POLIOMYELITIS

After about 3 days of prodromal manifestations, such as fever and gastrointestinal or upper respiratory symptoms, there occur signs of central nervous system invasion, such as irritability, drowsiness, headache, backache, stiffness of the neck and back, pain, tenderness of muscles and nerves, and acute onset of muscular paralysis. The paralysis is irregular, almost always asymmetrical, and may be unilateral. The legs are most frequently affected and, in decreasing incidence, the arms, trunk, and cranial nerves (seventh, sixth, third, fourth, tenth, and eleventh, resulting in weakness of the facial, extraocular, sternomastoid, and trapezius muscles, and of swallowing function). Respiratory paralysis may occur. The fifth and twelfth cranial nerves, supplying the jaws and tongue, are usually spared. Sensory nerves, including the optic nerves, are almost never affected. The muscular weakness becomes maximal in a few days, remains so for about 3 weeks, and recovery then usually occurs over a period of 3 to 6 months. The muscles innervated by the cranial nerves usually recover completely. Muscles innervated by the spinal nerves generally recover completely if their function was only partially impaired acutely, but if they were completely paralyzed only partial recovery is likely. In over 90 per cent of the patients the leukocytes in the spinal fluid are increased during the first 2 weeks of illness, usually to between 50 and 100/cu mm, with lymphocytes predominating. After the second week the cell count is usually normal.

ENCEPHALITIS

The manifestations of encephalitis vary to some extent depending on the etiologic agent, which is usually viral (mumps, measles, ECHO, Coxsackie, equine, St. Louis, Japanese B, etc.) or, less frequently, bacterial, fungal, or toxic (alcoholic or Wernicke's encephalitis).[8] There are usually prodromal symptoms lasting 1 to 7 days, with some symptoms, such as lethargy, drowsiness, headache, and occasionally radicular pains, myoclonic twitching, and ocular palsies, pointing to invasion of the nervous system, and other symptoms indicative of respiratory or gastrointestinal infection. There may be mild cervical rigidity, but fever is variable and may be absent. The majority of patients develop disturbance of consciousness, indicating cerebral dysfunction: somnolence is the most characteristic feature and this may progress to stupor or coma, but occasionally there is excitement and even hyperkinetic activity. The second most characteristic feature of encephalitis is the occurrence of palsies of the extraocular muscles. The third nerve nuclei are most frequently affected, but the nuclei of the fourth and sixth nerves are also commonly involved. The oculomotor palsies are usually bilateral, but often incomplete, and may be transient or persistent. Frequently one group of muscles is recovering while another group is being involved. Ptosis of one or both lids and diplopia are usually present. The pupils are often dilated, and the reaction to light and convergence diminished or lost. Facial palsies are next to oculomotor palsies in frequency, and are usually incomplete and transient. Dysphagia is uncommon. The optic nerve heads are almost always normal: optic neuritis and retrobulbar neuritis may occur, but are rare. Mild hemiparesis or monoplegia, accompanied by signs of upper motor neuron disease, occasionally occurs, but paralysis of the extremities is rare and, if present, is of brief duration. Evaluation of strength, however, is often difficult and the patient may appear to be weaker than he is. During deep coma or stupor the plantar reflexes are often extensor. Convulsions are unusual, and when present are usually focal rather than generalized. In the hyperkinetic form of encephalitis, lethargy and immobility are replaced by excitement, restlessness, and insomnia, and there may be involuntary movements such as tremors, choreiform movements, and myoclonic twitchings.

The *spinal fluid* contains increased lymphocytes, usually between 20 and 200/cu mm, but these may diminish after the first 2 weeks of disease. The *duration* of acute encephalitis varies from a few days to several weeks or even months. While most patients recover completely, some have residual signs of persistent oculomotor palsy, pupillary changes, extremity weakness, or alteration in behavior or personality. About 30 per cent of patients who have had epidemic encephalitis develop *sequelae* several months or years after apparent recovery. The commonest is the parkinsonian syndrome, consisting of muscular rigidity with cogwheel phenomenon, altered posture with flexion of the trunk and extremities, slowness of all movements, expressionless face, excessive salivation, rhythmical tremor at rest, and absence of arm swinging in gait. The rigidity may eventually become so severe that the patient is virtually paralyzed. Other sequelae include choreiform, myoclonic, or dystonic movements, tics, oculogyric crises, narcolepsy, and, particularly in children, reversal of sleep rhythm and personality changes with impulsive and destructive behavior.

Disease of Peripheral Nerves

Lesions of the peripheral nerves may occur acutely, as in peripheral neuritis or trauma, or more slowly, as in pressure due to cervical rib, carpal tunnel syndrome, hypertrophic osteoarthritis of the spine, spinal cord tumor, and hereditary diseases such as peroneal muscular atrophy and interstitial hypertrophic polyneuropathy. The peripheral neuropathies can be classified in several ways. They may be classified on the basis of etiology (Table 27), predominant symptoms (motor, sensory, and autonomic), distribution of nerves affected (mononeuritis, mononeuritis multiplex, and diffuse neuropathy), or course (acute, subacute, and chronic, or progressive and relapsing).[25]

The manifestations of peripheral neuropathy are due to lesions of the motor, sensory, and autonomic fibers of the peripheral nerves. In diffuse neuropathy the manifestations are usually symmetrical, and are more marked distally than proximally. Disease or injury of *motor nerve* fibers results in the characteristic manifestations of a lower motor neuron lesion: muscular weakness, flaccidity, softness, atrophy, and decreased tendon reflexes. If the disease or injury is slowly progressive, fasciculations may

TABLE 27

Causes of Peripheral Neuropathy

Infectious	Bacterial: leprosy
	Viral: infectious mononucleosis, herpes zoster
Hypersensitivity	Serum sickness, polyarteritis nodosa
Congenital	Peroneal muscular atrophy, hypertrophic interstitial polyneuropathy, hereditary sensory neuropathy
Deficiency	Thiamine deficiency, alcoholism, pellagra, pernicious anemia, sprue, pyridoxine deficiency
Toxic	Bacterial: diphtheria
	Tick: *Dermacentor andersoni*
	Chemical: heavy metals (As, Hg, Bi, Pb, Th), carbon monoxide, organic phosphates, sulfonamides, vincristine, vinblastine, isoniazid
Metabolic	Diabetes, uremia, porphyria, amyloidosis, Refsum's syndrome
Neoplastic	Pressure (e.g., Pancoast tumor), carcinomatous neuropathy
Vascular	Arterial or venous thrombosis
Trauma	Spondylosis, ruptured intervertebral disc, carpal tunnel syndrome, pressure, fracture, dislocation, wound
Unknown cause	Acute "infective" polyneuritis (Guillain-Barré), chronic polyneuritis

also occur, but they are less pronounced than in slowly progressive disease of the anterior horn cells. The functional loss differs from that which follows destruction of anterior horn cells in that it is usually not permanent, since regeneration of peripheral nerves and reinnervation of motor endplates occur if the cause of the interruption is removed before complete atrophy of the muscle has occurred. In addition, when the lesion is in the peripheral nerves, the motor loss is frequently accompanied by sensory loss, as both motor and sensory nerve fibers may be affected.

Lesions of the *sensory nerve* fibers result in paresthesias, sensations of pain, burning, and numbness, tenderness, hypo- or hyperesthesia, and loss of sensation for touch, pain, temperature, vibration, and position. The manifestations are predominantly distal, and are often of stocking and/or glove distribution. Vibratory sensation is usually impaired to a greater degree than position sense, in contrast to the effect of lesions of the spinal cord or brain, which tend to affect proprioception more than vibratory sensation.

Lesions of *autonomic nerve* fibers result in vasomotor changes (warmth or coolness, pallor or cyanosis) and trophic change, such as sweating and increased hair growth with incomplete lesions, or anhydrosis and decreased hair growth with complete lesions; pigmentation or depigmentation, irregular growth of nails, and skin ulcers also occur. Lesions of splanchnic nerves may result in postural hypotension, anhidrosis, impotence, and nocturnal diarrhea.

In diffuse neuropathy weakness and wasting are predominantly distal in distribution (Fig. 25), spinal fluid protein is usually increased, and sensory impairment is often present. These findings point to disease of the peripheral nerves or spinal cord rather than of muscle. However, if these findings are not present, it may not be possible to distinguish by clinical examination between weakness, atrophy, flaccidity, and diminished tendon reflexes due to disease of the lower motor neuron and the effects of primary muscle disease. The differentiation may be made by demonstrating in the patient with neuropathy delayed motor or sensory nerve conduction, spontaneous fibrillations, fasciculations, or giant potentials, normal serum levels of some of the enzymes present in muscle, and "neurogenic" distribution of muscle atrophy in the muscle biopsy (Table 26).

PERIPHERAL NEUROPATHY OF ACUTE ONSET WITH PREDOMINANTLY MOTOR
    MANIFESTATIONS

The most abrupt onset, occurring over minutes or hours and suggesting vascular occlusion, is seen in ischemic neuritis, periarteritis nodosa, and paralysis of the third cranial nerve in diabetes mellitus. A course with rapid onset over several days, a peak within about 2 weeks, and gradual improvement over several months is seen in the Guillain-Barré syndrome, porphyria, and reaction to toxic exposure.

Guillain-Barré Syndrome (Acute "Infective" Polyneuritis). This is the commonest type of diffuse, predominantly motor neuropathy of acute

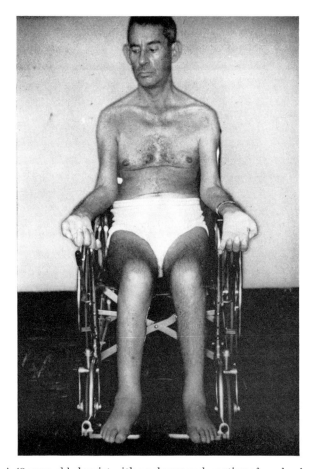

FIG. 25. A 48-year-old chemist with weakness and wasting of predominantly distal distribution due to peripheral neuropathy caused by organic phosphate compounds

onset.[53] It may occur at any age, but most often between 20 and 40 years. In two-thirds of the patients with this syndrome there is a prodromal illness, usually of the upper respiratory tract, less often of the gastrointestinal tract, and occasionally due to infectious mononucleosis. After a latent period of 5 to 18 days there occurs rapidly progressive, symmetrical weakness, usually beginning in the legs and ascending within 1 or 2 days to the arms and face. There is often low-grade fever, headache, pain in the limbs and back, and occasionally vomiting. The distribution of weakness differs from that seen in most other types of neuropathy, which involve predominantly the distal musculature, in that the proximal muscles may be involved to the same degree as the distal, or to even a greater degree, and over three-fourths of the patients have facial diplegia. Half the patients have weakness of the muscles of swallowing and speech, and one-fourth have respiratory weakness. Extraocular muscles are seldom impaired. Muscular weakness reaches its peak 2 to 21 (average, 12) days after onset. Muscle wasting occurs to a moderate degree, and tendon reflexes are diminished. Sensory manifestations usually occur, and are initially of stocking or glove distribution, with paresthesias, dysesthesias, pain, muscle tenderness, and impairment of all forms of sensibility. Occasionally sensory manifestations are minimal or absent. About 15 to 30 per cent of patients die of respiratory failure, aspiration, pneumonia, or pulmonary embolism. The remainder gradually improve over a period of 3 to 6 months, with most recovering completely, though some have residual disability or even chronic relapsing polyneuropathy.

Spinal fluid protein is characteristically elevated (50 to 1000 mg/100 ml), and there is usually no pleocytosis. However, in 25 per cent of patients the initial examination of the spinal fluid is normal, and the protein rises after the first week. In 20 per cent there is an increase in lymphocytes in the spinal fluid (10 to 100/cu mm). The cause of Guillain-Barré syndrome is not known, but an autoimmune mechanism is suggested by the reported occurrence of complement-fixing antibodies to nervous tissue in the sera of 50 per cent of patients.

Acute Intermittent Porphyria. The peripheral neuropathy that may occur in this disease resembles that of the Guillain-Barré syndrome, but the presence of porphyria should be suspected if there is familial disease (dominant, with variable penetrance) or a history of gastrointestinal symptoms (nausea, vomiting, cramping pain, constipation), hypertension, mental symptoms, or exacerbation following the administration of barbiturates, sulfonamides, fungicidal agents, or heavy metals. During acute attacks porphobilinogen is always present in the urine, and between attacks it is usually present.

Toxins: Diphtheritic Polyneuritis. One to three weeks after onset of diphtheria there occurs palatal weakness, with nasal voice and regurgitation and difficulty in swallowing. This is followed by palsy of the third cranial nerves, with weakness of extraocular muscles and paralysis of accommodation, resulting in blurring of near vision. Weakness then progresses over days or weeks to muscles innervated by other cranial nerves and by spinal nerves, and sensory manifestations may appear. Paralysis is maximal in several weeks, and recovery occurs over several months.

Tick Paralysis. The salivary glands of the Rocky Mountain wood tick, *Dermacentor andersoni*, secrete a toxin which produces weakness and sometimes ascending paralysis, resembling the Guillain-Barré syndrome.

Heavy Metals. Acute or chronic poisoning by lead, arsenic, thallium, mercury, bismuth, or gold may result in weakness and wasting, mainly in the extremities, due to peripheral neuropathy. In lead poisoning the extensors of the fingers and wrists are often involved, usually bilaterally, resulting in wrist drop, and sensory manifestations are usually slight. In arsenic poisoning sensory signs are more prominent. The occurrence of alopecia with motor and sensory neuropathy should alert the physician to the possibility of poisoning by thallium, a constituent of some rodenticides.

Organophosphorus Compounds. Some organophosphorus compounds, particularly tricresyl phosphates (TCP), including tri-*o*-cresyl phosphate (TOCP), have neurotoxic effects which give rise to severe polyneuritis, mainly motor in type, and involving both upper and lower extremities.[75] TOCP and TCP are constituents of some lubricating oils and plastics, and many instances of polyneuritis, some of epidemic proportions, have occurred from accidental or intentional contamination of cooking oils and other food or drink, or from industrial exposure. Some organophosphorus insecticides, such as mipafox, have also caused polyneuritis. While almost all the organophosphorus compounds that have neurotoxicity also have anticholinesterase activity, the neurotoxicity has been a late effect of these compounds, occurring after subsidence of any anticholinesterase effects and without any apparent relation to these effects.[21] Approximately 2 weeks after exposure there occur numbness, tingling, and crampy pains in the extremities. One or two days later weakness begins in the lower extremities, and about 1 week later in the upper extremities. Weakness becomes maximal in a few days and persists for many months. Sensory signs and symptoms are less marked than the motor changes, and usually disappear in 2 to 3 weeks. Bulbar and respiratory muscles are seldom severely affected, so that fatalities have been few. However, weakness and wasting of all extremities, particularly the lower extremities, persist for 6 to 18 months, following which there is slow improvement, in reverse order to the sequence of paralysis. Some patients have also had evidence of upper motor neuron lesion involving the pyramidal tracts. Twenty per cent of patients have still been paralyzed 6 years after poisoning (Fig. 25).

Trauma. Traumatic injury to a peripheral nerve or nerve root may result from bone fracture, joint dislocation (especially at the shoulder), protrusion of a cervical or lumbar intervertebral disc, carpal tunnel syndrome (median nerve palsy), pressure (Saturday night or bridegroom's radial nerve palsy), occupational trauma, as in prolonged squatting (external popliteal nerve palsy with foot drop), or knife or bullet wounds.

PERIPHERAL NEUROPATHY OF ACUTE ONSET WITH PREDOMINANTLY SENSORY
    MANIFESTATIONS

Infections. The neuritis produced by herpes zoster is readily recognized by the unilateral localization of pain in the distribution of the affected nerve, and by the vesicular skin eruption which occurs in this distribution, and which may occur some days after onset of the pain. In some patients the disease may be associated with an underlying lymphoma.

Leprosy could well be among the commonest causes of neuropathy in the world. While the disease is contracted in the tropics, it may not become manifest until 1 to 5 years after the patient has left the tropics. *Mycobacterium leprae* affects skin (often with leonine facies), mucous membranes of the respiratory tract, lymph nodes, bone (resorption), and nerves. Neuropathy is mainly sensory, resulting in numbness, paresthesias, and anesthesia. Muscle weakness and atrophy may also occur.

Dietary or Other Deficiency (Alcoholism, Pellagra, Malabsorption,

Pernicious Anemia). Among the more common causes of predominantly sensory neuropathy are alcoholism (thiamine deficiency), pellagra (multiple vitamin B deficiency), malabsorption syndrome (vitamin B_{12} and folic acid deficiency), and pernicious anemia (intrinsic factor deficiency leading to vitamin B_{12} deficiency). Symptoms of alcoholic neuropathy include burning, prickling, and jabbing discomfort in the feet and hands, often made worse by exercise. The muscles may be tender, and there may be associated weakness, atrophy, and areflexia. Improvement usually occurs after the administration of large doses of thiamine. In pellagra there is also photosensitivity dermatitis, with a scaly rash on the face and hands, glossitis, diarrhea, and psychiatric symptoms. In the malabsorption syndrome and pernicious anemia there may also occur evidence of posterior column injury (ataxia due to loss of proprioception, and decreased vibratory sensation) and of lateral (corticospinal) tract injury (upper motor neuron signs). Patients who receive isonicotinic acid hydrazide (INH) in the management of tuberculosis may develop sensory neuropathy which has been attributed to pyridoxine deficiency, and which is preventable by concomitant administration of pyridoxine to patients receiving INH.

Diabetes. Prolonged diabetes may result in several types of neuropathy.[17] The commonest is sensory neuropathy, manifested by aching or burning pain in the legs, especially the calves, and sometimes by paresthesias. The pain can be differentiated from intermittent claudication due to peripheral vascular insufficiency by the more striking relation of the latter to exercise. In sensory neuropathy examination will reveal hyperesthesia or hypoesthesia in the distal extremities, decreased vibratory sensation, and sometimes decreased proprioception. Motor neuropathy may or may not be present. Diabetes may also produce motor neuropathy, with or without sensory neuropathy. A single motor nerve may be affected, most commonly the third cranial nerve, resulting in ocular palsy, usually of acute onset, with or without ptosis and pupillary change. A number of motor nerves may be involved, as in mononeuritis multiplex or diabetic amytrophy,[50] or, less often, there may be widespread polyneuropathy resembling the Guillain-Barré syndrome, though of more gradual onset and longer duration (Fig. 26). Diabetes may also cause neuropathy affecting the sympathetic nervous system, resulting in decreased sweating in affected areas, nocturnal diarrhea, orthostatic hypotension, and impotence.

Toxins. A number of chemical agents may produce sensory neuropathy, with or without motor signs. These include vincristine and vinblastine as well as arsenic and other heavy metals. Endogenous toxins may be responsible for sensory and motor neuropathy in uremia, and for some remote neurologic effects of carcinoma (carcinomatous neuropathy).[12]

Disease of the Neuromuscular Junction or Muscle

The diseases of the neuromuscular junction or muscle that produce weakness of the extremities of acute onset, over minutes or hours, such as botulism, anticholinesterase intoxication, periodic paralysis, paroxysmal myo-

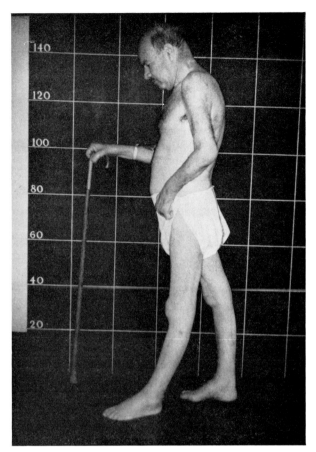

Fig. 26. A 59-year-old man with weakness and wasting due to peripheral neuropathy caused by diabetes mellitus. Note wasting of quadriceps muscles (diabetic amyotrophy).

globinuria, and, rarely, myasthenia gravis, do not cause muscular atrophy. Several diseases of muscle that produce weakness and atrophy of gradual onset, over weeks, such as polymyositis or hyperthyroidism, may occasionally begin more acutely, over a period of days. During the first few days after onset of weakness, before atrophy becomes evident, it may be difficult to distinguish some of these diseases of the neuromuscular junction or muscle from diseases of the lower motor neuron, such as acute polyneuropathy, unless the latter are accompanied by sensory signs or symptoms. The diagnosis of these diseases is discussed later.

Paraplegia or Quadriplegia with Atrophy: Gradual Onset

In paraplegia or quadriplegia of gradual onset, developing over a period of weeks, the presence of atrophy indicates that the lesion is in the lower motor neuron or in mucles. Lower motor neuron lesions may be in the anterior horn cells (progressive muscular atrophy, syringomyelia), in the ventral roots (spinal cord tumor, disc, or spondylosis), or in the peripheral nerves. Lesions restricted to the anterior horn cells (e.g., progressive muscular atrophy), muscle diseases, and some peripheral neuropathies produce only motor manifestations. Spinal cord lesions that affect sensory tracts or posterior roots, and most peripheral neuropathies, also result in sensory changes in which the cord lesions are usually manifested by a sensory level and the neuropathies by distal changes, often of stocking-glove distribution. Slowly progressive lesions of the anterior horn cells usually produce fasciculations, which are rarely present in diseases of muscle or of peripheral nerves. It is more difficult to distinguish among muscle disease, motor neuropathy, and anterior horn cell disease in the absence of fasciculations. Differentiation among these disorders is aided by measurement of motor nerve conduction (delayed only in neuropathy), electromyography (spontaneous fibrillations and fasciculations most pronounced in anterior horn cell disease), serum levels of some of the enzymes present in muscle (elevated in polymyositis and muscular dystrophy), and muscle biopsy (grouped atrophy of muscle fibers in anterior horn cell disease or neuropathy, diffuse atrophy in muscle disease).

Diseases of Anterior Horn Cells

PROGRESSIVE MUSCULAR ATROPHY

A number of chronic diseases affecting anterior horn cells and cranial motor nerve nuclei produce progressive weakness and atrophy of the extremities and of muscles innervated by cranial nerves (lower motor neuron signs), and occasionally upper motor neuron signs. It is not known whether these consist of several distinct diseases or of one disease with various manifestations. Classification is possible on the basis of age of onset, distribution of weakness, chronicity, and presence or absence of upper motor neuron signs, but there is considerable overlap. In adults the commonest form is *amyotrophic lateral sclerosis*, which is a combination in varying proportions of three diseases: *progressive spinal muscular atrophy*, affecting mainly muscles of the trunk and limbs, *progressive bulbar palsy*, affecting mainly muscles innervated by cranial nerves, especially the tongue and pharynx, and *primary lateral sclerosis*, affecting mainly the pyramidal tracts.[52] These diseases are only occasionally familial. The lower motor neuron lesion results in progressive weakness, decreased reflexes, atrophy and fasciculation of the muscles of the extremities, especially distally, and of the trunk and tongue, and impairment of swallowing and speech. The upper motor neuron lesion results in spasticity, mainly in the lower extremities, and extensor plantar reflexes. The mean duration of the disease to death is 3 years from the onset of peripheral muscle weakness, and $1\frac{1}{2}$ years from the onset of bulbar weakness. Five-year survival is only 10 per cent. The presence of fasciculations accompanying weakness and atrophy, and spontaneous electromyographic activity, aid in localizing the lesion to the lower motor neuron and to the anterior horn cells. Absence of sensory changes, of delayed nerve conduction, or of elevation of spinal fluid protein, and the progressive course of the disease, help to distinguish the disease from polyneuropathy. The normal or only slightly elevated levels of serum enzymes derived from muscle, and evidence of neurogenic muscle atrophy on biopsy, help to distinguish the disease from myopathy.

A less common lower motor neuron disease, *chronic proximal spinal muscular atrophy*, differs from amyotrophic lateral sclerosis and progressive spinal muscular atrophy in the following ways: familial incidence is much higher (60 per cent); juvenile onset is more common; proximal muscles are affected more than distal (Fig. 27); fasciculations are less common (50 per cent) and less pronounced; dysphagia and dysarthria are much less common (15 per cent) and life-threatening dysphagia is rare; extensor plantar reflex is much less common (6 per cent); and the course is much more prolonged (mean duration, 30 years).[60] Since the main manifestations

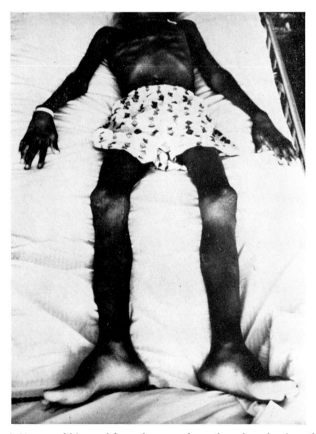

FIG. 27. A 16-year-old boy with weakness and wasting of predominantly proximal distribution due to chronic proximal spinal muscular atrophy. Note that the thigh muscles are more wasted than the calf muscles.

of the disease, slowly progressive proximal muscle weakness and atrophy with diminished tendon reflexes, resemble those of myopathy, diagnosis may be difficult when fasciculations are undetected. The electromyogram is helpful, revealing evidence of a lower motor neuron lesion in 97 per cent, with spontaneous discharges in 50 per cent and giant potentials in 90 per cent. The electromyogram shows nerve conduction to be normal. Spinal fluid is normal. The serum levels of enzymes derived from muscle are normal in 90 per cent, and slightly elevated in the remainder. Muscle biopsy shows neurogenic atrophy in 68 per cent, and both neurogenic atrophy and myopathic changes (probably secondary to atrophy) in 19 per cent.

SYRINGOMYELIA

This condition results from slowly progressive cavitation and gliosis of the cervical or lumbar cord and/or medulla (syringobulbia), beginning dorsal to the central canal and extending laterally and posteriorly to compress the posterior horns, anterior horns, and long tracts.[54] Destruction of anterior horn cells causes lower motor neuron signs, sometimes including fasciculations at the level of the lesion, usually in the hand, arm, and/or shoulder. The signs may be unilateral or bilateral, symmetrical or asymmetrical, depending on the location of the syrinx. There is decreased pain and temperature sensation at the level of the lesion, since decussating fibers are more likely to be destroyed by the syrinx, while light touch, vibration, and proprioception are initially intact (sensory dissociation). Loss of pain and temperature sensation results in burns and other trauma going unnoticed. Occasionally pain occurs. Trophic disturbances, including Charcot joints, may occur in the affected extremities (Fig. 28). Late in the disease damage to the corticospinal tracts may cause spastic paraplegia

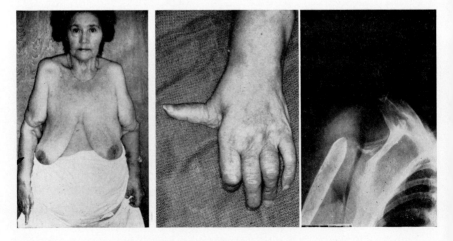

Fig. 28. A 67-year-old woman with weakness, wasting, joint deformity, and Charcot joint (note absence of head of humerus) due to syringomyelia.

with upper motor neuron signs below the level of the lesion, and sometimes bladder disturbance, and damage to the posterior columns may cause decreased proprioception and vibration sense below the lesion. The spinal fluid is occasionally xanthochromic, and its protein content may be elevated. Radiologic examination, including myelography, is necessary to exclude tumor, disc, and spondylosis. Subacute combined degeneration may also have to be excluded.

Disease of Spinal Nerve Roots (Radiculopathy)

SPONDYLOSIS (OSTEOARTHRITIS OF THE SPINE)

The spine is the commonest site of radiologic change due to osteoarthritis in men, and second in frequency only to Heberden's nodes in women. However, symptoms are usually absent or mild (backache, stiffness, limitation of motion), except in the minority of patients who develop compression of nerve roots (radiculopathy) or spinal cord (myelopathy).[14] The primary pathologic process is degeneration of the intervertebral discs, which results in increased stress at the lips of the vertebral bodies and zygapophyseal joints, leading to osteophyte formation and narrowing of the intervertebral foramina. Osteophyte formation or protrusion of intervertebral discs may cause compression of nerve roots or the spinal cord, especially in the cervical (C4–7) and lumbar spine. Symptoms may occur acutely, particularly after trauma, such as "whiplash" injury, or chronically. Compression of nerve roots results in pain, the distribution of which depends on the roots affected, and may include the head, neck, shoulders, arms, digits, or chest. The pain may be aggravated by active or passive movement of the spine, and may be accompanied by muscle spasm. There may also be sensory changes (paresthesias, dysesthesias, and hypesthesia) and signs of lower motor neuron lesion, occasionally including fasciculations, in the dermatome innervated by the affected root. When the sixth cervical root is involved the sensory symptoms are felt in the thumb and index finger, and when the seventh cervical root is affected, the middle finger. The spinalis, deltoid, biceps, brachioradialis, and supinator muscles are those most affected when there is compression of the fifth cervical root. In the case of the sixth cervical root the muscles involved are the triceps, extensors of the wrists and digits, pectoralis major, and latissimus dorsi.

Compression of the spinal cord may result in sensory symptoms and lower motor neuron signs at the level of compression, and upper motor neuron signs below the compression, mainly in the lower limbs. Occasionally tactile or postural sensibility may be diminished below the level of compression. Sphincter control is usually unaffected unless there is severe paraplegia or quadriplegia. The cerebrospinal fluid is usually normal, but occasionally the protein content is slightly elevated, and there may be delayed rise and fall of pressure in the Queckenstedt test when the neck is passively extended. The lower motor neuron signs of spondylosis may resemble those of progressive muscular atrophy, though fasciculations tend to be less pronounced, and the presence of upper motor neuron signs may lead to a mistaken diagnosis of amyotrophic lateral sclerosis. However, sensory manifestations occur in the majority of patients with spondylosis, and are very rare in the various forms of spinal muscular atrophy. When the sensory findings include loss of proprioception and vibratory sensation, and when these are accompanied by upper motor neuron signs, the clinical picture may resemble that of subacute combined degeneration.

The vertebral arteries enter the cervical spine at the level of the sixth cervical vertebra and pass upward through a canal in the transverse processes. Cervical osteoarthritis may thus result in symptoms of cerebral ischemia, particularly if collateral circulation through the circle of Willis is impaired by atheroma in the vertebral or carotid arteries. Transient episodes of giddiness or syncope may occur at rest, on standing, and particularly after rotation, extension, or, less frequently, flexion of the neck. A drop attack may occur, in which the patient suddenly falls, without impairment of consciousness. A persistent cerebral ischemic lesion (stroke) may occur after movement or manipulation of the neck.

The principal radiologic changes of osteoarthritis are joint narrowing (due to degeneration and disappearance of articular cartilage), sharpening of articular margins and intra-articular structures, bony sclerosis (eburnation), osteophytes and marginal lipping, and bone cysts. However, there is frequently no relation between the clinical and radiologic pictures, and the diagnosis should seldom be made on the roentgenographic findings alone. In a few patients focal changes may produce symptoms despite a normal roentgenographic appearance. Much more frequently there are radiologic changes of osteoarthritis without neurologic symptoms due to this cause. In evaluating a roentgenogram, the "normal" for the patient's age should be kept in mind. In the diagnosis of radiculopathy or myelopathy attributed to osteoarthritis of the spine, detection of posterior osteophytosis, reduction in diameter of the spinal canal and of spinal foramina, and diminution in the height of intervertebral discs are helpful. Myelography may be required.

INTERVERTEBRAL DISC PROTRUSION

Protrusion occurs most commonly in the fourth, fifth, or, rarely, third lumbar disc, and less commonly in the fifth, sixth, or, rarely, seventh cervical disc. The protrusion occurs posteriorly into the spinal canal, resulting in pressure on one or more nerve roots, or occasionally on the cervical cord.

Lumbar Disc Protrusion. The commonest symptom of lumbar disc protrusion is recurring attacks of low backache, with or without pain in sciatic distribution, usually unilateral.[73] The patient usually walks with a limp on the involved side. The erector spinae muscles are likely to be in spasm. Motion of the spinal column is limited and may aggravate the pain, and raising the extended leg on the involved side may reproduce the pain. The Achilles tendon reflex is usually diminished or absent, and there may

may be hypalgesia in the distribution of the first sacral root. If the protrusion is more marked, there is also weakness and mild atrophy of the lower leg. Severe weakness and wasting of the entire limb is rarely caused by disc lesions; only in the rarely seen massive disc protrusion is there flaccid paraplegia with or without loss of bladder and bowel control and extensive sensory loss, resembling the signs of tumor of the cauda equina.

Cervical Disc Protrusion. This is the commonest cause of root pain extending from the neck down an upper extremity.[85] It is accompanied by spasm of the neck muscles, loss of normal curvature of the cervical spine, and pain on motion of the neck. The tendon reflexes, particularly of the biceps or triceps, may be diminished, and paresthesias or dermatome hypalgesia may be present. If the disc protrusion is in the midline, which is uncommon because of the posterior longitudinal ligament, compression of the spinal cord may occur, producing upper motor neuron signs below the level of the lesion and other manifestations resembling spinal cord tumor, syringomyelia, or disseminated sclerosis[1].

The spinal fluid protein is usually elevated to between 40 and 100 mg/100 ml; higher concentrations are more suggestive of neoplasm. Radiologic examination may show narrowing of an intervertebral space; in the cervical region this is suggestive of disc protrusion, but in the lumbar or thoracic region it is of less significance. If bed rest and traction do not result in amelioration of symptoms, or if there are gross signs of nerve deficit, a myelogram should be performed to demonstrate and localize the lesion and to evaluate the desirability of surgical removal.

SPINAL CORD TUMOR

This is one-fourth as common as intracranial tumor, and, unlike the latter, is rare in children.[51] Manifestations depend on location. Extramedullary tumor initially produces compression of nerve roots and signs and symptoms of segmental distribution: posterior root compression causes pain, paresthesias, and sensory loss, while anterior root compression causes lower motor neuron signs of weakness with atrophy, diminished tendon reflexes, and occasional fasciculations.[7] Later extramedullary tumor produces compression of the long tracts of the spinal cord, resulting in motor and/or sensory changes, usually bilateral, below the level of the tumor; compression of corticospinal tracts produces upper motor neuron signs, including diminished bladder and rectal control; compression of sensory tracts produces diminished sensation to touch, pain, temperature, proprioception, and vibration with a sensory level near the tumor. Laterally placed tumors may cause the Brown-Séquard syndrome. Intramedullary tumor may produce long tract signs with or without segmental signs, resembling the manifestations of syringomyelia, but with more rapid progression.[11] Metastatic disease or epidural abscess of the spinal cord, or metastatic disease, lymphoma, or tuberculosis of the vertebral column may produce manifestations resembling those of spinal cord tumor.

Tumor or other disease causing compression of the spinal cord must be suspected whenever weakness or sensory signs or symptoms involve both legs or both arms or all four extremities; or are radicular in distribution or progressive; or when there is a sensory level, sphincter disturbance of the bladder (with urgency, frequency, incontinence, or retention), or less frequently of the rectum, loss of potentia without loss of libido, or tenderness to vertebral percussion. Radiologic examination of the spine is usually negative in spinal cord tumor, but may disclose evidence of metastatic disease or tuberculosis of the vertebrae. The spinal fluid protein is usually elevated, as in compression of the cord for any reason. The Queckenstedt test provides evidence of complete or incomplete subarachnoid block: complete if there is no rise in spinal fluid pressure with compression of the jugular vein (but a rise with compression of the abdomen to ensure patency of the recording system); incomplete block if there is a slow rise and slow fall, requiring more than 10 seconds, with compression of the jugular vein. A myelogram is essential to demonstrate a tumor or other lesion compressing the spinal cord.

Disease of Peripheral Nerves

An insidious onset and progressive course are seen in polyneuropathy due to diabetes mellitus, uremia, amyloidosis, carcinoma,[12] multiple myeloma, and various hereditary polyneuropathies, and in neuropathy due to the entrapment syndromes. A relapsing course is seen in Refsum's disease, Tangier disease, some cases of hypertrophic neuropathy, and some chronic neuropathies of unknown cause.

DIABETIC AMYOTROPHY

Weakness and wasting of the muscles of one or several extremities, usually involving the distal musculature first, is common in patients with prolonged diabetes mellitus.[17] Peripheral neuropathy is the commonest cause. Accompanying sensory changes may facilitate diagnosis. In some patients, however, the proximal muscles of the lower extremities are affected first (Fig. 26), and histologic studies have provided evidence that muscle as well as nerve may be affected.[50] These patients, who are mainly elderly male diabetics, have also had myalgia, with anterior thigh pain, marked muscle wasting, and weight loss. The disease is often "self-limited" and improvement or recovery may occur within a few months to several years.

HEREDITARY NEUROPATHIES

Peroneal Muscular Atrophy (Charcot-Marie-Tooth Disease). This condition, which begins during childhood or adolescence, is characterized by symmetrical weakness and atrophy of the distal muscles of the lower extremities, and occasionally, to a lesser extent, of the upper extremities. It is due to degeneration of the anterior horn cells, and to a lesser extent of the peripheral nerves. The atrophy of the calf and anterior tibial muscles results in "stork" legs. There is also foot drop deformity, with pes cavus or talipes equinovarus. Tendon reflexes in the affected extremities diminish and the ankle jerks disappear. Fasciculations may occur, but tend to disappear by the time atrophy is marked. Sensation to touch, pain, temperature, and vibration is either normal or slightly diminished in the distal lower extremities. Pain is rare.

Familial Interstitial Hypertrophic Polyneuropathy (Déjerine-Sottas Disease). This also begins during childhood or adolescence, and produces both motor and sensory neuropathy and palpable thickening of nerves, including the ulnar nerve. Motor changes include distal weakness, atrophy, diminished tendon reflexes, and, in one third, fasciculations. Sensory changes include pain, numbness, paresthesias, and sensory loss of stocking-glove distribution. In *Refsum's syndrome* hypertrophic neuropathy may be accompanied by ataxia, nystagmus, nerve deafness, retinitis pigmentosa, mental retardation, and increased serum levels of phytanic acid.

ENTRAPMENT SYNDROMES

These occur where a nerve passes over bone, tendon, or synovia; compression occurs as a result of bony overgrowth, tendonitis, or synovitis. Examples include the scalenus anticus (thoracic outlet), sciatic nerve, and carpal tunnel (median nerve) syndromes. In the thoracic outlet syndrome sagging of the shoulder causes compression of the brachial plexus against the first rib, scalenus anterior muscle, or a cervical rib, resulting in pain and paresthesias of ulnar distribution and sometimes weakness and atrophy of the small muscles of the hand. Compression of the sciatic nerve may occur as a result of fracture of the pelvis or upper end of the femur, injury to the hip joint, or pressure on the lumbosacral plexus by the fetal head during difficult labor. Sensory and motor manifestations occur, with difficulty in flexing the knee and dorsiflexing the foot, and with foot drop. Compression of the external popliteal branch may occur as a result of prolonged squatting, resulting in foot drop and in high-steppage gait necessary to enable the patient to clear the ground with his toes.

Disease of Muscle

Weakness and wasting result from many primary and secondary diseases of muscle. Mild to moderate weakness and wasting may occur in almost any acute or chronic debilitating disease associated with inanition or cachexia, and marked wasting may occur in some of these diseases and in senility. Often the mechanism of the alteration in muscle function is not clear, but in a few diseases, such as trichinosis, sarcoidosis, primary amyloidosis, and some of the glycogenoses, muscle biopsy shows histologic evidence of direct involvement of muscle by the systemic disease.

Weakness and wasting varying from mild degree to severe paraplegia or quadriplegia may be produced by inflammatory disease of muscle, particularly polymyositis, by an excess of thyroid or adrenal cortical hormone, and by muscular or myotonic dystrophy. In these diseases of muscle there is, in addition to weakness and wasting, muscular flaccidity and diminution of tendon reflexes, resembling the manifestations of lower motor neuron diseases of gradual onset. Identification of the muscle disease is aided by determination of the serum levels of enzymes derived from muscle (which are elevated in polymyositis and muscular dystrophy), by estimation of thyroid and adrenal cortical function, and by muscle biopsy.

CHRONIC INFECTIONS, NEOPLASTIC, AND MALABSORPTIVE DISEASES

Mild to moderate weakness and wasting may occur in almost any chronic disease associated with inanition or cachexia, especially tuberculosis, malnutrition, chronic hepatitis, neoplastic disease, and diseases associated with intestinal malabsorption. The muscle wasting is more severe than the weakness, which may be mild. Negative nitrogen balance and disuse atrophy are mainly responsible, but there may be other factors that are not understood. The muscle may show an unusual excitability to mechanical stimulus: a sharp blow to the belly of the muscle with a percussion hammer may cause an immediate local contraction in the form of a visible ridge, which persists for several seconds and may give rise to a small wave which moves along the muscle. This reaction is known as myedema or idiomuscular contraction. The propagated contraction wave is electrically silent.

INFILTRATIVE DISEASE

Skeletal muscle, like cardiac muscle, may be infiltrated by parasites (e.g., trichinae), granulomas (e.g., sarcoid), or deposits of an abnormal metabolic product, such as amyloid or glycogen. Weakness and wasting ensue; in trichinosis and sarcoidosis myalgia also occurs.

Sarcoidosis. This disease occasionally involves skeletal muscle, producing weakness, myalgia, and often wasting.[45] The biopsy of even clinically unaffected muscle often yields positive results, just as the biopsy of small lymph nodes is often positive.

Amyloidosis. The deposition of this material in skeletal muscle and in peripheral nerves occurs in primary amyloidosis, and only rarely in the secondary form of the disease, except for para-amyloidosis of multiple myeloma. However, it may not become manifest until late in life. There is often enlargement and firmness of the tongue (Fig. 29), and occasionally of other muscles. Generalized weakness may occur, and sometimes ophthalmoplegia is seen. Peripheral neuropathy may also occur. Rarely there is slowness of muscle contraction and relaxation that may simulate myotonia.

Glycogenosis. The utilization of intramuscular glycogen requires a number of enzymes, including debranching and branching enzymes and phosphorylase. Deficiency of debranching and branching enzymes results in glycogen deposition in skeletal and cardiac muscle and liver in early childhood (limit dextrinosis and amylopectinosis), while phosphorylase deficiency results in glycogenosis of skeletal muscle and the appearance of characteristic symptoms in later life (McArdle's syndrome). In classic von Gierke's disease, which is due to deficiency of glucose 6-phosphatase,

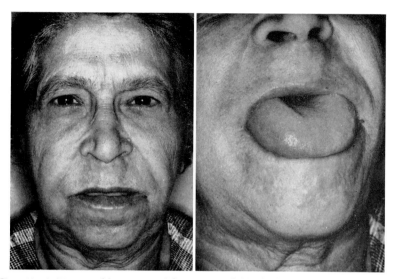

FIG. 29. A 72-year old woman with para-amyloidosis due to multiple myeloma. There is irregular thickening and enlargement and decreased mobility of the skin around the mouth, and of the lips and tongue.

massive deposition of glycogen occurs in early childhood in the liver and kidneys, but not in skeletal muscle, which normally lacks this enzyme.

EFFECT OF AGING: SENILE MUSCULAR WASTING

Wasting of skeletal muscles and general decrease in muscular strength, endurance, and agility are common in the aged. There is a decrease in the number of muscle fibers and in their individual bulk, which is merely part of a general atrophy of organs and tissues. The process of regeneration is not active. Fibrous tissue replacement occurs secondarily. The age at which these changes in the muscles begin is highly variable. The changes are particularly conspicuous in the small muscles of the hands, which become thin and bony, with deep interosseous spaces. The arm and leg muscles become thin and flabby. The atrophy may be so prominent as to suggest progressive muscular atrophy. However, this disease can be excluded by the absence of severe weakness, muscular fasciculations at rest, or progression of signs and symptoms. While some degree of weakness may occur in aged persons with senile muscular wasting, it is usually surprisingly little, and not proportionate to the degree of wasting.

INFLAMMATORY DISEASES WHICH MAY BE RELATED TO AUTOIMMUNITY

Varying degrees of muscle weakness and wasting, associated with round cell infiltration, perivascular collections of lymphocytes, and degeneration, necrosis, and atrophy of muscle fibers, may occur in association with any of the inflammatory connective tissue diseases which have been attributed to autoimmunity. The weakness and wasting are least marked in acute rheumatic fever, in which the skeletal muscle lesions are scattered; they are more marked in rheumatoid arthritis, in which muscle wasting is usually greater than would be expected from disuse alone; they are even more marked in some patients with disseminated lupus erythematosus, polyarteritis nodosa, or scleroderma; and they are most severe in dermatomyositis or polymyositis. Muscle pain and tenderness may occur, especially in the latter disorders.

Polymyositis. This is the commonest primary muscle disease of adults, and in children only muscular dystrophy is more frequent. It may begin at any age, though rarely before 4 years, with roughly equal distribution of onset from the first to sixth decades. In approximately one-third of patients polymyositis occurs alone; in 40 per cent it is accompanied by dermatitis (*dermatomyositis*), in 20 per cent by clinical and laboratory evidence of disseminated lupus erythematosus, polyarteritis, scleroderma, or, less often, rheumatoid arthritis, and in 15 per cent by a malignancy, usually of lung, gastrointestinal tract, breast, ovary, or uterus.[79] In patients whose disease begins after the age of 40 one-half have or develop a malignancy.

The disease may begin insidiously or acutely. The initial symptom is weakness, usually of the legs, in half the patients, dermatitis in one-fourth, and muscle or joint pain or Raynaud's phenomenon in one-fourth.[66] The main manifestation of the disease is muscular weakness, which occurs in all patients. Proximal muscles are affected more than distal. The proximal muscles of the legs are weak in almost all patients, and those of the arms in 80 per cent, while only 35 per cent have weakness of distal muscles. The neck flexors are weak in 65 per cent, and dysphagia occurs in 62 per cent. Facial and extraocular muscles are seldom affected. Pain or tenderness of muscles occurs in half the patients, but many with severe weakness have no other complaint. Severe atrophy and weight loss develop in half the patients (Fig. 30), and contractures in one-third. Tendon reflexes and the contractile response of affected muscle to direct percussion are usually diminished.

Approximately 40 per cent of patients have an erythematous eruption which usually begins on the face or upper trunk, with edema, erythema, and a pink "heliotrope" hue. The periorbital areas are particularly involved, and malar erythema may occur, as in lupus erythematosus. The hands are frequently involved, especially the extensor surfaces and nail beds, and sometimes the feet. In approximately half the patients the dermatitis precedes the weakness; in the others it accompanies or follows it. Pigmentation (Fig. 30), hardness, and even calcinosis of the skin and subcutaneous tissues may occur as a late development.

Approximately one-third of patients have Raynaud's phenomenon, one-third have joint pains, and a few have arthritis which may be indistinguishable from rheumatoid arthritis. About 8 per cent have significant intestinal hypomotility, and 2 per cent recurring pneumonitis. The heart is rarely affected. Fever is variable. Many patients have no fever, despite severe illness, while some, especially younger patients and those with an

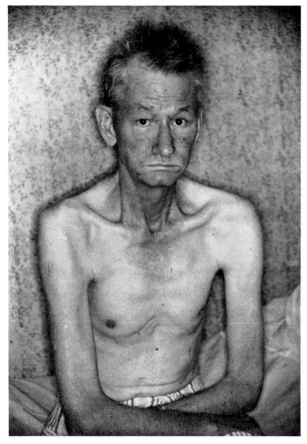

Fig. 30. A 60-year-old man with weakness and wasting of predominantly proximal distribution due to polymyositis. Note the erythema and bronzed pigmentation of the face and V area of the neck, resembling the effect of exposure to sunlight, despite confinement indoors for many months.

acute course, have either low-grade or high fever. The course of the disease is also variable, and may be progressive or characterized by "spontaneous" exacerbations and remissions.

During acute stages of the disease the erythrocyte sedimentation rate is elevated, and there may be a neutrophilic leukocytosis, but anemia is uncommon. The α_2- and γ-globulins are elevated in the serum of about half the patients, and the tests for circulating rheumatoid factor, antinuclear globulin, or lupus erythematosus factor are occasionally positive. There is usually increased creatinuria. The electromyogram is usually compatible with myopathy.

The *serum enzymes derived from muscle* are almost always elevated, sometimes markedly, during active stages of the disease, and usually decline toward normal levels with spontaneous improvement or following treatment with adrenal cortical steroids. The decline usually precedes by 3 to 4 weeks any improvement in strength, and relapse of the disease is often heralded by a rise in serum enzymes. The enzyme levels may be normal during chronic stages of the disease and, rarely, during active stages.

Muscle biopsy, if it includes an involved area, is almost always helpful in diagnosis. During acute stages there is usually degeneration of muscle fibers, with swelling, hyalinization, basophilia, vacuolization, granular degeneration, fragmentation, phagocytosis, and occasionally local hemorrhages. During both acute and chronic stages there is infiltration with round cells (lymphocytes, plasma cells, and histiocytes) and occasionally polymorphonuclear cells, and an increase in sarcolemmal nuclei (Fig. 31). During chronic stages there is diffuse atrophy of muscle fibers (Fig. 31) and there may be increased fibrous tissue and collagen, muscle regeneration, and, rarely, calcinosis. *Skin biopsy* of involved areas shows edema of the dermis, swelling of collagen fibers, and round cell infiltration, but these changes are not pathognomonic.

Disseminated Lupus Erythematosus. Three-fourths of patients with lupus, polyarteritis, scleroderma, or rheumatoid arthritis develop histologic evidence of nodular myosisis, but these lesions are usually without any clinical counterpart. However, about 20 per cent of those with lupus erythematosus develop weakness and atrophy due to polymyositis.[74] Usually clinical and laboratory evidence of lupus is already present: fever (90 per cent), arthralgia (90 per cent), polyarthritis (30 per cent), erythematous eruption (85 per cent), often of malar distribution (50 per cent), rena disease (65 per cent), pleurisy (55 per cent), pneumonitis (20 per cent)

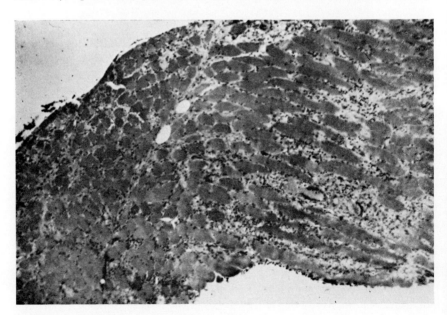

FIG. 31. Diffuse (nonfascicular) atrophy of muscle fibers, indicating myopathic disease, and round cell infiltration, due to active polymyositis. ×90.

heart disease (55 per cent), central nervous system disease (20 per cent),[32] anemia (78 per cent), leukopenia (70 per cent), thrombocytopenia (25 per cent), and lupus erythematosus factor in the serum (82 per cent). Since the patient may be receiving adrenal cortical steroids when weakness is noted, it is necessary to differentiate between steroid myopathy and other causes of weakness.

Polyarteritis Nodosa. Weakness and atrophy occur in over half the patients with this disease: in 10 per cent of patients it is due to polymyositis, and in 50 per cent to polyneuritis, which is usually localized, but occasionally involves all extremities.[31] Clinical and laboratory evidence of polyarteritis is usually already present: fever (85 per cent), weight loss (50 per cent), hypertension (60 per cent), albuminuria (60 per cent), hematuria (40 per cent), abdominal pain (50 per cent), asthma (20 per cent), albuminuria (60 per cent), hematuria (40 per cent), leukocytosis (80 per cent), and eosinophilia (20 per cent). Muscle biopsy usually reveals polyarteritic lesions, but this may require study of numerous serial sections and several biopsies.

Scleroderma (Progressive Systemic Sclerosis). Weakness and atrophy due to polymyositis occasionally accompany scleroderma, but in most patients the limitation of motion and weakness that occur are due mainly to induration and thickening of skin (95 per cent of patients), particularly of the hands and face (Fig. 32), and to arthritis (61 per cent). Other manifestations include Raynaud's phenomenon (83 per cent), symptomatic disease of the esophagus (50 per cent), lungs (30 per cent), heart (20 per cent), kidneys (20 per cent), and intestine (10 per cent), and gangrene of terminal digits due to arteritis (5 per cent) (Fig. 32).

Rheumatoid Arthritis. Most patients with rheumatoid arthritis develop weakness and atrophy, particularly of muscles near involved joints, more marked than would be expected from disuse alone. During acute stages of the disease joint pain usually limits motion and appears to aggravate weakness. In all stages of the disease there is histologic evidence of nodular myositis, but these lesions cannot be correlated with the degree or distribution of weakness and atrophy. Only a few patients develop polymyositis. While the muscular manifestations of rheumatoid arthritis appear to be mainly secondary to the joint disease, there may be an associated disturbance of muscle function of uncertain mechanism.

ENDOCRINE DISEASES

Weakness may occur when there is either deficient or excessive function of the thyroid, adrenal cortex, or anterior pituitary gland.[30, 39, 40] It may also occur when there is hypocalcemia (with tetany), hypercalcemia, or hypoglycemia, arising from any cause. The weakness is accompanied by muscle atrophy in excessive function of the thyroid or adrenal cortex, but not in deficient function of these glands or in acromegaly, calcium disorders, or hypoglycemia.

Hyperthyroidism. Skeletal muscle requires a normal state of thyroid

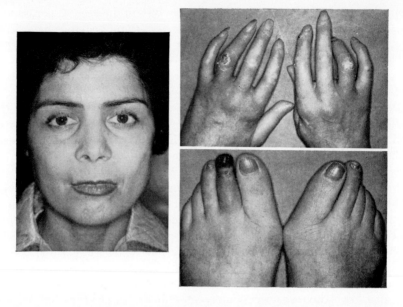

FIG. 32. A 30-year-old woman with scleroderma. There is tightness of the skin around the mouth and fingers, trophic changes over the phalangeal joints, and gangrene of a toe due to arteritis.

function for the preservation of normal function and bulk. When thyroid hyperfunction is present the majority of patients develop weakness and decreased muscle bulk, while in thyroid hypofunction the majority develop a mild degree of weakness accompanied by an abnormal slowness of muscle contraction and relaxation and by some increase in muscle bulk. Approximately 70 per cent of patients with hyperthyroidism have mild to moderate muscular weakness with easy fatiguability and a variable degree of muscle wasting and weight loss. Weakness is usually most prominent in the muscles of the pelvic girdle and upper legs, less often in the shoulder girdle and upper arms, with difficulty in climbing stairs or elevating the arms. The proximal muscles are affected to a greater degree than are the distal; the muscles of the face, tongue, and pharynx are seldom sufficiently affected to produce symptoms. Muscle wasting tends to be more generalized, involving distal as well as proximal muscles, but the quadriceps and temporal muscles are often involved to a greater degree than others. The tendon reflexes tend to be preserved, even in the presence of considerable weakness, and are usually brisk. The rate of muscle contraction and relaxation is normal or faster than normal.

While the majority of patients with hyperthyroidism have mild to moderate muscular weakness and wasting, a smaller proportion may have more pronounced evidence of a disturbance of muscle function.[39] The commonest generalized myopathy is the gradual development of a pronounced degree of muscle weakness and wasting (Fig. 33), to which the term chronic thyrotoxic myopathy has been applied. The commonest

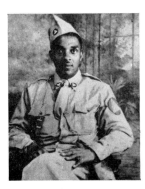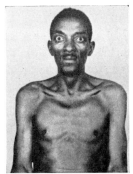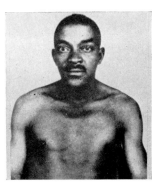

FIG. 33. Thyrotoxic myopathy and postoperative hypothyroidism. *Left,* patient at age 39, when he was in good health, at normal strength, and weighed 155 pounds. *Center,* patient at age 48, following appearance of hyperthyroidism, with marked muscular wasting and weakness, jitteriness, exophthalmos, and decline in weight to 100 pounds. *Right,* patient at age 49, 10 months after thyroidectomy which resulted in correction of the manifestations of hyperthyroidism, followed by development of hypothyroidism, with lethargy, dry, thickened skin, increase in muscle bulk and tone, muscle cramps, easy fatiguability, and weight gain to 163 pounds.

localized myopathy is weakness of one or more of the extraocular muscles, usually accompanied by exophthalmos, and in its most severe form manifested as exophthalmic ophthalmoplegia. Much less common is the acute onset in patients with fulminating hyperthyroidism of severe weakness, usually accompanied by evidence of central nervous system dysfunction, and termed acute thyrotoxic myopathy or encephalomyopathy. Occasionally hyperthyroidism occurs in association with myasthenia gravis or, more rarely, with hypokalemic periodic paralysis.

Chronic Thyrotoxic Myopathy. In chronic thyrotoxic myopathy there is more marked weakness and symmetrical muscle wasting than occurs in the great majority of patients with uncomplicated hyperthyroidism. There are no accurate figures on how often chronic myopathy complicates thyrotoxicosis, because there is no sharp dividing line from uncomplicated thyrotoxicosis. Chronic thyrotoxic myopathy has a higher incidence in males than in females (with a ratio of 60–40), in contrast with the much higher incidence of uncomplicated thyrotoxicosis in females (4.5:1). The average age at onset is slightly higher than in uncomplicated thyrotoxicosis (47 years compared with 40 years), but the range of onset is quite wide (from 18 to 69 years). Thyrotoxic myopathy is usually a complication of severe thyrotoxicosis, and seldom occurs in patients with milder degrees of increased thyroid activity. However, most patients with chronic myopathy differ in some ways from those with uncomplicated hyperthyroidism. Thus, in patients with thyrotoxic myopathy, exophthalmos is usually not prominent, the thyroid gland may or may not be grossly enlarged, and the usual manifestations of hyperthyroidism, such as tachycardia, sweating, heat intolerance, tremor, and hyperkinesis, may not be noted or may be overshadowed by the marked weakness, muscle wasting, and weight loss which are usually the principal symptoms. Some patients may actually be depressed and anorectic and may be said to have "masked" or "apathetic" hyperthyroidism.

The distribution of muscular weakness and wasting is constant. Weakness of the pelvic girdle and legs is usually the initial manifestation, with difficulty in walking, climbing stairs, getting up from a kneeling position, or rising from a chair. Weakness and wasting of the pelvic and shoulder girdles, quadriceps, temporalis, and muscles of the upper arms and hands are the main features (Fig. 33), while weakness of the neck and of trunk flexion is usually inconspicuous. The facial muscles may be affected, but rarely are the bulbar and ocular muscles involved. The tendon reflexes are usually normal, but may be more brisk than normal or, occasionally, diminished. There is no sensory loss. Muscle fasciculations occur occasionally, and may be pronounced. Most patients remain ambulatory, but in a few patients the weakness may be so severe as to render them bedridden; in rare instances death has been attributed to failure of the muscles of respiration.

The serum cholesterol level is usually within normal limits, although sometimes it is low. There is usually decreased tolerance to ingested creatine, but creatinuria is not constant and may even be absent, in contrast to the more marked creatinuria that occurs in hyperthyroidism without myopathy. It has been suggested that there may be decreased synthesis of creatine. The serum levels of enzymes derived from muscle are normal. Electromyography is usually normal. Histologic examination of muscle usually shows atrophy of the muscle fibers, some degeneration of fibers, and infiltration with fat and with collections of mononuclear cells called lymphorrhages. However, the muscle sometimes appears normal histologically, even in patients with pronounced weakness and wasting.

Patients with marked muscle wasting who do not have other signs of hyperthyroidism may be suspected of having polymyositis or cachexia due to neoplastic disease, and those with muscular fasciculations may be thought to have progressive muscular atrophy. Differential diagnosis is aided by determination of serum levels of enzymes derived from muscle (elevated in polymyositis), electromyography (abnormal in progressive muscular atrophy), and measurement of thyroid function.

Treatment of the thyrotoxicosis by any means, whether by radioactive iodine, drugs of the thiouracil type, or surgery, results in progressive improvement in the myopathy once normal thyroid function has been restored. Within a few months the muscle weakness and wasting disappear. This is in contrast to ophthalmoplegia, which usually does not improve with the restoration of normal thyroid function, or to concomitant myasthenia gravis, which responds much less well to restoration of normal thyroid function.

Acute Thyrotoxic Encephalomyopathy. This is a rare complication of hyperthyroidism, characterized by the acute development of severe weakness, dysphagia, and dysarthria simultaneously with all the nervous disturbances of thyroid "storm" or "crisis," such as impairment of consciousness and abnormalities of movement and posture. There is rapid progression of weakness of muscles innervated by the cranial nerves, with bulbar paralysis and weakness of the limbs and trunk. There may be marked tremor, agitation or depression, psychosis, delirium, and semicoma or coma. This disorder is more properly termed acute thyrotoxic encephalopathy or encephalomyopathy rather than myopathy, since it is probably due mainly to central neural dysfunction, although some patients described with bulbar paralysis may have had undetected fulminating myasthenia gravis appearing as a complication of hyperthyroidism. In the absence of treatment most patients with encephalomyopathy have died within 1 to 2 weeks after its onset, although a subacute form has been described.

Muscle Rigidity and Spasms. These may be myoclonic, and are a rare complication of hyperthyroidism. In some patients this has occurred in association with chronic myopathy, acute or subacute encephalomyopathy, choreiform movements, or parkinsonism. The muscular rigidity and painful spasms may be so severe as to resemble the "stiff man" syndrome.

Ocular Myopathy. This is the commonest myopathy associated with thyroid disease. The relationship to thyroid function is probably indirect, since the muscular symptoms may develop with or without thyrotoxicosis, and have been ascribed to increased activity of the thyroid-stimulating hormone (TSH), to some other secretion of the anterior pituitary gland, or to a serum globulin fraction. Eye signs may develop before there is evidence of hyperthyroidism, may be severe when there is minimal thyrotoxicosis, or may progress after amelioration of thyrotoxicosis. The most severe instances of exophthalmic ophthalmoplegia develop in older patients following the relief of hyperthyroidism by thyroidectomy.

In the milder ophthalmyopathy there may be weakness of convergence, infrequent blinking, tremor of closed lids, difficulty in everting the upper lid, absence of forehead wrinkling on upward gaze, palsy of one or more extraocular muscles, lid retraction with stare, and lid lag. Although some impairment of ocular motility may be present in as many as 20 per cent of patients with hyperthyroidism, ophthalmoplegia of a significant degree occurs in less than 0.5 per cent. In the more severe infiltrative ophthalmyopathy the lids become tense, bulging, and edematous, with conjunctival injection and edema; diplopia is common, often with inability to elevate the eyes; and retrobulbar resistance becomes increased, with exophthalmos. Ptosis does not occur, although edema of the lids may give the appearance of ptosis. Limitation of ocular movement may become evident in one or both eyes and in one or more directions, usually resulting in diplopia, which is a particularly significant indication of ophthalmyopathy. Limitation of elevation characteristically appears first, followed by decrease in lateral movement, while downward movement is seldom impaired. There is no relationship between the degree of ophthalmoplegia and the severity of weakness elsewhere in the body. Weakness of the ocular muscles usually occurs in the presence of exophthalmos, but occasionally develops in its absence or with minimal degrees of proptosis. It is only with extreme degrees of orbital pressure that all movements may be more or less uniformly restricted, in which case the eyes are usually fixed in depression. Marked exophthalmos may result in such an increase in orbital venous pressure as to cause edema of the optic nerve head and loss of visual acuity. Ulceration of the cornea may also impair visual acuity. The severe eye changes may be accompanied by localized pretibial myxedema and, more rarely, hypertrophic pulmonary osteoarthropathy.

Myasthenia Gravis. This condition occurs in approximately 1 per cent of thyrotoxic patients at some time in the course of the disease. Three per cent of patients with myasthenia gravis have or develop associated hyperthyroidism, and 2 per cent have exophthalmos in the absence of thyroid disease. The incidence of these associations is higher than would be expected to occur by chance. In slightly over half the patients with both diseases hyperthyroidism appears first, while in the remainder myasthenia gravis occurs first. Only occasionally do the two diseases have a simultaneous onset.

The manifestations of myasthenia gravis occurring in the presence of thyrotoxicosis do not differ from those which occur in euthyroid patients. The presence of myasthenia gravis is detected by improvement in muscle performance following the administration of an anticholinesterase compound, such as neostigmine or edrophonium. The weakness of thyrotoxicosis does not respond to the administration of these drugs.

In hyperthyroidism uncomplicated by myasthenia gravis there is no ptosis, the orbiculares oculi are usually fairly strong, and complete paralysis of extraocular movement is unusual unless the globes are fixed in a downward position by severe proptosis. The occurrence in a patient with thyroid disease or a history of thyroid disease of ptosis, weakness of the orbiculares oculi, or complete limitation of extraocular movement in the absence of severe proptosis is strongly suggestive of the presence of concomitant myasthenia gravis. This is confirmed by the response to neostigmine or edrophonium.

Hypopotassemic Periodic Paralysis. This also occurs with hyperthyroidism more frequently than would be expected from chance association. Periodic paralysis occurring in conjunction with hyperthyroidism has differed from the uncomplicated disease in only two respects: the patients have been older at the time of onset of attacks of paralysis, and a family history of the disease has usually been absent. In one-fourth of the patients with both diseases the periodic paralysis has begun before the onset of thyrotoxic symptoms. The relief of thyrotoxicosis has usually been followed by a subsidence of periodic attacks, but in some patients there has been only a decrease in their frequency.

Hyperadrenocorticism (Cushing's Syndrome). Weakness occurs in 80 per cent of patients with Cushing's syndrome, whether due to hyperplasia, adenoma, or carcinoma of the adrenal cortices, to basophilic adenoma of the pituitary, or to carcinoma of nonendocrine tissue, particularly the lung.[30] The weakness involves the extremities and trunk, and is usually accompanied by wasting of the muscles of the extremities. Cushing's syndrome is recognized by obesity, present in 97 per cent of patients, with characteristic distribution on the face, neck, and trunk, giving rise to moon facies, buffalo hump, and trunk obesity with sparing of the extremities. Hypertension is present in 85 per cent, and mild hirsutism, particularly of the face, amenorrhea or oligomenorrhea (or impotence in men), plethoric appearance, and purple striae, each in about 70 per cent. Mental symptoms, particularly depression, and purpura or easy bruising, occur in 60 per cent, poor healing of wounds or unusual failure to localize infections in 40 per cent, polyuria and polydipsia in 30 per cent, decrease in stature, kyphosis, and backache due to softening of vertebrae in 20 per cent, and exophthalmos in about 6 per cent.[70] Occasionally Cushing's syndrome may be manifested only by weakness and marked atrophy of muscle, skin, and bones, without the other features that are commonly observed.[56]

Reduced glucose tolerance is present in 94 per cent of patients with Cushing's syndrome, and glycosuria and diabetes, usually mild and without acidosis, in 15 per cent. The blood eosinophil count is below 100/cu mm in 80 per cent, and polycythemia, usually mild, is present in fewer than half. The serum concentration of potassium and chloride is reduced, and that of bicarbonate elevated (hypochloremic, hypopotassemic alkalosis), in less than half. The urinary excretion of 17-ketosteroids may be low, normal, or elevated, but the urinary and plasma levels of 11-oxysteroids and 17-hydroxycorticosteroids are usually increased, and the normal diurnal variation in their levels is usually absent. Urinary excretion of more than 12 mg of 17-hydroxycorticosteroids a day is suggestive of Cushing's syndrome. The syndrome is likely to be due to adenocortical hyperplasia if there is a greater than normal rise in plasma and urinary levels of 11-oxysteroids and 17-hydroxycorticosteroids following corticotropin administration, and a fall in these levels following suppression of the pituitary with a relatively large dose of dexamethasone (2 mg orally every 6 hours for 2 days), but not after attempted suppression with one-fourth this dose. The syndrome is likely to be due to a tumor of the adrenal cortex or of nonendocrine tissue if the steroid levels are not reduced after suppression of the pituitary with the larger dose of dexamethasone. A tumor of nonendocrine tissue is likely to produce more marked hypopotassemic alkalosis, greater urinary excretion of 17-hydroxycorticosteroids (over 50 mg/day), and more pigmentation.

Iatrogenic Hyperadrenocorticism and Steroid Myopathy. Administration of synthetic adrenal corticosteroids results in most of the clinical and metabolic features of Cushing's syndrome, except that there is usually no significant hypertension unless renal disease is present; diabetic glucose tolerance curves and temporary diabetes are less common than in naturally occurring Cushing's syndrome, and upper gastrointestinal ulceration is more common. A small proportion of patients develop weakness and wasting of skeletal muscles, especially of the pelvis and lower extremities, after prolonged administration of any of the synthetic adrenal cortico-steroids in clinical use, particularly triamcinolone, 9α-fluorohydrocortisone, and dexamethasone (Fig. 34). Weakness is most marked when large doses of steroid are administered for several months, but may occur after smaller doses and after a few weeks of administration. The earliest manifestation of this "steroid myopathy" is usually difficulty getting out of a chair or climbing stairs. There is usually increased creatinuria, but the serum levels of enzymes derived from muscle are normal. The electromyogram shows a myopathic pattern. Muscle biopsy shows minimal histologic changes in half of the patients, with increase in sarcolemmal nuclei, rowing of nuclei, central nuclei, and loss of cross-striations; necrosis of muscle fibers is seen in one-fifth.[5] Potassium administration does not affect the weakness or wasting, which are apparently due to an alteration of unknown mechanism in protein metabolism. Steroid myopathy is completely reversible following gradual withdrawal of the steroid, reduction in dosage without discon-tinuing the drug, or even substitution of prednisone or prednisolone for triamcinolone, 9α-fluorohydrocortisone, or dexamethasone, even though the former drugs may produce steroid myopathy in some other patients. Improvement may begin as early as 3 days or as late as 5 weeks, but usually

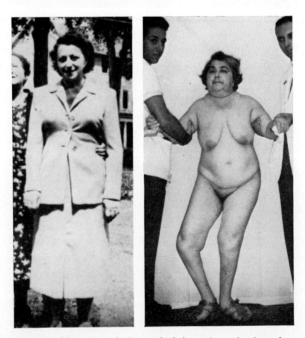

FIG. 34. A 48-year-old woman before administration of adrenal cortical steroid for management of rheumatoid arthritis, and after 5 years of steroid administration. The patient has developed moon facies, truncal obesity, and weakness and wasting of the muscles of the pelvic and shoulder girdles and extremities due to iatrogenic Cushing's syndrome.

within 2 to 3 weeks after institution of these measures. Complete recovery occurs in 2 to 12 months.

Since weakness may be a manifestation of the disease for which adrenal corticosteroid is being administered, as in polymyositis or lupus erythematosus, it may be difficult to decide whether an increase in weakness is due to steroid myopathy or to the underlying disease. If the disease is one that causes an increase in serum enzymes arising from muscle, such increase usually indicates exacerbation of the underlying disease. If weakness becomes worse despite normal or falling serum levels of enzymes, steroid myopathy must be considered.

MUSCULAR DYSTROPHY

This is the commonest primary muscle disease in children, and its incidence in the population (1:25,000) is second only to polymyositis among diseases of muscle. There are several types of dystrophy, including the severe, generalized, rapidly progressive type, the mild, restricted, slowly progressive facioscapulohumeral type (Fig. 35), the intermediate limb-girdle type, dystrophy of the extraocular muscles (Fig. 36), and myotonic dystrophy[80] (Fig. 38). All types are usually familial, though sporadic cases are not uncommon. All are degenerative diseases of muscle manifested by weakness. The tendon jerks of affected muscles are diminished or lost. Muscle atrophy, which may or may not be preceded by pseudohypertrophy, occurs, and later there may be contractures.

Electromyography of involved muscles usually shows a decrease in the average duration and amplitude of muscle action potentials, an increase in polyphasic potentials, and normal interference pattern.

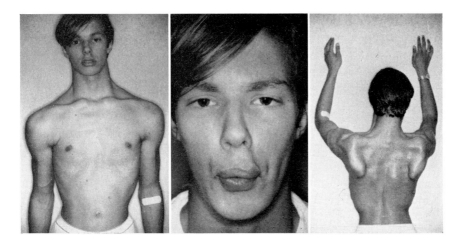

Fig. 35. A 16-year-old boy with facioscapulohumeral muscular dystrophy. There is asymmetric weakness and wasting of the orbicularis oris (patient is attempting to whistle) and of the muscles of shoulder girdle and upper arms, pseudohypertrophy of the deltoid muscles, and winging of scapulae.

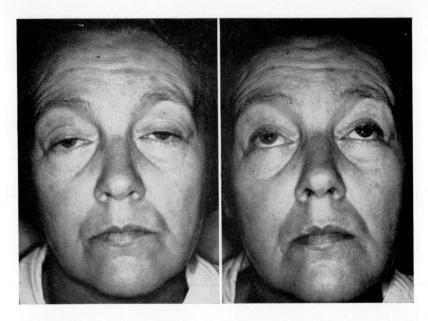

F IG. 36. A 48-year-old woman with ocular muscular dystrophy. There is ptosis and limitation of upward deviation of the eyes, as demonstrated by the patient's effort to look up.

If the *muscle biopsy* includes an affected area, histologic changes include atrophy of muscle fibers with varying degrees of fat deposition and connective tissue proliferation, and usually little or no leukocytic infiltration or evidence of regenerative activity (Fig. 37). Occasionally the latter changes occur, and may make histologic differentiation from slowly progressive polymyositis difficult.

Severe, Generalized, Rapidly Progressive (Pseudohypertrophic or Duchenne) Muscular Dystrophy. This is the commonest type. It is usually inherited as a sex-linked recessive trait, occasionally as an autosomal recessive, and is 6 times as common in males as in females. Onset is between the ages of 2 and 15 years, usually between 2 and 6. There is weakness and atrophy of the muscles of the pelvic and shoulder girdles and the proximal muscles of the limbs, usually symmetrical and progressive. The pelvic girdle and thigh muscles are usually affected first, resulting in a characteristic clumsy waddling gait and difficulty in getting up from a squatting position and in climbing stairs. Soon afterward the shoulder girdle and upper arm muscles become weak, resulting in difficulty in raising the arms and in winging of the scapulae. The quadriceps, hamstrings, glutei, deltoids, and pectorals usually atrophy, while pseudohypertrophy occurs in the gastrocnemii in 80 per cent, and occasionally in the deltoids, triceps, quadriceps, and glutei. The extraocular muscles and the muscles of the face and of swallowing are rarely affected. The course of the disease is inexorably progressive, and patients usually become bedridden before reach-

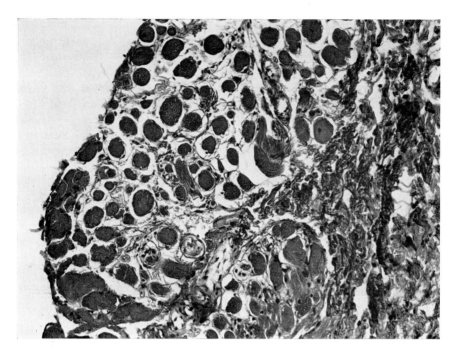

Fig. 37. Biopsy of the levator palpebrae of the patient shown in Figure 36. There is diffuse (nonfascicular) atrophy of muscle fibers, of the myopathic type, and some replacement by connective tissue and fat, compatible with muscular dystrophy. ×200.

ing adult life. Contractures may develop if movement is restricted. There is a high incidence of electrocardiographic abnormalities, particularly RSR complexes in the right precordial leads. Histologic examination of the heart muscle reveals changes similar to those seen in skeletal muscle in over 50 per cent of patients, and heart block or congestive heart failure may occur when the disease is advanced. Death usually occurs from respiratory infection or heart failure before the age of 20 years.

Creatine excretion and the *serum levels of enzymes derived from muscle* are increased. The serum enzyme levels tend to be highest in early, active dystrophy of childhood, though not as high as the peak levels observed in polymyositis, and may be in the normal range after a great deal of muscular wasting has occurred. The enzyme levels may be elevated years before the onset of symptomatic disease, as well as in carriers of the trait.[78]

Mild, Restricted, Slowly Progressive (Facioscapular or Landouzy-Déjerine) Type. This form of muscular dystrophy is usually inherited as an autosomal dominant disorder, and is equally common in males and females. Onset is usually between the ages of 6 and 20 years, though occasionally as late as middle age. There is almost always weakness and atrophy of muscles of the face, with "myopathic" facies, and usually of the shoulder girdle, with winging of the scapulae, and of the upper arms, pelvic girdle, legs, and trunk (Fig. 35). The changes may be asymmetrical. The muscles of swallowing and of the eyes are usually not involved. Pseudohypertrophy is rare. The course of the disease is slowly progressive, so that patients usually live to old age. There is usually increased creatinuria, but this is not as marked as in the severe, generalized form of the disease. The serum levels of enzymes derived from muscle are either normal or slightly elevated.

Intermediate Limb-Girdle (Erb) Type. This type of muscular dystrophy is usually inherited as an autosomal recessive trait, and occurs in either sex. It begins between the ages of 2 and 30 years, usually during the second or third decade. The distribution of weakness and atrophy resembles that of the severe, generalized type, but there is usually no pseudohypertrophy. The course of the disease is slowly progressive, resembling the mild, restricted form, but the facial muscles are spared. Mild creatinuria is usually present, and the serum levels of enzymes derived from muscle are either normal or slightly elevated.

Ocular Muscular Dystrophy. The extraocular muscles are seldom involved in the types of muscular dystrophy described above. There is, however, a less common type of dystrophy which affects mainly the extraocular muscles; this has been referred to as ocular myopathy, or progressive dystrophy of the external ocular muscles.[46] This disease, which usually starts before the age of 20, but may begin at any age, involves the extraocular muscles initially, with ptosis nearly always the first sign (Fig. 36). Progression is slow, but the muscles that move the eyeballs are next affected and complete external ophthalmoplegia usually occurs sooner or later. Diplopia is sometimes an early symptom, but usually soon disappears, owing to the slow and often symmetrical development of the ocular palsy. In most patients the disease is limited to the extraocular muscles, but in 25 per cent the orbiculares oculi and other facial muscles are involved. In 10 per cent the muscles of mastication and of the neck and limb girdles also become affected. In half the patients there is a positive family history, with a dominant mode of inheritance. Creatine excretion and the serum levels of enzymes derived from muscle are normal. The histologic changes in the eye muscles permit identification of the dystrophic process (Fig. 37).

Myotonic Form of Muscular Dystrophy. In this type, which is about one-fourth as common as the other forms, there is not only wasting and weakness, but also myotonia, and frequently frontal baldness, cataracts, evidence of testicular or ovarian atrophy, and hyperostosis frontalis. Inheritance is usually dominant, with variable penetrance. The muscular wasting is usually most marked in the facial muscles, sternomastoids, shoulder girdle, and extremities. Ptosis is present in nearly all patients, and oculomotor weakness in 50 per cent (Fig. 38). Weakness of the pharyngeal muscles may result in a weak, nasal voice. The heart may be involved and the electrocardiogram may be abnormal. The myotonia is manifested by slowness of muscle relaxation after voluntary contraction or after percussion with a reflex hammer. It is best seen in the muscles of the thenar emi-

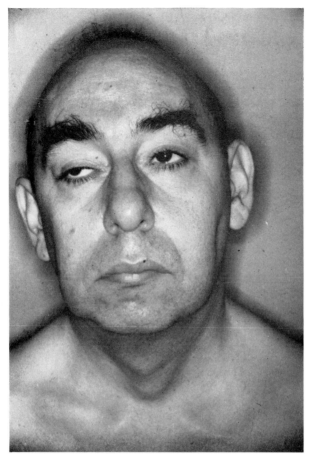

FIG. 38. A 46-year-old man with myotonic dystrophy. There is ptosis, limitation of ocular movement with divergent strabismus, myopathic facies with wasting of the temporal and facial muscles, and frontal baldness.

nence and in the tongue (Fig. 39), and may be recorded electromyographically as repetitive firing of muscle action potentials at a frequency of 25 to 100/second. The myotonia is increased by cold, and may be improved to some extent by the administration of 0.6 g of quinine sulfate every 4 to 8 hours. There is usually no increase in creatine excretion or in the serum levels of enzymes derived from muscle. The muscle biopsy usually shows centralization of muscle nuclei, and sometimes *ringbinden* and sarcoplasmic masses.

Deficiency of Vitamin E. This results, in some experimental animals, in a disease which has some similarity to human muscular dystrophy, but in man vitamin E deficiency, which may result from deficient absorption of tocopherols from the intestinal tract due to biliary tract disease or sprue, does not cause muscular dystrophy. An occasional patient may be seen with the malabsorption syndrome and low serum levels of tocopherols as

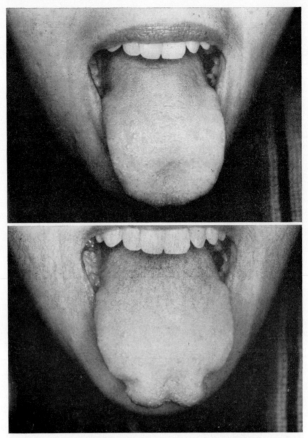

FIG. 39. Sustained contraction of muscles of the tongue of a 34-year-old woman with myotonic dystrophy after tapping with a reflex hammer.

well as weakness and wasting, which may improve following the administration of vitamin E or mixed tocopherols.

RARE MYOPATHIES

There are several rare myopathies, usually familial, which begin in early childhood and produce generalized weakness and atrophy that are non-progressive or very slowly progressive.[2, 4] The serum level of enzymes derived from muscle is normal. The electromyogram usually shows a decrease in the amplitude and duration of muscle action potentials and an increase in polyphasic potentials. In this group the diagnosis can be made only by muscle biopsy and histochemical examination.[28] In *nemaline myopathy* there are rodlike structures in the cytoplasm. In *central core disease* there is a unique degeneration, with abnormal staining, of the central "core" of muscle fibers, which lacks mitochondria, oxidative enzymes, and phosphorylase. In *myotubular myopathy* the central areas of muscle fibers lack myofibrils, resembling fetal muscle fibers.

WEAKNESS WITHOUT ATROPHY OR SIGNS OF
UPPER MOTOR NEURON LESION

When weakness is of acute onset it is often difficult to localize the site of the lesion. The signs indicative of an upper motor neuron lesion may not appear for several hours or days after onset, until spinal "shock" has worn off, but if these signs do not appear in 1 or 2 days it is unlikely that such a lesion is present. Muscle atrophy resulting from a lower motor neuron lesion may not be evident until 2 or 3 weeks after onset, or longer if weakness is mild or the patient obese, but if atrophy is not evident in several weeks it is unlikely that this lesion is present. Disorders affecting the neuromuscular junction (toxins, chemical agents, myasthenia gravis, carcinomatous myopathy) and some disorders affecting muscle (e.g., infections, hypothyroidism, adrenal insufficiency, disorders causing recurrent paralysis) are associated with little or no muscular atrophy unless this occurs as a result of prolonged disuse. Other disorders affecting muscle (e.g., hyperthyroidism, steroid myopathy, polymyositis, muscular dystrophy, myotonic dystrophy) are associated with muscular atrophy, but since this is slower to develop and less severe at comparable degrees of weakness than atrophy due to lower motor neuron disease, it may not be noted early in the course of the disease or in obese patients. Therefore, weakness without atrophy or signs of an upper motor neuron lesion may be due to almost any of the diseases of muscle or of the neuromuscular junction, and may be difficult to diagnose without laboratory studies, such as measurement of thyroid function, serum level of potassium and of enzymes derived from muscle, and muscle biopsy.

Acute Onset

Weakness of acute onset, over minutes or hours, may result from acute change in the chemical environment of the neuromuscular junction or muscle due to deficient or excessive concentrations of potassium, ionized calcium, magnesium, sodium, or glucose; poisoning by anticholinesterase compounds or the toxins of the botulinus or tetanus bacilli or black widow spider; or metabolic diseases such as the periodic paralyses, phosphorylase deficiency, or paroxysmal myoglobinuria. None of these disorders of the neuromuscular junction or muscle results in muscle atrophy.

The metabolic diseases mentioned above are characterized by recurring attacks of weakness, which in some instances follow exercise. Attacks of periodic paralysis are painless, while those due to phosphorylase deficiency or paroxysmal myoglobinuria are accompanied by muscle pain and tenderness which may arouse suspicion of poliomyelitis or polyneuritis. Periodic paralysis can be diagnosed if changes in the serum level of potassium or resultant changes in the electrocardiogram are detected, and an attack precipitated by appropriate means. Weakness and muscle cramps due to phosphorylase deficiency can be precipitated by ischemic exercise. Paroxysmal myoglobinuria is recognized by the appearance of myoglobin in the serum or urine. Botulism is readily recognized by the progression of ocular, bulbar, and then trunk and limb weakness. The association of hypocalcemia or alkalosis with tetany, of clonic and tonic muscular contractions with tetanus, and of local pain and abdominal rigidity with black widow spider bite enable these causes of weakness to be suspected.

Disorders of the Neuromuscular Junction

Weakness due to neuromuscular block occurs if there is either deficient or excessive action of the mediator of neuromuscular transmission (acetylcholine) on the motor endplate, or if drug action simulates these effects.

TOXINS

Botulism. The weakness produced by the toxin of *Clostridium botulinum* is due to deficient release of acetylcholine from the motor nerve endings. Both voluntary and smooth muscle are affected. Symptoms begin 12 to 48 hours after the ingestion of infected food. One-third of patients have nausea, vomiting, and diarrhea; the majority of patients have constipation, as well as urinary retention. The eye muscles are usually affected early, resulting in diplopia, ptosis, dilated and often fixed pupils, and blurring of near vision due to paralysis of accommodation. The bulbar muscles are affected next, resulting in difficulty in swallowing, speaking, and chewing. Finally the skeletal and respiratory muscles are affected, resulting in generalized weakness and respiratory distress. The course of botulism is brief. Patients with mild botulism recover in about 2 weeks. In former years patients severely ill with botulism died in 4 to 14 days of respiratory paralysis, aspiration, or pneumonia. Today, if patients can be kept alive by the use of tracheostomy, artificial respiration, and antibiotic treatment of pneumonia, function begins to return in 7 to 14 days and recovery is complete.

The weakness of botulism resembles myasthenia gravis in distribution, but is much more rapidly progressive, reaching a maximum within a few days; it is unaffected by anticholinesterase compounds, such as neostigmine and edrophonium, which produce some improvement in myasthenia gravis, and affects the smooth muscle of the iris, ciliary body, intestine, and bladder, unlike myasthenia gravis. The resulting dilated and often fixed pupils, blurring of near vision, constipation, and urinary retention enable botulism to be distinguished from other causes of weakness of acute onset. Furthermore, the spinal fluid is normal in botulism, in contrast to the pleocytosis that occurs in encephalitis and poliomyelitis, and the elevated spinal fluid protein seen in infectious polyneuritis. The tendon reflexes are normal in botulism and diminished in poliomyelitis and infectious polyneuritis. There are no central nervous system signs in botulism, unless these occur as a result of anoxia, while patients with encephalitis or poisoning due to centrally acting drugs, such as barbiturates or atropine, have drowsiness. Involvement of the eye and bulbar muscles is rare in periodic paralysis and paroxysmal myoglobinuria.

Snake Venoms. Some snake venoms, especially those of the cobra group, may produce generalized weakness involving the muscles of the extremities and eyes, and those of swallowing and respiration.

CHEMICAL AGENTS

Anticholinesterase Compounds. Some of the organic phosphate anticholinesterase compounds are highly toxic to animals of all species. Several of these compounds (parathion, tetraethyl pyrophosphate, hexaethyl tetraphosphate, mipafox, and, to a lesser extent, malathion) have been widely used as insecticides. They are highly toxic to man as well as to insects, and their indiscriminate use has resulted in a number of deaths. This group of compounds also includes the "nerve gases," which are among the most potent of the known chemical warfare agents.[34]

The mechanisms of action, effects, and prevention and treatment of symptoms are similar for the various organic phosphate anticholinesterase compounds. The effects are attributable to accumulation of acetylcholine 1) in smooth and cardiac muscle and secretory glands (muscarine-like effects), 2) in motor nerves to striated muscle and preganglionic nerves to autonomic ganglia (nicotine-like effects), and 3) in the central nervous system.[41] Exposure of the eyes and respiratory tract to the vapor or liquid forms of these compounds results in marked pupillary constriction, headache, rhinorrhea, and tightness in the chest. Systemic absorption by any route, including the respiratory tract and skin, results in sweating, nausea, abdominal cramps, increased salivation and bronchial secretion, muscular fasciculations, severe generalized weakness, including weakness of the muscles of respiration, giddiness, headache, drowsiness, confusion, ataxia, coma, and generalized convulsions. Poisoning by an anticholinesterase compound should be suspected when unexplained weakness or coma is accompanied by miosis, muscular fasciculations, and excessive sweating, salivation, and bronchorrhea.

Neuromuscular Blocking drugs. Curare, decamethonium, and succinylcholine are used to produce muscular relaxation during operative procedures, intubation, or convulsions. Since succinylcholine is hydrolyzed by plasma cholinesterase, its action is enhanced and prolonged in patients whose plasma cholinesterase activity is low because of liver disease, prior administration of anticholinesterase compounds, or familial deficiency of this enzyme.[43]

Antibiotics. Muscular weakness attributed to neuromuscular block has been reported to occur following the parenteral administration to patients with renal insufficiency of therapeutic doses of polymyxin B or E (colistimethate, colistin), neomycin, kanamycin, and streptomycin.[49] Manifestations have included paresthesias of the face and hands, ptosis, diplopia due to external ophthalmoplegia, dysarthria, dysphagia, ataxia, areflexia, dyspnea and other signs of respiratory insufficiency, and even complete respiratory paralysis, particularly following colistin. The weakness produced by neomycin, streptomycin, and possibly kanamycin is reported to be reversible by neostigmine, while that produced by the polymyxins is not.

Complete recovery occurs if the antibiotic is withdrawn and respiration maintained by mechanical means, if necessary.

Disorders of Muscle

DISORDERS OF ELECTROLYTES

Potassium Metabolism. *Hypokalemia* may develop when there is deficient intake or absorption of potassium, excessive loss in vomitus, stool, or urine, or excessive intracellular movement of the ion. The excretion of potassium by the distal tubules of the kidney, like the reabsorption of sodium, is under hormonal control. Aldosterone, cortisone, and deoxycorticosterone increase the tubular reabsorption of sodium and the excretion of potassium. Administration of these hormones, or their excessive endogenous production, as in primary or secondary hyperaldosteronism or hyperadrenocorticism, increases the excretion of potassium and may result in hypokalemia. Repeated administration of some diuretics, such as mercurial diuretics, acetazolamide (Diamox), and thiazide derivatives, as well as administration of sodium chloride and increased protein catabolism also increase the renal excretion of potassium. Renal tubular dysfunction may result in loss of potassium when the tubules are unable to secrete hydrogen or ammonium ions in exchange for reabsorbed sodium and must excrete potassium instead.

Hypokalemia may also occur as a result of excessive movement of potassium into cells of the liver following the administration of large amounts of glucose and insulin in the treatment of diabetic acidosis, into cells throughout the body in alkalosis, or into the muscle in *hypokalemic periodic paralysis*.[40] This rare disorder, which is usually familial, is characterized by periodic attacks of weakness. Onset of the disease usually occurs during puberty. Attacks almost always occur while the patient is asleep, 4 to 9 hours after supper, particularly after a meal high in carbohydrate. They can sometimes be provoked by insulin, epinephrine, adrenocorticotropic hormone, desoxycorticosterone, or 9α-fluorohydrocortisone. Muscle biopsy in some, but not all, patients reveals vacuoles containing granules consisting mainly of sodium, chloride, and water.[65]

The effects of hypokalemia on muscle are striking, and, if sufficiently severe, result in impairment of function of skeletal, cardiac, and, to a lesser extent, smooth muscle.[44] This is more likely to occur after rapid reduction in plasma potassium concentration than after gradual reduction. Weakness caused by hypokalemic periodic paralysis occurs following less marked depression of serum potassium (usually to less than 3 mEq/liter) than in other causes of hypokalemia (usually to less than 2 mEq/liter), and is much more severe at comparable levels of hypokalemia. Weakness arising from hypokalemia characteristically involves the muscles of one or all extremities and of the trunk and neck, and sometimes the muscles of respiration. The muscles innervated by the cranial nerves are rarely affected. Both the tendon reflexes and the muscle contraction in response to direct percussion are diminished. If weakness is severe, there may be flaccid paralysis of the extremities and trunk and, rarely, paralysis of the muscles of respiration.

The effect of hypokalemia on cardiac muscle may be recognized by electrocardiographic changes: first the appearance of a positive after-potential on the falling limb of the T wave with broadening, later lowering, and still later inversion of the T wave, and depression of the ST segment. The interval between the Q or S wave and the termination of the T wave may be prolonged, but the interval between the Q or S wave and the origin of the T wave is not prolonged, in contrast to the prolongation produced by hypocalcemia. Extrasystoles and other arrhythmias may develop. There is increased sensitivity to the arrhythmic effects of digitalis, and, when these are present, the possibility of hypokalemia should be investigated. In very severe hypokalemia cardiac dilation and even arrest of the heart in systole may occur.

The effect of hypokalemia on smooth muscle consists of relaxation and is often overlooked. Relaxation of muscle of the gastrointestinal tract results in anorexia, nausea, abdominal distension, and ileus. Bladder atony may occur. Vasodilation occurs, and may cause a fall in blood pressure, especially diastolic pressure.

Hypokalemia due to loss of potassium may be accompanied by metabolic alkalosis. When sodium ions are reabsorbed from the renal tubules they are normally exchanged for potassium and hydrogen ions, and if potassium is not available for this exchange an excess of hydrogen ions is lost. Furthermore, potassium ions lost from muscle are replaced by sodium and hydrogen ions from the extracellular fluid. The alkalosis that results from potassium loss is difficult to correct until potassium is replaced.

Primary Hyperaldosteronism. Increased urinary excretion of aldosterone has been classified as primary if caused by an abnormality of the adrenal cortex alone, and secondary if initiated by an abnormality outside the adrenal and unaccompanied by most of the specific features ascribable to aldosterone. Primary hyperaldosteronism is characterized by hypertension, muscular weakness, paresthesias, tetany, polyuria, thirst, polydipsia, and hypopotassemic, hypochloremic alkalosis.[35] In most patients with this disorder the adrenal cortex contains a benign tumor. Less often there is bilateral adrenal hyperplasia, occasionally a malignant tumor, and, rarely, morphologically normal adrenals.

Almost all patients with primary hyperaldosteronism have hypertension, but this rarely progresses to the accelerated (malignant) state. The blood pressure can often be reduced by antihypertensive medication, particularly ganglionic blocking agents. Periodic attacks of weakness, involving mainly the legs and arms, also occur, and are attributed to the disturbance in potassium metabolism. Less often there are paresthesias and tetany, with positive Chvostek and Trousseau signs, occurring with normal serum calcium concentration and without hyperventilation, and attributed to the alkalosis. There is usually no edema, although this may occur.

Primary hyperaldosteronism, as noted above, is characterized by hypopotassemia, alkalosis, and often by intermittent hypernatremia as well.

There is excessive renal loss of potassium, and the hypopotassemia usually responds poorly to the administration of large amounts of potassium. Weakness and paresthesias may become manifest when the renal loss of potassium is accentuated by the administration of a diuretic, particularly a thiazide derivative, or when supplementary potassium administration is stopped. There is usually persistently alkaline urine, mild proteinuria, and hyposthenuria unresponsive to pitressin. The occurrence of spontaneous hypoglycemia and hypomagnesemia, and even of hyponatremia, has been described. The urinary excretion of 17-ketosteroids and 17-hydroxycorticosteroids is normal, while the blood level and urinary excretion of aldosterone are elevated, usually to several times the normal values. (See Chapter on Systemic Arterial Hypertension.)

Secondary hyperaldosteronism occurs in patients with edema due to heart failure, nephrosis, cirrhosis, and possibly toxemia of pregnancy. Edema is present, but hypertension and most of the other manifestations of primary aldosteronism are usually absent.

Hyperkalemia results mainly from deficient renal excretion of potassium ions or from excessively rapid intravenous administration of potassium salts. The former usually occurs in association with anuria or oliguria, and is seen particularly in renal insufficiency. Hyperkalemia of moderate degree may also result from adrenal cortical insufficiency, hypoaldosteronism, or reduced renal blood flow. Movement of potassium out of the muscle into the extracellular fluid occurs in *hyperkalemic periodic paralysis* (adynamia episodica hereditaria), a heritable disorder even rarer than hypokalemic periodic paralysis, of which it is, in some ways, the opposite.[40] Attacks of weakness occur during the day rather than at night, often about 1 hour after exercise. There is slight to moderate elevation of serum potassium and reduction in muscle potassium during attacks, indicating leakage of potassium from muscle. The muscle becomes hyperirritable during attacks, and in some patients may undergo myotonic contraction. Attacks of weakness may be precipitated by oral administration of potassium. Attacks can often be prevented by the prior administration of diuretics such as acetazolamide and chlorothiazide, which increase excretion of potassium. Attacks can be terminated by the intravenous administration of calcium, glucagon, or epinephrine.

The effects of hyperkalemia, like those of hypokalemia, are exerted almots exclusively on muscle, and, if sufficiently severe, result in impairment of function of skeletal, cardiac, and, to a lesser extent, smooth muscle. This is more likely to occur after a rapid rise in serum potassium concentration than after a gradual rise. Weakness caused by hyperkalemic periodic paralysis occurs following a less marked elevation of serum potassium (usually to 5 to 6 mEq/liter) than in other causes of hyperkalemia (usually to more than 8 mEq/liter), and is much more severe at comparable levels of hyperkalemia. Weakness due to hyperkalemia characteristically involves the muscles of one or all extremities, the trunk and neck, sometimes the face and jaws, and sometimes the muscles of respiration. The oculomotor muscles are rarely affected. Tendon reflexes are diminished and the muscles are flaccid, except in the form of hyperkalemic periodic paralysis accompanied by myotonia.

The effect of hyperkalemia on cardiac muscle may be recognized by electrocardiographic changes: the T wave becomes elevated and peaked and the ST interval shortened, the R wave decreases and the S wave increases in amplitude, the QRS complex becomes widened to a biphasic curve, the PR interval is prolonged, and varying degrees of heart block occur; the P wave may disappear as a result of auricular standstill; ventricular extrasystoles and fibrillation may occur; and the heart may stop in diastole. Patients with atrioventricular block appear to be particularly susceptible to the cardiac effects of hyperkalemia, which may increase the block, retard impulse propagation, and depress the ventricular pacemaker, resulting in asystole.

The effect of hyperkalemia on smooth muscle is noted mainly on vascular muscle, which may contract, resulting in pallor, coldness, and pain. The concentration of potassium that produces severe vasoconstriction is higher than that ordinarily attained in the blood, but may be reached locally in the gastrointestinal tract following ingestion of tablets containing potassium salts, which can thus produce ulceration of the gastrointestinal mucosa.

A third type of hereditary *periodic paralysis (normokalemic)* resembles the hypokalemic type in onset during sleep, and the hyperkalemic type in onset following potassium administration, and differs from both in the normal level of serum potassium present during attacks and in the amelioration of weakness following sodium chloride administration.[65] The muscle contains vacuoles, and, during attacks, increased sodium concentration and decreased potassium. Attacks of normokalemic periodic paralysis appear to be preceded by urinary loss of sodium and retention of potassium, and have been prevented by high salt intake and by the administration of acetazolamide or 9α-fluorohydrocortisone, which causes renal retention of sodium and loss of potassium.

Hypercalcemia. Hypercalcemia occurs in hyperparathyroidism, in excessive administration of calcium and alkali (milk-alkali syndrome) or of vitamin D, in malignant disease with or without bony metastases, multiple myeloma, leukemia, sarcoidosis, hyperthyroidism, and following prolonged immobilization. Patients who are hypercalcemic often complain of lassitude and weakness; when the plasma concentration of calcium is above 12 mg/ 100 ml a moderate decrease in strength and tone of muscle may occur, presumably owing to decreased excitability of nerve and muscle. Hypercalcemia also reduces motility in the gastrointestinal tract, resulting in anorexia, nausea, vomiting, constipation, distension, abdominal pain, and even obstruction. It affects the heart, producing shortening of the QT (or ST) interval and an increase in the toxic effects of digitalis. It depresses the central nervous system, causing lethargy, mental depression, drowsiness, and even coma. It impairs renal concentrating ability, resulting in polyuria, thirst, polydipsia, and dehydration, and may cause nephrocalcinosis, renal stones, and azotemia. Hypercalcemia should be suspected when lassitude is accompanied by constipation, polyuria, polydipsia, or renal stones.

Hypermagnesemia. Increase in the plasma concentration of magnesium following administration of large doses of magnesium salts produces weakness resulting from decreased muscle excitability and contractility, as well as reduction in blood pressure resulting from vasodilation, and lethargy.

Sodium. Hyponatremia results from loss of sodium in the urine due to renal disease, diuretics, or hypoadrenalism, loss from diarrhea, vomiting, or excessive sweating, particularly if salt intake is restricted or water intake excessive, and, less commonly, from inappropriate excretion of antidiuretic hormone. Hypernatremia is less common, and may result from restriction of water intake, or from hyperaldosteronism or certain lesions in the brain. Either hyponatremia or hypernatremia may result in generalized lassitude and mild weakness. This may be related to the important role of sodium in depolarization of nerve and muscle. Excessive deprivation or loss may also result in muscle cramps, most commonly in the calf muscles and small muscles of the feet, probably owing to increased excitability of the peripheral parts of the motor nerves.

Gradual Onset

Weakness that occurs without the development of atrophy or signs of upper motor neuron lesion is usually due to a disorder of the neuromuscular junction or muscle, or to emotional causes. When the weakness is of gradual onset myasthenia gravis must be considered and investigated by pharmacologic tests, particularly if there is ptosis or weakness of the oculomotor muscles. If the weakness is of mild degree, deficient function of the thyroid or adrenal cortices should be excluded. If the weakness is of mild degree or short duration, or if obesity makes estimation of muscle bulk difficult, it is necessary to exclude diseases of the lower motor neuron as well as those disorders of muscle which eventually produce atrophy, such as hyperthyroidism, hyperadrenocorticism, polymyositis, and muscular dystrophy; this is best done by means of electromyography, electroneurography, tests of thyroid and adrenal cortical function, determination of the serum levels of enzymes derived from muscle, and muscle biopsy. Only after disease of the nervous system and of muscle has been carefully excluded can weakness be attributed to emotional cause. While emotional disturbance occasionally appears to cause objective weakness, as in hysterical loss of function, it is much more often associated with subjective weakness, and will therefore be discussed under that heading.

Disease of the Neuromuscular Junction

Myasthenia Gravis. This chronic disease is characterized by weakness and abnormal fatiguability of skeletal muscle due to neuromuscular block attributable to deficient action of the transmitter, acetylcholine, on the motor endplates. The symptoms are commonly ameliorated, although to a variable degree, by anticholinesterase compounds, which enhance the action of the transmitter by inhibiting muscle cholinesterase. This response serves as the basis for diagnosis and management of the disease.

The incidence of generalized myasthenia gravis is slightly higher in females, while localized ocular myasthenia gravis is slightly more common in males. Onset of the disease may occur at any age, but tends to be at an earlier age in female patients than in males, the average age of onset being 28 years in the former and 42 in the latter.

The disease results in either transient or persistent weakness and abnormal fatiguability. The initial manifestations are most commonly referable to the extraocular muscles. The initial symptom is ptosis in approximately 25 per cent of patients (Fig. 40), diplopia in 24 per cent, weakness of the legs in 13 per cent, and, in the remainder, blurring of vision, difficulty in swallowing or chewing, slurred or nasal speech, weakness of arms, hands, neck, face, or trunk, generalized fatigue, or shortness of breath.[37] The extraocular muscles are affected at some time in the course of the disease in almost every patient, and many have several episodes of transient weakness before the disease becomes persistent. Impairment of these muscles occurs unilaterally or bilaterally and in almost all combinations of functional disturbance. Elevation of the lids and upward deviation of the eyes are usually most affected, and downward deviation least affected. Occasionally there is complete limitation of extraocular movement. When ptosis is present, the orbicularis oculi is also usually affected, resulting in weakness of closure of the lid. This may persist even after remission of other symptoms of the disease, and is a very helpful sign in distinguishing between ocular palsy of

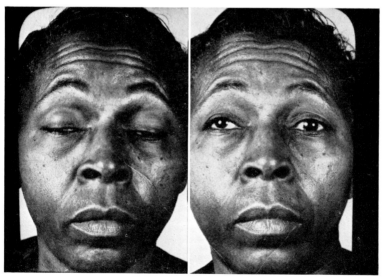

Fig. 40. A 62-year-old woman with myasthenia gravis whose severe ptosis, strabismus, and myasthenic facies were partially improved following the intramuscular administration of 2 mg of neostigmine methylsulfate.

neurogenic origin, which is usually not accompanied by orbicularis oculi weakness, and that due to myasthenia gravis or primary muscle disease. In about 20 per cent of patients with myasthenia gravis the disease remains localized to the extraocular muscles, except for concomitant involvement of the orbicularis oculi. In 80 per cent the disease progresses to involve numerous muscles, and usually becomes generalized within 2 years after onset. The commonest sequence is muscles of the eyes, face, swallowing, speech, jaw, tongue, neck, shoulders, arms, hands, hips, upper legs, lower legs, trunk, and respiration. Those patients who have had ocular symptoms for more than 2 years without evidence of extension beyond the orbicularis oculi usually continue to have the localized form of the disease. Smooth and cardiac muscle are not affected, and the pupils are normal. The tendon reflexes are usually normal, and it is only rarely possible to demonstrate fatigue of the muscle by tapping the tendon, as more rapid stimulation of the muscle is required. Persistent absence of tendon reflexes, or increase in the tendon reflex or muscle response to nerve stimulation following repetitive stimulation or exercise, should suggest that the weakness is due to carcinomatous myopathy rather than to myasthenia gravis.

There is usually no muscle atrophy or only mild wasting due to prolonged disuse. However, in some patients various muscles may develop severe wasting as a result of myopathic changes, usually after several years of disease. The extraocular muscles, including the levators, the triceps brachii, and the quadriceps femoris, are most often affected. Atrophy of the tongue occasionally occurs, giving rise to a triple longitudinal furrowing which is not seen in other diseases (Fig. 41).

Pain and tenderness of muscles are usually not present, but some patients complain of aching or soreness of weak muscles, especially of the neck and back. This usually occurs on exertion, and appears to be due to the effort required to maintain posture. Very rarely the patient may complain of paresthesias, loss of smell, or loss of taste.

The course of the disease is variable. In the majority of patients there is gradual extension of the involved areas, leading to a relatively steady state of weakness which remains unchanged for many years despite moderate fluctuations in severity. Exacerbation of the disease may occur during respiratory infection or emotional disturbance. Women are usually at their weakest for several days prior to the onset of each menstrual period. The basic level of weakness is usually reached within the first 3 years after onset, most often within the first year. In patients who develop severe myasthenia, the average interval between onset of the disease and the first severe episode is 8 months. Approximately 30 per cent of patients die of the disease, usually within 3 years after onset.

Symptoms of the disease tend to fluctuate in severity from day to day or at longer intervals in almost all patients, and approximately one-fourth have a remission lasting several months or longer, with complete or nearly complete disappearance of signs and symptoms. In some patients mild ocular symptoms persist during the remission; in others these symptoms recur

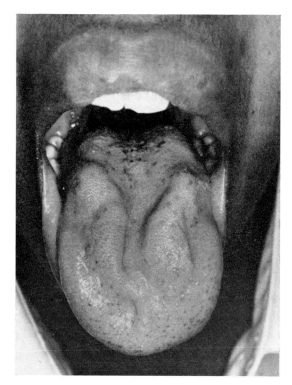

Fig. 41. Triple fissured tongue of a 9-year-old boy with myasthenia gravis.

from time to time, particularly after emotional stress or upper respiratory infection. Most patients have only one remission, while 10 per cent have two to four. Half of the remissions begin during the first year of illness, but others occur after as many as 17 years, with the average interval between onset of disease and remission being 4 years. The duration of remission varies up to 18 years, with an average of 4.6 years.

Children born of myasthenic mothers are usually normal, and never develop the progressive form of the disease, but approximately 10 per cent of such children have *neonatal myasthenia gravis* lasting from several hours to 7 weeks after delivery and usually requiring anticholinesterase medication during this period. Complete recovery then occurs.

Three per cent of myasthenic patients have associated hyperthyroidism, and 2 per cent have exophthalmos in the absence of thyroid disease. The incidence of these associations is higher than would be expected to occur by chance. While treatment of the hyperthyroidism is usually followed by improvement in the myasthenia, the relationship between the two diseases is quite variable. Myasthenia may have its onset during elevated thyroid activity or may appear after treatment, when the patient is euthyroid. It has been reported to have been both improved and made worse by treatment of existing hyperthyroidism or by administration of desiccated thyroid to a euthyroid individual. Because generalized muscular weakness and impairment of extraocular movements are common in hyperthyroidism it is probable that some instances of association of the two diseases are overlooked. In the great majority of patients with hyperthyroidism and weakness neostigmine administration does not produce any improvement in strength, excluding the presence of associated myasthenia gravis.

Pathologic changes in myasthenia are virtually limited to hyperplasia or tumor of the thymus gland, and scattered collections of lymphocytes (lymphorrhages) in some muscles. A tumor of the thymus (thymoma) is present in about 15 per cent of patients with myasthenia gravis. In approximately half of all myasthenic patients the thymus is hyperplastic, and in three-fourths contains numerous germinal centers, a rare finding in nonmyasthenic individuals. Thymic hyperplasia is more common in female patients, and thymoma in males.

Most patients who have a thymoma have a more severe and rapidly progressive myasthenia; thus, in patients demonstrating such a course, a thymic tumor should be searched for. However, there is no consistent correlation between the observed changes in the thymus and the clinical course of the disease; patients with no detectable thymus may have severe weakness, and occasionally patients with a thymoma have a mild form of the disease.

Thymomas can almost always be seen roentgenographically, best in the lateral view of the chest, in the anterior mediastinum, and occasionally with the help of lateral chest tomograms or following injection of air into the mediastinum. Thymus glands that are enlarged but free of tumor can rarely be seen. In spite of the large size of many tumors, only one-fourth invade adjacent structures and produce local symptoms, usually due to bronchial compression, pleural implants, or pleural effusion following tumor necrosis. While mitotic figures are occasionally seen and local implants may occur, distant metastases are extremely rare in myasthenic patients.

Three-fourths of the nonmetastasizing thymomas observed have occurred in myasthenic patients. The incidence of the tumor in nonmyasthenic subjects has been approximately 1/100,000 hospital admissions, compared to 15 per cent in myasthenic patients, and some of the former have developed myasthenia gravis years after the tumor was noted or even following incomplete or complete removal of the tumor. Malignant thymic tumors with distant lymphatic or blood-borne metastases occur almost exclusively in nonmyasthenic subjects, with approximately the same frequency as thymomas. These have been classified as carcinomas or seminomas, and are more likely to produce pain and evidence of compression of the trachea and superior vena cava.

Myasthenic patients should have annual roentgenologic examination of the chest, including a lateral projection. A mediastinal tumor occurring in a myasthenic patient is almost certain to be a thymoma. An extramediastinal intrathoracic tumor in such a patient is most likely to be an ectopic thymoma or, less often, a small-cell bronchogenic carcinoma which may occasionally be associated with a "myasthenic" syndrome, or some other tumor unrelated to myasthenia. An anterior mediastinal tumor occurring in a nonmyasthenic patient is more likely to be a lymphoma, bronchogenic or thymic carcinoma, teratoma, or substernal thyroid, rather than a thymoma.

While myasthenia gravis is the syndrome most frequently associated with thymic tumor, there have been a few reports of other associated disorders. Fifteen instances have been reported of the simultaneous occurrence of benign thymoma and refractory aregenerative anemia, accompanied in some by thrombocytopenia, hemolytic anemia, leukopenia, or aggammaglobulinemia. Four of these patients had myasthenia gravis.

Diagnosis. A presumptive diagnosis of myasthenia gravis can generally be made on the basis of the history, distribution, and fluctuating nature of the weakness, which usually increases following exercise of involved muscles. The diagnosis is confirmed by the improvement in strength which characteristically occurs following the administration of an anticholinesterase compound, such as neostigmine or edrophonium, when the patient is in a "basal" state at least 6 hours after the last medication (Fig. 40).[42] The improvement is often incomplete even after maximum doses, but careful measurement and recording of the level of strength reveals a significant change in all except a few patients with localized ocular myasthenia and a rare patient with generalized myasthenia. In these a response can sometimes be elicited later in the course of the disease. Unequivocal increase in strength of more than slight degree following neostigmine or edrophonium does not occur in patients who are not considered to have myasthenia gravis, with the exception of a few patients with polymyositis, disseminated lupus erythematosus, or carcinomatous neuropathy or myopathy, and with the exception of the extraocular muscles of a few patients with disseminated sclerosis or arteriosclerotic cerebral vascular disease. These responses, however, are sufficiently unusual to detract little from the diagnostic value of the test. In patients with a mild degree of weakness, and in those in whom emotional factors are thought to contribute to the subjective complaint, the effect of placebo administration on the level of strength should also be determined.

The anticholinesterase compound most widely used for the diagnostic test has been neostigmine, administered intramuscularly in a dose of 1 mg/100 pounds of body weight. Atropine sulfate (0.5 mg/100 pounds) should be injected intramuscularly before or with the neostigmine to prevent the muscarinic effects of the latter drug on smooth and cardiac muscle and secretory glands. Improvement in strength of involved muscles begins within 10 minutes, is maximal in 30 minutes, and lasts 3 to 4 hours. When the response is equivocal the test should be repeated on another day with a dose of 1.4 mg of neostigmine and 0.7 mg of atropine per 100 pounds. Neostigmine may also be administered intravenously in a dose of 0.5 mg following 0.5 mg of atropine. This produces a more dramatic response within a few minutes.

Nonmyasthenic subjects experience either no change in strength or mild weakness, and usually develop fasciculations in the muscles of the face, neck, and, to a lesser extent, trunk and extremities, although occasionally there are no fasciculations. In patients with generalized myasthenia neostigmine usually produces no fasciculations except in the least involved muscles, particularly in the lower extremities. In patients with localized ocular or oculobulbar myasthenia fasciculations frequently occur, but are usually less pronounced than in nonmyasthenic subjects. The latter are also more likely to experience gastrointestinal symptoms and occasionally a reduction in blood pressure, which in rare instances may lead to fatal termination unless atropine is administered with or preceding the neostigmine.

Another intravenous diagnostic test employs edrophonium, which has both an anticholinesterase and a direct depolarizing action on muscle. This drug is injected in an initial dose of 2 mg, followed in 30 seconds by an additional 8 mg if the first injection does not produce an increase in strength. Atropine need not be administered except in older patients, who are more likely to develop hypotension. For this reason, and because of its rapidity of action, edrophonium is now widely used as a diagnostic agent. However, the brief duration of its effect (1 to 3 minutes) necessitates speed in carrying out a detailed evaluation of muscle strength.

In the majority of patients the diagnosis of myasthenia gravis can be established or excluded with the help of the response to intramuscular neostigmine or intravenous edrophonium. In a few patients with predominantly ocular manifestations, and in a rare patient with generalized myasthenia, the response to these drugs is so meager that the diagnosis cannot be established. When the upper extremity is involved by the disease the intra-arterial injection of neostigmine in doses of 0.05 to 1 mg can be employed to elicit a local improvement in strength and in muscle response to nerve stimulation. In half the patients with localized ocular or oculobulbar myasthenia a latent myasthenic defect in the upper extremity can be brought out by the intra-arterial injection of acetylcholine or choline and identified by the reparative effect of neostigmine. On rare occasions it may be necessary to administer oral quinine (0.3 g., repeated in 3 hours) or intravenous or intra-arterial d-tubocurarine (0.1 to 0.5 mg) to bring about an aggravation of symptoms. d-Tubocurarine must be used with care, and muscle function promptly restored by intravenous neostigmine (with atropine), to avoid a critical exacerbation of symptoms with respiratory dysfunction.

Serologic Reactions. Approximately 50 per cent of patients with myasthenia gravis have increased serum titers of a globulin which binds to cross-striations of muscle, as demonstrated by immunofluorescent techniques.[61] This muscle-binding globulin is more likely to be present in patients with severe, generalized myasthenia than in those with mild or localized disease. It is rarely present in normal subjects or in patients with other diseases, except for benign thymoma. It is almost invariably present, usually in high titer, in patients with thymoma, whether or not myasthenia gravis is also present. Hence, the finding of an elevated serum titer of muscle-binding globulins indicates that the patient probably has myasthenia gravis or thymoma or both. A negative test for muscle-binding globulin in the serum makes it unlikely that the patient has a thymoma, but provides no information concerning myasthenia gravis, since half the patients with this disease, including some with severe weakness, have a negative test.

Approximately 15 per cent of patients with myasthenia gravis have antinuclear globulin in the serum. Occasionally the lupus erythematosus preparation is positive. While the association of myasthenia gravis and disseminated lupus erythematosus is rare, it is more common than would be expected by chance association.

Other Laboratory Studies. The serum levels of enzymes derived from muscle are normal. Urinary creatine excretion is usually normal or slightly increased in the few patients who develop muscle wasting. Muscle biopsy is normal except for scattered lymphorrhages, which may occur in a number of diseases of muscle. Specialized techniques are required to demonstrate abnormalities in the motor endplates.

Electromyography. When weakness of the muscle tested is severe, sustained maximal voluntary activity may result in decreasing muscle action potentials. Repetitive electrical stimulation of the motor nerve results in progressively decreasing response of the affected muscle (decrement), which is proportional to the rate of nerve stimulation. There is often a transient increase in muscle response shortly after repetitive nerve stimulation is begun (facilitation), but this is not as marked as in patients with carcinomatous myopathy (Eaton-Lambert syndrome), and is quickly followed by decrement. The administration of neostigmine or edrophonium, in doses employed for diagnosis, results in lessening or disappearance of decrement.

Carcinomatous Myopathy (Eaton-Lambert) and Other Myasthenic Syndromes. Muscular weakness and fatigue, with distribution and temporal characteristics similar to those seen in myasthenia gravis, but with little or no response to anticholinesterase compounds, occasionally occur without any detectable associated disease or in association with neoplastic disease, polymyositis, disseminated lupus erythematosus, peripheral neuropathy, and amyotrophic lateral sclerosis.[40, 84] The best studied of these myasthenic syndromes is the Eaton-Lambert syndrome, which is usually, but not always, associated with neoplasm, particularly small-cell bronchogenic carcinoma.[72] The muscular weakness and fatigue are usually most marked in the extremities, and may be accompanied by aching pain. The syndrome resembles myasthenia gravis in symptomatology, and usually in increased reactivity to *d*-tubocurarine and abnormal reactivity to decamethonium and succinylcholine. The syndrome differs from myasthenia gravis in that the muscle action potentials evoked by nerve stimulation are much smaller than normal, and increase markedly in amplitude following repetitive nerve stimulation or voluntary contraction. Furthermore, only a minority of patients with Eaton-Lambert syndrome respond to neostigmine or edrophonium, but most improve following the administration of guanidine sulfate (125 to 250 mg orally four times a day).

Diseases of Muscle

ENDOCRINE DISORDERS

Hypothyroidism. The slowing of physical activity that characterizes both juvenile and adult hypothyroidism is due not only to the lethargy and mental sluggishness that characterize this disease, but also to alterations in skeletal muscle (*hypothyroid myopathy*).[39] Almost all hypothyroid patients complain of subjective weakness, and nearly one-third have objective weakness, usually of mild degree, and primarily affecting the muscles of the shoulder and pelvic girdles. Slowness of movement is also common, and is due in part to retarded mental activity and also to actual slowness of muscular contraction and relaxation. Hypothyroid patients often complain of muscular stiffness and occasionally have muscular aching, spasms, and even painful cramps, especially in the calves and low back. The slowness of muscle movement that occurs in most hypothyroid patients is well seen in the characteristic retardation of the response in the tendon reflex, particularly of the relaxation phase. In three-fourths of the patients the relaxation phase is visibly prolonged, and the degree of change usually parallels the severity of the hypothyroidism. This easily elicited change is of considerable use as a diagnostic aid and in following the effect of replacement therapy. The contraction phase is prolonged in only half the patients, and to a lesser degree. The changes are best seen after percussion of the Achilles tendon.

In most patients there is also a visible delay in contraction and, to a greater degree, in relaxation, following direct percussion of the muscle with a reflex hammer (Fig. 42), or occasionally after pinching the muscle. This has been termed the "mounding phenomenon" or, less accurately, my-

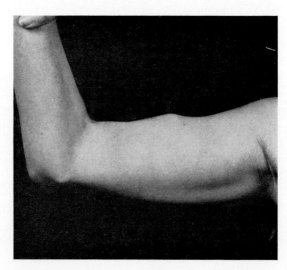

FIG. 42. Mounding of biceps of a 40-year-old man with hypothyroidism, lasting several seconds after tapping with reflex hammer.

edema. It, too, is a useful diagnostic sign and an aid in evaluating the effect of therapy. The delayed responses to percussion of the muscle and of its tendon are due to prolongation of muscular contraction and relaxation. The prolongation is not due to repetitive firing of the muscle fibers and is hence not true myotonia of the type seen in congenital myotonia or myotonic dystrophy. The *electromyogram* in hypothyroid patients does not show evidence of increased electrical activity of muscle, but may reveal a decrease in the size and duration of individual action potentials and an increased proportion of polyphasic potentials, which occur in many types of myopathy. It should be borne in mind that patients with myotonic dystrophy often have a basal metabolic rate that is below normal, probably owing to decreased metabolism of the diseased muscle, and they have an incidence of goiter that is above normal; however, they have normal serum protein-bound iodine concentrations and radioactive iodine neck uptakes, and there is no improvement in myotonia or strength following the administration of thyroid hormone.

In contrast to the muscular wasting that occurs in hyperthyroidism, hypothyroid patients have either normal or increased muscle bulk (Fig. 33). The increase in bulk is seen most easily in the hand, neck, and tongue. The patient may notice difficulty in closing the fist, an increase in neck size, and difficulty in articulating, with slow, thick speech, which may also be hoarse owing to thickening of the vocal cords. Enlargement of the calves may also be noted. The combination of muscle enlargement, slowness, and weakness has been called "Hoffmann's syndrome." Occasionally the muscle hypertrophy may be marked and generalized, a condition that has been termed "hypertrophia musculorum vera." The hypertrophied muscles are firmer than normal, and may become even harder and more swollen after exercise, with aching and local tightening; they are either of normal strength or are slightly to moderately weak. They are never of increased strength.

The muscle biopsy in hypothyroid patients may appear normal on histologic examination or may show abnormal variation in fiber diameter, as well as metachromasia and basophilism of sarcoplasm, increase and central invasion of sarcolemmal nuclei, segmental degeneration, phagocytosis, and collections of lymphocytes. In some patients there may be extracellular "mucinous" material composed of acid polysaccharides, chondroitin sulfate, and hyaluronic acid, similar to that found in other tissues of myxedematous patients.

Nervous System Effects. Alterations in central neural function of hypothyroid patients are responsible for the mental and psychomotor sluggishness that are characteristic of the disease, and probably for the chronic, recurring headaches that occasionally occur.[39] Over three-fourths of the patients have elevation of spinal fluid protein concentration due to increased permeability of the blood–cerebrospinal fluid barrier. A few instances of cerebellar ataxia have been reported. In patients with severe and protracted hypothyroidism coma may occur, accompanied by hypothermia and marked slowing of respiration and, in one-fourth, by convulsions. Artificial respiration may be required to prevent carbon dioxide narcosis. The mortality rate of patients with myxedema coma is extremely high. More common and less serious are peripheral nerve defects due to pressure from mucinous material, causing paresthesias, as in the carpal tunnel syndrome, and, less often, tinnitus, vertigo, or reduction in hearing, smell, or taste.

Hypoadrenalism (Addison's Disease). Generalized weakness of mild to moderate degree is usually present, and may be a prominent complaint.[40] Subjective complaints of asthenia and easy fatigue are usually more prominent than objective weakness, though some patients have decreased strength in the muscles of the extremities and trunk. Muscles innervated by the cranial nerves are not affected. The complaints are due in part to hypotension, especially postural hypotension, as well as hyponatremia, syncope, and hypoglycemia, but changes in muscle response to nerve stimulation may also occur, and have been attributed to glucocorticoid deficiency. The disease is recognized by the above manifestations and by the occurrence of gastrointestinal symptoms, increased pigmentation of exposed areas of skin and of pressure points, hyponatremia, and mild hyperkalemia. The diagnosis is confirmed by demonstration of reduced levels of plasma and urinary glucocorticoids and reduced response of these levels to administration of adrenocorticotropic hormone.

Hypopituitarism. The manifestations of secondary hypoadrenalism are similar to those of primary hypoadrenalism except for the absence of pigmentation and a lesser degree of electrolyte disturbance. Hypopituitarism also results in hypogonadism, manifested by amenorrhea, decreased libido and potentia, and hypothyroidism. Plasma and urinary levels of glucocorticoids are reduced, but these rise following the administration of adrenocorticotropic hormone. The urine and serum levels of gonadotropins and parameters of thyroid function are also decreased. It is important to recognize and treat hypoadrenalism when associated hypothyroidism is treated, since administration of thyroid hormone increases the requirement for adrenal cortical hormone and may precipitate a hypoadrenal crisis in patients with hypopituitarism.

Acromegaly. Weakness and fatigue are common complaints in patients with acromegaly, but are seldom severe and are overshadowed by other features. The cause of the disease is usually an adenoma of the pituitary, usually eosinophilic, but occasionally with chromophobe features, which produces systemic effects due to release of growth hormone and local effects due to the tumor. Growth hormone produces gigantism only if onset of the disease occurs before growth is completed (20 per cent of patients). In most patients onset occurs during adult life, so that there is no increase in height, but there is growth of bone and of all soft tissues, resulting in enlargement of hands, feet, supraorbital ridges, cheek bones, jaws, tongue, and viscera, as well as paresthesias and pain due to pressure on nerve trunks. The growth hormone also produces decreased glucose tolerance in most patients and insulin-resistant diabetes in 25 to 50 per cent. Enlargement of the pituitary results in headache, enlarged sella turcica (in 90 per cent), and, in some patients, pressure on the optic chiasm, causing upper bitemporal hemianopsia.

WEAKNESS WITH MUSCLE PAIN

Relatively few causes of weakness result in muscle pain or tenderness (Table 28), so that the presence of these symptoms facilitates diagnosis. Muscle pain, which must be distinguished from pain in the joints, tendons, bursae, or bones, may result from lesions in the brain, spinal cord, dorsal roots, peripheral nerves, or muscle. Disorders of the upper motor neuron, however, only rarely cause pain in the affected extremity, because of associated thalamic injury or vasomotor changes. Pain is more common in disorders of the lower motor neuron, particularly poliomyelitis, and in diseases affecting sensory roots (disc, tumor, spondylosis, or tabes) or peripheral nerves (neuropathy). Only a few disorders of muscle are accompanied by pain or tenderness. Several viral diseases are characterized by myalgia and subjective weakness, with little or no objective weakness. These include epidemic neuromyasthenia, epidemic myalgia, pleurodynia, Coxsackie viremia, and influenza. A few bacterial diseases cause prominent myalgia, especially brucellosis and leptospirosis. In acute trichinosis eosinophilia is almost invariably present, and there is often periorbital edema. In paroxysmal myoglobinuria and phosphorylase deficiency pain, tenderness, and weakness usually follow exercise and are frequently accompanied by painful muscle cramps. Vascular insufficiency of the extremities also results in pain and weakness after exercise (intermittent claudication). Approximately half the patients with polymyositis have muscle pain or tenderness, but this varies greatly in severity. The disease can be recognized by proximal weakness and wasting, associated with elevated serum enzymes derived from muscle, and by muscle biopsy. Some chemical agents, such as alcohol and clofibrate, may produce an acute myopathy with muscle pain and tender-

TABLE 28

Disorders Characterized by Weakness with Muscle Pain or Tenderness

Rare disorder of upper motor neuron	Thalamic syndrome, vasomotor
A few disorders of lower motor neuron:	
Anterior horn cells	Poliomyelitis
Nerve roots	Disc, tumor, spondylosis, tabes
Nerves	Peripheral neuropathy (sensory plus motor)
A few disorders of muscle	Some viral diseases (epidemic myalgia, epidemic neuromyasthenia, influenza), brucellosis, leptospirosis, trichinosis, paroxysmal myoglobinuria, phosphorylase deficiency, polymyositis, alcoholic or clofibrate myopathy, trauma, polymyalgia rheumatica, tension-anxiety state

ness, variable weakness, and elevation of serum enzymes derived from muscle. When muscle pain or tenderness is not accompanied by objective evidence of weakness, it is usually due to trauma (especially stretch), viral disease, polymyalgia rheumatica, or tension-anxiety states.

Infectious Diseases of Muscle

A number of viral, bacterial, and parasitic diseases produce muscle aching, pain, tenderness, and mild weakness as a result of either direct invasion or the action of toxins. The myalgia is usually increased by muscle contraction, leading to limitation of effort and activity, subjective weakness, and an exaggerated impression of objective weakness, which can usually be demonstrated to be mild if the patient is persuaded to maximal effort. The systemic manifestations of the infection facilitate diagnosis.

VIRAL DISEASES

Epidemic Myalgia and Pleurodynia (Bornholm Disease). The term Bornholm disease refers to infections with viruses of the Coxsackie B group in which myalgia is the main clinical feature. Epidemic pleurodynia includes those cases in which the thoracic musculature is chiefly affected, and epidemic myalgia consists of those in which other muscles are primarily involved. The disease is characterized by paroxysms of pain, most commonly localized to the lower part of the chest or upper part of the abdomen, and aggravated by anything that causes contraction of thoracic or abdominal muscles, such as deep breathing, coughing, or sneezing. The affected muscles may be tender. Fever and frontal headache are usually present and, less frequently, mild gastrointestinal or upper respiratory symptoms, hiccups, or pleural friction rub. The disease usually occurs in epidemics during the late summer or early fall. In some epidemics the neck muscles may be involved, giving rise to "stiff neck" or even torticollis. Occasionally the trapezius may be affected. The white blood cell count may be normal or moderately elevated, and the erythrocyte sedimentation rate is usually increased. The illness usually lasts from 2 to 7 days, but may last up to 3 weeks. Recovery is almost always complete, though patients sometimes feel fatigued and depressed for several months. Death from the disease has never been reported.

Epidemic Neuromyasthenia (Iceland Disease, Benign Myalgic Encephalomyelitis). This disease is characterized by myalgia, fever, and initial gastrointestinal symptoms (nausea, vomiting, diarrhea) or respiratory symptoms (coryza, cough). There is sometimes headache and pain and stiffness of the neck and back, which may arouse suspicion of meningitis, encephalitis, or poliomyelitis. The spinal fluid, however, is normal. There may be protracted fatiguability, lasting for months, with alterations in emotional status, and remissions and exacerbations, the latter often induced by exertion. Muscle atrophy does not occur.

BACTERIAL DISEASES

Bacterial diseases that produce myalgia and mild weakness include brucellosis, which may resemble influenza and epidemic neuromyasthenia, and leptospirosis, which may also cause jaundice, albuminuria, or lymphocytic meningitis.

PARASITIC DISEASE (TRICHINOSIS)

It is estimated that 10 to 20 per cent of the adult population of the United States have had trichinosis at some time, though only the more severe instances of infestation are detected clinically. Symptoms are due mainly to invasion of the muscles by trichinae, which results in muscle pain, especially on movement of the extremities, back, neck, masseters, and eyes, with tenderness and muscle stiffness and hardness. In addition, there may be edema of the eyelids and periorbital tissues, with conjunctivitis, chemosis, burning, and photophobia; there may be pain on swallowing, cough, dyspnea, hoarseness, and occasionally headache, limitation of extraocular movement, delirium, coma, or heart failure.[33] In 80 per cent there is fever, which in more severe infestations may persist up to 6 weeks; occasionally there is a rash, which may be pruritic, and sometimes subungual splinter hemorrhages and petechial skin lesions. The disease results from eating insufficiently cooked pork or pork products infested with trichina larvae. In about 40 per cent of patients diarrhea and abdominal cramps occur 2 to 7 days after ingestion of larvae, and in a few there is nausea and vomiting. The larvae infiltrate the muscles, nervous system, and heart 1 to 5 weeks after ingestion, resulting in acute symptoms, and then encyst, following which the acute manifestations subside, though the patient may have residual muscle aching, tightness and mild weakness and muscle atrophy for months or years.[24]

The most constant single finding in acute trichinosis, and the most important diagnostic aid, is eosinophilia, which occurs in nearly all patients, varying from 5 to 70 per cent of the peripheral blood leukocytes; thus, it may be more marked than in any other disease. The eosinophilia begins about 1 week after ingestion of larvae, reaches a peak in 1 month, and gradually declines over about a year, although on rare occasions it has been reported to persist up to 5 years. When the eosinophils first appear in the peripheral blood their granules may stain faintly and the cells may be mistaken for neutrophils. In 60 per cent of patients there is a leukocytosis (10,000 to 20,000). The skin test with trichina antigen becomes positive about 3 weeks after ingestion of larvae and remains positive for about 7 years. False-positive tests may result from intestinal infestation with trichiuris. Serologic tests for antibody to trichina, employing antigen from larvae and precipitin, flocculation, or complement fixation techniques, become positive 4 weeks after ingestion of larvae and remain positive for about 1 year. False-positive tests may occur in some other disorders, including Hodgkin's disease. Muscle biopsy, with demonstration of encysted larvae, is the definitive diagnostic test.

Chemical Agents

ALCOHOLIC MYOPATHY

An acute myopathy occasionally occurs in alcoholics who have been drinking for years and who drink continuously for a week or more.[67] These patients develop muscle pain and aching, which may be severe, mainly in the calves, thighs, and forearms. Muscles of the face and those involved in swallowing and respiration are not affected. The involved muscles and subcutaneous tissues may be swollen and tender, and there may be low-grade fever. Muscle cramps occasionally occur. Tendon reflexes may be normal, diminished, or absent. The serum enzymes derived from muscle are markedly elevated, including creatine phosphokinase, which is not present in liver and hence will not be elevated as a result of associated liver disease. Serum potassium (from muscle) rises, and myoglobinuria occurs and may darken the urine. The clinical and laboratory findings resemble those of paroxysmal myoglobinuria, and, as in this disease, acute renal failure may occur as a result of tubular obstruction and necrosis from myoglobin deposition. The electromyogram shows "myopathic" potentials, which are smaller and of shorter duration than normal, with more polyphasic potentials than normal. Muscle biopsy shows necrosis of muscle fibers, edema in the interstitial spaces, and infiltration with leukocytes, including polymorphonuclear cells.

In chronic alcoholic myopathy there is weakness, mainly in the shoulder and pelvic girdles, with some atrophy, and sometimes muscle tenderness and cramps. The serum enzymes derived from muscle are usually elevated. Muscle biopsy shows hyaline and granular degeneration of muscle fibers, diffuse atrophy, and increase in subsarcolemmal and central nuclei.

Alcoholic myopathy can be distinguished from alcoholic polyneuritis by the absence of sensory deficit, the presence of edema of muscle and of myoglobinuria, elevation of serum enzymes derived from muscle, evidence of myopathy in the electromyogram and muscle biopsy, and normal nerve conduction velocity. In both myopathy and polyneuritis improvement usually occurs over weeks to months if there is abstinence from alcohol.

CLOFIBRATE MYOPATHY

Clofibrate (Atromid-S) is a branched-chain fatty acid ester which has hypolipidemic action and has been used in the treatment of hyperlipidemic states. In approximately 8 per cent of patients administration of clofibrate produces elevation of serum enzymes derived from muscle, including transaminases and creatine phosphokinase, and in approximately 2 per cent there has also occurred severe myalgia, muscle cramps, stiffness, and tenderness that improved following discontinuation of the drug.[48]

Polymyalgia Rheumatica

This poorly understood syndrome, which is much more common in women than in men, is characterized by myalgia, arthralgia, and usually low-grade fever and increased erythrocyte sedimentation rate. There is often subjective weakness, but little or no objective weakness and no wasting. There is no elevation of serum enzymes derived from muscle; nor is there electromyographic abnormality or histologic change in muscle. The syndrome has a very protracted course and is accompanied by much emotional stress, but is not disabling. Since some patients eventually develop manifestations of rheumatoid arthritis, disseminated lupus erythematosus, polymyositis, temporal arteritis, or polyarteritis nodosa, the syndrome is thought by some to be related to autoimmunity. Specific diagnostic criteria are lacking, however, and it is often difficult to distinguish polymyalgia rheumatica from systemic infections and emotional disorders.

WEAKNESS WITH INCREASED TONE OR ABNORMAL MOVEMENTS

Weakness is accompanied by increased tone or abnormal movements in certain disorders of the motor system (Table 29), so that these signs often aid in diagnosis.

Spasticity of affected muscles results from upper motor neuron lesions. It is greater in flexors of the arms and extensors of the legs, absent at rest or

TABLE 29

Disorders Characterized by Weakness with Increased Tone or Abnormal Movements

Upper motor neuron	Spasticity, clonic movements, convulsions (cortex)
Extrapyramidal motor system	Rigidity
Basal ganglia	Resting tremor, chorea, athetosis, hemiballism
Cerebellum	Intention tremor
Olivary nucleus and tegmental and dentate connections	Myoclonus
Lower motor neuron	Reflex spasm (irritation of anterior horn cells in tetanus or poliomyelitis; of nerve roots in disc, tumor, or spondylosis; of nerves in tetany; or of muscles in myalgia or trauma)
	Fasciculations (slowly progressive injury of anterior horn cells in progressive muscular atrophy or syringomyelia; of nerve roots in disc, tumor, or spondylosis; or of peripheral nerves in chronic neuropathy)
Neuromuscular junction	Fasciculations (in anticholinesterase intoxication)
Muscle	Cramps in hyponatremia, vascular insufficiency, hypothyroidism, paroxysmal myoglobinuria, phosphorylase deficiency, black widow spider bite
	Stiffness in scleroderma, stiff man syndrome, myosclerosis, trauma, and occasionally in trichinosis, sarcoidosis, myalgia, and polymyositis
	Tremor or twitching in uremia, hypocalcemia, alkalosis, hyperthyroidism, alcoholism, drugs (barbiturate, bromide, penicillin), tension-anxiety state
	Myotonia in myotonic dystrophy and occasionally in hypothyroidism or hyperkalemic periodic paralysis

on slow movement, increased by rapid movement, and associated with increased tendon reflexes, extensor plantar reflex, clonus, and sometimes spontaneous *clonic movements* of the extremities. Other associated abnormal movements which may be seen include *myoclonic contractions* of any muscle or group of muscles, which may occur after lesions of the olivary nucleus or of its tegmental and dentate connections, and *convulsions*, which may occur in cerebral disorders of almost any etiology.

Rigidity of affected muscles results from diseases of the extrapyramidal motor system, especially the basal ganglia. It is greater in flexors of the arms and legs, is present at rest, and is not associated with increased tendon reflexes. It is often accompanied by *resting tremor*. Much less commonly lesions of the basal ganglia result in *chorea, athetosis,* or, rarely, *hemiballism*.

Lesions of the cerebellum or brain stem cause *intention tremor*. Each cerebellar hemisphere, through connections with the thalamus, influences the opposite motor cortex, which in turn controls movements of the opposite side of the body via the corticospinal tracts. Efferent cerebellar fibers also end in the red, vestibular, and reticular nuclei, from which descend the vestibulospinal and reticulospinal fibers, which eventually end on the anterior horn cells and cranial nerve nuclei and facilitate muscle tone. Each cerebellar hemisphere influences voluntary movement and muscle tone on the same side of the body. Cerebellar lesions may occur as a result of vascular disease (hemorrhage or thrombosis), tumor, abscess, disseminated sclerosis, or the hereditary ataxias, such as Friedreich's ataxia. Such lesions produce diminished tone and moderate weakness and slowness of movement on the same side of the body, with pendular tendon reflexes, ataxia, intention tremor, dysarthria, and nystagmus.

Ataxia may result not only from lesions of the cerebellum and its connections, but also from interruption of sensory proprioceptive pathways in the peripheral nerves (neuropathy), sensory roots (tabes dorsalis), or spinal cord (subacute combined degeneration, disseminated sclerosis, spondylosis, cervical disc protrusion, or syringomyelia), as well as from intoxication by alcohol, barbiturates, or bromides. Cerebellar ataxia, as well as that due to drug intoxication, is due to failure of central coordinating mechanisms, and is present with the eyes either open or closed. Sensory ataxia, on the other hand, is aggravated when the eyes are closed (positive Romberg sign), since the patient must rely on visual appreciation of the position of his extremities and body in space because of the absence of proprioceptive impulses.

Tetanic muscular *spasms* occur in tetany and tetanus. In the former there is carpopedal spasm and positive Chvostek and Trousseau signs, and in the latter tonic and clonic spasms, trismus, and sometimes seizures. Reflex spasm of muscle also occurs in poliomyelitis, pressure lesions of nerve roots due to disc, tumor, or spondylosis, and inflammatory or traumatic lesions of muscle.

Muscular *cramps* may result from hyponatremia, hypothyroidism, or black widow spider bite. Cramps occur following exercise in normal individuals, as well as in patients with vascular insufficiency, paroxysmal myoglobinuria, and phosphorylase deficiency.

Muscular *stiffness* or induration occurs in scleroderma, stiff man syndrome, myosclerosis, and trauma, and occasionally in trichinosis, sarcoidosis, epidemic myalgia, and polymyositis.

Resting tremor occurs in basal ganglia disease and hyperthyroidism. Intention or resting tremor, and sometimes *twitching*, occur in uremia, hepatic insufficiency, hypocalcemia, alkalosis, alcoholism, drug intoxication (barbiturates, bromides, massive doses of penicillin), and tension-anxiety states. In hepatic insufficiency, uremia, alcoholism, and barbiturate intoxication the tremor may be accompanied by flapping movements of the extremities and by inability to maintain them in a fixed posture (asterixis).

Myotonia is accompanied by weakness in myotonic dystrophy and hyperkalemic periodic paralysis, and by normal strength in congenital myotonia. Delayed relaxation of muscle is also encountered in hypothyroidism.

Fibrillations and *fasciculations* occur in slowly progressive lesions of the lower motor neuron, particularly of the anterior horn cells, and in poisoning by anticholinesterase compounds.

Rigidity

Disorders of the Extrapyramidal Motor System

The basal ganglia receive afferent fibers from the cerebral cortex and thalamus and send efferent fibers to the reticular and red nuclei, which in turn send fibers to the anterior horn cells. The basal ganglia function to reinforce movements and postural influences of cortical origin, and contribute to their automatic motor accompaniment. Lesions of the basal ganglia may occur as a result of arteriosclerotic cerebral vascular disease or senile or presenile degeneration (paralysis agitans), encephalitis (postencephalitic parkinsonism), rheumatic fever, certain tranquilizing drugs such as the phenothiazine compounds, poisoning by manganese, carbon monoxide, or rarely, mercury, or inherited metabolic defect (hepatolenticular degeneration). Impairment of function of the basal ganglia results in moderately increased muscle tone (rigidity), slowness and mild weakness of voluntary movement and of facial movements associated with emotion, abnormal movements (resting tremor, chorea, athetosis, dystonia, or hemiballism), and impairment of synergistic and semiautomatic movements (blinking, ocular convergence, and swinging of the arms in walking).[22] The increased muscle tone, or rigidity, is believed to result from release of lower centers which control tone and which are normally inhibited by the basal ganglia. In chorea or athetosis muscle tone may be decreased, owing to deficiency of the normal contribution of the basal ganglia to postural tone. Tremor is probably due to loss of regulating influence upon the rhythm of discharge of lower centers.

HEPATOLENTICULAR DEGENERATION (WILSON'S DISEASE)

This hereditary metabolic disorder affects the basal ganglia, liver, and cornea, and should be suspected whenever there is any association of rigidity and hyperkinesia with hepatic dysfunction or a pigmentary corneal ring.[23] Siblings are often affected. Symptoms usually begin between the ages of 10 and 25 years and consist of tremors, rigidity, and dysarthria in over three-fourths of the patients, and choreoathetoid movements and dysphagia in one-fourth. The tremor and choreoathetosis may be absent at rest, and tend to be evoked or augmented by voluntary efforts to maintain a posture. The rigidity and hyperkinesia interfere with voluntary activity, but weakness is not a prominent feature. Although a few patients have no clinical manifestations of liver disease, over three-fourths develop symptoms due to cirrhosis of the liver, and in some patients these symptoms predominate. In about one-fourth of the patients portal obstruction leads to ascites, esophageal varices, hematemesis, or tarry stools. In about 85 per cent of patients there are abnormalities of liver function, mainly sulfobromophthalein retention and lowered serum albumin concentration; liver biopsy usually reveals portal cirrhosis. Jaundice is rare. The renal tubules may be affected by the disease, resulting in aminoaciduria. The most distinctive feature of the disease is the Kayser-Fleischer ring, which does not occur in any other disorder. This consists of a brown, green, or yellow deposit of pigment in the cornea, in the form of either a complete or segmented ring 1 to 4 mm wide, with a clear zone between its outer margin and the limbus. Sometimes examination with a magnifying glass or slit lamp is necessary to identify the ring, which is present in about 85 per cent of patients with the disease and occasionally is the only manifestation. Most patients also have emotional disturbances and some show mental deterioration. The course of the disease is progressive, with death usually occurring from liver failure within 5 years, though a few patients live to old age.

The disease is due to an inherited deficiency in the plasma concentration of ceruloplasmin, a copper-binding protein. This results in deposition of copper in the tissues and decreased plasma concentration and increased urinary excretion of the metal. These chemical findings confirm the diagnosis. Increased hepatic concentration of copper can also be demonstrated. The disease should be excluded by appropriate chemical tests in any patient with unexplained tremor, rigidity, dysarthria, choreoathetosis, liver disease, or pigmentary corneal ring, since symptoms may be ameliorated to some extent by the administration of chelating agents such as penicillamine.

Effects of Aging

Changes in Posture. In old age the posture tends to become one of general flexion. The head and neck are held forward, the dorsal spine becomes gently kyphotic, the upper limbs are bent at the elbows and wrists, and the hips and knees are also slightly flexed. This flexed attitude of old age is due in part to changes in the vertebral column and in the intervertebral discs, to ankylosis of ligaments and joints, to shrinkage and sclerosis of tendons and muscles, and to degenerative changes in the extrapyramidal motor system. These factors also contribute to an increase in muscular rigidity, sometimes referred to as senile or arteriosclerotic rigidity. This is demonstrable clinically by resistance to passive movement, especially in the limbs and neck. The legs tend to be more affected than the arms, and the proximal segments of the extremities more than the distal. In its more severe form this increased rigidity may result in the aged individual's assuming catatonic postures and allowing his limb to remain in any position in which it is placed. Impairment of memory, especially for recent events, difficulty in concentrating, mental inattention, depression, apathy, perseveration, and dementia may also contribute to changes in posture and movement.

Disorders of Movement. The aged person usually shows a decrease in movement, attributable mainly to impairment of the extrapyramidal motor system. He may have an impassive facial expression, infrequent blinking of the eyes, and a decrease in spontaneous and associated movements. When they occur, movements are characteristically slow. At times a resting tremor may be present. The flexion attitude, rigidity, infrequency and slowness of movement, and tremor, when pronounced, constitute the parkinsonian state, attributable to degeneration of the extrapyramidal motor system. These signs are commonly seen in minor degree in normal old people, suggesting that this system is more vulnerable to the aging process than are other parts of the motor system.

Disorders of Eye Movements. Defective upward gaze and defective convergence of the eyes are common findings in the aged. It is not clear to what extent this is due to alterations in the central nervous system or in the muscles. The pupils tend to become miotic and sluggish in their reflex response to light and to accommodation. The pupils may even become unresponsive to light, while still contracting on accommodation (Argyll Robertson pupils). These changes are believed to be the result of fibrosis, hyalinization, and lipoid infiltration of the smooth muscle of the pupillary sphincter. Associated lipoid infiltration of the cornea may be seen, resulting in the presence of arcus senilis. There is, however, no clear relationship of the arcus senilis to chronologic age or to arterial degeneration, though it tends to occur at an earlier age in patients who are hypercholesterolemic.

Disorders of Reflexes. The tendon jerks tend to become decreased with advanced age, particularly the ankle jerks, which are often unobtainable. The arm reflexes (supinator, biceps, and triceps) are usually present, though diminished; the knee jerks are the most likely to be preserved. The loss of ankle jerks may be due mainly to inelasticity of the Achilles tendon. Less marked decrease in other tendon jerks is probably due more to shrinkage and sclerosis of tendons and muscles than to changes in the spinal reflex arc. Loss of the abdominal reflexes is common, and may occur as early in life as middle age. In some patients this may result from overstretching of the abdominal musculature by adiposity or childbearing. The plantar responses are often difficult to elicit, mainly because of deformities of the great toe, stiffness or ankylosis of the first metatarsophalangeal joint, and hardening of the sole. This results in a clear-cut flexor response being seen much less frequently than in younger individuals. However, a frank extensor response must always be regarded as an abnormal finding, usually indicating a lesion of the upper motor neuron.

Vascular Insufficiency of Extremities. The decrease in muscular power and endurance that occurs with advancing age is commonplace. Atherosclerosis of the larger arteries to the lower extremities may result in fatigue, weakness, and pain in the legs, which occurs on walking and is relieved promptly by rest (intermittent claudication). Muscle cramps and mild wasting are also sometimes seen. However, while atherosclerosis results in a decrease in endurance and work tolerance, it does not prohibit less strenuous muscular activity unless arterial occlusion or gangrene occurs. It is of interest that atherosclerosis seldom extends to the intramuscular arteries, and, when it does, only the larger arteries tend to be involved. This is because most of the intramuscular arteries are small, and atheromatous plaques are rarely seen in blood vessels less than 250 μ in diameter. However, occlusion of intramuscular blood vessels may occur in inflammatory disease of the arteries, as in polyarteritis nodosa and lupus erythematosus.

Myosclerosis. Widespread muscular wasting (senile atrophy), usually with little weakness, is common in the aged, as noted above. Some patients, particularly the elderly, who have been immobilized for a prolonged period for any reason develop progressive disuse atrophy and weakness of muscles, retraction of the wasted muscles and their tendons, and contractures of the limbs. The legs may be held in extreme flexion, and standing and walking may become impossible. The resulting picture, which has been termed myosclerosis, superficially resembles that produced by dermatomyositis. However, the disorder is probably not the result of a specific myopathy, but rather of immobility, disuse atrophy, and secondary contracture.

Spasm

Tetany

Hypocalcemia. Diminution in the concentration of ionized calcium in the plasma results in increased irritability and spontaneous discharge of sensory and motor nerves and of muscle, producing "tetany." Increase in plasma calcium concentration has the opposite effect, and results in hypotonia and weakness. Tetany may occur as a result of diminution of plasma calcium concentration, as in rickets, osteomalacia, hypoparathyroidism, steatorrhea, or uremic phosphorus retention, or as a result of diminution in the degree of ionization of plasma calcium without change in concentration, as in alkalosis due to hyperventilation or to the ingestion of excessive amounts of sodium bicarbonate. For tetany to occur as a result of hypocalcemia the serum level must usually be below 7 mg/100 ml. It is more likely to occur when the concentration of calcium is lowered rapidly. In chronic hypocalcemia adaptation occurs, and far lower concentrations of calcium can be tolerated without symptoms than in acute hypocalcemia.

When the concentration of ionized calcium is sufficiently reduced, sensory manifestations, consisting of tingling and a sensation of tension, begin in the face and hands and spread to the lower extremities and trunk. These are followed by muscular spasms and twitching in the same distribution. The spasms in the distal muscles of the extremities have a characteristic distribution which results in the typical attitude of carpopedal spasm. The hands are in the position of *main d'accoucheur*, with the fingers flexed at the proximal and extended at the distal joints, and the thumbs strongly adducted and opposed. The wrists and elbows may be flexed. The feet also show flexion of the proximal joints of the toes and extension of the distal joints, and concavity of the plantar surface. When there is marked reduction in plasma ionized calcium there may be facial spasm, laryngospasm, and occasionally convulsions. When tetany is latent, muscle spasm can be evoked locally by tapping a nerve, particularly the facial nerve (Chvostek's sign), by pressure and ischemia of a nerve following inflation of a sphygmomanometer cuff about the upper arm (Trousseau's sign), or by hyperventilation after removal of the cuff (von Bonsdorff's sign). Hypocalcemia and alkalosis also affect cardiac muscle, resulting in prolongation of the QT (or ST) interval, and decrease in some of the actions of digitalis.

Patients with hypocalcemia or tetany usually do not have objective weakness, but muscular spasms and twitching may interfere with motor activity, and may result in subjective weakness and a feeling of exhaustion. Hyperventilation in any individual often causes giddiness, and may cause subjective weakness.

Hypomagnesemia. Reduction in the plasma concentration of magnesium may result in muscle spasms and convulsions resembling tetany, probably because of increased excitability of nerve and muscle. This has been observed in experimental animals following magnesium deprivation. Reduced plasma concentration of magnesium has been reported to occur in some patients with hyperparathyroidism.

Tetanus

Clostridium tetani produces an exotoxin which is responsible for the clinical picture of tetanus. This is characterized by local and generalized muscular rigidity and generalized, reflexly induced, tonic and clonic convulsive seizures due to the action of the blood-borne toxin on the central nervous system, including the anterior horn cells of the spinal cord. The toxin appears to act on these cells and on internuncial neurons in a manner similar to strychnine, blocking the hyperpolarization normally produced by inhibitory synapses, with the result that excitatory impulses multiply through reflex pathways unchecked, and produce excessive discharges to the lower motor neurons. Muscular rigidity and stiffness usually begin in the muscles of mastication, resulting in trismus, and in the facial muscles, resulting in a characteristic facial expression termed risus sardonicus. This may be followed by rigidity of the muscles of the spine, resulting in opisthotonos; of the bulbar muscles, causing dysphagia; of the laryngeal muscles, causing laryngospasm; and of the muscles of the extremities, abdomen, and chest. Sustained contraction of the respiratory muscles may produce asphyxia, which is the usual cause of death. The convulsions occur both spontaneously and reflexly, in response to all types of sensory stimuli.

Cramps

Cramps are characterized by sustained involuntary and painful contractions of muscle which usually result from continuous firing of most of the motor units in the muscle at very high frequency, up to 300/second. This is much more rapid than the frequency of motor unit discharge (up to 50/second) that occurs in maximum voluntary contraction of peripheral muscle, and more rapid than that occurring in tetany. Cramps usually occur in one muscle group of the calf, foot, thigh, hand, or hip, following unusual muscular effort, and usually at night. They may also occur as a result of decrease in the plasma concentration of calcium, sodium deprivation or loss, peripheral vascular insufficiency, certain toxins, such as that of the tetanus bacillus and black widow spider, and, rarely, anterior horn cell or peripheral nerve disease. In uremia cramps and twitching may occur even in the absence of marked change in plasma calcium or sodium concentrations. Muscle cramps also occur in association with certain diseases of muscle, including the stiff man syndrome, McArdle's syndrome (phosphorylase deficiency), congenital myotonia, and, to a lesser degree, myotonic dystrophy, hypothyroid myopathy, and paroxysmal myoglobinuria. In the great majority of instances, however, cramps occur in apparently normal individuals, and their mechanism is unknown.

Stiff Man Syndrome. This rare syndrome is characterized by intermittent painful muscle cramps which may be precipitated by external stimuli or sudden voluntary or passive movement, and by gradually increasing rigidity which fluctuates in severity. Most patients with this disease do not have fasciculations or evidence of increased electrical activity of the muscle fibers, and the defect is thought to be either in the central nervous system or in the contractile mechanism. A few patients, however, do have fasciculations and continuous electrical activity of the muscle fibers resembling that seen in myotonia, but much more persistent.

Phosphorylase Deficiency. This rare disorder (McArdle's syndrome or McArdle-Schmid-Pearson disease) is characterized by the appearance of muscle pain, stiffness, cramps, and weakness within minutes after exercise is carried out, especially under ischemic conditions, such as after occlusion of the circulation of a limb. There is a fall in the concentration of lactate and pyruvate in the venous return from ischemic muscle performing work, in contrast to the rise which occurs in normal subjects under similar conditions. Exhausted muscle may continue in the contracted state, even at rest, owing to the persistence of localized contractures which are not accompanied by electrical activity. In half the patients, myoglobinuria occurs after exercise. The muscle contains excessive glycogen, and homogenates of muscle are unable to form lactate from endogenous or added glycogen unless muscle phosphorylase is added. This disorder is, so far, the only disease of muscle in which a specific metabolic defect has been demonstrated: a deficiency of muscle phosphorylase. There is no abnormality in the phosphorylase activity of other tissues, such as liver or leukocytes.

Paroxysmal Myoglobinuria. This rare disease is characterized by intermittent attacks of muscle pain and cramping, usually precipitated by exercise, and followed by muscle firmness, tenderness, weakness, and darkening of the urine as a result of excretion of myoglobin from degenerating muscle fibers.[27] The calf muscles are most often involved. Systemic manifestations, such as chills, fever, vomiting, abdominal pain, leukocytosis, and hypotension, may occur. Occasionally the muscles of respiration may be involved, leading to respiratory paralysis. The myoglobinuria usually does not cause renal impairment, but, when very marked and accompanied by hypotension, it may result in tubular damage, anuria, and renal failure. The disease appears to be caused by intermittent degeneration of muscle fibers of unknown cause, with release into the blood of muscle constituents, including myoglobin, potassium, creatine, amino acids, glutamic-oxalacetic transaminase, aldolase, and creatine phosphokinase. The serum levels of these enzymes increase markedly following attacks.

Myotonia

This is a painless, residual contraction of muscle which has been made to contract either voluntarily or by mechanical (percussion), electrical, or chemical means. The involuntary after-contraction lasts for several seconds and is accompanied by repetitive firing of muscle action potentials at a frequency of 25 to 100/second. Myotonia is increased by cold or by depolarizing compounds such as acetylcholine, decamethonium, neostigmine, and potassium, and is diminished by exercise, quinine, epinephrine, or calcium. The influence of neostigmine, potassium, exercise, and quinine on myotonia is opposite to their influence on myasthenia gravis. Since myotonia may be elicited by percussion even after complete curarization or after degeneration of motor nerves, the site of the disorder must be distal to the motor nerves and to the locus of action of curare on the endplate. Patients with myotonia have unstable muscle membranes which undergo spontaneous rhythmical depolarization, leading to repetitive spikes. There is thought to be a defect in membrane permeability, but the nature of the defect has not been identified.

Myotonia occurs in a congenital form (Thomsen's disease) and in myotonic dystrophy, both of which are often inherited as dominant traits, and in some patients with hyperkalemic peiodic paralysis. In congenital myotonia the disorder is more generalized than in myotonic dystrophy, in which the myotonia is usually localized to the muscles of the flexors of the fingers, the tongue (Fig. 39), jaws, and occasionally the legs. However, of greater significance to the patient is the fact that in congenital myotonia the muscles are strong and usually hypertrophied, possibly because of increased work caused by myotonia, while in myotonic dystrophy there is muscular weakness and wasting, often severe, caused by dystrophic changes in the muscle.

Fibrillations and Fasciculations

Within 3 weeks after denervation resulting from a lesion of the lower motor neuron there begin spontaneous electrical discharges of single muscle fibers or of groups of fibers constituting a fraction of a motor unit, giving rise to contractions called *fibrillations*. These discharges arise at the endplates and are believed to be due to increased reactivity of the denervated endplates to acetylcholine. The increased reactivity is an example of the general phenomenon that denervated structures become more responsive to their natural transmitters. The resulting muscle movements are very fine, visible only in the tongue except in very thin individuals, and usually detected by electromyography. They are increased by exercise, tapping the muscle, or the administration of depolarizing agents, such as anticholinesterase compounds.

Slow degeneration of the lower motor neuron, particularly the anterior horn cells, also results in spontaneous electrical discharges of single motor units or groups of motor units which produce visible muscular twitchings termed *fasciculations*. These are most striking in progressive muscular atrophy. They also occasionally occur when the anterior horn cells are slowly damaged by compression, as in syringomyelia or spinal cord tumor or disc, but they do not occur when these cells are rapidly injured or destroyed, as in poliomyelitis. They occasionally occur after slowly progressive injury to ventral roots, as in tumor or spondylosis, or to the motor nerves, as in interstitial hypertrophic neuropathy, but are seldom seen in the great majority of diseases of motor nerves, which are more rapidly progressive. Fasciculations and the potentials which precede them are greater in amplitude and duration than fibrillations, and are more regular in their rate and size. Like fibrillations, fasciculations are peripheral in origin, as they do not cease after nerve block or section. However, they do decrease in intensity, indicating that they are under the influence of the diseased anterior horn cells, though the mechanism of their production is not known. Like fibrillations, they are increased by exercise, by tapping the muscle, or by administration of depolarizing agents such as anticholinesterase compounds. When fasciculations are not observed in a patient in whom lower motor neuron disease is suspected it is sometimes helpful diagnostically to administer 1 mg of neostigmine (with 0.6 mg of atropine) intramuscularly. This results in visible fasciculations in the involved muscles of approximately 80 per cent of patients with lower motor neuron disease, generalized fasciculations in about 10 per cent of normal subjects, and few or no fasciculations in patients with muscle disease.[63] The test should not be performed in patients with dysphagia due to lower motor neuron disease, since it may cause an increase in pharyngeal weakness, with risk of aspiration.

Spontaneous fasciculations occurring in the presence of muscular weakness and wasting are a manifestation of slowly progressive destruction of any part of the lower motor neuron: anterior horn cells, cranial motor nerve nuclei, ventral nerve roots, or peripheral motor nerves. Occasionally spontaneous fasciculations occur in normal individuals. When marked, they are termed *myokymia*. These movements may resemble fasciculations due to lower motor neuron disease, but if the latter can be excluded by the absence of weakness and wasting, the movements are of no significance. Fasciculations occurring in normal individuals are usually more irregular in rate and size, and shorter in duration when observed electromyographically, than those due to lower motor neuron disease, but there is no reliable means of differentiation except by the presence or absence of weakness and atrophy.

Spontaneous fasciculations must be distinguished from *contraction fasciculations*, which may occur during voluntary contraction of atrophied muscle, regardless of the cause of the atrophy. These probably represent the contraction of isolated groups of motor units, which stand out because adjacent units are not responding.

SUBJECTIVE WEAKNESS

Acute or Recurrent

Subjective weakness, usually without objective evidence at the time of examination after subsidence of the episode, may occur acutely or recurrently when there is a decrease in the blood supply to the brain or skeletal muscles from any cause (Table 30). Sufficient decrease in blood supply to the brain results in giddiness and syncope, varying degrees of loss of consciousness, and finally convulsions. Observation or history of these complaints facilitates identification of cerebral ischemia as the cause, but when the ischemia is mild or transient the patient may complain only of weakness, and the cerebral origin of the symptoms may not be readily recognized.

Transient Cerebral Ischemia

This occurs most commonly as a result of vascular disease or decreased cardiac output, caused either by decreased venous return to the heart or, less commonly, by forward heart failure. It is most likely to occur in the standing position, and usually results in faintness as well as weakness. Postural (orthostatic) hypotension occurs when there is a decrease in the sympathetic vasoconstrictor reflexes which are necessary to maintain venous return in the erect position, resulting in pooling of blood in the periphery. It also occurs when there is a decrease in blood volume. Sympathetic vasoconstrictor tone may decrease as a result of heat, motionless standing, emotion (vasovagal syncope), disease of the midbrain or spinal cord, or sympathetic denervation from surgery, neuropathy (especially diabetic), or drugs (antihypertensive, antidepressant, or ataractic). Blood volume may decrease following blood loss, plasma loss into tissue, or dehydration and sodium loss from dietary restriction, sweating, diarrhea,

TABLE 30

Causes of Acute or Recurrent Subjective Weakness

I. Transient cerebral ischemia (usually accompanied by giddiness)
   A. Decreased cardiac output
      1. Decreased venous return (postural hypotension)
         a. Decreased sympathetic vasoconstrictor tone
            (1) Heat
            (2) Motionless standing
            (3) Emotion or pain (vasovagal)
            (4) Disease of midbrain (tumor, encephalitis, vascular)
            (5) Disease of spinal cord (disseminated sclerosis, trauma, inflammation)
            (6) Disease of nerve roots (tabes dorsalis)
            (7) Disease of peripheral nerves (neuropathy due to diabetes mellitus, porphyria, primary amyloidosis)
            (8) Surgical sympathectomy
            (9) Drugs (antihypertensive, antidepressant, ataractic)
            (10) Idiopathic ("primary")
         b. Decreased blood volume
            (1) Blood loss
            (2) Dehydration and sodium loss from dietary restriction, sweating, diarrhea, vomiting, diuretics, or renal or adrenal insufficiency
      2. Forward heart failure
         a. Heart block or tachyarrhythmia (Stokes-Adams)
         b. Bradycardia from hypersensitive carotid sinus or other cause
         c. Myocardial ischemia or infarction
         d. Myocarditis
         e. Mechanical obstruction due to aortic stenosis, mitral stenosis, auricular thrombus or myxoma, pulmonary emboli, or pericardial effusion
   B. Arterial disease (mainly atherosclerosis; rarely arteritis, embolic, congenital, tumor, trauma)
      1. Intracranial (cerebral, basilar)
      2. Extracranial (carotid, vertebral, subclavian)
II. Other cerebral causes
   A. Chemical
      1. Hyperventilation
      2. Hypoglycemia
   B. Irritant focus
      1. Akinetic epilepsy
      2. Brain tumor
      3. Labyrinthitis, Ménière's Syndrome (with vertigo)
   C. Narcolepsy
   D. Emotional
III. Peripheral arterial insufficiency
IV. Following recovery from episodic neuromuscular disease (myasthenia gravis)
V. Following recovery from episodic muscular disease
   A. Periodic paralysis (hypokalemic, hyperkalemic, normokalemic)
   B. Paroxysmal myoglobinuria
   C. Phosphorylase deficiency

vomiting, diuretics, or renal or adrenal insufficiency. A history of weakness on standing, with or without syncope, particularly on assuming the erect position, requires that the blood pressure be determined in the recumbent and erect positions.

A transient decrease in cardiac output may also result from heart block, ventricular tachyarrhythmia, bradycardia from hypersensitive carotid sinus or other cause, myocardial ischemia or infarction, or mechanical obstruction from aortic stenosis, mitral stenosis, auricular thrombus or myxoma, pulmonary emboli, or pericardial effusion. When cerebral ischemia occurs as a result of decreased cardiac output, whether due to decreased venous return, heart disease, or mechanical obstruction, syncope usually accompanies weakness. The most marked syncope, followed often by convulsions, occurs in the Stokes-Adams syndrome resulting from heart block or ventricular tachyarrhythmia. Syncope due to aortic stenosis generally follows exercise. When cardiac output is decreased as a result of myocardial ischemia or infarction, subjective weakness may occur without syncope, particularly if there is no fall in blood pressure. Occasionally subjective weakness is the sole or main complaint for several hours or days before a myocardial infarct occurs or is recognized. The patient may complain of heaviness and aching of his muscles, aggravated by exercise and relieved by rest, suggestive of decreased blood flow to muscles and intermittent claudication. Rarely, intermittent weakness may be the sole or main complaint in patients with angina pectoris. Like the pain of angina pectoris or the other concomitants or substitutes for pain, such as dyspnea, belching, nausea, or indigestion, the weakness may be brought on by exercise and relieved by rest or nitroglycerin. (See also the chapter on Episodic Unconsciousness.)

Transient cerebral ischemia may also result from *cerebral vascular disease or extracranial vascular disease*, particularly of the carotid, vertebral, or subclavian arteries.[3, 83] Generalized or localized weakness may occur, with or without syncope. Stenosis of the proximal subclavian artery may result in weakness or syncope following exercise of the upper extremity, owing to diversion of blood to the exercised limb and away from the vertebral artery (subclavian steal syndrome).[64]

OTHER CEREBRAL CAUSES

Acute or recurrent subjective weakness may also result from akinetic epilepsy, which may be recognized by electroencephalographic findings, or from hyperventilation, hypoglycemia, or emotional disturbances. In addition, weakness may be simulated by apraxia.

Apraxia. Loss of purposive movement without paralysis may occur following cortical, subcortical, or corpus callosal lesions.[62] If the lesion is in the dominant cerebral hemisphere (left in right-handed individuals), the apraxia is usually bilateral; if in the nondominant (right) hemisphere, the apraxia is in the left arm and leg. The patient is unable to execute certain acts in the correct context, although he can carry out the individual movements upon which such acts depend. There seems to be a loss of memory of how to perform a given act. Failure of the patient to follow a spoken request to imitate the examiner may also result from aphasia that prevents understanding of the spoken or written word, or agnosia that prevents recognition of the object to be used.

Hyperventilation. This produces giddiness, subjective weakness, and paresthesias of the face and extremities resulting from alkalosis due to removal of carbon dioxide from the blood. Symptoms are not improved by recumbency, in contrast to those produced by most causes of cerebral ischemia. Muscular twitching and carpal or pedal spasm occasionally occur. The hyperventilation usually results from anxiety, and may be accompanied by manifestations of an anxiety attack, including globus, fear, and the effects of epinephrine release: tachycardia, palpitations, sweating, and dilated pupils.

Hypoglycemia. Weakness is one of the commonest manifestations of hypoglycemia. Reduction in the blood glucose level results in symptoms due to compensatory hyperepinephrinemia (tachycardia, sweating, weakness, hunger) and, when severe and prolonged, symptoms referable to the central nervous system (headache, giddiness, confusion, visual disturbances including diplopia, weakness, hemiplegia, coma, and convulsions). Patients who complain of recurring episodes of weakness should have a determination of the blood glucose level during such episodes, as well as following a prolonged fast and for each of 5 hours after ingestion of 100 g of glucose. If those who are receiving antidiabetic drugs are excluded, approximately three-fourths of patients with symptoms due to hypoglycemia will be found to have functional (postprandial) hypoglycemia, as indicated by a blood sugar level which is normal after prolonged fasting but which falls below 40 mg/100 ml 2 to 5 hours after ingestion of 100 g of glucose.[18] These patients usually do not develop giddiness or other central nervous system symptoms, except for headache and mild confusion. The second commonest cause of hypoglycemia is alimentary hyperinsulinism, which occurs in about 5 per cent of patients who have had subtotal or total gastrectomy or gastroenterostomy. The next commonest cause is adenoma or carcinoma of the pancreatic islet cells, which causes low blood sugar both after prolonged fasting and after glucose ingestion and which may cause central nervous system symptoms. The administration of tolbutamide or leucine stimulates the islets of Langerhans and produces a greater fall in the blood sugar level and rise in the serum insulin level in patients with islet cell tumor than in normal subjects or patients with hypoglycemia due to other causes. The least common causes of hypoglycemia are hepatic insufficiency and adrenal cortical or anterior pituitary insufficiency, which cause low blood sugar after prolonged fasting but not after glucose ingestion.

Following Recovery from Episodic Neuromuscular or Muscular Disease

During episodes of weakness due to myasthenia gravis, periodic paralysis, paroxysmal myoglobinuria, or phosphorylase deficiency objective signs of weakness are present. However, if the patient is seen after recovery, or between attacks, the examination may be normal. The history of weakness due to these disorders is characteristic, and should aid in diagnosis.

Peripheral Arterial Insufficiency. This condition, which usually is due to atherosclerosis, results in pain and weakness of the muscles of the pelvic girdle or lower extremities on exercise, relieved promptly by rest. Occasionally pain may be minimal or absent, or described as muscle tightness, soreness, or cramps, and intermittent weakness of the lower extremities may be the main complaint.

Chronic Subjective Weakness

Subjective weakness, without clear-cut objective evidence, may occur in almost any acute or chronic illness, whether somatic or emotional. Many patients who consult a physician for any reason will include among their complaints weakness, fatigue, lack of energy, listlessness, or weariness. These symptoms may result from acute or chronic infectious diseases, anemia, nutritional deficiency, neoplastic disease, metabolic disease such as diabetes or uremia, disorders of the thyroid or adrenal glands, drug intoxication due to alcohol, barbiturates, or bromides, circulatory failure, senility, or emotional disorder. While emotional disorder is one of the more common causes of chronic subjective weakness, somatic disease must be carefully sought for, particularly since psychic and somatic disorders frequently coexist. A careful history and physical examination, including serial determinations of body temperature, as well as appropriate laboratory studies, will usually identify the presence of somatic disease. Only after somatic disease has been excluded should weakness be ascribed to emotional disorder.

Emotional Disorder

The impulse for voluntary motor activity arises in the frontal cortex, and any impairment of volition may result in symptoms of weakness or fatigue. Impairment of volition is almost always of emotional origin, but may occasionally result from organic disease of the frontal cortex, such as cerebral vascular disease, brain tumor, general paresis, or various cortical degenerative diseases such as Pick's, Alzheimer's, and Creutzfeldt-Jakob disease. Weakness of emotional origin may take the form of local weakness or paralysis, as in hysteria; generalized weakness and fatigue, as in neurasthenia; weakness with catatonia, as in schizophrenia; or weakness with wasting resulting from inanition, as in anorexia nervosa. The diagnosis of weakness or fatigue of emotional origin can be made only after careful exclusion of the many other causes, but is often suggested by a history of anxiety and increased muscle tension, fatigue on awakening, early evening drowsiness, and improvement in symptoms following suggestion or placebo administration. In the author's experience more than one-fourth of patients referred by physicians with the presumptive diagnosis of disease of the neuromuscular system have proved to have weakness of emotional origin. This has been much more common in women than in men. However, it must be kept in mind that emotional disorders do not protect the subject against disease of the motor system, and the disability of motor system disease may lead to emotional disorder. Weakness of emotional origin may then be superimposed on weakness due to other cause, and the distribution of the weakness of emotional origin may be determined by the underlying loss of function. In such instances the major part of the disability may be relieved following hypnosis, placebo, or other forms of suggestion, but evidence of the underlying disease process remains. The only conclusive demonstration that weakness is entirely of emotional origin is the complete amelioration of signs and symptoms following suggestion, persuasion, or more formal psychotherapeutic maneuvers.

Hysterical Paralysis. When paralysis of an extremity or part of an extremity is of emotional origin there may be accompanying decrease or increase in muscle tone. This change in tone may cause a difference in tendon reflexes between the two sides, and increased tone may cause pseudoclonus, resembling true clonus but less sustained. It is rare for hysterical palsy to persist more than a few months, but, if it does, disuse atrophy may ensue. The patient often shows calm indifference to his disability. A number of tests may be employed to demonstrate that the patient can make use of the affected muscles. With the forearms directed upward, the patient's fingers are interlocked, and the patient is asked to move each indicated finger promptly. It is difficult for the patient to decide at once whether the indicated finger is right or left, and the paralyzed finger may be moved. If the patient is told to press his hands or feet firmly together, and the examiner suddenly pulls them apart, it may be possible to detect contraction of the adductors on both sides. When the patient is supine and he is told to raise his normal leg, the examiner can detect downward movement of the opposite heel, since there is a normal associated movement.

Neurasthenia. This term is applied to generalized subjective weakness or fatigue of emotional origin. There is usually no clear-cut objective evidence of weakness, or the patient displays variable performance in tests of strength, reflecting lack of maximal effort and often improved by suggestion. There is no muscle wasting unless there is marked loss of appetite and weight. Neurasthenia is often associated with anxiety, irritability, emotional tension, worry, depression, difficulty in making decisions, and feelings of inadequacy.[19] It may occur in a setting of occupational or domestic problems. The emotional tension is frequently accompanied by a general increase in muscle tension, and by restlessness and incomplete muscle relaxation during rest or sleep. This undoubtedly contributes to the subjective weakness and fatigue. The increased muscle tension may cause pain in the back of the neck or head, headache, backache, pain in and around joints, simulating rheumatism, postural deformity, and even generalized muscle soreness. Some patients complain of difficulty in concentrating, early evening drowsiness, memory impairment, or symptoms attributable to disturbance of the

WEAKNESS 295

autonomic nervous system, such as spasticity of the gastrointestinal tract, gastric hyperacidity, or postural hypotension.

Anorexia Nervosa. The inanition resulting from starvation or self-induced vomiting may result in profound weight loss and muscle wasting. Generalized weakness may also occur, though this is usually less severe than the muscle wasting. Anorexia nervosa occurs more commonly in females than in males, and most often at puberty or during adolescence. Associated symptoms of psychiatric disorder may be profound, and differentiation from various endocrinopathies may be difficult. The improvement in body weight, muscle bulk and strength, and even appetite that follows forced feeding by nasogastric tube is often striking.

SUMMARY

Weakness is among the commonest complaints presented to the physician. The history will indicate whether the weakness is of acute or gradual onset, localized or generalized, intermittent or progressive. Physical examination will disclose the distribution and degree of weakness and the presence or absence of muscle atrophy, tenderness, alterations in tone and reflexes, abnormal movements, extensor plantar reflex, and sensory changes. The cause of weakness should first be localized anatomically, if possible, and then the etiology determined, with emphasis on the diagnosis of disorders amenable to specific management. Weakness occurs in the following settings.

Weakness with Signs of an Upper Motor Neuron Lesion. This condition is recognized by the presence of spasticity, increased tendon reflexes, clonus, extensor plantar reflex, and absence of atrophy. While the commonest cause of monoplegia, hemiplegia, or quadriplegia is arterial thrombosis in the cerebrum or brain stem, it is important to exclude extracranial arterial thrombosis, cerebral embolism, and bleeding berry aneurysms. Slowly progressive monoplegia or hemiplegia is suggestive of brain tumor. Examination of the pupils and spinal fluid will usually enable the physician to exclude central nervous system syphilis.

Paraplegia or quadriplegia of sudden onset, occurring in minutes, is usually due to traumatic or vascular necrosis of the spinal cord; fracture or dislocation of the spine should be excluded. When paraplegia or quadriplegia develops over hours or days, with signs of an upper motor neuron lesion, the cause is usually either disseminated sclerosis, subacute combined degeneration, or pressure on the cord from epidural abscess, Pott's disease, vertebral metastases, cord tumor, cervical disc, or spondylosis. If atrophy, rather than signs of an upper motor neuron lesion, develops, the lesion is in the lower motor neuron, and is usually due to peripheral neuropathy if symmetrical, or poliomyelitis if asymmetrical. If the paralysis is transient periodic paralysis or paroxysmal myoglobinuria should be excluded.

Weakness with Atrophy. Weakness with atrophy, flaccidity, and decreased tendon reflexes can result from any disease of the lower motor neuron or from most diseases of muscle. The distinction between neurogenic and myopathic disease is made by the more distal distribution of weakness and wasting and by sensory changes (if present) in neurogenic disease; by spontaneous electrical discharges from involved muscle in neurogenic disease and polyphasic potentials in muscle disease; by slow nerve conduction velocity in neuropathy; by increased serum levels of enzymes derived from muscle in some diseases of muscle; and by muscle biopsy, showing grouped atrophy in neurogenic disease and diffuse atrophy in myopathic disease.

Monoplegia with atrophy is usually due to lower motor neuron disease, and is usually the result of damage to the anterior horn cells by poliomyelitis, tumor, syringomyelia, or early progressive muscular atrophy, or damage to motor nerves from peripheral neuropathy, trauma, protruded intervertebral disc, spondylosis, or tumor. Paraplegia or quadriplegia with atrophy is usually due to these causes, especially peripheral neuropathy, if weakness develops over hours or days, or progressive muscular atrophy if it develops over weeks. The occurrence of a sensory level or paralysis of bladder or bowel sphincters indicates a lesion in the cord, while distal sensory or motor loss indicates a lesion in the peripheral nerves. Paraplegia or quadriplegia with atrophy, developing over weeks and of predominantly distal distribution, is likely to be due to progressive muscular atrophy or motor neuropathy if there are no sensory changes, or to spondylosis, disc, spinal cord tumor, syringomyelia, or motor and sensory neuropathy if there are sensory changes.

If the weakness and wasting are of predominantly proximal distribution and are unaccompanied by sensory changes, the patient is likely to have a disease of muscle, particularly polymyositis, muscular dystrophy, hyperthyroidism, hyperadrenocorticism, or wasting due to chronic infection, neoplasm, or malabsoprtion, though chronic proximal spinal muscular atrophy should be excluded.

Weakness without Atrophy or Signs of an Upper Motor Neuron Lesion. This type of weakness is usually due to disease of the neuromuscular junction or muscle, or to drugs or systemic diseases which affect the motor system. The physician should exclude myasthenia gravis by pharmacologic test, particularly if there is a history of ptosis or diplopia; chemical agents which affect neuromuscular transmission, such as botulinus toxin, polymyxin, and excess or deficiency of potassium or calcium; muscle diseases which are not associated with atrophy, such as hypothyroidism and hypoadrenalism; and drugs or diseases which affect central neural function, such as barbiturates, bromides, phenothiazines, uremia, and hepatic encephalopathy.

Weakness with Muscle Pain or Tenderness. This is generally due to trichinosis if accompanied by eosinophilia, to polymyositis or alcoholic myopathy if accompanied by increased serum levels of enzymes derived from muscle, to poliomyelitis, sensory root disease (disc, tumor, spondylosis, or tabes) or peripheral neuropathy if atrophy or sensory changes ensue, to viremia or bacteremia if the weakness is subjective only and is accompanied by malaise and fever, or to trauma (especially stretch), polymyalgia rheumatica, or tension-anxiety state if the weakness is subjective only.

Weakness with Increased Tone or Abnormal Movements. *Spasticity* is usually due to upper motor neuron disease; *rigidity*, to disease of the extrapyramidal system; *ataxia*, to disease of the cerebellum or proprioceptive pathways (sensory nerves and roots and the posterior columns); *spasms*, to tetany, tetanus, or pressure lesions on nerve roots; *stiffness*, to trauma, scleroderma, or polymyositis; *myotonia*, to myotonic dystrophy, hyperkalemic periodic paralysis, or hypothyroidism; *fasciculations*, to slowly progressive lesions of the lower motor neuron, especially progressive muscular atrophy, or to poisoning by anticholinesterase compounds; and muscular *cramps*, to hyponatremia, hypothyroidism, vascular insufficiency, paroxysmal myoglobinuria, phosphorylase deficiency, or unknown cause.

Subjective Weakness. Subjective weakness of acute or recurrent onset is usually due to transient reduction in the blood supply to the brain as a result of decreased cardiac output, cerebral or extracranial vascular disease, or hyperventilation. Another common cause is hypoglycemia. Subjective or objective weakness of the legs which recurs on walking, with or without pain, and is relieved by rest, is usually due to peripheral arterial insufficiency.

Chronic subjective weakness may occur in almost any acute or chronic illness, whether somatic or emotional. Only after somatic disease has been excluded should weakness be ascribed to emotional disorder.

REFERENCES

1. Adam, G. L., Finney, W., and Woodhall, B. Cervical disc lesions. J. Amer. Med. Ass. **166**:23, 1958.
2. Adams, R. D., Eaton, L. M., and Shy, G. M. *Neuromuscular Disorders.* The Williams & Wilkins Co., Baltimore, 1960.
3. Adams, R. D., and Vander Ecken, H. M. Vascular diseases of the brain. Ann. Rev. Med. **4**:213, 1953.
4. Adams, R. R., Denny-Brown, D., and Pearson, C. M. *Diseases of Muscle: a Study in Pathology*, 2nd ed., pp. 135, 329. Hoeber Medical Division, Harper and Row, New York, 1962.
5. Afifi, A. K., Bergman, R. A., and Harvey, J. C. Steroid myopathy. Clinical, histologic and cytologic observations. Johns Hopkins Med. J. **123**:158, 1968.
6. Altrocchi, P. H. Acute epidural abscess vs. acute transverse myelopathy. Arch. Neurol. **9**:17, 1963.
7. Auld, A. W., and Baermann, A. Metastatic spinal epidural tumors. Arch. Neurol. **15**:100, 1966.
8. Baker, A. B. Viral encephalitis and secondary forms of encephalitis. In *Clinical Neurology*, Baker, A. B., Ed., 2nd ed., Vol. 2, pp. 811, 859. Hoeber Medical Division, Harper and Row, New York, 1962.
9. Baldwin, J. W., and Dalessio, D. J. Folic acid therapy and cord degeneration in pernicious anemia. N. Engl. J. Med. **264**:1339, 1961.
10. Beerman, H., Nicholas, L., Schamberg, I. L., and Greenberg, M. S. Syphilis, review of the literature, 1960–61. Arch. Internal Med. **109**:323, 1962.
11. Benson, D. F. Intramedullary spinal cord metastases. Neurology **10**:281, 1960.
12. Brain, Lord, Croft, P. B., and Wilkinson, M. Motor neurone disease as a manifestation of neoplasm (with a note on the course of classical motor neurone disease). Brain **88**:479, 1965.
13. Brock, S. *Injuries to the Brain and Spinal Cord and Their Coverings*, 4th ed. The Williams & Wilkins Co., Baltimore, 1960.
14. Brooker, A. E. W., and Barter, R. W. Cervical spondylosis—a clinical study with comparative radiology. Brain **88**:925, 1965.

15. Chandor, S. B., Forno, L. S., and Wevel, N. A. Progressive multifocal leucoen-
    cephalopathy. J. Neurol. Neurosurg. Psychiat. **28:**260, 1965.
16. Cohen, C. Laboratory diagnostic measures in generalized muscular disease.
    Pediat. Clin. N. Amer. **14:**461, 1967.
17. Colby, A. D. Neurologic disorders of diabetes mellitus. Diabetes **14:**424, 516, 1965.
18. Conn, J. Hypoglycemia. Amer. J. Med. **19:**460, 1955.
19. Conn, J. Fatigue and inadequacy. Physiol. Rev. **37:**301, 1957.
20. Daniels, L., Williams, M., and Worthingham, C. *Muscle Testing: Techniques of
    Manual Examinations,* 2nd ed. W. B. Saunders Co., Philadelphia, 1956.
21. Davies, D. R. Neurotoxicity of organophosphorus compounds. In *Cholinesterase
    and Anticholinesterase Agents,* Koelle, G. B., Subed., p. 860. *Handbuch der
    experimentellen Pharmakologie Erganzungswerk,* Vol. 15. Springer-Verlag, Ber-
    lin, 1963.
22. Denny-Brown, D. Diseases of the basal ganglia. Their relation to disorders of
    movement. Lancet **2:**1099, 1155, 1960.
23. Denny-Brown, D. Hepatolenticular degeneration (Wilson's disease). Two differ-
    ent components. N. Engl. J. Med. **270:**1149, 1964.
24. Drachman, D. A., and Tuncbay, T. O. The remote myopathy of trichinosis.
    Neurology **15:**1127, 1965.
25. Dyck, P. J. Peripheral neuropathy: changing concepts, differential diagnosis and
    classification. Med. Clin. N. Amer. **52:**895, 1968.
26. Dyck, P. J., and Lofgren, E. P. Nerve biopsy: choice of nerve, methods, symp-
    toms, and usefulness. Med. Clin. N. Amer. **52:**885, 1968.
27. Elek, S. D., and Anderson, H. F. Paroxysmal paralytic myoglobinuria. Brit. Med.
    J. **2:**533, 1953.
28. Engel, W. K. Muscle biopsies in neuromuscular diseases. Pediat. Clin. N. Amer.
    14:963, 1967.
29. Fishman, R. A. Cerebrospinal fluid. In *Clinical Neurology,* Baker, A. B., Ed.,
    2nd ed., Vol. 1, p. 350. Hoeber Medical Division, Harper and Row, New York,
    1962.
30. Fitch, C. D. Muscle wasting disease of endocrine origin. Med. Clin. N. Amer.
    52:243, 1968.
31. Ford, R. G., and Siekert, R. G. Central nervous system manifestations of peri-
    arteritis nodosa. Neurology **15:**144, 1965.
32. Fulton, W. H., and Dyken, P. R. Neurologic syndromes of systemic lupus ery-
    thematosus. Neurology **14:**317, 1964.
33. Gould, S. E. *Trichinosis.* Charles C Thomas, Springfield, Ill. 1945.
34. Grob, D. The manifestations and treatment of poisoning due to nerve gas and
    other organic phosphate anticholinesterase compounds. Arch. Internal Med.
    97:221, 1956.
35. Grob, D. Diagnosis and management of the curable forms of hypertension. *Advan.
    Internal Med.* **10:**219, 1960.
36. Grob, D. Muscular disease. Bull. N. Y. Acad. Med. **12:**809, 1961.
37. Grob, D. Myasthenia gravis. A review of pathogenesis and treatment. Arch.
    Internal Med. **108:**615, 1961.
38. Grob, D. The neuromuscular system. In *Clinical Physiology,* Grollman, A., Ed.,
    p. 801. McGraw-Hill Book Co., Inc., New York, 1963.
39. Grob, D. Myopathies and their relation to thyroid disease. N. Y. State J. Med.
    63:318, 1963.
40. Grob, D. Metabolic diseases of muscle. *Ann. Rev. Med.* **14:**141, 1963.
41. Grob, D. Anticholinesterase intoxication in man and its treatment. In *Cholines-
    terase and Anticholinesterase Agents,* Koelle, G. B., Subed., p. 990. *Handbuch
    der experimentellen Pharmakologie Erganzungswerk,* Vol. 15. Springer-Verlag,
    Berlin, 1963.
42. Grob, D. Therapy of myasthenia gravis. In *Cholinesterase and Anticholinesterase
    Agents,* Koelle, G. B., Subed., p. 1029. *Handbuch der experimentellen Pharma-
    kologie Erganzungswerk,* Vol. 15. Springer-Verlag, Berlin, 1963.
43. Grob, D. Neuromuscular blocking drugs. In *Physiological Pharmacology,* Hoff-
    man, B., and Root, W., Eds., Vol. 3, p. 389. Academic Press, Inc., New York,
    1967.

44. Grob, D., and Johns, R. J. Disorders of the motor unit which may produce transient paralysis. Proc. Ass. Res. Nerv. Ment. Dis. 38:1001, 1960.
45. Hinterbuchner, C. N., and Hinterbuchner, L. P. Myopathic syndrome in muscular sarcoidosis. Brain 87:355, 1964.
46. Kiloh, L. G., and Nevin, S. Progressive dystrophy of the external ocular muscles (ocular myopathy). Brain 74:9, 1951.
47. Kurland, L. T. Studies on the natural history of multiple sclerosis. Acta Neurol. Scand. 42 (Suppl. 19): 157, 1966.
48. Langer, T., and Levy, R. I. Acute muscular syndrome associated with administration of clofibrate. N. Engl. J. Med. 279:856, 1968.
49. Lindesmith, L. A., Baines, R. D., Jr., Bigelow, D. B., and Petty, T. L. Reversible respiratory paralysis associated with polymyxin therapy. Ann. Internal Med. 68:318, 1968.
50. Locke, S., Lawrence, D. G., and Legg, M. A. Diabetic amyotrophy. Amer. J. Med. 34:775, 1963.
51. Lombardi, G., and Passerini, A. Spinal cord tumors. Radiology 76:381, 1961.
52. Mackay, R. P. Course and prognosis in amyotrophic lateral sclerosis. Arch. Neurol. 8:117, 1963.
53. Marshall, J. The Landry-Guillain-Barré syndrome. Brain 86:55, 1963.
54. McIllroy, W. J., and Richardson, J. C. Syringomyelia: a clinical review of 75 cases. Can. Med. Ass. J. 93:731, 1965.
55. McKissock, W., Paine, K., and Walsh, L. Further observations on subarachnoid hemorrhage. J. Neurol. Neurosurg. Psychiat. 21:239, 1958.
56. Mellinger, R. C., and Smith, R. W. Studies of the adrenal hyperfunction in two patients with atypical Cushing's syndrome. J. Clin. Endocrinol. Metab. 16:350, 1956.
57. Merritt, H. H., Adams, R. D., and Solomon, H. C. Neurosyphilis. Oxford University Press, New York, 1946.
58. Merritt, H. H., and Aring, C. D. The differential diagnosis of cerebral vascular lesions. Proc. Ass. Res. Nerv. Ment. Dis. 18:682, 1938.
59. Miller, H. G., Standton, J. B., and Gibbon, J. L. Acute disseminated encephalomyelitis and related syndromes. Brit. Med. J. 1:668, 1957.
60. Namba, T., Aberfeld, D. C., and Grob, D. Chronic proximal spinal muscular atrophy. J. Neurol. Sci. 11:401, 1970.
61. Namba, T., Himei, H., and Grob, D. Complement fixing and tissue binding serum globulins in patients with myasthenia gravis and their relation to muscle ribonucleoprotein. J. Lab. Clin. Med. 70:258, 1967.
62. Nielson, J. M. Agnosias, apraxias, speech, and aphasia. In Clinical Neurology, Baker, A. B., Ed., 2nd ed., Vol. 1, p. 433. Hoeber Medical Division, Harper and Row, New York, 1962.
63. Patel, A. N., and Swami, R. K. Muscle percussion and neostigmine test in the clinical evaluation of neuromuscular disorder. N. Engl. J. Med. 281:523, 1969.
64. Patel, A., and Toole, J. F. Subclavian steal syndrome—reversal of cephalic blood flow. Medicine 44:289, 1965.
65. Pearson, C. M. The periodic paralyses: differential features and pathologic observations in permanent myopathic weakness. Brain 87:341, 1964.
66. Pearson, C. M. Polymyositis and related disorders. In Disorders of Voluntary Muscle, Walton, J. H., Ed., 2nd ed., p. 501. Little, Brown and Co., Boston, 1969.
67. Perkoff, G. T., Dioso, M. M., Bleisch, V., and Klinkerfuss, G. A spectrum of myopathy associated with alcoholism. Ann. Internal Med. 67:481, 493, 1967.
68. Peterman, A. F., Yoss, R. G., and Corbin, K. B. The syndrome of occlusion of the anterior spinal artery. Proc. Staff Meet. Mayo Clin. 33:41, 1958.
69. Peyton, W. T., French, L. A., and Baker, A. B. Intracranial neoplasms. In Clinical Neurology, Baker, A. B., Ed., 2nd ed., Vol. 1, p. 460. Hoeber Medical Division, Harper and Row, New York, 1962.
70. Plotz, C. M., Knowlton, A. I., and Ragan, C. Natural history of Cushing's syndrome (review of 33 cases), coupled with an analysis of 189 cases culled from the literature. Amer. J. Med. 13:597, 1952.
71. Pool, J. L., and Potts, D. G. Aneurysms and Arteriovenous Anomalies of the Brain. Hoeber Medical Division, Harper and Row, New York, 1965.

72. Rooke, E. D., Eaton, L. M., Lambert, E. H., and Hodgson, C. H. Myasthenia and malignant intrathoracic tumor. Med. Clin. N. Amer. **44:**977, 1960.
73. Seemes, R. E. *Ruptures of the Lumbar Intervertebral Disc: Their Mechanism, Diagnosis and Treatment.* Charles C Thomas, Springfield, Ill., 1964.
74. Siebert, R. G., and Clark, E. C. Neurologic signs and symptoms as early manifestations of systemic lupus erythematosus. Neurology **5:**84, 1955.
75. Smith, H. V., and Spalding, J. M. K. Outbreak of paralysis in Morocco due to orthocresylphosphate poisoning. Lancet **2:**1019, 1959.
76. Van Pilsum, J. F., and Wolin, E. A. Guanidinium compounds in blood and urine of patients suffering from muscle disorders. J. Lab. Clin. Med. **51:**219, 1968.
77. Walshe, F. M. R. The Babinski response, its forms and its physiological and pathological significance. Brain **79:**529, 1956.
78. Walton, J. N. Muscular dystrophy: some recent advances in knowledge. Brit. Med. J. **1:**1271, 1344, 1964.
79. Walton, J. N., and Adams, R. D. *Polymyositis.* E. & S. Livingstone, Ltd., Edinburgh, 1958.
80. Walton, J. N., and Gardner-Medwin, D. Progressive muscular dystrophy and the myotonic disorders. In *Disorders of Voluntary Muscle,* Walton J. H., Ed., 2nd ed., p. 455. Little, Brown and Co., Boston, 1969.
81. Wartenberg, R. *Diagnostic Tests in Neurology.* Year Book Publishers, Inc., Chicago, 1953.
82. Weir, D. G., and Gatenby, P. B. B. Subacute combined degeneration of the cord after partial gastrectomy. Brit. Med. J. **2:**1175, 1963.
83. Williams, D., and Wilson, J. G. The diagnosis of the major and minor syndromes of basilar insufficiency. Brain **85:**741, 1962.
84. Wise, R. P., and MacDermot, V. A myasthenic syndrome associated with bronchial carcinoma. J. Neurol. Neurosurg. Psychiat. **25:**31, 1962.
85. Yoss, R. E., Corbin, K. B., MacCarty, C. S., and Love, J. G. Significance of symptoms and signs in localization of involved root in cervical disc protrusion. Neurology **7:**673, 1957.

Fever of Unknown Origin

ROBERT G. PETERSDORF and
JAMES F. WALLACE

INTRODUCTION

Fever of unknown origin (FUO) is a diagnostic and therapeutic challenge to all physicians from the family doctor to the specialist, and as a syndrome it encompasses diseases in all systems. Before considering the subject in detail, it seems appropriate to define FUO.

Several authors[5, 9, 10] have recently analyzed large groups of patients with FUO and have included in their series many patients who had fever for only a few days. Moreover, in many cases, elevations in temperature as low as 100.4°F were included in the analyses, resulting in a conglomeration of diagnoses without the formulation of significant concepts. In addition, in these series a large number of patients remained undiagnosed. This is not surprising, because many patients who have FUO for only a short time defervesce spontaneously or receive some form of therapy which leads to disappearance of fever. We contend that the clinical problem of FUO becomes much more meaningful when rigid criteria defining patients with FUO are employed. Over the past decade, the following definition has been useful to us:[16]

1. Continuous fever of 3 weeks' duration. This eliminates most viral and bacterial infections as well as other causes of fever, particularly those occurring in tandem, as happens when a patient with a myocardial infarction develops thrombophlebitis followed by a pulmonary embolus.

2. Daily elevation of temperature above 101°F.

3. Failure to make the diagnosis for at least the first week of intensive study. This criterion excludes many patients in whom the cause of pyrexia is obvious.

This definition of FUO will be employed throughout this presentation.

Neoplastic, inflammatory, infectious, hypersensitivity, and endocrine diseases may at times present as fevers of unknown etiology, and diseases as varied as melioidosis and gout may be associated with prolonged cryptic fever. It should be clear, however, that most diseases which present occasionally as FUO have other primary manifestations most of the time. For example, patients with renal cell carcinoma, which is often cited as a typical tumor presenting as FUO, much more commonly have flank pain,

ROBERT G. PETERSDORF, M.D. Professor and Chairman, Department of Medicine, University of Washington School of Medicine, and Physician-in-Chief, University Hospital, Seattle, Washington. JAMES F. WALLACE, M.D. Assistant professor of Medicine and Head, Division of Ambulatory Medicine, University of Washington School of Medicine, Seattle, Washington hematuria, or a palpable mass than fever. In many infections signs and symptoms pointing to the primary locus overshadow fever, and such patients, of course, do not have FUO.

It should also be clear that most patients with FUO do not have abstruse diseases. Rather, their fever is a manifestation of a common problem which presents in atypical fashion. For example, the classical patient with subacute bacterial endocarditis who is classified as having FUO does not have petechiae, splinter hemorrhages, Osler nodes, Janeway lesions, Roth spots, a diastolic murmur, splenomegaly, and clubbing; more commonly he simply has fever and a nondescript systolic bruit. Likewise, patients with leukemia who have FUO do not have telltale cells in the peripheral blood. Febrile patients with cancer are much more likely to have obstruction or infection secondary to a common tumor than a rare neoplasm such as diffuse fibrosarcoma of bone, which may cause fever by some unknown mechanism.

In general fever is an excellent objective mirror of organic disease and, among the vital signs, is a much more reliable indicator of illness than are the pulse, blood pressure, and respiratory rate. Stated differently, the temperature-regulating apparatus is relatively refractory to psychogenic stimuli. It is true, of course, that menstruation, ovulation, consumption of food, high external temperatures, and vigorous exercise may affect the temperature curve.[1] Usually, however, fever is a reflection of organic disease. One exception is a condition termed *habitual hyperthermia*,[18] which generally occurs in psychoneurotic, relatively young women, with vague complaints. These patients often have afternoon temperatures ranging between 100° and 100.5°F and exhibit other manifestations of vasomotor instability, including flushing, postural hypotension, and dermographia.[18] Often a change in life situation relieves the fever. These patients are prone to "doctor shopping" and must be identified early before they become victims of the intensive FUO work-up, which is often attended by iatrogenic disease.

A second psychodynamically determined form of FUO is *factitious fever*,[17] which is a form of malingering practiced by individuals who find that being hospitalized for fever of unknown origin satisfies personal needs. These patients have severe psychiatric disorders, and their methods for elevating temperatures falsely are both ingenious and varied. Holding light bulbs, matches, or lighters next to the thermometer, shaking the instrument in retrograde fashion, rubbing it against sheets, manipulating oral and even anal sphincters, or substituting a thermometer which has been elevated spuriously for one that has not are just some techniques practiced by these patients. When the ruse is discovered, they characteristically leave the hospital against medical advice, and they are notoriously averse to the psychiatrist's couch. A classic example of factitious disease has been set to verse by Bean.[2] Factitious fever is important primarily because it is incumbent upon all attending a patient with FUO to make the diagnosis, particularly if the fever is of long duration, lacks the normal diurnal variation, is excessively high (above 106° to 107°F in adults), and is associated with normal pulse and respiratory rates. Many a malingerer has been subjected to an extensive FUO work-up that has been traumatic to the patient, who generally doesn't seem to mind the trauma, and to the physician, who generally does.

It is also important to consider the patient's geographic locale in the differential diagnosis of FUO. Tuberculosis, neoplasm, and rheumatic fever are world-wide causes of fever, but melioidosis, relapsing fever, malaria, amebiasis, schistosomiasis, and other exotic diseases are unusual causes of prolonged undiagnosed fever in the continental United States. Recent studies of the causes of FUO in Viet Nam[8] attest to the importance of the environment in determining the cause of fever.

DIAGNOSTIC CONSIDERATIONS

Table 31 summarizes most of the diagnostic entities we have encountered in several hundred patients with FUO. This list is by no means complete, but contains most of the clinical situations in which FUO is seen. Some general comments on the table are pertinent.

Tumors

Many patients with cancer have fever, but in most instances the fever is short-lived and is related to secondary infection in adjacent organs, to surgical intervention or drainage procedures,[6] to defects in antibody synthesis, as in chronic lymphocytic leukemia,[20] or to compromised phagocytosis, as in acute leukemia.[21] Few tumors per se produce fever, and when they do they usually have metastasized, most commonly to the liver.

Patients with cancer who present with FUO usually do not have localizing signs on physical examination, and the laboratory data show only non-specific abnormalities. Hepatomegaly and palpable masses along with unexplained failure to clear sulfobromophthalein and an elevated alkaline phosphatase concentration in serum are important clues.

The diagnosis is most often made by biopsy of liver, lymph nodes, bone marrow, or tumor masses, and multiple biopsies may be necessary to obtain the answer.

Infections

Tuberculosis is a particularly common cause of FUO in relatively young, dark-skinned individuals—Negroes, American Indians, and Filipinos—and is usually disseminated. Cavitary lung disease is characteristically absent and the tuberculin test is often negative. The diagnosis is best made by demonstrating caseating granulomas in biopsies of liver, lymph nodes, and bone marrow; occasionally cultures of gastric aspirates or therapeutic trials with specific antituberculous agents—isoniazid and p-aminosalicylic acid—are helpful.

Granulomatous diseases other than tuberculosis often have precise localizing signs, such as thin-walled cavities in coccidioidomycosis or sinus tracts in actinomycosis.

Right upper quadrant infections causing FUO usually occur in patients with a history of calculous gall bladder disease, and are characterized by high fever, shaking chills, marked leukocytosis, chemical jaundice, abnormal liver function tests, and blood cultures positive for enteric organisms or salmonellae. A few patients with cirrhosis have bouts of "spontaneous bacteremia" with Gram-negative bacilli, presumably because portosystemic shunts bypass hepatic bacterial clearance mechanisms.[24]

Urinary tract infections rarely cause prolonged cryptic fever, and most patients with urinary tract infections defervesce spontaneously even without specific treatment.[14] Intra- or perirenal abscesses or obstruction are usually present in patients with pyelonephritis and FUO.

As mentioned previously, when patients with subacute bacterial endocarditis present with FUO, the typical picture of endocarditis is not in evidence. One source of confusion is that many patients have been treated with antibiotics during the "prodromal stages" of this infection. This does nothing more than to erect an obfuscatory facade between the patient and the diagnosis.

As will be shown subsequently, myxoma of the atrium may present in a fashion very similar to subacute bacterial endocarditis and can be diagnosed by angiocardiography.[25]

Most of the odd organisms causing FUO, such as *Listeria*, *Vibrio*, *Brucella, or Bacteroides*, are diagnosed principally because they appear in blood cultures taken from febrile patients.

Collagen Diseases

Rheumatic fever, disseminated lupus erythematosus, giant cell arteritis (temporal arteritis, polymyalgia rheumatica), and rheumatoid variants commonly present as FUO; scleroderma, dermatomyositis, and polyarteritis nodosa rarely do.

In collagen diseases abnormal physical findings play a relatively important role in making the diagnosis. In rheumatic fever, for example, there are usually heart murmurs, arrhythmias, pleural or pericardial rubs, arthralgias, and/or arthritis and skin rashes.

Conversely, biopsy is not particularly helpful in the diagnosis of collagen disease. We have seen patients with disseminated lupus erythematosus, for example, who have had miniature autopsies with biopsy of skin, muscle, lymph node, parotid gland, liver, and kidney, but in whom the diagnosis was not made until lupus erythematosus cells or antinuclear antibodies appeared.

Two of the most commonly encountered fever-producing collagen diseases are temporal arteritis (polymyalgia rheumatica) in older patients and atypical rheumatoid arthritis in young individuals.

Miscellaneous

In this day of polypharmacy drug fever remains an important cause of FUO. Furthermore, patients who respond with fever to one drug may do so to several drugs.

TABLE 31

Common Disease Entities Responsible for Fever of Unknown Origin

I. Neoplastic diseases
   A. Tumors of reticuloendothelial system
      1. Leukemia
      2. Lymphoma, Hodgkin's disease
      3. Multiple myeloma (rare)
   B. Metastatic tumors
      1. From gastrointestinal tract
      2. From lung, kidney, bone
      3. Melanoma
   C. Solid localized tumors
      1. Kidney
      2. Liver
      3. Lung
      4. Pancreas
      5. Atrial myxoma
II. Infections
   A. Granulomatous infections
      1. Tuberculosis
      2. Coccidioidomycosis
      3. Histoplasmosis
      4. Actinomycosis
      5. Nocardiosis
   B. Pyogenic infections
      1. Right upper quadrant infections
         a. Cholangitis
         b. Cholecystitis (stone)
         c. Liver abscess
         d. Subphrenic abscess
         e. Subhepatic abscess
         f. Lesser sac abscess
      2. Abscesses secondary to bowel diseases
         a. Diverticulitis
         b. Appendicitis
      3. Pelvic inflammatory disease
      4. Renal infections
         a. Pyelonephritis (rare)
         b. Perinephric abscess
         c. Intrarenal abscess
         d. Ureteral obstruction with infection
   C. Subacute bacterial endocarditis
   D. Additional bacteremias
      1. Meningococcemia
      2. Gonococcemia
      3. Vibriosis
      4. Listeriosis
      5. Brucellosis
   E. Miscellaneous
      1. Malaria
      2. Infectious mononucleosis
      3. Cytomegalovirus disease
      4. Coxsackie B diseases

TABLE 31—*Continued*

---

    5. Amebiasis
    6. Leptospirosis
    7. Trichinosis
    8. Q fever
III. Collagen diseases
    A. Rheumatic fever
    B. Disseminated lupus erythematosus
    C. Rheumatoid arthritis
    D. Giant cell arteritis (temporal arteritis, polymyalgia rheumatica)
    E. Rare
        1. Scleroderma
        2. Dermatomyositis
        3. Polyarteritis nodosa
IV. Unclassified
    A. Drug fever
    B. Multiple pulmonary emboli
    C. Thyroiditis
    D. Sarcoidosis
    E. Hemolytic anemia
    F. Cryptic trauma
    G. Regional enteritis
    H. Granulomatous hepatitis
V. Psychogenic fevers
    A. Habitual hyperthermia
    B. Factitious fever
VI. Periodic fevers
    A. Familial Mediterranean fever
    B. Etiocholanolone fever
VII. Undiagnosed FUO

Pulmonary embolization without infarction usually does not produce fever, and patients with solitary pulmonary infarcts remain afebrile unless cavitation and infection supervene. On the other hand, multiple pulmonary emboli may produce cryptic fever.

Pulmonary sarcoidosis is usually a nonfebrile disease; febrile patients with sarcoid tend to have hilar adenopathy, hepatosplenomegaly, and erythema nodosum.

Perisplenic and perivesical hematomas, with or without superimposed infection, are among the sites where accumulation of old blood and pus has resulted in foci responsible for prolonged fever.

When patients with regional enteritis present with FUO, their abdominal complaints are often notoriously vague, and fever and arthritis dominate the clinical picture.

Granulomatous hepatitis has been, in our experience, a not uncommon cause of FUO. It is probably a manifestation of hypersensitivity. Experimentally, sulfonamides and perhaps penicillin have been incriminated.[23] An example of this puzzling disease is given below.

The subject of "periodic fevers" remains in a state of confusion. It is

TABLE 32
Useful Diagnostic Maneuvers in Fever of Unknown Origin

I. Radiographic techniques	
A. Chest film	Tuberculosis, cavitary pulmonary infection, metastatic tumors, lymphoma, sarcoidosis
B. Bone films	Osteomyelitis, particularly *Salmonella;* primary and metastatic bone tumors
C. Contrast films	
1. Angiocardiography	Intracardiac tumors, cryptic pericarditis, pulmonary emboli
2. Lymphangiography	Abdominal lymphoma
3. Abdominal arteriography	Tumors of kidney and pancreas
4. Intravenous urography	Tumors of kidney, perinephric abscesses, intrarenal abscesses
5. Upper gastrointestinal x-rays	Rarely useful
6. Small bowel series	Regional enteritis
7. Barium enema	Diverticulitis with abscess formation
II. Radioactive scanning techniques	
A. Liver scan	Liver and subphrenic abscesses, tumors
B. Lung scan	Silent pulmonary infarcts, subphrenic abscess (combined with liver scan)
III. Examination of tissue	
A. Biopsies	
1. Liver	Granulomas and tumors
2. Bone marrow	Granulomas and tumors
3. Lymph node	Granulomas and tumors
4. Lung	Granulomas and tumors, interstitial processes
5. Pleura, pericardium, and peritoneum (hook needle technique	Granulomas and tumors
6. Skin and muscle	Collagen diseases
7. Kidney	Collagen diseases (rarely useful)
8. Temporal artery	Giant cell arteritis
9. Other masses	Tumors and infections
B. Peritoneoscopy	Tuberculous peritonitis, peritoneal carcinomatosis, cholecystitis, sometimes pelvic disease
C. Exploratory laparotomy or thoracotomy	
IV. Laboratory tests	
A. Cultures	
1. Blood	
2. Bone marrow	For intracellular organisms
B. Serum enzymes	
1. Alkaline phosphatase	
2. Glutamic-oxalacetic transaminase, glutamic-pyruvic transaminase, lactic dehydrogenase	
C. Bone marrow examination	Tumor cells, granulomas, and LE cells
D. Immunologic tests	Antistreptolysin O titers and other acute phase reactants; antinuclear factor, latex fixation tests; febrile agglutinins
E. Miscellaneous	Sulfobromophthalein retention

TABLE 32—*Continued*

V. Therapeutic trials	
A. Antituberculous therapy	
B. Aspirin	Acute rheumatic fever
C. Alkylating agents	Lymphoma
D. Heparin	Multiple pulmonary emboli
E. Adrenal steroids	Usually nonspecific
1. Polymyalgia rheumatica	
2. Rheumatoid disease	
3. Systemic lupus erythematosus	
F. Antibiotics	
1. Large doses of penicillin G plus streptomycin	Bacterial endocarditis
2. Ampicillin or chloramphenicol	Salmonellosis
3. Others according to most likely sensitivity of offending organisms	

clear that there is an entity, familial Mediterranean fever (FMF), in Turks, Armenians, Sephardic Jews, Syrians, and others residing in the Mediterranean basin. This genetically transmitted disease is characterized by bouts of fever, abdominal pain, and, less commonly, arthralgia, pleurisy, and rash. Between attacks the patients are well. A number of these patients develop renal and hepatic amyloidosis and die from chronic renal failure.[22] In the United States there are foci of FMF along the Eastern seaboard and in the Los Angeles area. In contrast to FMF, which is a well-defined clinical syndrome, the other periodic diseases described by Reimann,[19] as well as etiocholanolone fever,[4] are much less discrete nosologic entities. We agree with those who doubt that etiocholanolone fever is a specific biochemical disease,[27] and think that it is a genetically dilute form of FMF.

SOME USEFUL DIAGNOSTIC MANEUVERS IN FUO

Table 32 lists some of the procedures which have been most useful in the diagnosis of FUO, and their indications. This list is not complete, and is meant merely to highlight some features. As will be detailed below, angiocardiograms, arteriograms, and lymphangiograms are significant new radiographic techniques in the diagnostic approach to FUO.

Anteroposterior intravenous pyelograms may not detect renal cell carcinomas, particularly if the tumors are growing in an anteroposterior rather than a cephalocaudad plane. Lateral and oblique projections may be necessary. Actually, arteriography is the most useful technique for detecting renal masses, and has the additional advantage of separating carcinomas from cysts.

Among the various techniques available, histologic examination of tissue probably accounts for 50 per cent of diagnoses of patients with FUO, and liver biopsy is probably the single most productive diagnostic procedure.

Needle liver biopsies are often more accurate than open biopsies taken through a small incision; the latter often include too much capsular tissue and miss the lesion.

Multiple biopsies at the same or separate sites may be necessary to arrive at a diagnosis.

Needle biopsy of the lung has, in our experience, not been useful, while open lung biopsy via a limited thoracotomy has been helpful in detecting the cause of diffuse disease.

Similarly, renal biopsy has not been accurate in detecting either collagen disease or renal infection.

In attempting to diagnose collagen-vascular disease by muscle biopsy, it is essential to sample muscle at a site of tenderness or electromyographic abnormality.

Blood cultures should be incubated anaerobically, particularly to pick up *Bacteroides* and microaerophilic streptococci, and it is essential to save blood cultures for several weeks to isolate slowly growing and fastidious microorganisms.

In the nonjaundiced patient an elevated alkaline phosphatase concentration is an excellent clue to infiltrative liver disease; conversely, except for the occasional patient with chronic hepatitis, most patients with FUO have normal or nearly normal hepatocellular enzyme values in serum.

Abnormal sulfobromophthalein retention in a nonicteric patient is also helpful in screening patients for hepatic disease. It should be remembered, however, that fever per se may lead to a moderate (10 to 25 per cent) retention of the dye.

Therapeutic trials as a means for diagnosing FUO should be used only as a last resort and, when used at all, these trials should be as specific as possible. For this reason, trials with adrenal cortical steroids as well as with most antibiotics, are unlikely to provide a precise answer.

SOME LESSONS LEARNED FROM RECENT PATIENTS WITH FUO

Every patient with FUO teaches a clinical lesson, and in the section to follow we present a number of cases which have taught us how to approach patients with FUO more effectively.

Lesson 1: A Careful History, Including Particular Attention to Medications, Is Mandatory

Case 1

A 74-year-old woman had had occasional bouts of diarrhea for many years; she had not sought medical attention until 2 months before admission, when her symptoms became more severe. Her physician prescribed a bland diet and a course of Sulfasuxidine, which temporarily resulted in fewer loose stools. However, within several weeks the diarrhea increased again, and she began to have daily febrile spikes to 102°F. On admission to the hospital the physical examination was entirely normal except for a temperature of 101.4°F. The hematocrit was 36 per cent, white cell count 3900 cu mm, with a normal differential, and the sedimentation rate was 112 mm/ hour. Chest x-ray was normal.

All medications were witheld when the patient was admitted to the hospital, and, as her work-up proceeded, the fever disappeared. During that time she underwent sigmoidoscopy and rectal mucosal biopsy, which established the diagnosis of idiopathic ulcerative colitis. The barium enema showed minimal but typical mucosal abnormalities in the rectosigmoid. Before the fever disappeared she had several negative blood cultures and negative stool examinations. The alkaline phosphatase was 176 units (normal <90), but all other liver functions tests were normal.

At the time of discharge she was afebrile and was having only an occasional loose stool. It was felt that the fever had most likely been caused by a small abscess associated with the colitis, which had resolved spontaneously.

Upon leaving the hospital she was given Azulfidine (salicylazosulfapyridine) and felt well for approximately 1 month before noting fever once again. She was readmitted to the hospital for further studies and again found to have a normal physical examination except for fever of 101.2°F.

The white cell count was 5000/cu mm, but now 72 per cent of the cells were eosinophils. The alkaline phosphatase was 250 units; other liver function tests, hepatic scan, and liver biopsy disclosed no abnormality. Cranial artery biopsy was normal.

For 2 weeks the patient continued to have fever ranging between 101.4° and 104°F as the negative results of the various studies accumulated. On the 15th hospital day Azulfidine was discontinued, and within 24 hours she became afebrile and remained so until time of discharge.

COMMENT

Common things are common, and drug fever due to sulfonamides should be considered in all patients receiving this class of drugs.

Lesson 2: Consider the Social History in Approaching the Diagnosis

Case 2[3]

A 36-year-old professional gambler was admitted to the hospital complaining of fever and malaise which had been present for 2 weeks. Twenty-one months earlier, during a game of cards, he had sustained a gunshot wound causing a laceration of the liver, retroperitoneal bleeding, and damage to the cauda equina. Afterward, in addition to a neurogenic bladder, he experienced severe muscle cramps in the legs, attributed to arachnoiditis, for which he received analgesics and sedatives. Subsequently he became addicted to a morphine derivative, codeine, and barbiturates, which he injected intravenously with nonsterile equipment. During the 1½ years prior to admission he had noted frequent skin infections, had several episodes of thrombophlebitis, and had a suprapubic cystostomy because of persistent urinary tract infections and vesical calculi. Two days before the current admission he had been seen in the emergency room because the suprapubic catheter was obstructed. The history of a 2-week febrile illness was obtained, and pyrexia was attributed to a urinary tract infection. Treatment with sulfisoxazole was initiated, but the fever persisted and he was admitted to the hospital 2 days later.

Physical examination revealed an acutely ill young man with a blood pressure of 180/90 mm Hg, a bounding pulse with a rate of 100 beats/ minute, and a temperature of 103°F. The antecubital areas showed several erythematous puncture sites and firm venous cords. The precordium was hyperdynamic and there was a grade 2 systolic ejection murmur at the base. A harsh, continuous bruit with systolic accentuation was audible over the entire abdomen, but was loudest in the right upper guadrant. The liver and spleen were not palpable and there were no petechiae. Pertinent laboratory data included a hematocrit value of 38 per cent, leukocyte count of 14,000/ cu mm with a shift to the left, bacteriuria, pyuria, and hematuria. Roentgenogram of the chest was normal.

The initial impression was that he had a urinary tract infection, and because significant numbers of *Proteus mirabilis* were cultured from the urine, treatment with ampicillin was instituted. However, when blood cultures taken on admission were positive for a penicillin-resistant, coagulase-positive strain of *Staphylococcus aureus*, cephaloridine was substituted. At this time the working diagnosis was changed to staphylococcal endocarditis related to intravenous administration of narcotics. Although the staphylococcus was sensitive to antibiotics employed, bacteremia and fever persisted. After a 10-day course of cephaloridine, methicillin was substituted and there was gradual defervescence despite detectable bacteremia for 5 additional days following therapy. In view of the persistent bacteremia and the history of a gunshot wound to the abdomen, the possibility of bacterial endarteritis involving a traumatic arteriovenous fistula was raised, and an aortogram confirmed the diagnosis. Excision of the fistula, which showed a large vegetation containing staphylococci, resulted in complete cure.

COMMENT

Several salient features of this patient's problem were ignored. First, fever of 2 weeks' duration was attributed to a urinary tract infection, a most unusual occurrence. Since the patient was a known drug user, endocarditis should have been considered much earlier.[7] Second, the history of abdominal trauma, the abdominal bruit, the high output state, and the persistent bacteremia in the face of adequate antimicrobial therapy should have pointed to the source of the infection much earlier. This surely was an infection of our urban culture!

Lesson 3: When Approaching Patients with FUO, Consider the Geography, But Bet on the Home Front

Case 3

A 45-year-old seaman presented with fatigue, chills, fever up to 103°F, diarrhea, and a dry cough for 2 weeks. Two weeks before he became ill he had had an infected sebaceous cyst on his chest wall treated by incision, drainage, and soaks, with apparent cure. He had previously been healthy except for amebic dysentery on one occasion 8 years before. On admission to the hospital he appeared only moderately ill and, except for a temperature of 103°F, had an entirely normal physical examination. The admitting diagnosis was influenza despite a white blood cell count of 17,800/cu mm with a left shift. The admission hematocrit, urinalysis, and chest x-ray were normal.

During the next 8 days he continued to have daily fevers up to 104°F and intermittent diarrhea. Five blood cultures were negative, as were cultures of urine and stool. No amebic cysts were found in the stool, and the hemagglutination test for amebiasis was negative. *Salmonella* and *Brucella* agglutinins were not present. Skin tests for tuberculosis and common fungal diseases were negative. Serum bilirubin, glutamic-oxalacetic transaminase, and lactic dehydrogenase were not elevated; the sulfo-bromophthalein retention was 7.1 per cent. The alkaline phosphatase concentration in serum was 26 King-Armstrong units (normal, 13).

On the ninth hospital day a liver scan was performed, primarily because of the past history of amebiasis. It revealed a normal-sized liver containing a 6-cm defect in the dome of the right lobe. Subsequently a large abscess was drained, from which *Bacteroides* and anaerobic streptococci were cultured. Following surgery the patient was given a 4-week course of tetracycline and made an uneventful recovery.

Case 4

A 63-year-old oil company executive and world traveler was hospitalized because of fever and right upper quadrant and right shoulder pain of 2 weeks' duration. He had previously enjoyed excellent health except for one bout of diarrhea while in the West Indies several years before. He had last been out of the country 2 years previously.

On examination the liver was palpable 10 cm below the costal margin, smooth, and somewhat tender. The spleen was also just palpable. The remainder of the examination was normal except for the temperature, which was 103°F.

The white blood cell count was 12,100/cu mm with normal differential, and the urinalysis and chest film were normal. Stool examinations for ova, parasites, and enteric pathogens were negative. Skin tests, febrile agglutinins, and many blood cultures were also negative. The serum glutamic-oxalacetic transaminase, glutamic-pyruvic transaminase, and lactic dehydrogenase concentrations were all modestly elevated, but alkaline phosphatase and bilirubin were normal. An oral cholecystogram was normal, but a liver scan showed many small filling defects.

The patient continued to have spiking, high fevers, his liver increased in size, and a hepatic friction rub appeared. He was given chloroquine as a therapeutic trial for the possibility of amebic hepatic abscess, and after no improvement was noted within 48 hours he underwent exploratory laparotomy. At surgery multiple hard nodules were found in the liver and spleen, which proved to be anaplastic carcinoma from an indeterminate primary source.

COMMENT

Because of their peripatetic backgrounds, both these patients were thought to have amebiasis; yet one turned out to have a bacterial liver abscess and the other cancer. These histories also point out the value of the liver scan in finding answers to cryptic sources of fever. It can be argued that these patients were really occasional travelers and that the emphasis on amebic disease was misplaced. But what about the many Viet Nam war veterans who are coming to our hospitals with FUO?

Case 5

A 23-year-old veteran had recently returned from Viet Nam. He presented to the hospital with a 2-week history of fevers over 105°F. The only other symptoms were mild arthralgias in the right shoulder and both knees, but there was no redness, swelling, or heat. Except for fever, physical examination was entirely normal. The white blood cell count was 5000 and 4000/cu mm on two occasions, and there was a slight shift to the left. While in Southeast Asia he had been well except for a brief bout of diarrhea and a 1-week febrile illness which subsided spontaneously. There was no history of malaria.

He remained hospitalized for approximately 2 months, during most of which he remained febrile. Numerous laboratory tests, including blood cultures, bone marrow culture, liver biopsy, malaria smears, acid-fast studies, heterophil and cold agglutinins, antistreptolysin titer, rheumatoid factor, antinuclear factor, and liver function tests, as well as complete x-ray studies, were entirely negative. While in the hospital he developed splenomegaly but, except when he was febrile, felt quite well. After much discussion of the differential diagnosis, he was treated with aspirin and defervesced slowly. More significant was the prompt return of fever when aspirin therapy was discontinued. During and after aspirin therapy he continued to have arthralgias but had no evidence of arthritis. The only laboratory abnormalities were mild anemia and mild hyperglobulinemia. While still receiving aspirin, he eventually became entirely afebrile and 6 months later was feeling well.

COMMENT

Here was a patient who could have had any one of several exotic diseases, but who most likely had Still's disease, an entity upon which we shall comment further. When patients who have been in endemic areas have malaria, the diagnosis is usually fairly obvious. However, when the fever is prolonged, malaria is unlikely, and the diagnosis usually turns out to be a disease which is as common in the United States as anywhere else.

Lesson 4: There Is Nothing Like a Thorough Physical Examination

Case 6

Following a normal pregnancy a 33-year-old mother of 10 children was delivered of a normal infant. Shortly after delivery she had a fever spike which was treated with penicillin. On the third postpartum day she had a severe shaking chill and developed right upper quadrant and right flank pain. Therapy with multiple antibiotics was instituted. During the next 6 weeks she continued to have spiking fever and shaking chills. Several blood cultures taken at another hospital were positive for *Escherichia coli*. It was felt that the urinary tract was the focus of this infection, and she was given several antibiotics. Because fever and chills persisted, she underwent an abdominal and pelvic exploration 1 month after the onset of her illness. No abnormalities were found, and the fever continued despite therapy with chloramphenicol, to which the *E. coli* were sensitive *in vitro*. When she was admitted to our hospital physical examination, including rectal and pelvic, was negative except for slight right upper quadrant tenderness. The hematocrit was 40 per cent, and the white blood cell count 13,600/cu mm with a normal differential. Urinalysis as well as chest and abdominal films were normal. Because of the right upper quadrant tenderness and a sulfobromophthalein retention of 19 per cent, the diagnosis of liver abscess was considered, but a liver scan was normal. On the third hopsital day the patient began to complain of discomfort over her right buttock; on examination there was a raised area of deep cellulitis with central fluctuation. Incision and drainage were performed, and 20 ml of pus appeared, from which the same *E. coli* which had been cultured from the blood was isolated. She was treated with a 5-day course of kanamycin and continued drainage. Following these therapeutic maneuvers she recovered completely.

COMMENT

Res ipsa loquitur.

Lesson 5: In Patients Who Are Thought to Have Rheumatic Fever or Bacterial Endocarditis But Who, with Prolonged Study, Turn out to Have Neither, Angiocardiography Should Be Performed

Case 7

A 32-year-old woman with a long-standing diagnosis of rheumatic heart disease was hospitalized for the fourth time in 5 years because of recurrent fever, fatigue, and cardiac enlargement. On each previous occasion she was felt to have had "atypical rheumatic fever" following extensive evaluations, including multiple blood cultures, serologic tests for infectious agents, batteries of tests for collagen-vascular diseases, and, on one occasion, a laparotomy. Each time, with rest, salicylates, corticosteroids, and specific measures for congestive heart failure, she had gradually become afebrile and was able to return to work.

Physical examination at the time of admission showed a thin woman with a temperature of 101°F and several splinter hemorrhages beneath the nails of the right hand, but no rash. The chest was clear and there was a holosystolic murmur at the cardiac apex, radiating into the axilla. The liver was palpable 2 cm below the right costal margin, but the spleen could not be felt. Slight pedal edema was present bilaterally. Laboratory studies on admission included a hematocrit of 36 per cent, white blood cell count of 8200/cu mm, and a sedimentation rate of 50 mm/hour. The urinalysis was normal.

The admitting diagnosis was bacterial endocarditis, and once again a series of blood cultures was obtained, all of which were negative. Liver function tests and a hepatic scan disclosed no abnormalities. No group A β-hemolytic streptococci were cultured from the throat, and the antistreptolysin O titer was not elevated.

The patient continued to have daily temperature elevations of 101.5°F and on the fifth hospital day, in the absence of a definitive cardiac diagnosis, cardiac catheterization was performed. The angiograms demonstrated radiolucent areas in both atria which proved to be myxomas attached to both sides of the atrial septum. These tumors were resected, and for the next 2 years she remained well. Following this she had a recurrence of atrial myxoma and died following another exploratory cardiotomy.

Case 8

A 43-year-old university professor was hospitalized because of progressive congestive heart failure. A year previously his physician had noted a murmur of mitral stenosis during a routine physical examination. The patient, who was then asymptomatic, did not recall having had rehumatic fever as a youth. A few months later he began to experience exertional dyspnea and orthopnea for which he was given digitalis and diuretics, with only modest improvement. The day he was hospitalized he had a syncopal attack while climbing stairs. Since the onset of his illness he had lost 35 pounds, but had not been aware of fever.

He appeared as an orthopneic man with a blood pressure of 96/70, pulse of 130/minute, and temperature of 101°F. Rales were present bilaterally throughout the chest; there was a right ventricular heave, accentuated pulmonic second sound, and a right ventricular gallop, but no definite murmur could be heard. The liver was enlarged to 8 cm below the costal margin, and hepatojugular reflux could be demonstrated. There was no splenomegaly, pedal edema, or evidence of systemic embolization.

Laboratory studies included a white blood cell count of 14,000/cu mm, hematocrit of 33 per cent, and erythrocyte sedimentation rate of 120 mm/ hour. The urine contained 20 to 30 white blood cells per high-power field, but was sterile. The bilirubin level was slightly elevated, but other liver function tests were normal. Chest x-ray showed left atrial enlargement and pulmonary vascular congestion.

It was felt that he most likely had either bacterial endocarditis or active rheumatic carditis, but six blood cultures showed no growth, and the antistreptolysin O titer was not elevated. Despite vigorous attempts at diuresis and large doses of salicylates, the patient remained febrile for 4 weeks and continued to have severe dyspnea. Because of his failure to respond to treatment, the possibility of a semiemergency mitral commissurotomy was considered, and for this reason he underwent cardiac catheterization. The hemodynamic findings were those of severe mitral stenosis, but on angiography a constant filling defect was seen in the left atrium, extending into the ventricular cavity during each diastole. At open heart surgery a large myxoma was removed from the left atrium. The patient did well postoperatively and became afebrile within a week.

COMMENT

The ability of atrial myxomas to mimic subacute bacterial endocarditis, rheumatic fever, and occasionally even collagen disease is well known,[15] but we have not appreciated until recently how common an occurrence this is. For example, we have seen five patients with atrial myxomas in the past 2 years, two of whom had marked fever.

Lesson 6: The Technique of Lymphangiography Probably Represents a Diagnostic Advance, But Not Always

Case 9

For a year a 59-year-old man had been having bouts of chills, fever as high as 104°F, and drenching night sweats, recurring regularly every 4 to 6 weeks and lasting approximately a week before remitting spontaneously. Between episodes he felt well except for the occurrence of severe occipital headaches after ingestion of small amounts of alcohol. Nine months earlier, while he was undergoing diagnostic tests for the fever, a large left renal calculus had been found, for which nephrectomy was performed. The kidney was said to have shown chronic pyelonephritis. Several months before his admission to the hospital his physician had prescribed chloramphenicol on an empiric basis, and the patient had taken this nearly daily without noticeable effect on the pattern of the fever.

At the time of admission he was an obese man who did not appear ill, and whose physical examination was normal except for the nephrectomy scar. The hematocrit was 35 per cent, white blood cell count 7900/cu mm with a normal differential, and erythrocyte sedimentation rate 40 mm/hour. The urinalysis was normal and urine culture was negative.

On the evening of the sixth hospital day his temperature rose to 1084.°F and remained in this range for the next 5 days before gradually returning to normal. Coincident with the defervescence a vesicular rash over the distribution of the inferior division of the left trigeminal nerve appeared. The rash was typical of herpes zoster.

Many tests, including 14 blood cultures, febrile agglutinins, liver function studies, lupus erythematosus preparations, and tuberculin and fungal skin tests, all failed to indicate the source of the patient's fever. Because lymphoma was strongly suspected, bilateral percutaneous lymphangiograms were performed; these showed several large femoral, iliac, and peri-aortic nodes as well as multiple smaller nodes in the same regions, all of which contained filling defects with ill-defined margins, and which were felt to be consistent with Hodgkin's disease. Subsequently biopsies of superficial femoral and iliac nodes showed only hyperplasia and moderate eosinophilia and were nondiagnostic. The patient was discharged to the care of his private physician with the presumptive diagnosis of Hodgkin's disease and the recommendation that he receive a course of nitrogen mustard after the herpetic lesions had resolved. Before this recommendation could be carried out, the patient again became febrile and was given a 3-week course of tetracycline by his physician, who felt that he had acute seminal vesiculitis. With this treatment the fever resolved in a week and did not recur. Five years later the patient was well except for mild maturity-onset diabetes mellitus.

COMMENT

This case contained enough red herrings to go on sale at a fish market. The Pel-Ebstein fever (which in our experience is most often not due to Hodgkin's disease), sensitivity to alcohol, and development of herpes zoster all supported the lymphangiogram, which was felt to be the definitive diagnostic study. The nonspecific histologic findings were not surprising, because in Hodgkin's disease this is not uncommon. The best bet is that this patient probably developed a urinary tract infection, perhaps with prostatitis and seminal vesiculitis, following nephrectomy. Perhaps the almost continuous therapy with chloramphenicol intermittently suppressed the symptoms.

Case 10

A 53-year-old Indian woman with a 4-month history of daily fever up to 104°F, 25 pound weight loss, and leukopenia had had an extensive work-up in another hospital, including many cultures, x-rays, and a variety of serologic studies, which had failed to reveal the cause of her illness. For several weeks before admission she had received high doses of prednisone, aspirin, and many antibiotics, including streptomycin, kanamycin, and chloramphenicol, with no response.

On admission she was a semiobtunded, wasted woman appearing acutely ill. Her temperature was 104°F, and physical examination revealed oral moniliasis, a small right supraclavicular lymph node, no hepatomegaly, a palpable spleen tip, and a questionable mass deep in the left epigastrium.

Laboratory studies showed a hematocrit of 23 per cent, white blood cell count of 3900/cu mm, a normal differential, a platelet count of 77,000/cu mm, and a normal urinalysis. Chest x-ray was normal. Blood and bone marrow cultures were negative for acid-fast bacilli, fungi, and bacteria. Throat and stool cultures yielded *Candida albicans*. *Salmonella* agglutinins were absent. Lumbar puncture was normal, and bone marrow biopsy was nondiagnostic. An intravenous pyelogram revealed slight depression of the left kidney due to an enlarged spleen, and a question of medial displacement of the right upper ureter by a mass.

On the fourth hospital day lymphangiography was performed; this showed obstruction above the inguinal regions, with increase in the number and size of the nodes. The periphery of some of the nodes filled, but 24 hours after injection of the dye normal nodal architecture was absent. A diagnosis of lymphoma was made on the basis of this study. Four days later the right supraclavicular node was biopsied, and a diagnosis of Hodgkin's disease established.

She failed to respond despite a course of nitrogen mustard and died on the 10th hospital day. Autopsy confirmed extensive Hodgkin's disease involving liver, spleen, lymph nodes, and bone marrow.

COMMENT

This time the study was accurate, but unfortunately it was carried out too late to help the patient.

Lesson 7: Most FUO Work-ups Should Contain a Liver Scan

Case 11

A 25-year-old, insulin-dependent diabetic was hospitalized because of nausea, vomiting, generalized malaise, and weight loss of 4 weeks' duration. He had had a "flu-like" illness at the onset, but was unaware of fever for several weeks prior to admission. On physical examination he was a thin, moderately dehydrated man with a temperature of 101°F and a tachycardia of 120/minute. The remainder of the examination was unremarkable. Laboratory studies included a normal hematocrit and white blood cell count of 10,900/cu mm with a left shift. The urine showed 4+ glucose and contained 0 to 3 white cells per high-power field. Blood sugar was 525 mg/100 ml, and serum acetone was detectable in trace amounts.

The initial diagnostic impression was ketoacidosis, and the fever was attributed to the metabolic abnormality. However, despite adequate control of the diabetes in the hospital, he continued to have fevers between 101° and 102°F for the next 3 weeks. During that time many studies, including urine and blood cultures, skin tests, febrile agglutinins, heterophil and cold agglutinins, lupus erythematosus cell preparations, stool examinations for ova and parasites, and serologic studies for amebiasis and echinococcosis, were obtained, all of which were normal. Liver function studies, including sulfobromophthalein retention, glutamic-oxalacetic transaminase, alkaline phosphatase, and bilirubin, were also entirely normal.

Three weeks after admission, because of a questionably palpable spleen, a radioactive gold hepatic scan was obtained; this disclosed a 6-cm filling defect in the upper lateral aspect of the right lobe of the liver. At surgery a large abscess was drained through a posterior, extraperitoneal approach. Although no microorganisms were grown from the pus, the patient was treated with both cephalothin and tetracycline, and after several additional aspirations of the abscess he became afebrile.

COMMENT

This patient's liver function tests were entirely normal and his physicians were alerted to the possibility of disease below the diaphragm by discovering the enlarged spleen—again emphasizing the value of repeated physical examinations. The liver scan was particularly helpful here, because it guided the surgeon to the lesion. In former days this patient might have had an anterior laparotomy, and with this anatomic approach the abscess might well have been missed.

Case 12

A 30-year-old housewife was hospitalized because of a 6-week illness during which she had fever up to 101°F, increasing weakness, and a dull right upper quadrant pain. Five years earlier she had had a darkly pigmented nevus removed from her back by her father, who was a physician. Otherwise she had enjoyed good health all her life. On admission examination showed a small scar on the middle of her back, a 1 × 2-cm nodule in the left breast, and a firm, easily palpable liver, extending 5 cm below the costal margin. The temperature was 101°F. Laboratory studies included a normal blood count, urinalysis, chest x-ray, and liver function studies.

Twenty-four hours after entering the hospital she suddenly developed a severe, left retro-orbital headache, anisocoria, and right hemiparesis. Lumbar puncture was normal and cerebrospinal fluid was sterile on culture. Other studies, including electroencephalogram, brain scan, and carotid arteriograms, indicated the presence of a left temporal lobe mass lesion. Twist drill biopsy was promptly performed, yielding a large intracerebral hematoma which was sterile on culture. The patient showed dramatic neurologic improvement following this, but fever persisted. She then had an excisional biopsy of the nodule in her left breast, which showed an undifferentiated malignant tumor of indeterminate source. A liver scan was performed next, and disclosed a large lesion at the lower border of the right lobe. Needle biopsy of this area was carried out, and tissue containing amelanotic melanoma was obtained. Despite continued neurologic improvement, she remained febrile and died at home 6 weeks later.

COMMENT

In this instance the liver scan permitted accurate biopsy, which led to a prompt diagnosis. As a result prolonged hospitalization, innumerable therapeutic trials, including treatment for subacute bacterial endocarditis for presumed ruptured mycotic aneurysm, and exploratory laparotomy, were avoided.

Lesson 8: Observe Sutton's Law:* Go Where the Money Is

Case 13

A 49-year-old man had an 18-month illness characterized by fever, myalgias, lymphadenopathy, and hepatosplenomegaly. Late in the course of the illness extensive pulmonary nodular lesions also appeared, and inappropriate antidiuretic hormone secretion was demonstrated.

The illness had been present for 13 months before he came to our attention. An extensive work-up, including lymph node, muscle, and liver biopsies, had not provided the diagnosis. A trial of adrenal steroids was not effective. Because of the nodular infiltrate, a senior consultant recommended a limited thoracotomy but was outvoted, and 1 week after admission an exploratory laparotomy was performed which showed only congestive hepatosplenomegaly. The lung lesions were biopsied 3 weeks later, using the percutaneous needle technique. Inadequate tissue for diagnosis was obtained, and a pneumothorax resulted, which was difficult to re-expand. The patient died 2 weeks later, despite intensive pharmacologic efforts. At no time did he receive antineoplastic drugs. Autopsy revealed histiocytic medullary reticulosis.

COMMENT

If Sutton's law had been observed a limited open thoracotomy would have been performed 6 weeks before this patient died. Gaensler et al.[12] have pointed out the value of this procedure in diffuse lung disease, particularly when re-expansion of the lung following pneumothorax may be difficult because of poor compliance. Our experience with needle biopsy of the lung leaves something to be desired, and this case is no exception. Histiocytic medullary reticulosis is a rare disease,[11] which probably is best classified with the lymphomas, and usually responds poorly to treatment. It is conceivable, however, that this patient would have benefited from cancer chemotherapy had the diagnosis been made before death. If the case proves nothing else, it shows again that Willie Sutton is right, and also that we run a democratic service.

---

* In the middle 1940's a series of spectacular bank robberies took place in the New York area. When the culprit, whose name was Willie Sutton, was apprehended, like all celebrities he had a press conference, and a reporter asked, "Willie, why do you rob banks?" Sutton looked at him incredulously and answered, "Why, that's where the money is." Readers will be pleased to know that Willie Sutton was paroled in late 1969, and is now employed by a bank.

Lesson 9: Don't Perform an Exploratory Laparotomy Unless There Are Clues Pointing to the Abdomen

Case 14

A 56-year-old farmer, who had previously enjoyed good health, developed diffuse bilateral thoracolumbar muscular tenderness and generalized malaise over a 2-week period and then began to have chills and daily fever to 102°F, associated with increasing myalgias in the left shoulder and both thighs. Brief courses of erythromycin, tetracycline, and penicillin had no effect on his symptoms, and he was referred for further evaluation. On examination he did not appear chronically ill. Except for fever of 103°F, which persisted throughout his hospital stay, the physical examination remained entirely normal. The initial hematocrit was 41 per cent, the white blood cell count was 17,300/cu mm with a normal differential, and the erythrocyte sedimentation rate was 100 mm/hour. The urine contained 3 to 4 white blood cells per high-power field, but was sterile. A chest x-ray showed minimal discoid atelectasis, but was otherwise normal. Ten blood cultures, as well as bone marrow cultures, were negative. Liver function tests were normal except for a slight elevation of the alkaline phosphatase concentration. Liver scan and percutaneous liver biopsy yielded no abnormalities. Febrile agglutinins were negative, as were tests for antinuclear and rheumatoid factors and lupus erythematosus cells. Serum aldolase and creatine phosphokinase tests were normal. An intravenous pyelogram, renal scan, and renal arteriogram failed to show a hypernephroma.

After 2 weeks the patient's fever had still not been explained, and, despite the absence of abdominal signs, he underwent laparotomy, which also failed to result in a diagnosis. Next he was treated empirically with methicillin and ampicillin for 6 days without effect on the fever. Finally he was given prednisone, 100 mg daily, and the pyrexia and myalgias promptly vanished. The steroid dosage was tapered rapidly, and after 6 weeks these drugs were discontinued altogether. The patient continued to feel well and has remained free of fever for over 3 years.

COMMENT

When the diagnosis of FUO does not become apparent after the usual barrage of laboratory tests and biopsies, it has become almost a routine procedure to explore these patients empirically. Often laparotomy is carried out even before evaluation of the abdominal contents with liver function tests, hepatic scan, needle liver biopsy, and appropriate x-rays has been completed. It has been our uniform experience that laparotomy will not reveal abnormalities unless the patient's symptoms, signs, or laboratory data point to the abdomen as the source of fever. In case 14 this clearly was not so. This patient tolerated the operation well, but others often do badly. Actually the patient probably had polymyalgia rheumatica, which is much more common than generally appreciated.[26]

Lesson 10: Despite Complaints Which May Be "Crocky" on the Surface, Fever Remains a Good Objective Sign of Disease

Case 15

A 27-year-old nurse was admitted to the hospital for the first time in September 1967 with fever and diarrhea of 6 days' duration. Not long before the onset of these symptoms she had been in Mexico, and several others in the party with whom she had traveled had had similar symptoms. She was hospitalized briefly, and, in addition to the diagnosis of viral gastroenteritis, was thought to have had a superficial thrombophlebitis.

Three months later she was again hospitalized with fever, lower abdominal crampy pain, malaise, myalgia, and diarrhea tinged with blood. Her temperature was 101.6°F. Extensive evaluation turned up only a mild peripheral blood eosinophilia (3 to 6 per cent). Negative studies included febrile agglutinins, stools for amebae and other parasites, throat cultures, electrocardiogram, chest film, upper gastrointestinal series, small bowel series, barium enema, intravenous pyelogram, brain scan, electroencephalogram, and urine porphobilinogen. The tuberculin test (PPD) was positive. During her hospital stay her temperature ranged between 100° and 101°F. She was given a trial of tetracycline, but did not defervesce.

Because of her persistent fever she was transferred to another hospital, where physical examination, including pelvic examination, was entirely normal. During this hospitalization she had the following normal studies: electrocardiogram, sinus films, upper gastrointestinal series, small bowel x-ray, barium enema, intravenous pyelogram, lymphangiogram, white cell counts, febrile agglutinins, antinuclear factor, iron, protein-bound iodine, serum electrophoresis, cold agglutinins, malaria smears, Sabin-Feldman dye test, blood cultures, bone marrow, including culture, serum electrolytes, urinalyses, urine for 17-keto- and hydroxysteroids, viral studies of the urine, cytomegalic inclusion bodies in urine, nose, throat, and five stool cultures, gastric cultures for acid-fast bacilli, 12 stools for ova, parasites, and guaiacs, and PPD, coccidioidin, blastomycin, histoplasmin, and atypical mycobacteria skin tests. Mumps skin test was positive. The sulfobromophthalein retention was 2.5 per cent; the hematocrit ranged from 34 to 41 per cent, and eosinophils from 6 to 9 per cent. A Kveim test was negative, and pulmonary function tests were normal.

There was no response to chloroquine and diodoquine. Liver scan and bone marrow biopsy were normal. Other negative studies included antibody titers to adenoviruses, psittacosis and lymphogranuloma venereum, influenza A and B, herpes simplex, mumps, Q fever, Eastern, Western, and St. Louis encephalitis, rickettsialpox, and Rocky Mountain spotted fever. Two liver biopsies were performed. The first showed no evidence of liver tissue, but the second showed granulomatous disease of unknown etiology.

During her 6-month stay in the hospital the only abnormalities were persistent mild eosinophilia and a low-grade fever, with temperatures between 99° and 100.6 F, usually between 4 and 8 p.m. Following the needle liver biopsy, which showed granulomatous disease, an open liver biopsy with a limited exploratory laparotomy was performed. The liver looked normal grossly, but histologically again showed granulomatous hepatitis. No cultures were obtained from the liver biopsy.

The patient gradually became asymptomatic, and her temperature tended to drift toward normal. However, treatment was begun with isoniazid and p-aminosalicylic acid, and 3 days after initiation of these drugs she became completely afebrile. Skin tests remained negative.

She was transferred to a tuberculosis hospital, where physical examination was unchanged, and she again showed a mild iron deficiency anemia. The serum glutamic-oxalacetic transaminase level was elevated to 118 units on two occasions. Many laboratory tests were repeated, again without showing any abnormalities. The liver biopsies were reviewed, and showed granulomatous hepatitis with well-defined giant cells, but no caseation or other abnormalities. She was afebrile in the tuberculosis hospital and the diagnosis of tuberculosis was questioned. Two months after institution of antituberculous therapy these drugs were discontinued, the liver function tests returned to normal, and the patient was discharged afebrile. When seen 10 months later she was entirely well.

COMMENT

Because of this patient's many psychosomatic complaints, consideration was given to habitual hyperthermia or factitious fever. However, the temperature elevations were thought to be real and the eosinophilia showed objective evidence of disease. The most reasonable conclusion is that the patient had nonspecific granulomatous hepatitis, related to an unknown allergen, perhaps one of the drugs which she was given early in her illness. The case is also of interest because it probably represents one of the most exhaustive fever work-ups ever recorded.

Lesson 11: Collagen Diseases Remain a Surprisingly Common Cause of FUO, and Patience Usually Results in the Diagnosis

Case 16

A previously healthy 15-year-old high school student had sudden onset of muscle pains, localized initially to the thighs, and daily fever, ranging between 103° and 104°F. Six weeks later he developed a generalized rash and pain and swelling in both knees and the joints of both hands.

At the time of admission to the hospital he was a pale, thin youth whose temperature was 100.4°F. There was a faint but diffuse, macular, erythematous rash over his trunk. Several moderately tender lymph nodes between 1 and 3 cm in diameter were present in the axillae and left supraclavicular region. The heart and lungs were normal. The spleen was palpable 4 cm below the costal margin, but the liver was not enlarged. There were pain and limitation of motion at the wrists and metacarpophalangeal joints bilaterally and in both knees. The hips demonstrated diminished internal rotation, but were not painful.

The hematocrit was 38 per cent, white blood cell count 19,400/cu mm with a slight left shift, and erythrocyte sedimentation rate 76 mm/hour; the urinalysis and chest and joint films were normal. Urine and blood cultures were sterile and a bone marrow sample was normal, as were febrile agglutinins, liver function tests, and tuberculin and fungal skin tests. The Coombs test, rheumatoid and antinuclear factors and lupus erythematosus cell preparations were negative. Biopsy of an axillary lymph node showed only reactive hyperplasia.

During the first week in the hospital the patient's daily temperature spikes ranged from 101° to 103°F. He was given intermittent doses of salicylates. When the results of the many studies became known, most observers felt that the patient represented a fairly typical case of juvenile rheumatoid arthritis in the form usually seen in younger patients. Accordingly, he was given large doses of salicylates, and was discharged afebrile with considerable improvement in his articular symptoms. When seen 9 months later, he was asymptomatic and had gained 30 pounds.

Case 17

A 26-year-old man was admitted because of fever and joint pains of 6 weeks' duration. Six weeks before admission he had noticed a sudden onset of fever, chills, myalgias, and arthralgias involving the elbows, back, and wrists. He was admitted to another hospital, where he had fevers to 105°F, shaking chills, and drenching sweats. He had lost 30 pounds. Pertinent laboratory findings included an elevated sedimentation rate, a leukocytosis between 20,000 and 38,000/cu mm with a shift to the left, and mild anemia. All cultures, studies for collagen diseases, and x-rays were negative. He was given a course of penicillin and developed a skin rash. Indomethacin and tetracycline did not affect the fever. There was slight improvement with low doses of adrenal steroids. The electrocardiogram was consistent with myocarditis or pericarditis. During the week before admission he developed tender nodules over both malleoli.

Physical examination showed a pale, sick man with a temperature of 102°F and pain in the right knee and back. There was marked tenderness over the spine in the thoracic region and spasm of the paraspinal muscles. There was bilateral epitrochlear lymphadenopathy. The remainder of the examination was normal. The laboratory data again demonstrated anemia, a rapid sedimentation rate, and leukocytosis. There was mild hyperglobulinemia. All tests for collagen diseases were negative, as were all x-rays. Liver and spleen scans were normal. During his stay in the hospital he continued to have fever to 105°F; the pyrexia was not influenced by low doses of aspirin, although doses in the neighborhood of 6 to 8 g/day resulted in some blunting of the febrile spikes. He developed a subcutaneous nodule over the sternum, biopsy of which was not diagnostic. Tuberculin (PPD) and fungal skin tests were negative.

The working diagnosis was juvenile rheumatoid disease. When he had not improved 2 months later he was given adrenal steroid hormones and improved dramatically. The hormones were tapered off slowly after several months. Two years after the onset of this illness he was symptom-free except for occasional arthralgias, for which he took aspirin.

COMMENT

Both these patients probably had juvenile rheumatoid arthritis (Still's disease). As is usual in this syndrome, the younger the patient the milder the disease, and the better the prognosis. Hence it is not surprising that the patient described in case 16 had a relatively benign course. In contrast, the patient described in case 17 was severely ill and recovery was much more prolonged. It would not be surprising if this patient should develop more definitive changes of rheumatoid arthritis, or if his symptoms returned.[13]

Case 18

A 59-year-old woman complained of recurrent right-sided headaches and fever of 3 months' duration. Nine years previously she had undergone segmental colonic resection for an adenocarcinomatous polyp, with apparent cure. She had had several urinary tract infections 2 years before, which had not recurred following urethral dilations. For at least a year her hematocrit had been in the mid-30s and the erythrocyte sedimentation rate between 50 and 100 mm/hour. Physical examination at the time of hospitalization was normal except for conjunctival pallor and a temperature of 101°F. Initial laboratory studies included a hematocrit of 27 per cent, a normal white blood cell count, urinalysis, and chest x-ray. The sedimentation rate was 63 mm/hour.

For the next 2 weeks the patient had daily temperature elevations between 101° and 103°F. During that time cultures of urine, blood, and bone marrow were sterile. No pathogens were demonstrated in the stool, and serum agglutinins for *Salmonella* and *Brucella* were not found. A lumbar puncture revealed no abnormalities. Several lupus erythematosus cell preparations as well as liver function tests were normal. In view of the past history of genitourinary and gastrointestinal difficulties, complete x-ray studies of these areas were obtained, but were normal.

On the 15th hospital day a biopsy of the right temporal artery was performed, and disclosed chronic inflammatory changes and multinucleated giant cells, with some intimal proliferation and fibrosis, consistent with the diagnosis of giant cell arteritis. The patient was given prednisone, 30 mg daily, and promptly became afebrile. Within 2 weeks the hematocrit and sedimentation rate returned to normal and the headaches disappeared.

COMMENT

This is a classical case of temporal arteritis, and the prolonged work-up is an example of *Jeff's law*.* In this instance the "routine" FUO work-up was assumed to shed more light on the problem than the obviously indicated temporal artery biopsy. The very brisk response to steroids was typical of this disease, and confirmed the diagnosis.

Case 19

A 38-year-old housewife was well until 3 years before admission, when she developed pain and swelling of the ankles, knees, and distal interphalangeal joints. She was treated with adrenal steroids, but continued to have pain and stiffness in the fingers. At that time she also developed generalized petechiae, but had no further systemic symptoms. A laboratory work-up showed no bleeding abnormalities, and cryoglobulins were absent. The petechiae cleared, and a subsequent flare-up of her joint symptoms responded to adrenocorticotropin. Five months before admission she was found to be anemic, and 8 days before entry she developed arthralgias and fever between 102° and 104°F with several shaking chills. She was treated with penicillin with some improvement. Other medications included chloramphenicol and Panalba. On the day before admission she developed a rash. Previous laboratory data showed only an elevated erythrocyte sedimentation rate, but were otherwise normal. Physical examination showed a temperature of 101°F and a generalized maculopapular rash. There was cervical lymphadenopathy, and on the dorsal surfaces of the distal interphalangeal joints there were firm 1- to 2-cm nodules. Laboratory examination showed a hematocrit of 29 per cent, a very rapid sedimentation rate, and a leukocyte count of 20,000/cu mm with a slight shift to the left. The anemia was typical of iron deficiency. Urinalysis showed red blood cell casts on a few occasions, but otherwise was not remarkable. All bacteriologic examinations were normal. The serum globulin was 4.7 g/100 ml with a broad γ-band on electrophoresis. Liver scan and liver biopsy were normal. Lupus erythematosus cell preparations, antinuclear factor tests, and examinations for rheumatoid disease were negative. Kidney, lymph node, and muscle biopsies were normal.

During the first 3 weeks in the hospital her temperature ranged between 103° and 104°F and several courses of antibiotics did not alter the fever. After that she was given prednisone in dosage of 60 mg/day and became afebrile. Following institution of steroid therapy she remained afebrile. The steroids were tapered off during the next 3 months, and when seen 5 years after her hospitalization (and 8 years after the onset of her illness)

---

* Mutt and Jeff are on a street and Jeff is under a street lamp on all fours looking for something. Mutt asks what the problem is. Jeff says he is looking for a cuff link which he had lost some 100 yards up the street. Mutt asks, "But why are you looking here?" Jeff replies, "Because it's lighter here."

she had only minimal changes in the hands and occasional arthralgias, which responded promptly to aspirin.

COMMENT

This case again points up how difficult it is to make the diagnosis of collagen vascular disease by examination of tissue. It shows further, as do all of the other cases in this group, that the prognosis in collagen diseases is relatively good as long as renal involvement is absent. Although these patients are often desperately ill when they are febrile, they tend to improve after the acute inflammatory response is suppressed.

Lesson 12: When in Doubt, Disseminated Tuberculosis Remains a Good Bet

Case 20

A 56-year-old Filipino man was admitted complaining of weakness and generalized body aches for two months. Two months before admission he had sustained several stab wounds in the neck, but these were healing satisfactorily with local treatment. He had been an alcoholic for many years. Physical examination showed a chronically ill man with a temperature of 101°F and marked hepatomegaly, but no other evidence of cirrhosis. Laboratory data showed mild anemia and a white cell count which varied between 19,000 and 24,000/cu mm. Liver function tests showed a serum bilirubin of 1.0 mg/100 ml and an alkaline phosphatase between 20 and 50 Bodansky units (normal < 5). The chest x-ray showed a suggestion of hilar adenopathy. During the first 10 days in the hospital his temperature spiked to 103°F daily. At that time treatment with tetracycline, 2.0 g/day, was instituted, and with this therapy his temperature fell to 100°F and remained there. After 2 weeks tetracycline was discontinued, and fever to 103°F recurred promptly. During the fourth week in the hospital supraclavicular nodes were felt for the first time and were biopsied. At the same time bone marrow and liver biopsies were performed. All showed evidence of miliary tuberculosis.

COMMENT

The clinicians taking care of this patient were led astray by the good response to tetracycline. This is not unusual in tuberculosis. On the other hand, they ignored this patient's race and hilar adenopathy. Earlier liver biopsy clearly would have made the diagnosis.

Case 21

A 79-year-old rancher was hospitalized for evaluation of fever and chills. Four months before admission he was thought to have had biliary colic, but a gall bladder x-ray was normal. At that time an effusion in the right knee joint was noted, and this was aspirated several times; 20 to 100 ml of sterile fluid was obtained. Two months before admission, because of the persistent effusion, the knee was placed in a cast, and shortly thereafter the patient had shaking chills, fever, and sweats. These would last 1 to 2 days and during the ensuing 2 to 4 days the patient would be afebrile. He was tested perfunctorily for a variety of diseases and was treated empirically with many antibiotics, to which the fever did not respond. He also received adrenal steroids in low doses intermittently, without improvement. A scalene node biopsy was said to show nonspecific inflammation. No cultures for acid-fast bacilli were taken, and he received no antituberculous therapy.

Physical examination revealed an acutely and chronically ill, disoriented old man whose temperature was 103°F. Except for an enlarged prostate, a cast on the right leg, and disorientation, the examination was negative.

Although the patient's diagnosis had not been made during a month-long hospitalization elsewhere, the admitting chest x-ray showed a fine miliary infiltrate, and liver and bone marrow biopsies showed caseating granulomas with acid-fast bacilli, which subsequently were grown on culture. The patient was treated with isoniazid and p-aminosalicylic acid and improved promptly.

COMMENT

This case illustrates the point that miliary tuberculosis should also be considered in elderly Caucasians. The diagnosis is usually easy to make, and the only reason it was missed here was the slovenly approach to this patient's fever. At no time did he had a skin test, cultures of gastric aspirates or joint fluid, chest x-rays of good quality, or biopsy of liver or bone marrow.

Lesson 13: When a Patient Has Fever Postoperatively It Is Usually Related to the Surgical Procedure, Not to Some Unrelated Disease. For Want of a Better Eponym We Have Called This Petersdorf's Law

Case 22

A 19-year-old basketball player was admitted with fever of 2 weeks' duration. Three weeks before admission he suffered an injury to his right knee while playing basketball, and on the following day underwent surgical repair of a ligamentous tear. Postoperatively he was febrile, and when the fever failed to respond to aspirin he was treated with cloxacillin. He was discharged 10 days after his operation, but, because of continued fever to 101°F, antimicrobial therapy was continued. Physical examination on admission showed a healthy-looking boy with a temperature of 102°F. The right leg was in a cast and there was mildly tender right inguinal and femoral adenopathy. The cast was opened, revealing a swollen, somewhat warm and tender knee without fluctuation. Aspiration of the knee joint showed only a small amount of fluid, which was sterile on culture. The laboratory data showed mild anemia. The white blood cell count was normal but the sedimentation rate was elevated. Multiple cultures were negative.

When the patient was first admitted to the hospital antibiotics were withheld, and the temperature averaged 103°F. Another aspiration of the knee and a synovial biopsy were negative. Inasmuch as infection was thought to be absent, antibiotics were withheld initially. However, because of persistent fever after a week's "watchful waiting," a course of cephalothin was instituted, and concurrently he became afebrile. Therapy with cephalothin was discontinued after 1 week, and the patient remained free of fever and improved symptomatically.

COMMENT

Although there was little objective evidence of inflammation, the response to antibiotics was sufficiently impressive to convince most observers that he had a postoperative infection.

Lesson 14: *Primum Non Nocere*

Case 23

A 57-year-old farm worker was first seen by her physician 1 year before admission because of a rash which was presumed to be an allergic phenomenon. At that time she also had fever and right upper quadrant pain, and was presumed to have chronic cholecystitis and cholangitis. A cholecystectomy was performed; the common duct was not dilated and there were no stones. The postoperative course was stormy, and there was again a good deal of fever, presumably associated with a reaction to penicillin. The temperature subsided following therapy with chloramphenicol. Shortly after discharge, while still receiving this drug, she developed pruritus and a recurrence of fever, and was referred for evaluation. Upon physical examination she was chronically ill, but there was no jaundice. The spleen was enlarged 2 cm below the costal margin and the rest of the examination was negative. The white blood cell count was 4000/cu mm and the hematocrit 30 per cent. She had sterile effusions of both knee joints. The liver function tests were not significantly deranged. All tests for collagen disease were negative. On intravenous pyelography the right kidney was small, presumably because of chronic pyelonephritis, but renal function was normal. Although she was neither acutely ill nor excessively febrile, it was felt that the cause of her fever had not been elucidated, and 3 weeks after admission she had another exploratory laparotomy with open liver biopsy and splenectomy. At operation the liver was normal and the spleen showed only reactive hyperplasia. No other abnormalities were noted. Histologically the liver biopsy showed scattered foci of inflammation. She remained afebrile for 10 days after operation but then again had fever and for the first time developed a rise in alkaline phosphatase and serum glutamic-oxalacetic transaminase. The fever again responded to chloramphenicol, but because she had received so much of this drug therapy was changed to tetracycline and chloramphenicol was discontinued. In the meantime there was progressive deterioration in liver function, with a rise of the serum glutamic-oxalacetic transaminase to 1130 units. Liver failure progressed, and she died 2 weeks later. At autospy there was massive hepatic infiltration with fat as well as acute necrosis of liver cells.

COMMENT

This patient's primary problem was never resolved. She could have had a collagen disease or perhaps sclerosing pericholangitis. In any event she died of hepatic failure which almost surely was iatrogenic. Grounds for an exploratory laparotomy—while she was improving—were questionable, and her terminal hepatic failure may have been due to Halothane anesthesia during the second procedure, or perhaps was a consequence of tetracycline therapy given when her liver function was already compromised. In this case we clearly would have been wiser had we been "watchers" rather than "treaters."

Lesson 15: Sometimes the Diagnosis Is Not Forthcoming—Even in the Best of Hands

Case 24

A 57-year-old salesman was admitted for work-up of fever of unknown origin which had been present for 1 month. He was well until 2 days after he returned from a 2-week vacation in Mexico, when he developed severe shaking chills, sweats, and fever to 103°F. He was hospitalized by his private physician and treated with penicillin, streptomycin, and chloramphenicol for 2 weeks, but fever and chills continued unabated. During the ensuing several weeks he became profoundly weak, lost 30 pounds, and developed severe dyspnea, associated with a large right pleural effusion. A liver biopsy was reported as normal. On admission physical examination revealed a chronically ill, dyspneic man with poor skin turgor, dry mucous membranes, several old splinter hemorrhages under the nails, and dullness over the right chest posteriorly. There were neither murmurs nor cardiomegaly. The abdomen was protuberant, and the liver was palpable 8 cm below the right costal margin. The spleen tip was palpable, and moderate scrotal and pretibial edema was present. Laboratory data included mild leukopenia with a shift to the left, an elevated alkaline phosphatase, which rose from 28 King-Armstrong units on admission to 60; and a serum glutamic-oxalacetic transaminase level which increased from 103 to 1200 units. A liver scan was normal, as were lumbar puncture and bone marrow aspiration.

Despite restoration of extracellular fluid volume he became progressively obtunded and developed deep jaundice, uremia, and intractable bleeding from the gastrointestinal and urinary tracts. He died 48 hours after admission to our hospital, and 5 weeks after onset of his fever. Autopsy revealed Hodgkin's disease involving the liver, spleen, and lymph nodes, including nodes in the porta hepatis.

COMMENT

This patient's problem was approached carefully and thoroughly by his physician, but clues were scanty and neither biopsy nor therapeutic trials provided the answer. When we saw him multiple coagulation defects precluded further biopsies or surgery. Moreover, it is likely that chemotherapy would not have been effective even if the diagnosis had been made. Fortunately, this type of patient represents the exception rather than the rule, and in good hands the diagnosis of FUO should be made in 90 per cent of patients.

CONCLUDING REMARKS

It is our hope that these cases will be instructive; if they teach anything at all, it is that no one patient resembles another, and that each patient must be approached individually. No FUO work-up should be done "by the numbers"; each patient must be considered a unique intellectual challenge. More importantly, however, we must remember that these patients are sick and distressed, and that the needle, the x-ray tube, and the scalpel should be used with that in mind. Each of these patients deserves the most thoughtful and compassionate diagnostic approach of which we are capable.

REFERENCES

1. Atkins, E. Fever. In *Signs and Symptoms*, MacBryde, C. M., Ed., 4th ed. J. B. Lippincott Co., Philadelphia, 1964.
2. Bean, W. B. The Munchausen syndrome. Trans. Amer. Clin. Climatol. Ass. **70:** 236, 1958.
3. Belcher, D., and Turck, M. Staphylococcal endarteritis in a renal artery-inferior vena cava fistula. Arch. Internal Med. **119:**198, 1967.
4. Bondy, P. K., Cohn, G. L., and Gregory, P. B. Etiocholanolone fever. Medicine **44:**249, 1965.
5. Brewis, E. G. Undiagnosed fever. Brit. Med. J. **1:**107, 1965.
6. Browder, A. A., Huff, J. W., and Petersdorf, R. G. The significance of fever in neoplastic disease. Ann. Internal Med. **55:**932, 1961.
7. Cherubin, C. E., Baden, M., Kavaler, F., Lerner, S., and Cline, W. Infective endocarditis in narcotic addicts. Ann. Internal Med. **69:**1091, 1968.
8. Deller, J. J., Jr., and Russell, P. K. An analysis of fevers of unknown origin in American soldiers in Vietnam. Ann. Internal Med. **66:**1129, 1967.
9. Effersoe, P. Fever of unknown origin. A follow-up study of 34 patients discharged without diagnosis. Dan. Med. Bull. **15:**240, 1968.
10. Fransen, H., and Bottiger, L. E. Fever of more than two weeks' duration. Acta Med. Scand. **179:**147. 1966.
11. Friedman, R. M., and Steigbigel, N. H. Histiocytic medullary reticulosis. Amer. J. Med. **38:**130, 1965.
12. Gaensler, E. A., Moister, M. V. B., and Hamm, J. Open-lung biopsy in diffuse pulmonary disease. N. Engl. J. Med. **270:**1319, 1964.
13. Jeremy, R., Schaller, J., Arkless, R., Wedgwood, R. J., and Healey, L. A. Juvenile rheumatoid arthritis persisting into adulthood. Amer. J. Med. **45:**419, 1968.
14. Lindemeyer, R. I., Turck, M., and Petersdorf, R. G. Factors determining the outcome of chemotherapy in infections of the urinary tract. Ann. Internal Med. **58:**201, 1963.
15. MacGregor, G. A., and Cullen, R. A. The syndrome of fever, anemia, high sedimentation rate with atrial myxoma. Brit. Med. J. **2:**991, 1959.
16. Petersdorf, R. G., and Beeson, P. B. Fever of unexplained origin: report of 100 cases. Medicine **40:**1, 1961.

17. Petersdorf, R. G., and Bennett, I. L., Jr. Factitious fever. Ann. Internal Med. 46:1039, 1957.
18. Reimann, H. A. Habitual hyperthermia. J.A.M.A. 99:1860, 1932.
19. Reimann, H. A. Periodic disease. Medicine 30:219, 1951.
20. Shaw, R. K., Szwed, C., Boggs, D. R., Fahey, J. L., Frei, E., III, Morrison, E., and Utz, J. P. Infection and immunity in chronic lymphocytic leukemia. Arch. Internal Med. 106:467, 1960.
21. Silver, R. T., Utz, J. P., Frei, E., III, and McCullough, N. B. Fever, infection and host resistance in acute leukemia. Amer. J. Med. 24:25, 1958.
22. Sohar, E., Gafni, J., Pras, M., and Heller, H. Familial Mediterranean fever. Amer. J. Med. 43:227, 1967.
23. Tisdale, W. A. Focal hepatitis, fever and skin rash following therapy with sulfa-methoxypyridazine, long-acting sulfonamide. N. Engl. J. Med. 285:687, 1958.
24. Tisdale, W. A. Spontaneous colon bacillus bacteremia in Laënnec's cirrhosis. Gastroenterology 40:141, 1961.
25. Wight, R. P., Jr., McCall, M. M., and Wenger, N. K. Primary atrial tumor: evaluation of clinical findings in 10 cases and review of the literature. Amer. J. Cardiol. 11:790, 1963.
26. Wilske, K. R., and Healey, L. A. Polymyalgia rheumatica: a manifestation of systemic giant cell arteritis. Ann. Internal Med. 66:77, 1967.
27. Wolff, S. M. Familial Mediterranean fever. In *Principles of Internal Medicine*, 6th ed. McGraw-Hill Book Co., Inc., New York. In press.

Acute Inflammatory Disease
of the Lung

EDWARD W. HOOK

INTRODUCTION

The patient with an acute febrile illness, respiratory symptoms, and abnormal pulmonary densities on roentgenography presents a common and challenging diagnostic problem. Virtually any microbe capable of causing disease in man can produce inflammatory changes in the lung as a result of primary invasion via the tracheobronchial tree or as a metastatic manifestation of a systemic infection. Furthermore, innumerable non-infectious diseases may involve the lungs and mimic in a striking fashion pneumonia caused by microbial agents.

Modern therapeutic measures, not only for infectious diseases, but also for many other problems, have become increasingly specific. If the physician is to avoid continuous utilization of a "shotgun" approach in therapy, he must, in each instance, be aware of all of the diagnostic possibilities and take the necessary steps as indicated to arrive at a specific diagnosis. He will frequently be required to establish a presumptive diagnosis based on data from the history, physical examination, and simple laboratory procedures that can be applied at the bedside. Immediate presumptive diagnosis is required because in many instances, especially in patients with bacterial pneumonia, antimicrobial therapy will have to be initiated immediately, before the results of laboratory procedures designed to produce a definitive diagnosis become available.

Despite the large number of processes that can be manifested by fever and pulmonary infiltrates, the clinical features of some diseases are specific enough to permit a relatively accurate presumptive clinical diagnosis.

The purpose of this chapter is to consider the differential diagnosis of diseases which present as acute inflammation of the lungs. Attention obviously will be focused on disease caused by microbial agents, but non-infectious causes will also be considered. Since there may be considerable overlap among acute, subacute, and chronic pulmonary diseases, the information presented in the present chapter should be considered with that in the following chapter, "Poorly Resolving Pneumonias."

ETIOLOGY OF ACUTE INFLAMMATORY DISEASES OF THE LUNGS

The major categories of etiologic possibilities in the patient with acute inflammatory disease of the lungs are shown in Table 33, which lists dis-

EDWARD W. HOOK, M.D. Henry B. Mulholland Professor and Chairman, Department of Medicine, University of Virginia School of Medicine, Charlottesville, Virginia

TABLE 33

Acute Inflammatory Diseases of the Lungs
Diseases of Microbial Origin in Adults

I. Bacteria
    A. Frequently encountered
        1. Pneumococcal pneumonia
        2. Staphylococcal pneumonia
        3. *Klebsiella* pneumonia (Friedlander's pneumonia)
        4. Necrotizing or aspiration pneumonia, including lung abscess
        5. Pneumonia caused by Gram-negative enteric bacilli
    B. Infrequently encountered
        1. Anthrax
        2. Brucellosis
        3. Glanders
        4. *Hemophilus* pneumonia
        5. Melioidosis
        6. Mimeae pneumonia
        7. Meningococcal pneumonia
        8. *Pasteurella multocida*
        9. Pertussis
      10. Plague
      11. Salmonellosis other than typhoid fever
      12. Streptococcal pneumonia
      13. Tularemia
      14. Typhoid fever
II. Bacteria-like agents
    A. *Mycoplasma* pneumonia
    B. Psittacosis
III. Mycobacteria
    A. Tuberculosis
IV. Spirochetes
    A. Leptospirosis
V. Viruses
    A. Adenoviruses
    B. Coxsackie, ECHO, and polioviruses
    C. Cytomegalovirus
    D. Influenza
    E. Measles
    F. Parainfluenza viruses
    G. Respiratory syncytial virus
    H. Rhinoviruses
    I. Varicella
VI. Fungi
    A. Aspergillosis
    B. Blastomycosis
    C. Candidiasis
    D. Coccidioidomycosis
    E. Cryptococcosis
    F. Histoplasmosis
    G. Mucormycosis
    H. Other fungus infections
VII. Actinomycetes (fungus-like bacteria)
    A. Actinomycosis
    B. Nocardiosis
VIII. Rickettsiae
    A. Q Fever

TABLE 33—*Continued*

IX. Protozoa and other parasites
    A. Amebiasis
    B. Ascariasis
    C. Creeping eruption
    D. Echinococcosis
    E. Malaria
    F. Paragonimiasis
    G. *Pneumocystis carinii*
    H. Schistosomiasis
    I. Strongyloidiasis
    J. Toxoplasmosis
    K. Trichinosis
    L. Visceral larva migrans

eases of microbial origin, and in Table 34, which lists diseases of nonmicrobial origin. No effort has been made to list every disease capable of producing acute pulmonary disease. However, the tables do include the most common causes of acute pulmonary inflammation and, in addition, a number of rare pulmonary processes which are of unusual interest or about which specific diagnostic information is available. In the paragraphs that follow, most of these specific diagnostic possibilities are discussed briefly, with emphasis on the main clinical features useful in differential diagnosis.

CLINICAL FEATURES

Pneumonia Caused by Microbial Agents

Bacteria—Frequently Encountered

PNEUMOCOCCAL PNEUMONIA

Diplococcus pneumoniae is the most common cause of acute bacterial pneumonia, and is responsible for more than 90 per cent of such infections in otherwise healthy persons in the general population. Thus, if it is relatively certain that a patient has bacterial pneumonia, the diagnosis of a pneumococcal etiology is probably correct simply on the basis of the prevalence of the disease. Nevertheless, in the individual case all aspects should be considered to differentiate pneumococcal pneumonia from other bacterial pneumonias and from the multiple causes of the nonbacterial or atypical pneumonia syndrome.

Pneumococcal pneumonia frequently occurs in persons who have had an identifiable preceding event which alters the defense mechanisms of the lower respiratory tract and predisposes to infection. The most important respiratory defense mechanisms are the epiglottal and cough reflexes, the ciliated epithelium, the mucous blanket of the trachea and bronchi, phagocytic cells, and specific antibody. Any process which interferes with any of these protective mechanisms can predispose to pulmonary infection.

In previously normal individuals the most frequently recognized predis-

TABLE 34
*Diseases of Nonmicrobial Origin Which May Mimic Acute
Pulmonary Infection*

I. Cardiovascular diseases
   A. Pulmonary infarction
   B. Pulmonary edema
II. Chemical and physical agents
   A. Berylliosis
   B. Acute heroin intoxication
   C. Hydrocarbon pneumonitis
   D. Pulmonary lesions associated with irradiation
   E. Lipoid pneumonia
   F. Pneumoconiosis
   G. Silo filler's disease
III. Diseases of presumed or proven immunologic origin
   A. Allergic alveolitis or hypersensitivity pneumonitis; inhalation of im-
      munogenic dusts, especially organic dusts (farmer's lung, pigeon breeder's
      disease, bagassosis, maple bark disease, etc.)
   B. Pulmonary reactions to drugs
   C. Collagen-vascular diseases, including rheumatic fever, systemic lupus
      erythematosus, polyarteritis, Wegener's granulomatosis, Goodpasture's
      syndrome, systemic rheumatoid disease, etc.
   D. Loeffler's syndrome
IV. Neoplastic diseases
   A. Tumors of lung
   B. Leukemias
V. Miscellaneous diseases
   A. Atelectasis
   B. Desquamative interstitial pneumonia
   C. Hamman-Rich lung (diffuse idiopathic interstitial pulmonary fibrosis)
   D. Idiopathic pulmonary hemosiderosis
   E. Inflammatory diseases below the diaphragm (such as acute pancreatitis,
      splenic abscess or infarction, cholecystitis, or subdiaphragmatic abscess)
   F. Intrapulmonary hemorrhage
   G. Pneumonia of the cholesterol type
   H. Pulmonary alveolar proteinosis
   I. Sarcoidosis

posing factor is infection with a respiratory virus, which accounts for the
high incidence of the disease in winter and early spring. For example, influenza virus causes desquamation of the ciliated epithelium of the trachea
and bronchi, inhibits phagocytosis of bacteria by leukocytes, and is associated with a high incidence of bacterial pneumonia. Other factors
which predispose to infection in previously normal individuals include
ethanol, anesthesia, or opiates, all of which enhance the possibility of
aspiration, decrease the likelihood that aspirated material will be expelled,
and, in the case of ethanol, decrease mobilization of leukocytes. In some
instances the predisposing event may be quite simple and may go unnoticed; for example, localized trauma to the thorax, such as a blow with a
baseball, may lead to splinting, atelectasis, and local fluid accumulation,

all of which may set the stage for the development of pneumonia. Pneumococcal pneumonia also occurs with surprising frequency in persons with major underlying diseases. Austrian and Gold, in an extensive study of pneumococcal pneumonia with bacteremia at the Kings County Hospital in Brooklyn, New York, found a significant predisposing illness in 56 per cent of their patients. The most common underlying conditions were cardiac decompensation, delirium tremens, carcinoma, blood dyscrasias, pulmonary tuberculosis, asthma, cirrhosis of the liver, and diabetic acidosis.

The clinical manifestations of pneumococcal pneumonia are well known. The onset of infection is usually *abrupt*, with a *single* chill, followed by fever, cough, chest pain, and *diffusely* bloody or *rusty* sputum. Manifestations of a preceding virus infection of the respiratory tract are often present, but can usually be distinguished from the striking signs and symptoms that appear with the onset of pneumococcal infection.

The initial major symptom is usually a chill, which occurs in about 80 per cent of the patients. Multiple chills may be observed, but their occurrence should suggest the possibility of another etiology, especially staphylococcal, Friedlander's, or other necrotizing pneumonia. Multiple chills are also frequently iatrogenic, related to the administration of antipyretics.

Fever is present in almost all patients with pneumococcal pneumonia, and is characteristically sustained. Wide swings in the temperature should suggest another etiology or a localized suppurative complication, but are usually caused by administration of antipyretics or anti-inflammatory corticosteroids. Absence of fever in untreated pneumococcal pneumonia is almost nonexistent, although the temperature response may be diminished in elderly individuals and in patients with major underlying diseases, especially renal insufficiency. Although the usual antipyretics, such as aspirin, are not capable of completely suppressing the temperature response in patients with pneumococcal pneumonia, active pneumococcal infection may actually progress in the absence of fever in patients receiving substantial doses of corticosteroids.

About 75 per cent of patients produce a diffusely bloody or rusty sputum. In pneumonia caused by type III pneumococcus, the sputum may be very sticky and stringy because of the large amount of polysaccharide produced by this organism.

Pleural pain, which occurs in about 70 per cent of patients with pneumococcal pneumonia, may cause confusion in diagnosis by suggesting the possibility of acute intra-abdominal disease. In patients with lower lobe pneumonia, pain may be referred to the shoulders or abdomen, and may suggest the possibility of acute appendicitis or acute cholecystitis. The ileus and abdominal distension which are so common in acute pneumococcal infection add to the diagnostic difficulties. The occasional problem of differentiation of infection above and below the diaphragm is further complicated by the fact that subdiaphragmatic abscess, liver abscess, or other infections in the upper abdomen may produce local diaphragmatic inflammation, small collections of pleural fluid, chest pain, and atelectasis secondary to decreased respiratory excursions. Diseases below the diaphragm can usually be distinguished from pneumonia by careful history, physical examination, roentgenograms, and simple laboratory procedures.

Herpes simplex infections of the mucocutaneous junctions of the mouth are quite frequent during pneumococcal infection, and their presence has been suggested as being helpful in differentiating pneumococcal pneumonia from pulmonary processes of other etiology. Although "fever blisters" occur in one-fourth to one-third of patients with pneumococcal pneumonia, they also occur in other febrile states and are not of genuine aid in diagnosis.

Mild icterus is not unusual in patients with severe pneumococcal pneumonia, and results from destruction of red blood cells in consolidated lung and the occurrence of focal areas of necrosis in the liver, as well as the effects of hypoxia on liver function. As long as the physician recognizes that elevation of total bilirubin, usually not exceeding 2 or 3 mg/100 ml, may be a component of the pneumococcal disease, the icterus does not create diagnostic difficulties. The unconjugated bilirubin is elevated to a greater extent than the conjugated bilirubin.

Physical findings of lobar consolidation are typical of pneumococcal pneumonia, and occur in this disease more often than in any other type of pulmonary infection. However, lobar consolidation also occurs with considerable frequency in pneumonia caused by other bacteria, and is not of aid in differentiating among the various bacterial pneumonias. In contrast, lobar consolidation is uncommon in nonbacterial pneumonias, and is one of the many factors to be considered in distinguishing bacterial from non-bacterial pulmonary infections. The pulmonary process is limited to a single lobe or a single pulmonary segment in slightly more than two-thirds of patients with pneumococcal pneumonia.

It is important to note that, early in the course of pneumococcal pneumonia, physical and radiographic examination of the chest may occasionally be normal despite the presence of fever, cough, and hemoptysis. Patients who present in this manner almost always develop definite physical and radiographic signs of disease within 24 hours.

Leukocytosis occurs in the majority of patients with pneumococcal pneumonia, usually in the range of 15,000 to 25,000 cells/cu mm, and a shift to the left is characteristic. However, counts below 5000 cells/cu mm occur in about 5 per cent of patients, and counts exceeding 25,000 cells/cu mm are noted in about 10 per cent of patients.

One of the most helpful laboratory aids for the rapid diagnosis of pneumococcal pneumonia is the Gram-stained smear of sputum. Demonstration of large numbers of Gram-positive, lancet-shaped diplococci in sputum, especially when associated with pus cells, permits a presumptive diagnosis of pneumococcal pneumonia.

The sputum specimen should also be cultured. The finding of a predominance of pneumococci on culture of sputum from a patient with pneumonia is excellent presumptive evidence of pneumococcal etiology. A culture of the nasopharynx should be obtained if it is impossible to obtain sputum. There is a high positive correlation between the types of pneumococci isolated from nasopharynx and sputa of patients with pneumococcal pneumonia. Nevertheless, there are definite limitations of sputum and nasopharyngeal cultures as diagnostic aids. Isolation of pneumococci from the secretions of the upper respiratory tract does not constitute conclusive proof that the organisms are responsible for disease existing in the lower respiratory tract, because the nasopharyngeal carrier rate for pneumococci in the general population may be quite high (5 to 50 per cent).

False-negative cultures also occur, although the frequency of this phenomenon obviously depends on the competence of the laboratory involved. In a recent study at the Baltimore City Hospital by Rathbun and Govani, 45 per cent of patients with pneumococcal pneumonia and bacteremia had negative sputum cultures for pneumococci! Although this proportion of false-negative cultures seems unusually high, these investigators showed that it was possible to increase recovery of pneumococci markedly by inoculating sputum into a mouse. This old technique, uncommonly utilized by diagnostic laboratories at present, probably should be employed more often in the diagnosis of pneumococcal infections.

One or two blood cultures should be obtained in every patient suspected of having pneumococcal pneumonia. Pneumococci can be isolated from the blood of about 30 per cent of the patients, and this finding constitutes definitive proof of etiology.

About 10 per cent of patients with pneumococcal pneumonia develop small pleural effusions, sufficient to be detected on radiographic examination. This fluid contains large numbers of leukocytes and has other characteristics of an exudate, but on culture is usually sterile. Actual infection of the pleural cavity leading to empyema now develops in less than 2 per cent of patients.

Abscess formation in the lung is not a characteristic feature of pneumococcal pneumonia. In fact, one of the most remarkable features of pneumococcal infection of the lungs is that complete resolution of the process without tissue necrosis or scarring usually occurs by 21 days after onset. An occasional exception to this generalization occurs with type III pneumococcal infections, which may be associated with lung necrosis and abscess formation. Other complications that occur in patients with pneumococcal pneumonia include pericarditis, meningitis, endocarditis, arthritis, and peritonitis. About 20 per cent of cases of pneumococcal meningitis develop secondary to pneumococcal infection of the lungs. The manifestations of meningitis usually overshadow those of the pneumonia, and the pneumonia may be overlooked unless roentgenograms are obtained. When meningitis complicates pneumococcal pneumonia endocardial localization is quite common. Pneumococci usually localize on the aortic valve and lead to ulceration of the margins of the valve or perforation of a cusp, both of which lead to aortic insufficiency. Systolic murmurs are frequent during the febrile phase of pneumococcal pneumonia, but a diastolic murmur is indicative of endocarditis or pre-existing valvular heart disease. Peritonitis, a rare complication, usually occurs in patients with the nephrotic syndrome or postnecrotic cirrhosis.

It is of interest that mixed bacterial infections of the lung may occur occasionally. A few patients with pneumonia caused by multiple pneumococcal types have been described, and simultaneous infection of the lungs by pneumococci and *Klebsiella* has been reported. Diagnostic difficulties may be encountered when pneumococcal pneumonia complicates pulmonary tuberculosis.

The response to therapy of the patient suspected of having pneumococcal pneumonia has important diagnostic implications. If the diagnosis is correct and no complications have occurred, response to antimicrobial therapy should be dramatic. Marked improvement almost always takes place during the initial 24 to 48 hours, with a decrease in fever, malaise, and toxemia. Objective evidence of response as indicated by a *decrease* in temperature usually occurs within 24 hours after starting penicillin. In about two-thirds of the patients the temperature returns to normal in 48 hours or less. In about one-third the temperature response is not so striking, and the temperature gradually returns to normal over a period of 3 to 7 days after beginning therapy. The return of temperature to normal is delayed in patients with multiple lobe involvement, bacteremia, or alcoholism, and in patients with extrapulmonary suppuration.

Pneumonia developing in patients who are receiving full doses of penicillin, erythromycin, chloramphenicol, a cephalosporin derivative, or several other antibiotics is probably not pneumococcal in origin. Although the same comments probably apply to the tetracycline derivatives, these antibiotics were omitted because a number of intrahospital outbreaks of infection with tetracycline-resistant pneumococci have been described in which infection developed and progressed during tetracycline therapy. Tetracycline-resistant pneumococci are widespread at the present time, but their incidence is still relatively low, at about 3 per cent of isolates. Erythromycin-resistant pneumococci have been described, but appear to be exceedingly rare at the present time.

STAPHYLOCOCCAL PNEUMONIA

Staphylococcus aureus accounts for 1 to 5 per cent of cases of acute bacterial pneumonia. These organisms gain access to the lungs by way of the tracheobronchial tree to produce primary staphylococcal pneumonia, or by way of the bloodstream to produce metastatic staphylococcal pneumonia. The hallmark of staphylococcal disease is abscess formation, an event which strikingly differentiates staphylococcal from pneumococcal pneumonia.

Primary staphylococcal pneumonia, like pneumococcal pneumonia, is usually preceded by an identifiable event which alters the normal defense mechanisms of the respiratory tract. Influenza virus infection is one of the most common predisposing events, even though pneumococcal pneumonia is much more common after influenza than is staphylococcal pneumonia.

Staphylococcal pneumonia also occurs as a complication of measles, whooping cough, and other bronchial infections, and is relatively common in infants, patients with fibrocystic disease of the pancreas, and patients with other major diseases such as carcinoma, bronchiectasis, emphysema, and diabetes mellitus. Staphylococcal pneumonia is a relatively frequent terminal infection. Therapy with antibacterial drugs, especially broad-spectrum antibiotics, enhances the possibility of staphylococcal pneumonia by suppressing the normal flora of the upper respiratory tract, which in turn favors implantation and overgrowth of antibiotic-resistant staphylococci.

Metastatic staphylococcal pneumonia occurs as a blood-borne extension of staphylococcal disease at another site. Thrombus formation, perhaps consequent to coagulase activity, is frequent in blood vessels around staphylococcal lesions; small infected emboli presumably break away and eventually lodge at multiple foci in the lungs. In about 40 per cent of patients with metastatic pneumonia the skin is the primary site of infection, although staphylococcal infection at any location may serve as the source of emboli. The most common source of metastatic staphylococcal pneumonia in recent years has been infection of venous cutdowns or sites of insertion of indwelling intravenous devices. Cutdowns or intravenous devices must always be suspected as a source of metastatic pulmonary infection, even though the surrounding skin shows little or no cellulitis and the cutaneous site is not obviously infected.

The pattern of onset and the clinical manifestations of primary staphylococcal pneumonia are quite variable. There may be a history of an influenza-like illness with fever, headaches, general malaise, muscle aching, and dry cough. Staphylococcal pneumonia may occur at any time during the course of influenza, although usually the patient is improving when the bacterial complication develops. Nevertheless, at the onset of bacterial infection, the patient usually becomes obviously much more ill, with an increase in temperature, repeated chills, and an increase in cough productive of purulent, blood-streaked sputum. Pleural pain is common, and if the disease is progressive, dyspnea and cyanosis may develop.

The onset of primary staphylococcal pneumonia is not always so striking, and may be manifested only by moderate fever, cough, and purulent sputum in patients who are ill with another underlying disease or who are receiving antimicrobials or chemotherapeutic compounds that alter host resistance to infection.

Patients with metastatic pneumonia are usually extremely ill. Chills and fever are prominent, and dyspnea secondary to multiple emboli is frequent. As indicated previously, symptoms related to the extrapulmonary focus of staphylococcal disease may be evident.

The physical findings in staphylococcal pneumonia are not very helpful in diagnosis. However, the finding of an indwelling intravenous device or some other peripheral staphylococcal infection in a febrile patient with pneumonia should strongly suggest the diagnosis.

The Gram-stained smear of sputum from a patient with staphylococcal pneumonia usually reveals numerous leukocytes, red blood cells, and *spherical* cocci in small clusters or within leukocytes. Sputum culture from a patient with staphylococcal pneumonia almost always reveals many colonies of staphylococci after 24 hours, and frequently the staphylococcus is the predominant organism. The diagnosis of staphylococcal pneumonia should be made with caution if staphylococci are not isolated in large numbers in the sputum culture. This restraint in the interpretation of the significance of staphylococci isolated from sputum is related to the fact that *S. aureus* can be cultured from the anterior nares of 30 to 60 per cent of the general population, and an even larger proportion of hospital personnel. These organisms frequently appear in small numbers in sputum cultures from individuals without evidence of pulmonary disease.

The blood culture is positive in only about 20 per cent or less of patients with primary staphylococcal pneumonia. In contrast, the presence of metastatic pneumonia is itself evidence of bacteremia at some time in the past; thus it is not surprising that the blood culture is usually positive in these patients. Endocarditis should be suspected in all patients with staphylococcal bacteremia. Even in the absence of obvious pre-existing valvular disease, endocardial localization occurs in about 20 per cent of patients with staphylococcal bacteremia.

Empyema is a relatively frequent complication of staphylococcal pneumonia, and definitive etiologic diagnosis may be established in some patients by isolation of staphylococci from the pleural fluid.

The leukocyte count in patients with staphylococcal pneumonia is usually between 15,000 and 25,000 cells/cu mm. Occasionally the leukocyte count may be normal, and rarely leukopenia is observed.

The chest roentgenogram may be helpful in suggesting the diagnosis. Primary staphylococcal pneumonia is usually patchy in distribution, and the areas of consolidation are usually not as dense as in pneumococcal pneumonia. Dense lobar consolidation is distinctly unusual. In metastatic pneumonia multiple lesions may be scattered throughout the lung fields. Irrespective of the route of infection, cavity formation occurs frequently as the contents of abscesses are evacuated. The occurrence of cavities in areas of consolidation should always suggest the possibility of staphylococcal pneumonia. Pneumatoceles, small cystlike air sacs which appear with great rapidity and apparently result from ball-valve obstructions in the smaller radicles of the tracheobronchial tree, occur in as many as 60 per cent of cases of staphylococcal pneumonia in infants and young children. These lesions also occur occasionally in adults with staphylococcal pulmonary infections. Pneumatocele formation, although characteristic of staphylococcal pneumonia, is not an exclusive property of this organism, and can be seen at times in other types of pulmonary infection.

Although the presence of certain host and environmental factors, the course of illness, or the radiographic findings may suggest the diagnosis of staphylococcal pneumonia, and although presumptive evidence of etiology may be obtained by isolating staphylococci in large numbers from the sputum, the only definitive proof of etiology is isolation of the organism from blood or pleural fluid of patients with pneumonia.

The response of staphylococcal pneumonia to antimicrobial therapy is not dramatic. There may be no evidence whatever of response within 48 or 72 hours after beginning appropriate therapy, but then the temperature usually decreases slowly toward normal. The patient may not become afebrile for 3 to 7 days after initiation of therapy, even in the absence of extrapulmonary complications.

KLEBSIELLA PNEUMONIA (FRIEDLANDER'S PNEUMONIA)

Klebsiella pneumoniae accounts for 1 per cent or less of the cases of acute bacterial pneumonia. Members of the genus *Klebsiella* can be subdivided into at least 77 different types on the basis of specific capsular polysaccharides. About two-thirds of the cases of acute pneumonia caused by these organisms developing outside the hospital—the typical *Klebsiella* or Friedlander's pneumonia—are caused by type 1 (A) strains; the second most frequent strain responsible for pulmonary infections is type 2 (B). These organisms are usually sensitive to a number of antibiotics and are highly virulent for mice. Members of the genus *Klebsiella* are also relatively frequent causes of nosocomial infections and superinfections of the lungs in patients receiving antibiotic therapy. The *Klebsiella* strains responsible for infection in these patients are types other than 1 (A) or 2 (B), are usually resistant to multiple antibiotics, are frequently not virulent for mice, and produce a less fulminating type of pulmonary disease than the typical "respiratory" *Klebsiella*. Nosocomial infections and superinfections with Gram-negative enteric bacilli are discussed in a subsequent section.

Acute *Klebsiella* pneumonia usually develops in persons between the ages of 40 and 60 years; over 70 per cent of the patients are 50 years of age or older. Factors which predispose to infection are usually present; the most common conditions are chronic alcoholism and malnutrition, but almost any debilitating disease may be present. Antecedent upper respiratory tract infection is not a frequent predisposing event, in contrast to pneumococcal pneumonia.

The manifestations of acute *Klebsiella* pneumonia are quite similar to those of pneumococcal pneumonia. The onset of illness is usually abrupt, with chills, fever, pleuritic pain, cough, and bloody sputum. A characteristic feature present in some patients is the production of large amounts of brick-red or bloody, gelatinous sputum, sometimes described as "currant jelly" sputum. Patients may have difficulty in coughing up sputum because of its sticky, gelatinous character, a quality related to the large amount of polysaccharide formed by the organisms in the lungs. Frank hemoptysis occurs in the majority of patients, and jaundice is observed in about 20 per cent. Despite radiographic evidence of pulmonary consolidation, the classic physical signs of consolidation are frequently absent, and only dullness and muffled breath sounds may be detected. The absence of physical signs over areas of consolidation is presumably due to plugging of bronchi with the voluminous mucoid sputum. Fever may be sustained, as in pneumococcal pneumonia, but more often is remittent. In elderly individuals fever may be low and sometimes is absent. *Klebsiella* pneumonia is a severe disease which may progress with amazing rapidity, occasionally running a course from onset to death in 36 to 48 hours.

Dense lobar consolidation visible on roentgenograms develops very early in the course of *Klebsiella* pneumonia. There is a strong predilection for involvement of the upper lobes, occurring in as many as 80 per cent of the patients. An increase in volume of the involved lobe or lobes occurs with considerable frequency, and may give rise to a convex bulging of the interlobar fissure toward the uninvolved lobe. A bulging interlobar fissure should always suggest the possibility of *Klebsiella* pneumonia, but also may occur with other types of pulmonary infection, notably severe pneumococcal lobar pneumonia. The pulmonary lesions frequently undergo necrosis and form abscesses. Abscess formation may be extensive, with virtual complete destruction of a lobe.

The Gram-stained smear of the sputum from a patient with *Klebsiella* pneumonia usually reveals large numbers of short, plump, Gram-negative diplobacilli. A clear space around each bacillus can often be seen, representing the area of the capsule. The sputum smear in patients with *Klebsiella* pneumonia is often misinterpreted. The stain is usually incorrectly decolorized, and elongated-diplobacillary forms of the organism are thought to be lancet-shaped diplococci or pneumococci. This error can be prevented by including on every Gram stain of sputum a control of a small amount of tartar from around the teeth; observation of both Gram-negative and Gram-positive organisms in this material provides assurance that the stain has been correctly prepared.

The sputum culture reveals many large mucoid colonies of *Klebsiella*, sometimes almost in pure culture, and the blood culture is positive in 50 to 70 per cent of the cases. Empyema is a relatively frequent complication, and provides another source of material from which organisms can be isolated.

Most patients with *Klebsiella* pneumonia have a moderate leukocytosis, but the leukocyte count is below 6000 cells/cu mm in about one-third of the cases.

The diagnosis of acute Friedlander's pneumonia should be considered in any patient with acute bacterial pneumonia, and should be suspected especially in patients over 50 years of age with remittent fever, bloody gelatinous or mucinous sputum, abscess formation, or a history of chronic alcoholism or evidence of other debilitating disease. Recognition of *Klebsiella* pneumonia is very important, since antimicrobial therapy for this disease differs considerably from that for pneumococcal and staphylococcal pneumonia. Even in the presence of appropriate antimicrobial therapy the mortality rate runs between 25 and 50 per cent. If the diagnosis is established and appropriate therapy initiated, response is characteristically slow; the patient may show no definite decline in temperature for 48 to 72 hours, and convalescence is slow.

NECROTIZING PNEUMONIA; LUNG ABSCESS

Necrotizing pneumonia follows aspiration of infectious material from the mouth and upper respiratory tract into the tracheobronchial tree. The bacterial pneumonia may be preceded by an acute chemical pneumonia if gastric contents have been aspirated.

Multiple organisms characteristic of mouth flora can be isolated from sputa or bronchial washings of patients with necrotizing pneumonia. Difficulties are encountered in defining the pathogenetic significance of these organisms, but there is evidence that anaerobes, especially anaerobic streptococci and *Bacteroides* species, act synergistically with other organisms to produce the necrotizing pulmonary infection. Synergism between bacteria may explain the effectiveness of treatment with an antibiotic active against some but not all of the infecting microorganisms. Foreign materials, such as acid gastric contents and organic debris, aspirated into the lungs with bacteria, are probably also of great importance in the pathogenesis of necrotizing pneumonia. In addition, bronchial obstruction by neoplasms, foreign bodies, or constricting scars may play a role in some cases.

The event leading to aspiration of material from the upper respiratory tract may be evident, and may provide a clue to the correct diagnosis. Recent loss of consciousness (e.g., coma from alcohol, epilepsy, opiates, anesthesia, diabetes, stroke, or head trauma) is a common event prior to onset of pneumonia. Repeated aspiration may occur in patients with obstructing esophageal lesions and in certain neuromuscular diseases. It is of interest that severe gingivodental disease with advanced oral sepsis is present in about half the patients. In this regard, lung abscess is unusual in edentulous adults. Sometimes a history of oropharyngeal surgery, dental manipulation, or some other procedure on the mouth or upper respiratory tract is obtained. Severe lung abscess may be seen in patients with carcinoma of the larynx undergoing radiotherapy. However, despite a most careful history and physical examination an occasional patient will show no evidence of an event or condition that might have been associated with aspiration.

In contrast to most other types of bacterial pneumonia, the onset usually is gradual, with fever and cough coming on several days after the event leading to aspiration. The cough is productive of mucoid or mucopurulent sputum which is usually not foul initially. Patients are not ordinarily seen by physicians at this stage of the disease, but if they are, physical findings are not striking, and the chest roentgenogram shows atelectasis and pneumonia. During the next 4 to 10 days, as the necrotizing process develops and abscess formation occurs, fever becomes increasingly prominent, pleurisy may develop, and sputum production may increase. Systemic symptoms and spiking fever may be marked, especially in patients with undrained abscess cavities. When the abscess ruptures into the tracheobronchial tree, sputum production may become voluminous. Although there are many exceptions, the sputum at this stage may have a foul, putrid odor characteristic of necrotizing pneumonia with abscess formation.

The physical examination of the chest is usually not helpful in differential diagnosis, but merely indicates that an active process is occurring in the pulmonary parenchyma. Examination may reveal rales over the involved area, typical signs of consolidation, or occasionally findings indicative of abscess formation. Extrapulmonary physical findings may have great diagnostic value. There may be evidence of recent dental work or evidence of marked disease of the mouth, gums, or teeth. Neurologic examination may reveal an absence of the gag reflex or other evidence of neurologic disease that might provide the basis for aspiration. Clubbing of the fingers or painful pulmonary hypertrophic osteoarthropathy is rarely present early in the course of uncomplicated necrotizing pneumonia. This finding should suggest the possibility of carcinoma of the lung or that the abscess has been present for a considerable period of time.

The usual result of sputum cultures in patients with necrotizing pneumonia is to isolate "the usual mouth flora." If anaerobic cultures are performed, anaerobic streptococci and *Bacteroides* can be isolated from sputa of almost all such patients, though this finding is of no help diagnostically because these organisms are part of the normal flora of the mouth. In some patients suspected of having necrotizing pneumonia and lung abscess the sputum culture may reveal a predominance of staphylococci or *K. pneumoniae*, a finding which would strongly indicate an unrecognized staphylococcal or Friedlander's pneumonia with an atypical onset.

In addition to routine culture, sputum should be examined by smear and culture for tubercle bacilli and fungi, since tuberculosis and a number of different fungus infections can mimic lung abscess. The sputum should also be routinely examined for malignant cells. Bronchoscopy is probably indicated in all patients with necrotizing pneumonia and abscess formation; bronchial washings should be collected for routine bacterial and acid-fast smears, cultures, and cytology. Amebic abscess of the liver perforating the diaphragm should also be considered when the pulmonary process involves the right lower lobe, and appropriate parasitologic examinations should be performed on sputum and pleural fluid.

The radiographic findings consist of an area of pneumonitis, often with a single cavity with an air-fluid level, located most often in the posterior segment of the right upper lobe or the superior segments of the lower lobes. Lung abscesses are more common on the right (75 per cent) than on the left (25 per cent), and are more often single (75 per cent or more) than multiple (25 per cent or less). Multiple abscesses should suggest the possibility of staphylococcal or Friedlander's pneumonia. Although the thickness of the wall of the cavity may vary widely, a very thin-walled cavity should suggest the possibility of infection within a pre-existing lung cyst, and a cavity with very thick, irregular walls should suggest the possibility of excavation of a bronchogenic carcinoma.

PNEUMONIA CAUSED BY GRAM-NEGATIVE ENTERIC BACILLI

Although enteric bacilli have low virulence for the lungs, the frequency of pulmonary infections with these organisms has increased dramatically during the past two decades. Pierce and associates observed a 10-fold increase in fatal pneumonia caused by these organisms between 1952 and 1963 in Dallas, Texas, and the data recently gathered by Tillotson and Lerner at the Detroit Receiving Hospital showed that Gram-negative enteric bacilli accounted for about 4 per cent of all bacterial pneumonias at that hospital.

Any of the so-called Gram-negative enteric bacilli can produce infection of the pulmonary parenchyma. The organisms usually responsible, listed in order of decreasing importance, are *Klebsiella-Aerobacter*, *Escherichia coli*, *Pseudomonas aeruginosa*, and *Proteus* species.

Several factors account for the increased prevalence of serious pulmonary infections caused by enteric bacilli. Of obvious importance is the increasing proportion of patients with serious underlying diseases which alter the capacity of the host to resist bacterial invasion. Although pneumonia caused by enteric bacilli may develop rarely in previously healthy persons, the vast majority of infections occur in patients with major underlying diseases, including alcoholism, malignancy, diabetes mellitus, or chronic cardiovascular, pulmonary, renal, or central nervous system diseases. Host defense mechanisms may be further impaired in these patients by drugs, such as corticosteroids and antimetabolites. Although by no means a prerequisite of infection, the vast majority of patients who develop pneumonia with enteric bacilli are receiving or have recently received antimicrobial therapy, usually penicillin in large doses, a tetracycline, or a combination of antibiotics. In fact, about 10 per cent of the cases of pneumonia caused by enteric bacilli develop as a complication during therapy of pneumococcal pneumonia. Antimicrobial therapy suppresses the normal flora of the upper respiratory tract and fosters the overgrowth of antibiotic-resistant enteric bacilli from the patient's flora or from exogenous sources. In an occasional patient these organisms gain access to the lower respiratory tract and find the conditions there favorable for multiplication. In some patients enteric bacilli or other organisms may actually be introduced into the respiratory tract by certain therapeutic measures. Organisms may contaminate ventilatory equipment or fluid placed in reservoirs of nebulizers and, under these conditions, the aerosol created may contain millions of bacteria incorporated into small particles capable of reaching the smallest radicles of the lungs during inspiration. A number of sporadic cases and several outbreaks of severe and even fatal pneumonia due to *Klebsiella*, *Pseudomonas*, or other organisms have been described which were caused by utilization of contaminated aerosol solutions or ventilatory equipment.

Pneumonia caused by enteric bacilli does not have a seasonal prevalence, and the vast majority of these infections are acquired within the hospital.

The clinical manifestations of pneumonia caused by enteric bacilli are extremely variable and have no pathognomonic features. The onset is usually gradual, but the patients are frequently extremely ill, sometimes as much from an underlying disease as from the pulmonary infection. Tillotson and Lerner noted a reversal in the usual diurnal variation in the temperature curve in about 80 per cent of their patients with *Pseudomonas* pneumonia, and indicated that this curious phenomenon was very unusual in patients with pneumonia caused by other enteric organisms. It is doubtful that this finding is of diagnostic significance.

Empyema is a common complication of pneumonia caused by enteric bacilli. The figures from the Detroit Receiving Hospital give an incidence of 18 per cent in pneumonia caused by *Proteus* species, 40 per cent in *E. coli* pneumonia, and 80 per cent in *Pseudomonas* pneumonia.

The sputum of patients with pneumonia caused by enteric bacilli usually reveals a predominance of Gram-negative bacilli on smear, and the culture shows many colonies of the causative organism. The blood culture is positive in 15 to 20 per cent of the patients. Leukocytosis in the range of 15,000 to 20,000 cells/cu mm is usually present. However, about two-thirds of the patients with *Pseudomonas* pneumonia have normal leukocyte counts.

The roentgenogram reveals either a patchy bronchopneumonia or a lobar type of consolidation. *Klebsiella-Aerobacter* and *Proteus* species are more often responsible for lobar or confluent lobular consolidation than other enteric organisms, and a nodular or patchy bronchopneumonia is more often associated with *Pseudomonas* or *E. coli* infections than with other enteric organisms. The lower lobes are involved more often than the upper. Abscesses visible on roentgenogram occur in about 10 per cent of the patients, and are more frequent with *Pseudomonas, Klebsiella-Aerobacter,* and *Proteus* than with *E. coli.*

The diagnosis of pneumonia caused by enteric bacilli should be considered whenever a large number of Gram-negative bacilli are demonstrated on smear or culture of sputum from a patient with pneumonia. If the patient has been on antimicrobial therapy, interpretation of the significance of a large number of enteric organisms in cultures of material from the upper respiratory tract is difficult because of the frequency of antibiotic-induced overgrowth of these organisms. Complete clinical evaluation is required to detect such events as recurrence of fever or alterations in an existing febrile pattern that might indicate that lower respiratory tract infection has occurred. Radiographic examination may reveal a pulmonary infiltrate or, in patients with pneumonia, may reveal evidence of new areas of involvement at a time when pre-existing lesions are clearing.

Pneumonia caused by enteric bacilli should always be considered when patients receiving aerosol therapy develop fever, respiratory symptoms, or unexplained pulmonary infiltrates, or when similar findings occur in hospitalized patients receiving antimicrobial drugs. A diagnosis of pneumonia caused by enteric bacilli should be viewed skeptically if the patient has had no previous contact with the hospital, has no major underlying disease, or has not recently received antimicrobial therapy.

Bacteria—Infrequently Encountered

ANTHRAX

Pulmonary anthrax is usually related to the inhalation of anthrax spores, residing on imported animal hides or hairs. Improvement in working conditions in processing plants has resulted in a marked decrease in incidence of inhalation anthrax in the United States because of reduced exposure to spore dust. However, the disease has not been eliminated and occasional cases continue to occur.

Inhalation anthrax begins abruptly, has a short duration, and frequently terminates in death. Very few symptoms are apparent until the systemic stage of the disease is reached, and the diagnosis is rarely established until it is too late to save the patient from a fatal outcome. High fever and prostration develop rapidly, and the patient may have a sense of suffocation, severe dyspnea, and cyanosis. It is important to emphasize that pneumonic lesions are usually minimal or absent. The most significant lesion is an acute hemorrhagic mediastinitis secondary to multiplication of bacilli in regional lymph nodes. The leukocyte count may be moderately elevated. Roentgenograms usually reveal widening of the mediastinum and occasionally pleural effusion. The mortality rate is quite high, approaching 80 per cent.

Anthrax should be suspected in patients with appropriate occupational exposure who develop cutaneous lesions, febrile illnesses, or signs of mediastinitis. In pulmonary or inhalation anthrax the sputum is rarely positive because the spores usually do not germinate until the organisms have been carried to mediastinal nodes in alveolar macrophages. However, the blood culture is usually positive.

BRUCELLOSIS

Acute pneumonia is exceedingly unusual during the course of brucellosis. Single and multiple infiltrates in the lungs and a clinical picture resembling atypical pneumonia have been described, but such reports are rare. In a series of 244 cases of brucellosis, Spink did not encounter in a single patient pulmonary consolidation sufficient to yield a suitable specimen of sputum for study.

GLANDERS

Glanders is a rare disease of animals, primarily horses and donkeys, which is occasionally transmitted to man. Involvement of the respiratory tract is frequent. The disease is world-wide in distribution, but has been largely eradicated from the United States. The glanders bacillus apparently enters the body in man through abrasions in the skin or through the mucous membranes, but infection may be acquired by inhalation. Glanders in man may occur as an acute fulminating infection or may follow a chronic indolent course. The disease may be characterized by nasal cellulitis and necrosis, ulceration of the palate and pharynx, cellulitis and ulceration of the skin at sites of invasion, and regional lymphadenitis and nodular abscesses along lymphatics. The patient is often febrile. Pneumonia is common in glanders, and may be complicated by abscesses, pleural effusion, and empyema. Leukopenia or a normal leukocyte-count is the rule.

The diagnosis of glanders should be suspected on the basis of the clinical course and a history of exposure to horses. Confirmation may be obtained by culture of the organism, *Pseudomonas mallei*, and by serologic tests.

HEMOPHILUS INFLUENZAE

Pneumonia caused by *Hemophilus influenzae* is not unusual during infancy and early childhood. However, in adults, pneumonia caused by this organism and documented by isolation of the bacterium from blood is exceedingly unusual. At the New York Hospital–Cornell Medical Center only five cases were counted between 1932 and 1967. Most of the cases reported in the literature have been in alcoholics or in patients with chronic pulmonary or other debilitating diseases. However, some of the patients have been healthy, without underlying problems. The clinical findings do not distinguish *H. influenzae* pneumonia from other bacterial pneumonias, and the diagnosis must be sought by bacteriologic means. *H. influenzae* not infrequently can be isolated from the upper respiratory tracts of normal individuals. Therefore, isolation of the organism from the sputum of patients with acute pneumonia does not constitute proof of etiology. Definitive diagnosis is established by isolating the organism from the blood of a patient with pneumonia, but, as mentioned above, this is an unusual occurrence.

H. influenzae strains are commonly isolated from sputum or bronchial washings of patients with chronic pulmonary disease, such as chronic bronchitis or bronchiectasis. These organisms apparently play a role in the pathogenesis of the acute exacerbations, characterized by fever, increase in cough, purulent sputum, and at times pulmonary infiltrates, that punctuate the lives of these individuals. Many other organisms can be isolated from the respiratory tracts of patients with chronic bronchitis, and it is frequently difficult to assess the exact role of any one organism in the pathogenesis of the recurrent episodes of acute bronchitis and bronchopneumonia.

MELIOIDOSIS

Melioidosis, a rare disease which man acquires from wild rodents and some domesticated animals, has been observed primarily in Southeast Asia. The disease has been recognized a number of times in soldiers returning to the United States from these areas, especially from Viet Nam. The causative organism, *Pseudomonas pseudomallei*, a bipolar, poorly staining, Gram-negative bacillus, grows well on ordinary culture media.

Acute melioidosis is rapid in onset, with fever, chills, and malaise. Presenting symptoms include cough, hemoptysis, pleurisy, skin ulcerations with cellulitis, regional lymphangitis and lymphadenitis, diarrhea, and abdominal pain. The most striking manifestations are usually pulmonary. Multiple fluffy or nodular infiltrates may be disseminated throughout both lungs or may be evident only in one lobe on roentgenograms. Hematogenous spread of the organism leads to the production of pyogenic arthritis, meningitis, and abscesses, not only in the lungs but also in the skin, subcutaneous tissue, liver, spleen, bone marrow, lymph nodes, and other organs. Although findings vary from one patient to another, physical examination may reveal signs of pneumonia, empyema, lung abscess, hepatomegaly, jaundice, or splenomegaly. The acute phase of the disease is usually fatal, but if the patient survives, the infection may become subacute or chronic.

The subacute form of the disease is a less fulminating form of the acute systemic disease. These patients present with fever, cough, and occasionally hemoptysis, of several weeks' duration. The roentgenogram shows a fibronodular infiltrate, usually involving a single lobe, frequently an upper lobe, and often associated with cavitation; the process may be confused with tuberculosis.

Chronic melioidosis is characterized by osteomyelitis, suppurative lymphadenitis, and abscesses in the lung, muscle, subcutaneous tissue, liver, spleen, or kidney. The chronic disease may develop without preceding acute illness. Patients with chronic melioidosis may survive for months, and may occasionally recover.

The clinical and epidemiologic history may suggest the diagnosis. In the United States the occurrence of an obscure febrile illness associated with pulmonary lesions in a person recently returned from Viet Nam should certainly suggest the possibility of melioidosis. Confirmation can be obtained by isolating the organism from sputum, blood, urine, pus, joint fluid, or cerebrospinal fluid. Serologic methods of diagnosis are available, but are of no value in diagnosis of the acute form of the disease.

INFECTIONS CAUSED BY TRIBE MIMEAE (HERELLEA)

Several fatal cases of acute bacterial pneumonia with bacteremia caused by these highly pleomorphic, Gram-negative bacilli have been described. Members of the tribe Mimeae may also be isolated from the sputa of patients with chronic pulmonary infections. Although these organisms cannot be dismissed as nonpathogens, they are in general opportunistic in behavior, like other Gram-negative organisms. Evaluation of their role as etiologic factors in patients with pulmonary disease is difficult.

MENINGOCOCCAL PNEUMONIA

Although meningococci are common inhabitants of the upper respiratory tract, they rarely gain access to the lower respiratory tract to produce acute bacterial pneumonia. According to Paine and colleagues, who reported a case in 1967, the medical literature at that time contained only three reports of primary meningococcal pneumonia without meningitis during the previous 20 years. In these patients the manifestations of the

pulmonary infection were typical of those of acute pneumococcal pneumonia. Diagnosis was made by demonstrating Gram-negative diplococci of
typical morphology on sputum smear, and by culture of the organism from
the upper respiratory tract and blood.

Patients with meningococcemia occasionally develop pulmonary infiltrates secondary to hemorrhage from vascular lesions in the lung. These
lesions are apparently similar in pathogenesis to hemorrhagic lesions developing elsewhere in patients with meningococcemia.

PASTEURELLA MULTOCIDA

The most common type of *Pasteurella multocida* infection in man is local
cellulitis around the bite of an animal, most often the cat. However, this
organism may involve the respiratory tract, usually when another respiratory infection or some other physiologic disturbance markedly decreases
the natural resistance of the host. The organism may rarely cause acute
pneumonia and empyema, but more often appears as a secondary invader
along with other organisms in patients with bronchiectasis. Many of the
cases of empyema or bronchiectasis associated with *P. multocida* have been
reported in farmers or other persons who have had abundant exposure to
various animals. The diagnosis is sometimes suggested by a history of
animal contact, although not all infections are associated with animal
exposure. Gram staining of infected material may reveal pleomorphic
Gram-negative bacilli; definitive diagnosis must be based on isolation of
the organism on culture.

PERTUSSIS PNEUMONIA

Pertussis in children is frequently complicated by bacterial pneumonia.
In fact, this complication is responsible for 90 per cent of the deaths from
pertussis in children under 3 years of age. Although the pulmonary infection
may be due to the pertussis bacillus, it is usually caused by other organisms,
such as the pneumococcus or the staphylococcus. *Hemophilus pertussis* has
not been recognized as a significant cause of pneumonia in adults.

PLAGUE

Plague is an infection of rodents and their ectoparasites, primarily fleas,
in many areas of the world. Metastatic pneumonia may develop in patients
with bubonic plague, or a primary pneumonia may occur secondary to
inhalation of plague bacilli.

Plague has been recognized in the United States since 1900. It occurs as a
sylvatic infection of wild rodents, such as rats, mice, marmots, gophers,
badgers, rabbits, prairie dogs, squirrels, and chipmunks, and in owls.
The disease is limited to the western third of the United States. A few infections in man are recognized each year in the United States, usually in
individuals who have come in contact with wild rodents.

The incubation period is usually 6 days or less. Bubonic plague, by far
the most common type, is characterized by enlargement of regional lymph

nodes, with marked local pain and tenderness and edema of surrounding structures. About 5 per cent of patients with bubonic plague develop metastatic pulmonary lesions which are characterized by patchy infiltrates scattered throughout the lungs. In these patients myriads of plague bacilli are present in the sputum, and may be transmitted via the respiratory route to close contacts. Inhalation of plague bacilli results in a primary pneumonia, with a clinical picture quite similar to that of severe pneumococcal pneumonia.

The recognition of sporadic or sentinel cases of plague is difficult, although the diagnosis does not remain in doubt very long if the disease reaches epidemic proportions. The history of a febrile illness associated with lymphadenopathy or pulmonary lesions in a patient in recent contact with wild rodents, patients with plague, or cultures of the organism in a laboratory should arouse suspicion regarding the possibility of plague. A tentative diagnosis can be established if sputum or fluid obtained from puncture of an involved lymph node shows short, thick bacilli with bipolar staining. Sputum or material aspirated from lymph nodes should be cultured and perhaps inoculated into suitable laboratory animals. Rapid definitive diagnosis may be obtained by staining organisms with specific antibody labeled with fluorescein if this technique is available. The organism may also be isolated by blood culture. Retrospective diagnosis may be established by serologic means. Agglutinins can be detected during the second week of the disease, and reach a peak titer 4 to 5 weeks after onset.

Patients with plague in whom therapy with tetracycline or chloramphenicol is initiated early in the course of the disease should respond rapidly, with a decrease in fever.

SALMONELLOSIS OTHER THAN TYPHOID FEVER

In *Salmonella* infections pulmonary involvement may occur as a consequence of hematogenous spread of the organisms. Multiple areas of metastatic pneumonia may develop and lead to the formation of lung abscess or empyema. Infection with *Salmonella choleraesuis*, one of the most virulent serotypes, is more often associated with pulmonary lesions than infections with other serotypes. Diagnosis must be established by bacteriologic means.

PNEUMONIA CAUSED BY GROUP A STREPTOCOCCI

More common in the past than at present, streptococci of group A now account for only a small proportion of cases of bacterial pneumonia, perhaps less than 1 per cent of the total.

Streptococcal pneumonia may occur as a complication of pharyngitis, but this is unusual. Measles, pertussis, influenza, other virus infections of the respiratory tract, or chronic pulmonary diseases are more frequent antecedent illnesses. Once group A streptococci have entered the lower respiratory tract, the organisms produce a bronchopneumonia. Rapid spread of infection, so typical of streptococcal disease at other sites, also occurs in the lungs. The organisms quickly reach regional lymph nodes and may proceed in a retrograde direction to reach the pleural surfaces.

The onset of streptococcal pneumonia is usually quite sudden, with fever, chills, malaise, cough, and chest pain. Pleurisy is the most striking symptom, and has been reported to occur in as many as 75 per cent of patients. The sputum may be quite profuse and thin. Spread of infection is rapid, and dyspnea and cyanosis may appear early in the course of the disease. Rapid spread of streptococci to the pleural surfaces with the production of effusion or empyema is characteristic, and has been reported in 20 to 50 per cent of various groups of patients. Involvement of the pleural space develops early, usually within 48 to 72 hours of onset, and is slightly more frequent on the left side. The fluid is often present in large amounts, is thin, serous, or serosanguinous, and contains many streptococci.

The leukocyte count is usually quite high, often in the range of 20,000 to 30,000 cells/cu mm. The sputum may show large numbers of streptococci on smears and in culture. The blood culture is positive in 10 to 15 per cent of cases. The roentgenogram of the chest shows extensive bronchopneumonia; lobar consolidation is not common.

Streptococcal pneumonia should be suspected in patients with pneumonia who rapidly develop pleural effusions. However, differentiation on the basis of clinical findings is impossible in the individual case. Demonstration of group A streptococci in the sputum by culture does not establish a definitive diagnosis, since the organisms isolated may represent streptococci from the nasopharynx of a carrier. However, definitive bacteriologic diagnosis is established by demonstrating the organism in blood or pleural fluid. The diagnosis may be strongly supported in retrospect by the results of immunologic studies designed to detect the antibody response to any one of several streptococcal antigens; determination of the titer of antistreptolysin O is the technique most commonly utilized. A titer rising to or exceeding 250 Todd units is considered indicative of recent streptococcal infection. A low titer of antistreptolysin O several weeks after onset is evidence against the diagnosis of group A streptococcal pneumonia, although early antimicrobial therapy may delay or suppress antibody response.

TULAREMIA

Tularemia is characterized by a febrile course, by a local lesion at the site of entry of the organism in the majority of cases, and by pulmonary involvement in up to 50 per cent of the cases. The most common mode of infection of man is by direct contact with an infected rabbit, although other animals may be involved. The disease can also be transmitted to man by insect vectors, such as ticks and deer flies, or by the inhalation of infected aerosols. The disease occurs in all seasons and is common in hunters and trappers.

The incubation period is 3 to 10 days, with an average of 7 days. All forms of the disease are associated with a systemic reaction varying from mild to severe and characterized by prominent headache, chills, fever, and general toxemia. The site of invasion of the organism determines the clinical type of disease. Cutaneous invasion gives rise to ulceroglandular tularemia, the most common type, which occurs in about three-fourths of the patients. The initial lesion begins as small papules which ulcerate after several days. The local lesion may not be prominent and usually is not very painful. Regional lymphadenopathy is the other characteristic feature of this form of the disease; the nodes become enlarged and tender and eventually undergo fluctuation after 2 to 3 weeks. When invasion occurs through the conjunctiva, the term oculoglandular tularemia is applied. This form is quite similar to ulceroglandular tularemia except for the local reaction in the eye, which may produce serious ulceration of the cornea. These patients have prominent enlargement of the preauricular nodes. The term typhoidal tularemia is applied when a local lesion is not evident or when the portal of entry presumably has been the gastrointestinal tract or oropharynx.

Pulmonary involvement is secondary to hematogenous spread of the organism, and is common in all clinical types of the disease. Signs of respiratory tract involvement usually begin several days after onset and may be overshadowed by other manifestations of the disease, such as fever, delirium, and regional lymphadenopathy. Patients with pulmonary involvement frequently have nonproductive cough, substernal discomfort, and, late in the course of the disease, moderate amounts of mucoid or bloody sputum. Severely ill patients with pneumonia may show dyspnea, tachycardia, and cyanosis. Pleural involvement is common, and is manifested as pleurisy and small pleural effusions containing a predominance of mononuclear cells. Despite extensive pulmonary involvement visible on roentgenogram of the chest, there may be a paucity of physical signs of pneumonia.

The leukocyte count is usually normal or low, although a moderate leukocytosis is observed occasionally. The chest x-ray usually reveals bilateral involvement of the lungs, with small, irregular, oval lesions and hilar lymphadenopathy initially. In the later stages the infiltrates may be quite large. True abscess formation is rare.

Antimicrobial therapy is quite effective in tularemia, and a prompt response should be obtained with streptomycin, tetracycline, or chloramphenicol. If a dramatic response is not evident by 48 hours after initiation of therapy, the diagnosis of tularemia is unlikely.

Tularemia should be suspected in any patient with a febrile illness and an ulcerative skin or mucous membrane lesion with regional lymphadenopathy. Contact with rabbits or ticks or other pertinent epidemiologic data should also suggest the diagnosis. The greatest diagnostic difficulties occur in patients who have the typhoidal form of the disease or in patients with prominent pulmonary involvement but minor skin or lymph node involvement.

Cultures may provide definitive diagnostic information but require special media and are dangerous. Serologic methods provide the easiest means of establishing the diagnosis. Agglutinins against *Pasteurella tularensis* develop within 8 to 10 days after onset of infection, and reach a maximum titer within 4 weeks. A single specimen is not of great value, although a titer of 1:160 should arouse strong suspicion of the diagnosis.

TYPHOID FEVER

Pneumonia is a well-recognized complication of typhoid fever and usually develops during the second or third week of illness. In Huckstep's series lobar pneumonia occurred in 2.4 per cent of the patients. Other symptoms of typhoid fever occurring during the first several weeks of illness usually direct attention to the correct diagnosis, which is confirmed by isolation of the organism or by demonstration of a 4-fold or greater increase in titer of agglutinins against the somatic (O) antigen. Although it is clear that *Salmonella typhosa* can produce pneumonia, the physician should be aware that other bacteria, such as the pneumococcus, may be responsible for the pulmonary complications observed in typhoid fever.

Bacteria-like Agents

MYCOPLASMA PNEUMONIA

Mycoplasma pneumoniae is a common cause of pneumonia. Most cases are sporadic, but epidemics occur in families, military bases, schools, and other institutions. Individuals of any age may become infected, but the majority of infections are recognized in children and young adults under the age of 30 years. Although this organism may produce a spectrum of illness ranging from the common cold to severe pneumonia, involvement of the lower respiratory tract with the production of pneumonia or bronchitis is much more typical of *Mycoplasma* infection than involvement of the upper respiratory tract with manifestations of pharyngitis and rhinorrhea.

Mycoplasma pneumonia usually has a gradual onset, with fever, cough, headache, and malaise. Constitutional symptoms are prominent, as in a number of systemic virus infections. Chilly sensations are frequent, but shaking chills are unusual. Sore throat is common, although less frequent than in adenovirus infections of the respiratory tract. Headache may be quite distressing and severe. The outstanding symptom is cough, which is often severe and paroxysmal; if cough is absent the diagnosis should be viewed with skepticism. During the early phases of illness the cough may be dry but, contrary to popular concepts, is frequently productive of mucoid sputum. Blood-streaked sputum is observed in about 10 per cent of the patients. Substernal chest pain or soreness accentuated by coughing is common but pleurisy is distinctly unusual, although it does occur in 3 to 5 per cent of patients.

On physical examination the patient is acutely but rarely critically ill.

The temperature may range from 99° to 105°F, but is usually in the range of 102° to 104°F. The temperature may be sustained or remittent. Although not widely appreciated, an erythematous maculopapular rash on the trunk occurs in about 10 per cent of the patients. Bullous myringitis, in which small vesicles form on the ear drums, occurs in an occasional patient and is quite characteristic of mycoplasma infection. A relative bradycardia occurs in about 50 per cent of patients. The significant feature on examination of the chest is that the physical findings of pulmonary disease are fewer and less impressive than expected on the basis of the roentgenographic findings. A few fine or medium rales are frequently heard over the areas of involvement, but typical signs of consolidation are very unusual.

An acute hemolytic anemia occasionally complicates *M. pneumoniae* infections, and is related to the formation of cold agglutinins. Hemolysis may be precipitated or accentuated by chilling, and occasionally occurs after mild, almost unrecognized respiratory infections.

Aseptic meningitis with several hundred mononuclear cells per cubic millimeter of cerebrospinal fluid develops in an occasional patient, and well-documented examples of severe meningocncephalitis with profound neurologic deficits but with subsequent complete recovery have also been reported.

Most patients with *Mycoplasma* pneumonia have normal leukocyte counts, but moderate leukocytosis to 15,000 or even 20,000 cells/cu mm develops in 15 to 20 per cent of patients, especially during convalescence. A slight shift to the left may be observed in the differential count, but it is usually not as marked as in bacterial pneumonia.

M. pneumoniae can be isolated from the sputum and the pharynx of infected patients, but special techniques are required which are not available in most hospital laboratories. A complement fixation test which detects antibody to a species-specific surface antigen of the mycoplasma is the best method of diagnosis. With this antigen a significant rise in antibody titer can be detected in virtually all patients with *Mycoplasma* pneumonia. Because of accuracy and specificity, this technique is the best method for diagnosis. Although not now generally available, this technique will eventually replace the cold agglutination test for diagnosis. Cold agglutinins for human O cells develop only in about 55 per cent of patients with *Mycoplasma* pneumonia. This technique is unreliable because of the frequency of false-negative results and because cold agglutinins also develop in a number of other conditions.

The roentgenogram is not especially helpful in differential diagnosis. The lower lobes of the lungs are involved more often than the upper lobes, with mottled, feathery, or uniformly opaque infiltrates. About 50 per cent of patients show involvement of only one lobe, but in the remainder there is multiple lobe involvement. Sometimes the lesions are migratory, clearing in one area as new lesions develop elsewhere. The radiographic abnormalities usually clear in an average of 11 days, and are almost always resolved within 25 days after onset.

Mycoplasma pneumonia should be suspected on the basis of the clinical findings. The diagnosis is suggested by gradual onset, fever, relative bradycardia, normal respiratory rate, paroxysmal cough, and radiographic findings of pneumonia with concomitant paucity of physical findings. Lack of response to penicillin, a normal leukocyte count, and failure to demonstrate bacterial pathogens on routine culture of sputum provide additional support for the diagnosis. The disease may respond to therapy with tetracyclines or erythromycin, but return of fever to normal is gradual.

The diagnosis is almost always established in retrospect after the acute illness has subsided. The demonstration of a 4-fold or greater increase in titer of cold agglutinins is presumptive evidence of *M. pneumoniae* infection in a patient with respiratory symptoms. Definitive diagnosis is dependent on the demonstration of a significant rise in titer of antibodies against the species-specific antigen in complement fixation tests.

PSITTACOSIS

Psittacosis or ornithosis (the terms are used synonymously) is world-wide in distribution. Psittacine birds, especially parrots and parakeets, are the usual sources of infection of man, but finches, pigeons, sea gulls, and domestic fowl, especially turkeys and ducks, may be incriminated. Dried bird fecal material spread by the airborne route is probably the major method of infection in man. However, psittacosis is an important occupational disease in persons working with domestic fowl in poultry-processing plants, especially turkey-processing plants. The majority of patients with psittacosis give a history of bird exposure, but the source of infection is not determined in at least 25 per cent of the patients.

The incubation period of psittacosis varies from 1 to 3 weeks. The majority of infections are mild, but illness may be severe, even fatal. The onset of the disease may be insidious, but is often abrupt, with chills, fever of 103° to 105°F, intense headache, myalgias, and arthralgias. The first evidence of respiratory involvement is usually cough, which becomes prominent in most cases. However, cough may not appear until late in the first week of the disease or, in some patients, may even be absent throughout the entire illness. A small to moderate amount of sputum, occasionally streaked with blood, may be observed. Pleural pain is rare, but does occur in a small proportion of cases. Delirium, stupor, cyanosis, and dyspnea may be observed in severe infections.

The physical examination in a typical case shows a febrile patient with muscle pain, an increase in respiratory rate, and relative bradycardia. A macular rash resembling the rose spots of typhoid fever may be observed, and jaundice has been described in severe cases. Fine rales may be present, but frank signs of consolidation are not common. Mild hepatomegaly may be observed, and the spleen is palpated in perhaps one-third of the cases.

The course of the illness varies from a mild, influenza-like illness to a severe fulminating pulmonary infection. Patients with mild illnesses show defervescence in about 1 week, but patients with severe illness may continue febrile for as long as 3 weeks if antimicrobial therapy is not administered.

The leukocyte count is usually normal, although about 25 per cent of patients show leukopenia and a few patients show leukocytosis as high as 15,000 cells/cu mm. Moderate leukocytosis is not unusual in the late stages of the disease. The roentgenogram of the chest shows patchy infiltrates, usually involving both lungs and radiating from the hilum. The lesions are more prominent in the lower portions of the lungs than the upper portions. Occasionally a miliary type of infiltrate may be observed and, rarely, lobar consolidation or small pleural effusions may be evident.

Psittacosis is characteristically manifested as a primary atypical pneumonia syndrome, but may occasionally mimic acute bacterial pneumonia in all respects. A history of contact with birds in a patient with pneumonia should bring to mind the possibility of psittacosis. If the patient is seen before manifestations of pulmonary involvement have appeared, the febrile illness must be differentiated from typhoid fever, brucellosis, infectious mononucleosis, infectious hepatitis, miliary tuberculosis, and other causes of obscure febrile illnesses.

The diagnosis can be established by isolation of the psittacosis agent from blood or sputum during the acute phase of illness, but this should be attempted only by laboratories specially trained to work with the agent. The diagnosis is usually established by serologic means. Complement-fixing antibody begins to appear during the second week of the disease, and reaches a maximum titer by about 30 days after onset; a 4-fold increase in titer is required for diagnosis. Antimicrobial therapy may weaken and delay the antibody response, so that a significant rise in titer is not obtained for as long as 3 months after onset. It should also be noted that persons frequently exposed to birds may have an elevated titer of 1:8 to 1:32 in the absence of acute infection. The usual antigen employed in the complement fixation test does not differentiate between psittacosis and lymphogranuloma venereum, and positive sera must be tested with specific antigens to establish conclusively the significance of an increase in titer.

Mycobacteria

PULMONARY TUBERCULOSIS

Tuberculous disease of the lung usually follows a chronic course, but an acute respiratory illness may result when hematogenous dissemination develops or when bronchogenic spread occurs. Miliary tuberculosis involving the lungs does not produce impressive respiratory manifestations until late in the course of the disease. However, bronchogenic spread may lead to extensive lobar pneumonia with typical signs and symptoms of acute bacterial pneumonia. Patients with extensive acute tuberculous disease frequently have fever to 105° to 106°F and may be quite ill. At times, however, despite extensive consolidation and marked fever, the clinical condition of the patient remains relatively good. Many patients with tuberculous pneumonia are treated initially with antibiotics because of the possibility of another type of bacterial pneumonia. The lack of response may lead to further studies, which in turn establish the correct diagnosis. The leukocyte count is not helpful in differentiating tuberculous pneumonia from that caused by the usual bacteria; in florid tuberculous infection the total leukocyte count may be as high as 15,000 or even 20,000 cells/cu mm and there may be a shift to the left. The tuberculin test is a valuable diagnostic aid. Although the test may be negative in extensive disease, a negative intermediate or second-strength tuberculin response is a strong point against a tuberculous etiology.

It should be recalled, as noted previously, that on rare occasions tuberculous and pyogenic infections may coexist in the same pulmonary segment or lobe. Such a combined infection may be suspected when clinical and radiographic clearing is incomplete despite adequate therapy of the pyogenic component; under such circumstances appropriate additional studies should be done.

The most important laboratory aid for the rapid presumptive diagnosis of tuberculosis is examination of the sputum for acid-fast bacilli. The demonstration of morphologically characteristic acid-fast bacilli in smears virtually establishes the diagnosis, because acid-fast saprophytes are rare in sputum. Nevertheless, definitive diagnosis depends on showing that the bacilli in sputum are *Mycobacterium tuberculosis*, and this requires culture or animal inoculation.

If cavitation has occurred tuberculosis may be confused with lung abscess. Differentiation of pyogenic abscess and tuberculosis depends in the final analysis on whether tubercle bacilli can be isolated from sputum, but the history and the physical signs as well as the character of the sputum are helpful. In suppurative lung disease there is often a history of a predisposing factor, such as aspiration of a foreign body or an episode of unconsciousness, and on standing the sputum characteristically separates into three layers (pus at the bottom, middle watery zone, mucoid material on top).

Tuberculosis may also be confused with fungus infections of the lungs. The epidemiologic history and skin and serologic tests are helpful in differential diagnosis, but the final diagnosis depends on culture of the etiologic organism.

Spirochetes

LEPTOSPIROSIS

Cough with production of blood-streaked sputum occurs in about 25 per cent of patients with severe leptospirosis. Hemoptysis may be profuse, and in these patients physical and roentgenographic evidence of pneumonitis may be observed. The pneumonitis is characterized by extensive alveolar hemorrhage, and is probably a consequence of the bleeding tendency observed in patients with severe leptospirosis.

Viruses

ADENOVIRUS INFECTION

Adenoviruses infect virtually all persons early in childhood, but the majority of these infections are apparently asymptomatic. Adenoviruses account for about 6 per cent of respiratory illnesses among children, but in civilian adults the proportion is even less, perhaps in the range of 2 to 3 per cent. In contrast to the situation in civilians, adenoviruses are often responsible for respiratory disease among military recruits, accounting for 15 to 50 per cent of all acute respiratory disease in this population.

The respiratory syndromes resulting from infection with adenoviruses include 1) an influenza-like illness, termed acute respiratory disease of recruits, 2) pharyngitis, sometimes with pharyngeal exudate or conjunctivitis, and 3) pneumonia, which is discussed below. Although adenovirus infections in man are grouped into different clinical syndromes, it is important to emphasize that this division is somewhat artificial, and that there is considerable overlap.

Patients with adenovirus pneumonia have a grippelike illness in which pharyngitis is frequent. The pneumonia is often discovered incidentally on roentgenograms obtained because of respiratory symptoms and fever or because of the detection of rales on physical examination. Radiographic evidence of pneumonia has been observed in as many as 10 per cent of the cases of adenovirus infection observed during an epidemic.

In patients with pneumonia the onset is gradual, with fever, chilliness, headache, malaise, and anorexia. Nasal obstruction and slight nasal discharge occur in about half the patients. Sore throat is the most prominent localizing symptom. Almost all patients have a cough, but this is productive in less than half the patients. Substernal chest pain is common.

On physical examination these patients appear acutely ill but rarely severely ill. Nasal obstruction, mild injection of the pharynx, and lymphoid hyperplasia on the pharyngeal wall are the most common findings. Exudates may be present on the pharyngeal wall. Mild cervical lymphadenopathy is present in about 10 per cent of patients.

The febrile illness lasts from 2 to 7 days. A temperature of 103° to 104°F may be reached, but usually the temperature does not exceed 100°F. There is no temperature-pulse disproportion. Respiratory tract symptoms may persist for 1 or 2 weeks after the fever subsides.

The leukocyte count and differential are usually normal, although leukopenia may occur in some patients. The roentgenogram may show patchy, ill-defined densities, usually in the basilar segments; hilar adenopathy and pleural effusions occur rarely.

Adenovirus infection may be associated with conjunctivitis; this presentation, termed pharyngoconjunctival fever, is characterized by the respiratory symptoms described above and acute follicular conjunctivitis, which is usually unilateral. The eye is swollen and suffused, and preauricular lymphadenopathy is often prominent.

Definitive diagnosis of adenovirus infection depends on isolation of the virus from the respiratory tract, eye, or stool in a patient with typical symptoms, and the demonstration of a significant increase in antibody during the course of infection. The infection should be suspected in patients with exudative pharyngitis and pneumonia in whom other causes have been excluded, especially group A streptococci. Adenovirus infection should also be suspected in patients with conjunctivitis and respiratory tract infection. Adenovirus pneumonia can be grouped among the atypical pneumonias, and on clinical grounds in the individual patient cannot be distinguished from pneumonia caused by *Mycoplasma pneumoniae*, the agent of psittacosis, Q fever, or pneumonia caused by other viruses.

RESPIRATORY INFECTIONS ASSOCIATED WITH COXSACKIE, ECHO, AND POLIO-VIRUSES

These viruses of the picorna group frequently produce minor respiratory illnesses but do not contribute significantly to severe respiratory diseases in man.

CYTOMEGALOVIRUS INFECTION

Cytomegalovirus may occasionally be responsible for subacute or chronic pulmonary infection in man but is not usually a cause of acute infections of the lower respiratory tract.

This virus is widely disseminated among the population. The majority of infections appear to be asymptomatic; serologic studies indicate that as many as 80 per cent of persons over 35 years of age have been infected with cytomegalovirus.

Cytomegalic inclusion disease in the newborn or young infant is usually the result of intrauterine infection, and leads to the involvement of many organs, including the lungs. A more common occurrence, however, is reactivation of latent virus, an event which occurs almost exclusively in children or adults with generalized malignancy (such as leukemias and lymphomas) or in subjects of renal transplantation operations who have received massive immunosuppressive therapy with corticosteroids or metabolic inhibitors. Reactivation of the virus may be associated with evidence of generalized cytomegalovirus disease (hepatosplenomegaly, thrombocytopenic purpura, hepatitis, jaundice, etc.) but is more frequently expressed as an interstitial pneumonia. *Pneumocystis carinii* frequently coexists in the lungs of these patients, and probably represents reactivation of another ubiquitous latent infection. Bacterial infection is also common in this type of patient with depressed host resistance, and it is frequently difficult to determine which pathogen is playing the dominant role in the pulmonary disease.

The diagnosis of cytomegalovirus infections can best be established by recovery of the virus from urine, saliva, or other body fluids or tissues. At times typical cytomegalic cells (cytomegaly and prominent intranuclear inclusions) may be demonstrated in various body fluids. However, caution is required in interpretation of the results, since failure to demonstrate typical cells does not rule out cytomegalovirus disease, nor does demonstration of virus or typical cells clearly indicate that the pathologic process is related to infection with cytomegalovirus.

INFLUENZA VIRUS INFECTION

Influenza recurs in epidemics which start abruptly at about the same time in many places in a country. The disease spreads rapidly, a characteristic which was evident even before the age of modern rapid transportation. Epidemics occur in cycles (type A every 2 to 4 years, type B every 4 to 6 years), but the intervals are not always predictable. Sporadic infections occur continuously, and the virus may be maintained in this manner during interepidemic periods.

Influenza occurs, as a rule, in the fall and spring. The incidence of infection is highest in children 5 to 9 years of age and decreases progressively above the age of 35.

Influenza in man follows a variable course. It may be asymptomtic or may vary from a slight fever with minor respiratory symptoms to fatal influenza virus pneumonia. Subclinical infection is common; the ratio of infection to disease in several studies has ranged from 3:1 to 9:1. Influenza virus infection also results in an increase in susceptibility to secondary bacterial pneumonia, which may occur concomitantly with the illness caused by the virus or may follow it.

Uncomplicated influenza is an acute, self-limited tracheobronchitis with fever, which usually lasts 3 to 5 days. Typical influenza is associated with fever, generalized muscular aching, headache, prostration, and anorexia. Substernal pain consequent to tracheitis is common and sometimes severe, but pleuritic pain does not occur with uncomplicated influenza. Chilly sensations are common, but frank rigors are unusual. Even in uncomplicated influenza the temperature may vary from low-grade to 106°F in the absence of bacterial infection. The disease lasts only 2 to 5 days, and all symptoms have usually abated by 7 to 10 days. Any striking deviation from this pattern should suggest another diagnosis or a complication.

Extensive diffuse pneumonia, a serious complication with a high mortality rate, may occur rarely as a result of infection with influenza virus. Although there are exceptions, this disease is almost restricted to persons with pre-existing cardiac or pulmonary diseases or to patients who are pregnant, especially in the last trimester. The cardiac lesion is usually rheumatic heart disease with mitral stenosis. Pneumonia usually develops within 24 hours after onset of symptoms of influenza. The patients have a very high fever, profuse bloody sputum, dyspnea, and intense anxiety, and are usually cyanotic. Diffuse, moist rales are present throughout the lungs, but signs of consolidation are not common. The roentgenogram reveals diffuse, bilateral nodular infiltrates that radiate from the hilum. The course of illness is one of unremitting fever, progressive pulmonary involvement, and vascular collapse. Death usually occurs within 5 to 10 days, as a result of progressive cardiopulmonary failure.

Influenza virus may also produce a less extensive pulmonary consolidation than that just described. These patients do not usually have underlying diseases, show no evidence of bacterial complications, and have a good prognosis.

Secondary bacterial pneumonia accounts for the majority of deaths from influenza, and is not unusual during influenza outbreaks. During recent epidemics the pneumococcus and *Staphylococcus aureus* have been the most frequent causes of bacterial pneumonia, although other organisms may be responsible. The onset of bacterial pneumonia occurs, as a rule, late in the course of influenza. Some patients are improving from influenza when "relapse" occurs at the onset of the bacterial infection. In a typical case cough becomes noticeably more productive, the sputum becomes purulent, and shaking chills and pleurisy develop. All these manifestations are much more characteristic of bacterial pneumonia than of influenza. In addition, the roentgenogram is more likely to show segmental, lobar, or focal pneumonia than the diffuse process characteristic of influenza virus pneumonia. The nature of the bacterial pathogen may be suspected on the basis of the sputum smear, and the causative organism can be isolated from sputum as well as from the blood in some patients.

The blood leukocyte count in patients with uncomplicated influenza is usually normal, but may range from 2,000 to 14,000 cells/cu mm. Lymphocytopenia is frequent during the first 4 days of the disease. In patients with influenza virus pneumonia there is usually leukocytosis, even in the absence of bacterial infection. In these patients the arterial oxygen saturation is usually low, ranging from 46 to 85 per cent; the partial pressure of CO_2 in plasma is increased, and the blood pH is lowered.

A presumptive diagnosis of influenza during epidemic periods is usually made accurately on the basis of the clinical picture and the epidemiologic data. Laboratory confirmation of the diagnosis, although relatively simple, is too costly and troublesome for general application to all patients during an outbreak. Definitive diagnosis can be made by isolation of the virus from nasal or throat washings inoculated into chick embryos, but the results are not available for 2 to 3 days, even under optimal circumstances. Immunofluorescent techniques for demonstrating viral antigens in desquamated cells from the nasopharynx may give a definitive diagnosis in about 50 per cent of infected individuals, but this technique is not generally available. Specific diagnosis is usually made by complement fixation or hemagglutination inhibition tests. Because many people have antibodies that react with the virus, a 4-fold or greater rise in antibody titer is required for diagnosis.

Influenza must be differentiated from other causes of respiratory infection and fever. In adenovirus infection fever and prostration are usually less marked than in influenza, and the onset is usually less sudden. In addition, sore throat and laryngitis are usually more prominent in adeno-virus infection than in influenza. Infection with respiratory syncytial virus and with various arbo- or enteroviruses may simulate influenza. In some patients influenza must be differentiated from streptococcal pharyngitis and from all of the causes of the primary atypical pneumonia syndrome.

MEASLES VIRUS INFECTION

Respiratory manifestations are invariably encountered in uncomplicated measles as a result of widespread involvement of the respiratory mucosa by the virus. In children an increase in the severity of the laryngitis and tracheitis which normally accompany measles may result in sufficient airway obstruction to produce typical croup. In small children and infants edema and local secretions in small air passages (i.e., bronchiolitis) may produce severe illness with cyanosis, dyspnea, and rales. Measles virus also produces giant cell pneumonia, a rare and nearly always fatal disease characterized by formation in the lungs of multinucleated giant cells with intranuclear and intracytoplasmic inclusion bodies. Almost all children with this process also have an underlying condition, in most instances leukemia. The disease is characterized by prolonged persistence of measles virus and by marked depression of production of specific antibodies. Some of these patients do not have rash or other typical manifestations of measles, but usually have clinical findings of severe respiratory infection and radio-graphic evidence of bronchopneumonia or interstitial pneumonia.

Bacterial pneumonia is a frequent and serious complication of measles. Most of the mortality consequent to measles results from bacterial infec-tions, primarily pneumonia, in children less than 5 years of age, and in the aged. The bacterial pathogens usually responsible are the pneumococcus, *S. aureus*, group A streptococcus, and *H. influenzae*. The pathogenesis of bacterial pneumonia complicating measles is quite similar to that of bacterial pneumonia complicating influenza virus infection. Measles virus is destructive to respiratory mucosa, and disrupts normal ciliary action and the intact cellular lining.

Bacterial complications of the lower respiratory tract in measles are sometimes difficult to detect because of the prominence of respiratory symptoms directly related to the virus infection. The acute stage of measles, with its accompanying bronchitis, cough, and fever, ordinarily has begun to subside by the third day of the rash. An increase in respiratory symptoms with a second fever spike after this time should alert the physician to the possibility of bacterial pneumonia. In addition, the persistence of fever for longer than 6 days or the occurrence of leukocytosis should lead to sus-picion of a bacterial complication. A chest roentgenogram may prove helpful if the physical examination is not revealing.

PARAINFLUENZA VIRUSES

The four types of parainfluenza virus are common causes of respiratory illness in children and adults. Few individuals, if any, escape infection and reinfection with these viruses, and antibodies against more than one type are present in about 70 per cent of children by 6 years of age. The initial infections in childhood tend to be more severe than those encountered later in life after previous contacts with these agents.

Parainfluenza viruses make a significant contribution, estimated at 4 to 17 per cent, to respiratory illness in children, and account for an estimated 5 per cent of common colds and upper respiratory illness in adults.

The most characteristic infection with parainfluenza viruses in children is croup. These viruses account for one-third to one-half of the cases of severe croup in children. Although croup is the most distinctive syndrome, these agents also cause rhinitis or pharyngitis about twice as often as croup, and bronchitis, bronchiolitis, or pneumonia about as often as they cause croup.

In adults the common cold syndrome, sometimes associated with hoarseness and cough, is the predominant expression of infection. Fever, sore throat, and headache also occur in some patients, but pneumonia is not a part of the clinical spectrum of diseases produced in adults by these agents.

RESPIRATORY SYNCYTIAL VIRUS

Respiratory syncytial virus is a common cause of serious respiratory disease in children, accounting for 20 per cent of pediatric patients hospitalized with respiratory infections. During the first year of life respiratory syncytial virus is the single most prevalent infection causing lower respiratory illness. In one study of children under 8 years of age the syndrome produced by infection with this agent was classified as the common cold in about one-half, as bronchitis in about 15 per cent, as bronchiolitis in about 10 per cent, and as bronchopneumonia in about 20 per cent.

In adults the entire spectrum of viral respiratory illness may be produced, but, because of previous infections earlier in life, illness is much less severe than in children. The most common manifestation in adults is acute coryza or the common cold, but occasionally the virus may produce an acute exacerbation of chronic bronchitis, bronchopneumonia, or an influenza-like syndrome. In patients with chronic respiratory disease the infection may be quite severe.

Diagnosis is established by serologic methods or isolation of the agent from respiratory secretions during the acute illness.

RHINOVIRUSES

Rhinoviruses, of which there are more than 75 serotypes, are the most common cause of the common cold syndrome. In adults about 95 per cent of symptomatic infections are typical common colds, but occasionally these agents also cause acute bronchitis and pneumonia. In contrast, in children only about 50 per cent of symptomatic rhinovirus infections are common colds; about 25 per cent are classified as acute bronchitis, and the remaining 25 per cent of infections are characterized as croup, bronchiolitis, or bronchopneumonia. The distribution of illness caused by rhinoviruses is somewhat similar to that observed with respiratory syncytial virus infection; however, rhinovirus infections are in general milder than those caused by respiratory syncytial virus. Diagnosis must be established by isolating the agent and by specific serologic response; evaluation of the significance of a viral isolate is difficult because these agents can be isolated at times from normal individuals.

VARICELLA (CHICKENPOX)

Varicella is usually a benign disease in children, but in adults may be a much more severe illness with an extensive eruption and marked constitutional symptoms. Pneumonia is the most frequent serious complication of varicella in adults, and is responsible for most fatalities from this disease. Although varicella pneumonia may occur at any age, about 90 per cent of cases develop in patients older than 19 years. The true incidence of varicella pneumonia is difficult to assess, but is probably about 10 to 15 per cent of cases of varicella in adults and less than 1 per cent in children.

The generalized rash of chickenpox or the localized eruption of herpes zoster is always present in patients with varicella pneumonia. Symptoms of pneumonia develop within 1 to 6 days after the onset of rash; in 70 per cent the onset occurs within the first 3 days. Symptoms vary from a slight cough in a patient with radiographic evidence of pneumonia to a progressive severe disease with dyspnea, cyanosis, and death. However, the majority of patients are quite ill. The cardinal manifestations are cough, dyspnea, hemoptysis, and pleuritic chest pain. The chest pain is thought to be secondary to involvement of the pleural surfaces with vesicles.

In adults with varicella pneumonia the temperature is usually elevated. However, in 10 to 15 per cent of the reported cases, the temperature is less than 100°F orally, and in only 15 per cent is the temperature more than 104°F. Examination of the chest is often unimpressive, and correlates poorly with the severity of pneumonia as judged by the general appearance of the patient and the roentgenogram.

The most frequent abnormalities found on roentgenography of the chest are scattered nodular pulmonary infiltrates, often with a peribronchial distribution, varying from a few small nodules to extensive bilateral infiltrates. The nodules are rarely greater than 0.5 cm in diameter and are denser near the hilum. There is a tendency for coalescence of lesions at the lung bases. Minimal pleural effusions occasionally occur, and hilar adenopathy may be observed.

The blood leukocyte count is usually normal or slightly increased. In a review of the literature, Triebwasser and associates found the blood leukocyte count in adults with varicella pneumonia to be 10,000 or more cells/cu mm in 37 per cent of the cases. Thrombocytopenia may be observed. The sputum culture usually reveals normal respiratory flora.

The diagnosis of varicella pneumonia is usually not difficult, because the typical rash is always present. However, confusion may be encountered in differentiating primary varicella pneumonia from secondary bacterial pneumonia. The occurrence of pulmonary infiltrates in children immediately suggests the possibility of bacterial pneumonia, since clinically apparent varicella pneumonia is rare in this age group. In addition, the occurrence of segmental or lobar consolidation, in contrast to the diffuse nodular infiltrates usually observed in varicella, favors a diagnosis of bacterial pneumonia. Because reliable differentiation of varicella from bacterial pneumonia is not possible in the individual patient, it is advisable to administer antimicrobial therapy to all patients with varicella and pneumonia until the diagnosis of viral pneumonia is quite clear.

The mortality rate in patients with varicella pneumonia admitted to the hospital varies from 10 to 30 per cent. The highest mortality occurs in patients with underlying diseases, especially those receiving cortiocosteroids or antimetabolites, or in patients who are pregnant.

Fungi

ASPERGILLOSIS

Although more likely to be confused with chronic pulmonary diseases, aspergillosis may occasionally be confused with an acute pulmonary infection. Although it is extremely uncommon, a primary acute pneumonia may occur in persons exposed to a high concentration of spores (agricultural workers who handle grain, squab feeders who take grain in the mouth, chimney sweeps). Lesions vary from localized, small, pneumonic infiltrates to diffuse, bilateral, confluent lesions in which abscesses may be found. Loeffler's syndrome related to multiplication of *Aspergillus* in the lungs of patients with chronic pulmonary disease may also occur, producing fever, eosinophilia, and fleeting infiltrates. Aspergillosis may also be manifested as a secondary infection in patients with major underlying diseases who have received extensive antimicrobial or corticosteroid therapy. In this type of patient findings vary widely, but chest roentgenograms may show isolated nodules or areas of pneumonia, sometimes accompanied by abscess formation. Finally, one of the most common types of pulmonary aspergillosis, the fungus ball, results from growth of *Aspergillus* in a cavity due to tuberculosis, histoplasmosis, sarcoidosis, or neoplastic disease.

The diagnosis of pulmonary aspergillosis or Loeffler's syndrome related to this organism should be suspected on recovery of the organism from the sputum. However, the organism is widespread and is often recovered from the sputum of normal individuals. Repeated recovery of the organism or demonstration that it is present in large numbers adds support, but is not confirmatory. The only completely convincing way to establish the diagnosis is by lung biopsy. Skin and serologic tests have not been adequately standardized to be of value in diagnosis.

An aspergilloma in a cavitary lesion can be suspected by the characteristic roentgenographic appearance. It appears as a solid mass within a cavity, surrounded partially by a crescent of air. The mycetoma can often be shown to move within the cavity if x-rays are taken in different positions.

BLASTOMYCOSIS

Blastomycosis may begin insidiously or sometimes abruptly. Although the lungs are almost always the portal of entry, about half the patients show little evidence of pulmonary involvement during the early phase of illness but instead have evidence of infection at some distant site. Initial pulmonary manifestations may be fever, chills, chest pain, dyspnea, and cough. Physical findings are variable, but most commonly there is focal consolidation. Erythema nodosum may accompany the acute pulmonary disease. On roentgenography a dense area of consolidation involving part of a single lobe is characteristically found, but multilobar or lobar consolidation may be noted; enlargement of mediastinal modes is common. These acute lesions may resolve completely, progress relentlessly or become chronic.

The majority of patients with untreated blastomycosis have evidence of extrapulmonary spread of the infection at some time during the course of the illness. Lesions resulting from hematogenous dissemination are usually found in the skin, but bones and/or joints are frequently affected.

Routine laboratory studies are not helpful diagnostically. In tissues the dimorphic fungus grows entirely in the yeast phase, and yeast cells can often be visualized by careful examination of sputum or exudate from draining subcutaneous lesions. Sputum specimens should be mixed with an equal amount of 3 to 10 per cent sodium or potassium hydroxide and examined with the low-power microscope lens. The fungi appear as spherical cells 5 to 20 μ in size, which may have a single bud. The cells have a thick, double-contoured, refractile wall, and give a "figure eight" appearance when single buds are present. Cultures should be made on Sabouraud's glucose agar. A presumptive diagnosis of blastomycosis can also be made by histologic study of tissues obtained by biopsy, although cultural confirmation is required. Blastomycin is the least reliable of the three major fungal skin test materials. As many as 50 per cent of patients with blastomycosis have negative skin tests. Serologic tests are also unreliable, but recent results with precipitin tests show promise.

CANDIDIASIS

Candida organisms are frequently present in the mouth, vagina, and stools of normal individuals. These organisms may become invasive under conditions of lowered host resistance, such as in patients with debilitating diseases or those receiving corticosteroid or antibiotic therapy. Pulmonary involvement may occur consequent to spread of infection from the oral cavity or may be secondary to hematogenous dissemination of the organism. If invasion has occurred from the upper respiratory tract the bronchi may be involved but either route of invasion may lead to a patchy bronchopneumonia. In patients with hematogenous dissemination manifestations related to extrapulmonary sites of infection, especially in the kidneys, are usually the dominant aspect of the disease. The possibility of pulmonary candidiasis arises frequently, but diagnosis is difficult. A definitive diagnosis cannot be established merely by isolating *Candida* from the sputum, because the organism is frequently found in the upper respiratory tracts of normal individuals or patients receiving antimicrobial therapy. Positive blood cultures are clearly indicative of systemic *Candida* infection and constitute excellent evidence, although no proof, that a pulmonary lesion is related to *Candida*. Histologic evidence of actual lung invasion by the fungus is definitive if coupled with isolation of the agent from the tissue. Because of the toxicity of available, effective antimicrobials, therapy in suspected cases should be initiated only if the fungus is cultured repeatedly in almost pure culture from both sputum and bronchial washings and if the pulmonary disease is progressing relentlessly.

COCCIDIOIDOMYCOSIS

Infection with *Coccidioides immitis* may be manifested by acute or chronic pulmonary disease; in some patients hematogenous dissemination may occur.

The endemic area for human coccidioidomycosis is geographically limited to certain areas of Mexico and the southwestern United States. States lying in part within the endemic region are California, Nevada, Arizona, Texas, Utah, and New Mexico. Sporadic cases outside the endemic area have been attributed to transportation of the fungus on various objects. The infectious arthrospores are present in soil and are easily inhaled. Residence in one of the endemic areas is followed by development of a positive skin test in many individuals; only transient exposure may be required.

About 80 per cent of persons whose skin tests convert from negative to positive give no history of illness that might be readily related to coccidioidal infection. The majority of those who develop symptoms have only an influenza-like illness of short duration 1 to 4 weeks after exposure. Symptoms are fever, cough, myalgia, and at times arthralgias and conjunctivitis. A roentgenogram of the chest may show hilar adenopathy or infiltrates which are usually in the upper lobes; the lesions clear rapidly.

A very small proportion of infected individuals have an illness of greater severity. Respiratory symptoms are more marked, pleurisy may be present, and shaking chills, headaches, myalgias, and arthralgias occur. Erythema nodosum is a frequent finding, and erythema multiforme-like lesions and urticaria may be observed rarely. The physical findings are variable, ranging from no abnormalities to extensive signs of consolidation. About 3 per cent of the patients develop pleural effusions large enough to be detected on physical examination. Roentgenograms of the chest may show soft perihilar infiltrates, patchy pneumonic infiltrates, nodular densities, or miliary lesions.

Most patients with pulmonary coccidioidomycosis recover completely in 1 to 3 weeks, but about 5 per cent develop serious residua or progressive disease, including cavitation, fibrosis, or persistent pleural effusion.

The routine laboratory findings are not helpful in the diagnosis of coccidioidomycosis. The blood leukocyte count is normal or elevated, and mild to moderate eosinophilia may be observed, especially if erythema nodosum is present. The diagnosis can be established by isolation of the fungus and by skin and serologic tests. Spherules may be seen in the sputum of patients with acute pulmonary coccidioidomycosis, but these are usually difficult to find; the fungus is more readily found in abscess, biopsy, or resection specimens. Exudates or tissue specimens should be cultured on Sabouraud's glucose agar, on which colonies may appear in 2 to 8 days. Ninety-nine per cent of patients with acute nondisseminated coccidioidomycosis develop positive skin tests within 3 weeks, but the skin test remains negative in 70 per cent of patients with disseminated disease. Significant cross-reactions occur with histoplasmin and blastomycin, but almost invariably a reaction of greater size and intensity is observed with the homologous antigen. The precipitin and complement fixation tests are helpful in diagnosis. The precipitin test becomes positive earlier than the complement fixation test, antibodies usually appearing in the second or third week of illness. One or the other of these tests is positive in about 90 per cent of patients with acute pulmonary coccidioidomycosis and in virtually all individuals with extra-pulmonary infection. The height of the titer of the complement fixation test is also of value. Higher titers are obtained in patients with disseminated disease; the presence of a titer of 1:16 or greater in association with a negative skin test is indicative of a diagnosis of disseminated disease.

CRYPTOCOCCOSIS

The most characteristic feature of infection with *Cryptococcus neoformans* in man is meningeal disease. However, the primary site of invasion is virtually always the lungs, and pneumonia may occur. The fungus can be isolated from soil and is found frequently in association with pigeon droppings. Most cases of cryptococcosis occur in persons who have previously been in good health. However, susceptibility to cryptococcal infection is increased in patients with certain neoplastic diseases, especially those of the reticuloendothelial system, and also perhaps in patients who are receiving therapy with corticosteroids or who have hypogammaglobulinemia or diabetes.

There is nothing characteristic about the signs and symptoms of pulmonary cryptococcosis. Fever may be very slight or even absent. Exposure to pigeons or severe headache or other evidence of meningeal disease should heighten suspicion of the possibility of cryptococcosis. The roentgenographic manifestations vary from a single coin lesion to extensive nodular infiltrates.

Cryptococci occasionally can be seen in the sputum; the specimen should be mixed with equal parts of 10 per cent sodium or potassium hydroxide. The organisms appear as round yeasts, the total size of the cell and the capsule ranging from 4 to 20 μ. The organism grows rapidly, and can be isolated on Sabouraud's or blood agar. Although serologic tests are available, these are not well standardized; definitive diagnosis depends on isolation of the organism.

HISTOPLASMOSIS

Histoplasma infection may be associated with a variety of pulmonary syndromes, including acute or chronic, localized or disseminated pneumonia, chronic cavitary disease, localized nodular lesions, miliary lesions, or single or multiple pulmonary calcifications. In addition, in a small number of patients, progressive extrapulmonary infection ensues, with involvement of liver, spleen, lymph nodes, bone marrow, and adrenal glands. The oropharynx, tongue, and larynx are also frequently affected by an ulcerative or granulomatous lesion.

Pneumonic histoplasmosis may simulate acute exudative tuberculosis, acute bacterial pneumonia, or pneumonias of viral origin. Fever, cough, shaking chills, sweats, anorexia, headache, and weakness are all common symptoms. Cough may be productive of mucopurulent sputum, and as many as one-third of the patients have hemoptysis. Chest pain is frequent and may be pleuritic. The upper lobes are more commonly involved, but any area of the lung may be diseased. Physical examination of the lungs is not helpful in differential diagnosis because the findings are quite variable; however, it is important to note that signs of consolidation indistinguishable from those in acute bacterial pneumonia may be present. Friction rubs may be heard, and occasionally there is pleural fluid. Roentgenograms of the chest show one or more areas of soft infiltrates, patchy coalescent densities, or consolidation, occasionally accompanied by pleural reaction. Hilar adenopathy is frequently present. The pulmonary lesions may cavitate as the process progresses.

Although pneumonia caused by *Histoplasma* may initially be confused with bacterial or viral pneumonia, the lack of response to the usual antimicrobial agents and the course of the disease soon make it evident that the process probably is not caused by viruses or bacteria. Epidemiologic factors may suggest the diagnosis. The fungus is easily isolated from infected soil; soil around chicken coops or from the habitats of birds, such as starlings, may be heavily parasitized. Although the disease is of world-wide distribution, it is especially prevalent in certain areas in the central and eastern United States, the largest number of cases being reported from Kentucky, Illinois, Kansas, Indiana, Iowa, Missouri, Ohio, Tennessee, Maryland, and Virginia.

The fungus rarely may be seen within mononuclear cells in Giemsa- or Wright-stained smears of sputum of patients with pulmonary histoplasmosis. However, the diagnosis is more often established by isolation of the organism from the sputum cultured on Sabouraud's agar. Blood cultures should be obtained if there is evidence of disseminated disease, since the organism occasionally can be isolated in this manner. *Histoplasma capsulatum* can also be seen in histologic sections of tissues obtained by biopsy or at necropsy.

Serologic techniques are helpful in diagnosis, and sera should be collected as soon as the diagnosis is suspected. The complement fixation test becomes positive in most patients with pulmonary histoplasmosis. About 90 per cent of persons with acute histoplasmosis develop positive skin tests to histoplasmin within 2 to 4 weeks after onset. However, about two-thirds of patients with progressive or disseminated disease have negative skin tests. Skin tests may evoke the formation of complement-fixing antibodies and should not be performed until serologic studies have been made.

MUCORMYCOSIS

This infection almost always develops in patients with severe underlying disease, such as diabetic ketosis, lymphoma, leukemia, carcinoma, or extensive burns. In its most typical form mucormycosis is manifested by orbital cellulitis and meningoencephalitis in a patient with diabetic acidosis. However, the lungs may be involved by an acute inflammatory process, either as a primary pneumonia or secondary to disease at another site. Whereas meningoencephalitic mucormycosis is more common in diabetics, pulmonary involvement is the predominant form in patients with lymphoma or leukemia. Pulmonary mucormycosis may also be associated with pulmonary infarction consequent to invasion of blood vessels by the fungus. In addition, the broad hyphae may act as a nidus for bacterial growth which leads to necrotizing pneumonia and abscess formation. There is no distinctive clinical pattern in pulmonary mucormycosis. Cough, chills, hemoptysis, and pleural pain have all been described. Roentgenograms of the chest show areas of pneumonia or pulmonary infarction, occasionally with cavitation or pleural effusion.

The organism can be isolated readily on Sabouraud's glucose agar. Mere demonstration of the organism in sputum does not establish the diagnosis, because species of mucor are widespread and may be present in the sputum without evidence of pulmonary infection. Although a series of positive cultures is highly suggestive of pulmonary mucormycosis, definitive diagnosis can only be established by isolation of the organism from lung and demonstration of fungal invasion in sections of tissue.

OTHER FUNGUS INFECTIONS

Other fungus infections that might rarely be confused with acute pulmonary inflammation are sporotrichosis, South American blastomycosis, and geotrichosis, even though the pulmonary disease produced by these fungi is usually chronic. Diagnosis is made by isolation of the fungus.

Actinomycetes (Fungus-like Bacteria)

ACTINOMYCOSIS

There are three major forms of actinomycosis: cervicofacial, abdominal, and thoracic. The thoracic form is associated with pulmonary involvement, which apparently results from aspiration of infected material from the pharynx. Once established, there is a striking tendency for the process to burrow from one tissue to another without respect for anatomic barriers.

The onset of illness may be rapid, but is usually insidious. Symptoms include low-grade fever and cough, sometimes productive of purulent or blood-streaked sputum. The course of the disease is characterized by pulmonary consolidation, the formation of abscesses, pleurisy, and chest wall fistulae. The disease in its early stages may be confused with acute inflammatory disease of the lungs, but because of the chronic course, which soon becomes evident, is more often mistaken for tuberculosis, other fungus infections, or malignancy. Roentgenograms of the chest show focal infiltrates, areas of consolidation, abscesses, or pleural effusions.

There is no reliable skin or serologic test for the diagnosis of actino-mycosis. The diagnosis is supported by the finding of typical sulfur granules in sputum, pus, or histologic sections, and confirmed by isolation of the fungus from infected material. Caution in interpretation of results is required, because *Actinomyces* can be isolated from the mouths of normal persons and granules can be expressed from normal tonsils. The organism grows only anaerobically, and is thus distinguished from species of *Nocardia*.

NOCARDIOSIS

Nocardia asteroides is world-wide in distribution, grows aerobically, and is Gram-positive. Unlike *Actinomyces*, this organism is not ordinarily a saprophytic inhabitant of the upper respiratory tract. Therefore, recovery of the organism in culture from sputum, tonsils, bronchial washings, or gastric aspirates is almost always indicative of active infection. About half the cases of nocardiosis occur in patients with significant underlying illnesses, including lymphoma, leukemia, carcinoma, sarcoidosis, and tuberculosis. The disease has been reported in association with pulmonary alveolar proteinosis, and about 20 per cent of the cases have occurred in patients receiving adrenal glucocorticoids.

Pulmonary involvement occurs in the majority of patients, and may mimic acute bacterial pneumonia or tuberculosis. The process usually begins insidiously with cough, which may be productive of purulent or bloody sputum, fever, and occasionally shaking chills. Pleural pain is common. Physical findings are very variable. Some patients may have a few rales, whereas other have extensive consolidation. About 25 per cent of patients develop empyema. The disease may extend through the pleural space to subcutaneous tissues, with the formation of draining chest sinuses, but this is uncommon. Hematogenous spread occurs in some patients; a characteristic consequence is brain abscess, although localization may occur in any organ. Chest roentgenogram shows patchy nodular or fluffy infiltrates, focal areas of consolidation with abscesses, cavities without surrounding pneumonia, or dense infiltrates fanning out from the hilar areas.

As in actinomycosis, there is no reliable skin or serologic test. Granules indistinguishable from those observed in actinomycosis may be seen in exudate or sputum. Some strains of *Nocardia* are acid-fast. Diagnosis depends on isolation of the fungus on culture.

Rickettsiae

Q FEVER

Q fever, a self-limited rickettsial infection caused by *Coxiella burnetii*, is characterized by abrupt onset of fever, headache, muscle pain, and severe malaise. The febrile course may continue for 1 to 3 weeks. Approximately half the patients have roentgenographic evidence of pneumonitis, which is manifested clinically as slight, nonproductive cough, usually developing in the second week of illness.

The principal reservoirs of Q fever are animals domesticated by man, primarily cattle, sheep, and goats. The disease has been recognized throughout the United States. In animals, rickettsiae are excreted in placental tissue, milk, or feces. Man acquires infection from aerosols emanating directly from cattle or from contaminated clothing, wool, hides, bedding, or soil. The rickettsiae are resistant to prolonged drying, and may be transported on fomites, such as wool or hides, over long distances from infected cattle.

Q fever should be suspected in patients with febrile illnesses for which no obvious cause can be found, especially if the patient's occupation involves contact with sheep, cattle, or goats, or their by-products, such as wool or hides. The diagnosis also should be suspected in patients with the atypical pneumonia syndrome. The physician should bear in mind that this rickettsia may produce vegetative endocarditis, and that Q fever may be associated with hepatitis with or without jaundice.

Attempts to isolate the organism should not be undertaken because of the danger of laboratory-acquired infection. Complement fixation or agglutination tests may be employed in diagnosis; with either test a 4-fold or greater rise in antibody titer can be demonstrated to occur between the first and fourth weeks of illness.

The response to antimicrobial therapy may be helpful in differential diagnosis. The disease responds promptly to tetracycline or chloramphenicol, and the patient usually becomes afebrile within 48 hours after the initiation of therapy.

Protozoa and Other Parasites

AMEBIASIS

Amebic abscess of the liver, with or without perforation of the diaphragm, may simulate right lower lobe pneumonia.

Liver abscess may occur without preceding intestinal symptoms, is usually solitary, and involves the right lobe of the liver more often than the left. Abscesses may become quite large and produce marked elevation of the hemidiaphragm. As this occurs, pulmonary manifestations, such as cough, pleurisy, and rales, may develop because of inflammation of the diaphragmatic pleura and basilar atelectasis secondary to the elevated diaphragm. Pain in the right shoulder or scapula or pleurisy in the region of the right lower hemithorax may be prominent. Fever and leukocytosis are usually present.

In some patients the amebic abscess of the liver perforates the diaphragm, infects the pleural space, burrows into the lung, and eventually may rupture into a bronchus. The perforation occurs on the right side in the vast majority of cases. Because of the proximity of the pericardium, pericarditis is not unusual, and in some cases pericardial effusion develops. The pleural reaction may result in the formation of large amounts of thick, chocolate-colored pus; if rupture into a bronchus occurs, a bronchopleurohepatic fistula may be formed. In such patients an air-fluid level in an abscess cavity below the diaphragm may be seen occasionally on chest roentgenography. Patients with bronchopleurohepatic fistulae may complain that their sputum tastes like liver.

The clinical picture of a febrile patient with a tender liver, elevated hemidiaphragm, right pleural effusion, and atelectasis or rales at the right base should suggest the possibility of amebic liver abscess. A history of recent foreign travel is common, and most of these patients look quite ill. Aspiration of thick, chocolate-colored pus from the right pleural space or expectoration of similar pus obviously should also suggest the diagnosis. An attempt should be made to confirm the clinical diagnosis by demonstration of the parasites. However, trophozoites are difficult to find in typical material aspirated from liver abscesses or in sputum or pleural fluid from patients with lung involvement. It is sometimes possible to demonstrate trophozoites or cysts of *Endamoeba histolytica* in stools, but usually the strongest support for the diagnosis of amebic hepatic or pulmonary abscess is obtained from hepatic scanning techniques, which reveal a filling defect in the liver, or from the clinical response to a therapeutic trial of emetine or chloroquine. Response to specific therapy is relatively rapid, and usually occurs in 24 to 48 hours if no other complications are present. However, differential diagnosis is often complicated by secondary bacterial infection of the amebic hepatic or lung abscess. Specific evidence of amebiasis may be obtained by the complement fixation test, which is positive in almost all patients with amebic hepatic abscesses.

PNEUMOCYSTIS CARINII PNEUMONIA

This ubiquitous organism, presumably a protozoan, possesses low virulence for man, and produces disease which is almost always limited to the lungs of patients with major defects in host resistance. *Pneumocystis* pneumonia has been observed in newborn and premature infants, patients with immunoglobulin deficiencies, leukemia, or lymphoma, recipients of organ transplants who are treated with corticosteroids and immunosuppressive drugs, and patients with other severe debilitating disease.

Pneumocystis pneumonia usually follows a subacute or chronic course over a period of 4 to 6 weeks or longer. The disease is not usually confused with acute inflammatory diseases of the lungs except in rare instances in which the course is rapidly progressive. The disease begins slowly, with low-grade fever, cough, tachypnea, and eventually dyspnea and cyanosis. Hemoptysis and pleural involvement are rare. As the disease progresses these patients develop an alveolar-capillary block syndrome and die of progressive hypoxia. Physical findings are usually minimal or unimpressive, especially in view of the striking symptoms and radiographic manifestations that may be present. The roentgenogram shows a finely granular, diffuse parenchymal infiltrate, sometimes with areas of dense consolidation or atelectasis.

Pneumocystis has not been isolated *in vitro* and no satisfactory serologic test is available; therefore, the diagnosis has to be confirmed by demonstration of the parasite.

The diagnosis is suggested by the occurrence of progressive pulmonary disease in a host with markedly impaired resistance. Although there are occasional reports of demonstration of the organism in sputum or tracheal aspirates, these techniques are notoriously poor. Examination of lung tissue obtained by needle or open biopsy and stained by methenamine silver stain is almost always required for antemortem diagnosis. These rather extreme measures required to establish diagnosis are indicated in some patients, because effective antimicrobial therapy is available in the form of pentamidine isethionate.

It should be emphasized that the majority of patients with fatal *Pneumocystis* pneumonia have been shown to have additional pathogenic microbes in the lungs, including cytomegalovirus, *Aspergillus*, *Nocardia*, *Histoplasma*, or bacteria. It is frequently difficult to determine which pathogen is playing the dominant role in the pulmonary process.

ASCARIASIS

Ascariasis is an infection which may be associated with an intense acute pulmonary reaction during the phase of larval migration. *Ascaris lumbricoides* is widespread throughout the world and is one of the most common parasitic infections of man. The adult worms live in the small intestine, where females produce large numbers of eggs. Eggs excreted in feces undergo a developmental phase in soil, and then, as embryonated eggs, are ingested in contaminated food or directly from dirty fingers. The eggs hatch in the upper intestine, liberating larvae which penetrate the intestinal wall, enter the bloodstream, and are carried to the lungs, where they penetrate alveolar septae and evoke a marked allergic response. The larvae migrate up the tracheobronchial tree to the esophagus and are swallowed and returned to the small intestine, where they mature. The pulmonary phase lasts about 10 days.

Pulmonary manifestations ranging from mild cough to fatal bronchopneumonia occur during the phase of migration of larvae through the lungs. Most patients with relatively heavy infection have fever of 99° to 101°F; temperature above 102°F is distinctly unusual. Symptoms, variable in degree, consist of cough, hemoptysis, substernal pain, and dyspnea. Physical examination may reveal musical rales or wheezing. Some patients have a pruritic skin eruption. Eosinophilia is present in most patients, and ranges from 20 to 60 per cent. Occasionally counts of 40,000 cells/cu mm with 50 per cent eosinophils are observed. Eosinophilia may not be present or may be minimal in patients observed early during the illness. The chest roentgenogram reveals scattered soft densities of variable location and extent; in severe cases there may be confluent densities involving large areas of lung.

Specific diagnosis is made by demonstrating *Ascaris* larvae in the sputum or gastric contents. *Ascaris* ova may also be detected in the feces at the time of onset of the pulmonary problem, but it is not unusual for the stools to be negative. However, patients with negative stools when first seen may begin to excrete eggs after a few weeks, upon maturation of the adult worms. The sputum frequently contains large numbers of eosinophils.

There is considerable controversy regarding the pathogenesis of this disorder. It seems unlikely that the mechanical effect of larvae per se is responsible for the symptoms, even though larvae in large numbers are present in the lungs of some patients with *Ascaris* pneumonia. It seems reasonable to assume that the pulmonary process is largely an allergic response to the presence of the worm or its products, quite analogous to other types of hypersensitivity pneumonitis.

It may be helpful in diagnosis to be aware of the fact that, irrespective of management and therapy, the majority of patients with *Ascaris* pneumonia recover within 2 weeks after onset.

SCHISTOSOMIASIS

Pulmonary involvement may occur during the course of schistosomiasis, but is rarely confused with acute microbial disease of the lung. Early in the disease, shortly after cercariae have penetrated the skin, cough and asthmatic symptoms may develop as the larvae pass through the pulmonary vasculature. However, the major pulmonary involvement occurs later, follows a chronic course, and is related to metastatic spread of ova produced by adult worms residing intravascularly at other sites. The ova reach the lungs by the hematogenous route and produce an obliterative granulomatous arteritis which leads to fibrosis, pulmonary hypertension, and cor pulmonale. The process is slowly progressive and characterized by cough, dyspnea, diffuse interstitial fibrosis, and fine parenchymal mottling. Hepatosplenomegaly and eosinophilia are present in most patients. Occasionally, apparently in response to the release of a large number of ova, an intense inflammatory reaction develops which produces an acute exacerbation of the chronic pulmonary process with severe respiratory distress, productive cough, hemoptysis, bilateral rales, and an increase in pulmonary infiltrates. Acute episodes of cough, wheezing, widespread infiltrates, and eosinophilia may also complicate therapy with trivalent antimonials; these manifestations are presumably secondary to a hypersensitivity reaction consequent to release of schistosomal antigens during therapy.

The diagnosis of pulmonary schistosomiasis is suggested by epidemiologic observations. *Schistosoma mansoni* is endemic in Africa, the Middle East, South America, and the Caribbean, *S. hematobium* in Africa and the Middle East, and *S. japonicum* in Japan, the Philippines, and the Chinese mainland. Pulmonary reactions to ova are most frequent in *S. hematobium* infections and are rare in *S. mansoni* and *S. japonicum* infections. This is related to the fact that the adult worms of *S. hematobium* reside in and release eggs into the systemic venous drainage of the bladder, whereas the adult worms of the other types are found for the most part in the portal circulation.

The diagnosis of schistosomiasis can be confirmed at times by demonstration of ova in sputum, but usually these are found only in feces, urine, or rectal biopsy tissue.

TRICHINOSIS

Most of the clinical manifestations of trichinosis are related to invasion and encystment of larvae in skeletal muscle. However, in massive infections large numbers of larvae may migrate through the lungs and produce petechiae and foci of acute pneumonitis. Pulmonary symptoms may include cough, blood-streaked sputum, dyspnea, and chest pain; blood-tinged pleural effusions and bronchopneumonia have been reported. The diagnosis is suggested by the findings of fever, myalgia, periorbital edema, subungual hemorrhages, and eosinophilia in a patient who gives a history of ingestion of raw pork. Specific diagnosis is made by detecting encysted larvae in muscle obtained by biopsy. The diagnosis can also be established by serologic means, although this approach will not be of value early in the infection.

STRONGYLOIDIASIS

During the pulmonary migration of the larvae of *Strongyloides stercoralis* pneumonitis may occur. This is characterized by fever, wheezing, productive cough, and patchy or diffuse infiltrates on chest roentgenography. Blood and sputum eosinophilia are common, and larvae may be detected in the sputum at times. Fresh stools should also be examined for larvae and eggs.

CREEPING ERUPTION

During the cutaneous migration of larvae of the dog and cat hookworm, some patients develop a transitory patchy infiltration of the lungs accompanied by marked eosinophilia in the blood and sputum. The intense itching and the erythematous, serpiginous skin lesion migrating 1 cm or so each day direct attention to the correct diagnosis.

VISCERAL LARVA MIGRANS

An interstitial pneumonitis or bronchopneumonia may occur during the course of visceral larva migrans. During pulmonary migration of larvae patients may have wheezing, cough, cyanosis, and even dyspnea, but these are only rarely the major manifestations of the disease. Hepatomegaly is a uniform finding, and splenomegaly is frequent. The syndrome is also characterized by fever, cutaneous eruptions, marked hypereosinophilia, leukocytosis in the range of 12,000 to 100,000 cells/cu mm, and hyperglobulinemia. The course of the disease may extend over a period of months.

This disease usually results from the ingestion of embryonated ova of the dog or cat roundworm, *Toxocara canis* or *T. mystax*, and occurs predominantly in young children who have close contact with dogs or cats and who eat dirt. The diagnosis is suspected on the basis of the clinical picture and a history of pica. The diagnosis can be established by liver biopsy, which reveals eosinophilic granulomas and larvae.

ECHINOCOCCOSIS

Echinococcal larvae may implant in the pulmonary parenchyma or, less commonly, in the pleura, especially the mediastinal pleura. Cyst formation occurs slowly, and clinical manifestations may not be observed for as long as 10 to 20 years after initial ingestion of eggs. Manifestations of *Echinococcus* cysts are usually those of a space-occupying lesion, and the signs and symptoms are related to slow compression or infiltration of adjacent tissues. Symptoms such as cough, hemoptysis, and pleurisy may be observed, but the clinical picture is usually not confused with pulmonary infection because there is little fever and the radiographic findings are not indicative of diffuse disease. Chest roentgenography shows one or more discrete, round lesions, usually sharply defined, without surrounding inflammatory response, and sometimes with a thinly calcified wall. These lesions are usually confused with metastatic carcinoma.

Rupture of an *Echinococcus* cyst into the tracheobronchial tree may give rise to an acute inflammatory reaction in the lungs. If rupture occurs there may be severe manifestations of hypersensitivity, including severe itching, urticaria, and vascular collapse. Once rupture of cysts into the tracheobronchial system has taken place, secondary infection is common.

Definitive diagnosis depends on recovery of hydatid elements from biopsy material or sputum. Serologic tests are available, but false-positive and false-negative tests occur. An epidemiologic history may be helpful in diagnosis. Hydatid disease is prevalent in the Middle East, Australia, New Zealand, Central Europe, and parts of Latin America, areas in which sheep are an important part of the economy. The disease is uncommon in North America except in certain areas of Canada and Alaska.

PARAGONIMIASIS

Paragonimus westermani, the adult lung fluke, may produce striking pulmonary disease. This infection is widespread in the Orient, especially in Japan, Taiwan, Korea, China, the Philippines, and Indonesia, and is usually acquired by eating uncooked crabs or crayfish harboring metacercariae, or by drinking water or other liquids harboring the detached organism. The metacercariae excyst in the duodenum, migrate through the intestinal wall, burrow through the diaphragm, and enter the lungs, where they develop to mature worms. Inflammation and fibrosis develop around the worms and lead to the formation of pulmonary cysts. These lesions are frequently found in the lower and midlung fields, and are associated with inflammation, consolidation, or abscess formation. Atelectasis and bronchiectasis are also common. Most of the pulmonary cysts eventually rupture into the tracheobronchial tree, giving rise to cough and blood-stained or purulent sputum. The roentgenogram shows nodular densities up to 4 cm in diameter. Secondary bacterial infection is common. The disease may resemble tuberculosis, pneumonia, or bronchiectasis.

The diagnosis should be suggested by the clinical picture in a person with appropriate epidemiologic background. The diagnosis is established by finding the eggs of the parasite in the sputum or feces. Aberrant worms sometimes wander into other parts of the body; subcutaneous creeping tumors in patients from endemic areas are strongly suggestive of paragonimiasis.

TOXOPLASMOSIS

Acquired disseminated toxoplasmosis, a rare disease, may be associated with pneumonitis as a component of the generalized organ involvement in this disease. The clinical picture is characterized by lymphadenitis, meningoencephalitis, hepatitis, myocarditis, maculopapular skin rash, high fever, and extreme prostration. The lung is rarely the focal point for diagnosis, and confusion with acute viral or bacterial pneumonia is unlikely. The diagnosis is established by isolation of the parasite from diseased tissue, or by serologic methods.

MALARIA

Respiratory symptoms and signs may occur in *Plasmodium falciparum* malaria, but these are usually overshadowed by the systemic manifestations of the disease. Cough, rales, rhonchi, and interstitial infiltrates may develop, and pulmonary edema has been reported as a complication. At least some of these findings are related to changes in the microcirculation in severe malaria. In the unlikely event that the pulmonary manifestations of malaria are confused with other types of acute inflammatory disease, epidemiologic circumstances should suggest the proper diagnosis, which should be rapidly confirmed by the presence of parasites in thick and thin blood films stained with Giemsa's stain.

Diseases of Nonmicrobial Origin

Cardiovascular Diseases

PULMONARY INFARCTION

The differential diagnosis of pulmonary infarction and bacterial pneumonia may be exceedingly difficult. The correct diagnosis can best be established by considering all aspects of the case. One of the best diagnostic clues may be the presence of a concurrent condition which predisposes to pulmonary thromboembolism or to bacterial pneumonia. Factors suggesting pulmonary infarction are venous disease of the legs, obesity, carcinoma, trauma to the legs or pelvis, or immobility. On the other hand, the presence of influenza, other virus infections of the respiratory tract, chronic lung disease, or bronchial obstruction should suggest the diagnosis of bacterial pneumonia. Some diseases predispose to both pulmonary infarction and pneumonia, the outstanding example being congestive heart failure with pulmonary congestion.

The presence of a shaking chill, especially in a patient with symptoms of a preceding upper respiratory infection, points strongly to the diagnosis of bacterial pneumonia. Shaking chills are rare in patients with pulmonary infarction.

The abrupt onset of dyspnea and tachypnea is suggestive of pulmonary infarction. In this situation cough is rarely present at the beginning of the illness, in contrast to most patients with bacterial pneumonia.

The height of the fever is not a good differential feature in the diagnosis of pulmonary infarction and pneumonia. Although it is true that a temperature above 102°F is not common in patients with pulmonary infarction, such temperatures occur with sufficient frequency to make the finding nonspecific. Other aspects of the physical examination may be helpful in differential diagnosis. Patients with pulmonary infarction rarely exhibit classical signs of pulmonary consolidation, whereas such findings are, of course, common in patients with bacterial pneumonia. A friction rub is common in both conditions, but a rub in the absence of radiographic manifestations of pulmonary consolidation is suggestive of pulmonary infarction.

The appearance of the sputum may be of diagnostic value. A purulent sputum containing large numbers of polymorphonuclear leukocytes shortly after the onset of symptoms, or the presence of a foul sputum, is highly suggestive of bacterial pneumonia. Although the sputum in patients with pulmonary infarction is frequently bloody, it usually does not contain large numbers of inflammatory cells. The total leukocyte count in patients with pulmonary infarction is usually normal; however, in some patients striking leukocytosis may be seen, with elevations as high as 40,000 cells/cu mm. In the individual patient the presence or absence of leukocytosis is not of diagnostic value.

Elevation of the serum lactic dehydrogenase, a normal serum glutamic-oxalacetic transaminase, and an elevated serum bilirubin level form a triad which was once considered to be a sensitive indicator of pulmonary infarction. Subsequent studies have shown that this is not the case, and that such findings are not of value in differential diagnosis of pulmonary infarction, pneumonia, or a host of other diseases.

The presence of bloody pleural effusion is suggestive of pulmonary infarction. However, it should be emphasized that many patients with pulmonary infarction have small accumulations of pleural fluid which are not bloody.

The radiographic manifestations may be of help. In patients with pulmonary infarction the lesion almost always impinges against the pleural surface. Pulmonary infarction predominates in the lower lobes of the lung, especially on the right side. The presence of multiple lesions is not helpful in differential diagnosis.

An electrocardiogram revealing evidence of right ventricular strain (right axis deviation, right ventricular conduction defects) is highly suggestive of a diagnosis of pulmonary infarction if one can be sure that such changes are new and correspond in time to the pulmonary process.

Scintillation scanning may be of help in diagnosis. However, any process responsible for parenchymal abnormalities in the lungs may result in decreased radioactivity within the involved region of the lung. A characteristic finding of pulmonary infarction, however, is the demonstration of a cold area in a portion of the lung in which the roentgenogram reveals no abnormality.

Arteriography probably constitutes the most specific means for differentiating pulmonary infarction from bacterial pneumonia. Patients with pulmonary infarction may show filling defects or vascular obstructions, findings which are not encountered in patients with pneumonia. Areas of vascular obstruction may undergo resolution rapidly, and an arteriogram may be normal if performed a week or more after an embolic episode.

PULMONARY EDEMA

Lobar pulmonary edema, with radiographic densities confined to a single lobe, may occasionally be confused with acute pulmonary infection. However, in most patients the history, physical findings of heart disease, and the absence of fever point to the correct diagnosis. When considering this differential diagnosis, the physician should recall that congestion in the lungs, irrespective of etiology, predisposes to bacterial pneumonia, and that pulmonary congestion and bacterial pneumonia not infrequently coexist.

Chemical and Physical Agents

BERYLLIOSIS

Beryllium may produce an acute pneumonitis which develops within hours or days after inhalation of the compound, or it may produce a chronic granulomatous disease of the lungs which develops months or years after the provoking event. The acute chemical pneumonitis may resemble pneumonia caused by microbial agents. Exposure is usually related to industrial use of the substance, and, for example, was relatively common in plants manufacturing fluorescent lamps prior to 1949. Industrial safety measures during recent years have greatly decreased the possibility of new cases. A careful history provides the information leading to diagnosis.

ACUTE HEROIN INTOXICATION

Ill-defined, fluffy, coalescent densities may develop throughout the lungs of patients with acute heroin overdosage. These edema-like changes usually clear within 24 to 48 hours. These lesions, which may be associated with fever and leukocytosis, may be confused with bacterial pneumonia, especially if the infiltrates are lobar in distribution. The diagnosis is usually established by the history and associated findings, such as stupor, coma, decreased respiratory rate, and constricted pupils. The pathogenesis of the lesions is not clear; they may represent pulmonary edema on a central basis, or may be a pulmonary reaction to foreign materials injected intravenously.

HYDROCARBON PNEUMONITIS

Acute pneumonitis may develop in patients who have ingested kerosene, gasoline, lighter fluid, furniture polish, or various cleaners. Turpentine, although not a petroleum product, behaves in the same way. Although these compounds or products of them may reach the lungs by way of the bloodstream, the pulmonary lesions usually result from inhalation or aspiration of the chemical. In these patients bilateral lung infiltrates visible on roentgenograms may develop within 30 minutes after ingestion of the compound. The vast majority of cases are observed in young children. The diagnosis is usually established by history.

PULMONARY LESIONS ASSOCIATED WITH IRRADIATION

Pulmonary changes secondary to irradiation for neoplastic disease usually consist of fibrosis. However, in some patients a transient form of pulmonary disease, characterized by slight fever, cough, chest pain, and radiographic changes of bronchopneumonia, may result from irradiation therapy. Diagnosis is suggested by the history of neoplastic disease under therapy with irradiation, but exclusion of pulmonary infection is difficult.

LIPOID PNEUMONITIS

Although cases of acute diffuse pulmonary disease resembling acute bacterial pneumonia have been reported after aspiration of large quantities of lipoid material, lipoid pneumonia usually follows a chronic course. The disease is most often seen in chronically ill and debilitated patients in whom aspiration is common. Ingestion of mineral oil or application of salves or other lipids to areas of the upper respiratory tract is followed by aspiration of the oil, which results in the formation of inflammatory foci, granulomas, and fibrosis. Cough, sputum, and dyspnea may be present in advanced cases, but symptoms are only occasionally acute. The diagnosis is suspected on the basis of the history. Lipid-laden macrophages can be demonstrated in the sputum weeks or months after the last known intake of lipoidal material.

PNEUMOCONIOSES

Pneumoconioses such as silicosis and asbestosis are characterized by pulmonary fibrosis and eventual pulmonary insufficiency. These diseases per se are rarely confused with acute pulmonary infection. Acute bacterial infection of the lungs is a common complication in these patients, because the distorted tracheobronchial architecture results in an increase in susceptibility to bacterial invasion.

SILO FILLER'S DISEASE

An acute pulmonary syndrome characterized by cough, dyspnea, and pulmonary infiltrates may develop after exposure to nitrogen dioxide gas. The acute process may be confused with pneumonia of microbial origin during the initial phases of illness. Exposure to the gas usually occurs in farmers working in a silo a few days after it has been filled; the nitrogen dioxide is a product of the fresh silage. This gas may also be formed after breakage of bottles of nitric acid or burning of nitrocellulose film. The clinical spectrum of the disease ranges from acute to chronic. A history of exposure to nitrogen dioxide is required for diagnosis.

Diseases of Presumed or Proven Immunologic Origin

ALLERGIC ALVEOLITIS OR HYPERSENSITIVITY PNEUMONITIS

Inhalation of protein-containing dusts of vegetable, microbial, or animal origin may produce impressive pulmonary manifestations in hypersensitive individuals. Farmer's lung is caused by inhalation of fungal spores on moldy hay, grain, or silage; bagassosis results from inhalation of dust of sugar cane pulp; byssinosis results from breathing dust created during blowing and carding raw cotton; maple bark stripper's lung is apparently the result of inhalation of fungal spores liberated in large numbers during stripping or sawing maple logs; and pigeon breeder's and budgerigar fancier's lung apparently result from hypersensitivity to feathers or droppings. Similar situations have been described in patients using pituitary snuff prepared from porcine and ox pituitaries, in mushroom pickers and malt workers, and in persons exposed to hen litter and redwood dust. Although precipitins against specific antigens have been demonstrated in some situations, in most it is unclear whether the hypersensitivity reaction is the result of exposure to contaminating microbes, such as fungi, to animal proteins, or to other antigens.

The clinical manifestations in these patients may be confused with those of acute microbial infection of the lung. Shortly after exposure, usually within hours, these patients develop breathlessness, cough, malaise, chills, fever, and rales, without wheezing, and exhibit diffuse macronodular densities on roentgenograms of the chest. Chronic illness may be observed in patients with prolonged or repeated exposure. Eosinophilia may be observed in some patients. Diagnosis is established by a history of respiratory exposure to allergenic agents such as those mentioned above. Precipitins to appropriate antigens may be demonstrated in the sera from some patients.

PULMONARY REACTIONS TO DRUGS

An acute illness characterized by chills, fever, cough, dyspnea, malaise, pleurisy, rales, and diffuse or localized pulmonary infiltrates may result from the ingestion of certain therapeutic agents. Drugs that have been incriminated include nitrofurantoin, sulfonamides, mecamylamine, mephenesin, aminosalicylic acid, and penicillin. In some instances the symptoms may be typical of Loeffler's syndrome, with marked eosinophilia and migratory flocculent infiltrates; in others eosinophilia is not prominent. Pleural effusions may occur, and are especially common in reactions to nitrofurantoin.

The diagnosis, which may be suggested by the presence of eosinophilia, depends on an accurate history which links the onset of pulmonary symptoms to drug ingestion. Nitrofurantoin seems especially likely to produce the syndrome. Strauss and Griffin reported one patient with recurrent "pneumonitis" on each of five occasions when she took nitrofurantoin for urinary tract infection. Another of their patients complained, "Doctor, why do I get fever and cough every time I come from the urologist?" The process should subside within a few days after stopping the drug, or should respond to corticosteroid therapy.

COLLAGEN-VASCULAR DISEASES

Systemic lupus erythematosus may be associated with pulmonary lesions which are confused with microbial infection; the problem of differential diagnosis is further complicated by the fact that bacterial infection of the lungs is common in these patients. Lupus pneumonitis, which often resembles atypical pneumonia, may be associated with dyspnea, rales, scattered infiltrates, and areas of atelectasis. Pleurisy and small effusions are quite common. The pulmonary process is rarely the primary manifestation of the disease, and the diagnosis is usually suggested by the presence of associated clinical or serologic findings of lupus.

Although the lungs are spared in most cases of necrotizing angiitis (including polyarteritis nodosa, hypersensitivity angiitis, and granulomatous arteritis), pulmonary lesions do occur occasionally, and may even precede the onset of manifestations resulting from involvement of other organs. The pulmonary involvement may be evident as asthma, chronic bronchitis, or pneumonitis which does not respond to antimicrobial drugs. The lung damage may be extensive, and may lead to fibrosis, bronchiectasis, and cavitation. Roentgenograms may reveal coarse miliary foci, transient infiltrations of the Loeffler type, or changes that may be mistaken for fibrocaseous tuberculosis. There may be striking eosinophilia. The multiplicity of signs and symptoms suggests the correct diagnosis, which is usually established on the basis of biopsy of muscle, skin, or other tissue.

Wegener's granulomatosis is characterized by the triad of necrotizing giant cell granulomatosis of the upper respiratory tract and lungs, widespread necrotizing vasculitis of small arteries and veins, and focal glomerulitis. The onset is usually suggestive of infection of the respiratory tract. Rhinorrhea, antral pain, epistaxis, cough, hemoptysis, pleurisy, mucosal ulceration, and widespread pulmonary consolidation are common. Severe renal disease is an almost uniform feature. Diagnosis is suggested by the presence of nasal or pulmonary infection which continues without response to antimicrobial therapy together with evidence of widespread organ involvement, especially renal dysfunction. Diagnosis is established by biopsy of the respiratory tract lesions or kidney. Differential diagnosis between this disease and pulmonary infection is compounded by the fact that secondary bacterial infection is common in Wegener's granulomatosis.

Pulmonary involvement is frequent in scleroderma. However, this fibrotic process is chronic in course and is rarely confused with acute microbial infection.

Goodpasture's syndrome might be confused with pulmonary infection, but this is unusual. This disease is characterized by pulmonary hemorrhage with hemoptysis and dyspnea, and evidence of glomerulonephritis. The pulmonary manifestations usually precede and overshadow the renal changes, but the latter suggest the diagnosis. The illness is rapidly fatal. Cough, chills, and fever may occur, but are much less common than hemoptysis.

Rheumatoid arthritis may be associated with nodular or fibrosing lesions in the lungs. These are not usually confused with acute microbial infections.

Acute rheumatic fever may be associated with lung involvement. Rheumatic pneumonia is most common in severe and fulminating cases, and the clinical or roentgenographic evidence of the pneumonic process is usually obscured by acute congestion of the lungs resulting from cardiac failure.

LOEFFLER'S SYNDROME

Loeffler in 1932 described a process characterized by patchy and fleeting pulmonary infiltrates and eosinophilia. The pulmonary infiltrates in this process may be unilateral or bilateral, are of short duration, and are frequently recurrent. Systemic symptoms are not usually marked; many patients have cough and some have fever, although most patients remain afebrile. Eosinophilia as high as 60 per cent is not unusual during an acute episode. Many different causes of this syndrome of pulmonary infiltrates with eosinophilia have been identified. Present concepts are that the pulmonary process represents an allergic response to a variety of antigens.

This syndrome is sometimes confused initially with viral or even bacterial pneumonia, but when the recurrent nature of the process is recognized, or when eosinophilia is detected, the problem becomes one of determining the etiologic basis for the pulmonary reaction. Many of the etiologic possibilities have been discussed elsewhere in this chapter; they are, broadly grouped, 1) various parasitic diseases in which parasites may be present in lung tissue or only in extrapulmonary tissues; 2) acute or chronic allergic states, including asthma, hay fever, and serum sickness; 3) a variety of drugs; 4) collagen-vascular disorders; 5) neoplastic diseases such as lymphomas, eosinophilic leukemia, and eosinophilic granuloma; 6) hypersensitivity states related to certain infections, such as tuberculosis, brucellosis, and fungal infections; and 7) idiopathic forms, in which no etiologic basis has been established.

Neoplastic Diseases

TUMORS OF THE LUNG

Primary or metastatic neoplastic disease of the lung is rarely confused per se with acute pulmonary infection. However, when the neoplasm produces bronchial obstruction acute bacterial infection distal to the obstruction is a frequent occurrence. In fact, bacterial pneumonia is frequently the initial manifestation of lung tumors producing bronchial obstruction. The conventional symptomatic, bacteriologic, or radiologic response to antimicrobial therapy may occur in these patients. However, in some patients the roentgenogram fails to clear because of the underlying neoplasm, an abscess forms distal to an obstructing tumor, or necrosis of a large tumor leads to cavity formation.

The possibility of lung carcinoma as a predisposing factor should always be considered in patients with pneumonia, especially if the pneumonia is recurrent, if the patient is a heavy smoker, if respiratory symptoms, notably cough or hemoptysis, were present before the onset of acute infection, if there is a history of wheezing before the onset of infection, or if there is a poor response to antimicrobial therapy with incomplete clearing of the infiltrate.

Diagnosis can be established by cytologic study of sputum or bronchial washings, bronchoscopy, or exploratory thoracotomy.

LEUKEMIA

Although pulmonary infiltrates and symptoms and signs of lung infection are common in patients with leukemia, these are not usually the result of leukemic infiltration of the lungs, but are caused by a complicating microbial infection of the pulmonary parenchyma. Microscopic evidence of leukemic infiltration of the lungs has been reported in as many as one-third of patients with leukemia of all types coming to autopsy. However, only about one-fifth of these have shown roentgenographic evidence of leukemic infiltration. Radiographic findings usually include diffuse peribronchial infiltrations which are not localized, or nodular lesions; consolidation caused by the leukemic process is exceedingly rare.

Miscellaneous Diseases

ATELECTASIS

Collapse of the lung, irrespective of etiology, may be associated with dyspnea and cough. However, this condition does not cause fever, leukocytosis, and purulent sputum, and should not be confused with acute pneumonia. These findings in patients with clinical or radiologic evidence of lung collapse are usually related to bacterial infection in the atelectatic area.

DESQUAMATIVE INTERSTITIAL PNEUMONIA

This chronic disease may be confused in its early stages with microbial infection of the respiratory tract. An upper respiratory infection precedes the onset of illness in many patients. Patients complain of cough and progressive shortness of breath. The roentgenogram shows a ground glass opacification of the bases of the lungs radiating to the hila. Lung biopsy is required for diagnosis.

HAMMAN-RICH LUNG (DIFFUSE IDIOPATHIC INTERSTITIAL PULMONARY FIBROSIS)

Patients with this syndrome usually show relatively rapid onset, over days to weeks, of progressive dyspnea, orthopnea, minor degrees of hemoptysis, constricting chest pain, increasing cyanosis, persistent unproductive cough, and diffuse pulmonary shadows of interstitial fibrosis. The majority of patients are afebrile at first. In patients with rapid onset of symptoms the process may be confused occasionally with acute pulmonary infection. The disease does not respond to antimicrobial therapy and usually follows a chronic progressive course.

IDIOPATHIC PULMONARY HEMOSIDEROSIS

This rare disease of unknown etiology results from recurrent pulmonary hemorrhages from small blood vessels, presumably pulmonary capillaries. The recurrent febrile episodes of hemoptysis associated with cough, dyspnea, and diffuse pulmonary mottling on roentgenography may be confused with acute pulmonary infection. Although difficulty may be encountered in the differential diagnosis of a single episode, consideration of all aspects of the case should indicate clearly that an underlying process other than infection is present. In the vast majority of reported cases the onset of the disease is before the age of 16 years, and almost always before the age of 30. Hypochromic anemia is present because of blood loss, and hepatosplenomegaly, clubbing of the fingers, and eosinophilia are relatively common. The diagnosis is suspected on the basis of the history and physical examination and confirmed by the demonstration of hemosiderin-laden macrophages (siderophages) in the sputum. Although the pulmonary lesions clear completely during the initial phases of the disease, repeated hemorrhages over months or years lead to hemosiderosis and fibrosis, and permanent changes characterized by miliary stippling and linear striations in the lungs on roentgenography.

INFLAMMATORY DISEASES BELOW THE DIAPHRAGM (ACUTE PANCREATITIS, SPLENIC ABSCESS OR INFARCTION, CHOLECYSTITIS, OR SUBDIAPHRAGMATIC ABSCESS)

Any inflammatory process below the diaphragm but near enough to involve that structure can lead to small accumulations of pleural fluid on the involved side and areas of atelectasis secondary to elevation and immobility of the diaphragm. These changes, especially in patients with underlying diseases associated with fever, may lead to confusion with pneumonia of microbial origin. Signs of the basic condition are usually more prominent than those of the pulmonary process, and point to the correct diagnosis. However, respiratory symptoms may, on rare occasions, overshadow the abdominal complaints. In patients with pancreatitis and pleurisy it is of interest that pancreatic enzyme concentrations are higher in the pleural effusion than in simultaneously obtained serum. Pancreatic enzymes are thought to reach the pleural space from the abdominal cavity via lymphatic channels.

INTRAPULMONARY HEMORRHAGE

Moderate to large intrapulmonary hemorrhage, irrespective of etiology, may give rise to pulmonary densities simulating pneumonia. Alveoli in an area of lung are filled with blood, which evokes a moderate inflammatory response and leads to fever, dyspnea, cough, and, of course, bloody sputum. Vascular erosion in tuberculous cavities was a relatively common cause of hemorrhage in the past; a similar event may occur rarely in a lung abscess or any other cavitary disease. Intrapulmonary hemorrhage may also occur as a rare complication of anticoagulant therapy; Reussi and associates recently reported on two patients receiving anticoagulant therapy for coronary artery disease who developed fever, dyspnea, cough, and bloody sputum in association with diffuse densities on chest roentgenograms.

The magnitude of the hemoptysis, the relatively minor nature of the constitutional symptoms, and the rapidly changing radiographic picture make differentiation of intrapulmonary hemorrhage from acute pulmonary infection relatively easy.

PNEUMONIA OF THE CHOLESTEROL TYPE

Cholesterol pneumonia often starts abruptly, and in about half the cases is mistaken for either influenza or lobar pneumonia. Other cases pursue a more chronic course characterized by fever, cough, pleuritic pain, and hemoptysis, and are frequently misdiagnosed as bronchial carcinoma, lung abscesses, or unresolved pneumonia. The diagnosis is usually established on the basis of pathologic examination of lung tissue, showing marked fibrosis and deposits of cholesterol and cholesterol esters within enlarged macrophages.

PULMONARY ALVEOLAR PROTEINOSIS

This disease, in which large groups of alveoli are filled with proteinaceous material, is characterized by progressive dyspnea, expectoration of sputum containing gelatinous material which may be blood-streaked, chest pain, fatigue, and weight loss. Some patients have persistent pyrexia. The roentgenogram reveals diffuse, soft densities radiating from the hila of the lungs, suggestive of pulmonary edema. The disease is chronic and is rarely confused for very long with acute pulmonary infections. However, it should be noted that alveolar proteinosis may be complicated by terminal nocardial infection.

SARCOIDOSIS

Sarcoidosis involves the lungs with the formation of granulomas which eventually lead to fibrosis. Fever of slight to moderate degree, weight loss, and fatigue occur in about 40 per cent of the patients. These symptoms, coupled with diffuse pulmonary granulomas or fibrosis, may lead to confusion with pneumonia of microbial etiology. However, the chronic nature of the process, the frequency of lymph node involvement, and manifestations related to involvement of other organs usually lead to the correct diagnosis. The not infrequent late complication of pulmonary aspergillosis has been referred to previously.

AN APPROACH TO DIAGNOSIS

Diagnosis at the Bedside

The physician who is responsible for the care of a patient with acute inflammatory disease of the lungs—a patient with fever, respiratory symptoms, and pulmonary infiltrates on roentgenogram—must promptly establish a presumptive etiologic diagnosis. This approach is necessary because certain acute inflammatory processes—notably the bacterial pneumonias—must be treated promptly with antimicrobial agents if morbidity and mortality are to be reduced. Although definitive diagnostic procedures (e.g., isolation of the etiologic agent, serologic tests) may be initiated shortly after the initial history and physical examination, the results of these tests will probably not be available for some time; thus, the initial diagnosis upon which therapy is based must be formulated from data obtained from the history, physical examination, and a few simple procedures, such as the sputum smear, leukocyte count, and chest roentgenogram.

Many etiologic possibilities, as listed in Tables 33 and 34, must be considered in a patient with acute inflammatory disease of the lungs. In actual practice most physicians, either consciously or unconsciously, group the etiologic possibilities into broad categories by asking, "Is the process infectious or noninfectious?" The immediate clinical decision whether a respiratory illness is infectious or noninfectious is made on the basis of many factors; however, the most important ones which point toward an infectious etiology are as follows.

1. The history of an event or the presence of another disease which favors aspiration of upper respiratory or stomach secretions or which enhances susceptibility to infection (e.g., premonitory upper respiratory infection, acute alcoholism, epilepsy, achalasia of the esophagus, acute leukemia).

2. An epidemiologic history indicating susceptibility and exposure to a specific infectious agent (e.g., varicella, tularemia, measles, psittacosis).

3. Clear-cut signs of infection at extrapulmonary sites which suggest the possibility of metastatic infection to the lungs (e.g., staphylococcal cellulitis).

4. Infection at a distant site which appears to have originated from a pulmonary lesion (e.g., pneumococcal meningitis).

5. The presence of a generalized infection which can be diagnosed on the basis of the clinical evidence and which is known to be associated with pulmonary involvement (e.g., varicella, measles).

6. The presence of purulent sputum.

7. The presence of definite chills and high fever (above 104°F).

8. The presence of pleural fluid shown to be purulent or containing microorganisms on staining.

9. Physical and roentgenographic findings of lobar consolidation.

10. Failure to demonstrate the presence of noninfectious diseases which could account for the pulmonary lesions.

The factors mentioned in the preceding paragraphs are, of course, not absolute, and many exceptions exist. However, if, after weighing the evidence for and against microbial or nonmicrobial disease, the decision is made that the etiology of the pulmonary process is infectious, the physician must then go further to make a presumptive microbiologic diagnosis, for this will form the basis for initial antimicrobial therapy. One approach would be to review the causes of pneumonia of microbial origin as listed in Table 33 and formulate a list of the most likely etiologic possibilities. Although this approach has merit, it is more common for the physician at first to group the etiologic possibilities by asking, "Is the process bacterial or nonbacterial in origin?" and then consider the most likely etiologic agents within these major subdivisions. This approach takes advantage of the fact that the common bacterial pathogens of the lung, notably pneumococci, staphylococci, *Klebsiella*, the enteric bacilli, and the organisms associated with necrotizing pneumonia, produce, in general, a relatively characteristic clinical picture—"the bacterial pneumonia syndrome" (Table 35). The majority of these patients have abrupt onset of fever associated with cough productive of purulent sputum which frequently contains blood. Shaking chills and pleuritic chest pain are common, and a history of some predisposing event, such as an upper respiratory infection, is often present. Pulmonary consolidation can be demonstrated by roentgenography, and leukocytosis frequently occurs.

TABLE 35

Features Differentiating Bacterial from Nonbacterial Pneumonia

Parameter	Bacterial Pneumonia*	Nonbacterial Pneumonia†
Age	Frequently over 50 years	Usually young adults
Health status before onset	May obtain history of underlying condition favoring aspiration or increasing susceptibility	Underlying diseases usually not present; however, heart or lung disease or pregnancy common in influenza virus pneumonia
Animal exposure		Exposure to birds raises possibility of psittacosis; cattle, sheep, and goats, the possibility of Q fever
Onset	Usually rapid	Slower than in bacterial
Shaking chills	Characteristic	Not characteristic; usually chilly sensations
Myalgias	Not characteristic	Characteristic
Hemoptysis	Rusty sputum frequent	Rusty sputum not characteristic; sputum may be blood-streaked
Substernal pain	May occur, but is not characteristic	Burning substernal pain with severe cough is common
General appearance	May be quite ill, even moribund	Usually not critically ill
Respirations	Increased respiratory rate; may be dyspneic	Respiratory rate usually normal
Pulse	Tachycardia frequent	May see bradycardia
Cyanosis	Not unusual	Quite unusual
Delirium	Not unusual	Quite unusual
Dehydration	Frequent	Infrequent
Temperature-pulse disproportion	Rare	Relatively common
Signs of consolidation	Common	Not as common as in bacterial pneumonia
Location of pulmonary findings	Frequently unilateral	Often bilateral, diffuse
Splenomegaly	Rare	Not unusual in psittacosis and Q fever

TABLE 35—*Continued*

Parameter	Bacterial Pneumonia*	Nonbacterial Pneumonia†
Skin rash	Not characteristic	May suggest varicella, measles, etc.
Fever	Frequently over 104°F except in the elderly or persons with chronic disease	Generally below 103°F, but children may have temperature to 105°F
Tonsillar exudate	Not characteristic but may occur rarely in streptococcal pneumonia	Suggests adenovirus infection
Fever blisters	Common	Not common
Leukocyte count	Characteristically high, but may be low in patients critically ill or in those with *Klebsiella* or *Pseudomonas* pneumonia	Leukocytosis not characteristic during acute phase; however, may increase to 15,000–20,000 cells/cu mm in second week of disease
Sputum	Shows polymorphonuclear leukocytes and perhaps intracellular bacteria	Sputum more likely clear without pus cells
Eosinophilia	Not characteristic	Not characteristic, but may suggest pulmonary disease of immunologic origin
Evidence of meningitis	Purulent meningitis present occasionally	Lymphocytic meningitis or meningoencephalitis present occasionally
Response to therapy	Specific therapy may be followed by dramatic improvement within 24–48 hours	Response is characteristically slow or does not occur

* Especially pneumococcal, staphylococcal, *Klebsiella*, necrotizing, and Gram-negative bacillary pneumonias.
† Especially viral, mycoplasmal, and rickettsial pneumonias and psittacosis.

In contrast, certain of the "nonbacterial" agents, notably viruses, mycoplasmas, rickettsiae, and the agent of psittacosis, produce a clinical syndrome after invasion of the lower respiratory tract which is usually different from that caused by the ordinary bacteria (Table 35). This "nonbacterial or atypical pneumonia syndrome" is characterized by insidious onset, fever, anorexia, headache, and myalgia, followed by a hacking, irritating cough which is occasionally productive of sputum streaked with blood. On physical examination the chest is frequently normal or shows minimal signs of pneumonia, but roentgenographic examination of the lungs demonstrates hazy, patchy areas of infiltration which often involve more than one lobe.

Although utilization of the concept of "bacterial pneumonia" and "nonbacterial pneumonia" syndromes is worthwhile in establishing a presumptive etiologic diagnosis, it should be emphasized that the distinction is not absolute. Ordinary bacteria may occasionally produce the picture of "atypical pneumonia," and rarely viruses or mycoplasmas may cause a picture closely resembling acute bacterial pneumonia.

On the basis of this approach and other information obtained from the history, physical examination, and routine laboratory and roentgenographic examinations, the physician may be able to develop a relatively accurate presumptive etiologic diagnosis. If the findings are indicative of bacterial pneumonia, the results of Gram or other stains of the sputum obviously will be considered in further subdividing the etiologic possibilities; the role of the sputum smear in diagnosis is discussed in a subsequent paragraph.

Role of Previous Antimicrobial Therapy in Diagnosis

Previous antimicrobial therapy may be a factor of considerable importance in diagnosis in a patient with pneumonia. If a patient has shown a dramatic response to therapy within 24 to 36 hours, a diagnosis of bacterial pneumonia, probably pneumococcal, is quite likely. However, if fever and systemic symptoms continue despite the administration of an antimicrobial agent, several possibilities should be considered: 1) superinfection of the lungs may have taken place with bacteria resistant to the antibiotic administered; 2) the pneumonia may be related to a microbial agent insensitive to the antibiotic administered; 3) persistent fever may represent an allergic reaction to the antibiotic; 4) fever may be caused by a coexistent process unrelated to the pneumonia; 5) the diagnosis of pneumonia may be incorrect, the pulmonary manifestations representing an expression of a systemic noninfectious disease; 6) the antibiotic may not have been given sufficiently long to obtain a response; this might occur in staphylococcal pneumonia or other suppurative processes characterized by abscess formation; 7) a localized suppurative complication of bacterial pneumonia may have developed; or 8) the dose of the antimicrobial agent may be inadequate, or the history of antimicrobial therapy may be incorrect.

Roentgenographic Findings in Diagnosis

The information obtained from chest roentgenograms in a patient with acute inflammatory disease of the lungs must be integrated with all the other findings in arriving at a correct diagnosis. A posteroanterior view and lateral film should be obtained if possible; portable films are frequently of poor quality, and should be obtained only as a last resort. Right or left lateral decubitus views should be obtained if the diagnosis of pleural effusion is in doubt, because layering may provide conclusive proof of the presence of fluid.

Dense lobar consolidation is more characteristic of bacterial pneumonia than of pneumonia caused by other microbial agents. Viral or mycoplasmal pneumonia is usually less dense than bacterial pneumonia, and often gives the appearance of an interstitial or diffuse process. Pleural reactions and pleural effusions are definitely more suggestive of bacterial than viral or mycoplasmal pneumonia. Pneumatoceles are characteristic of staphylococcal pneumonia, but also occur occasionally in *Hemophilus influenzae* and group A streptococcal pneumonia. Pneumatoceles are exceedingly unusual in viral or mycoplasmal pneumonia.

The occurrence of pneumothorax in a patient with pneumonia, especially pyopneumothorax, suggests a staphylococcal etiology; this complication occurs primarily in infants, but may be seen occasionally in adults.

Radiolucent areas may indicate early abscess formation and point to a diagnosis of staphylococcal, *Klebsiella*, type III pneumococcal, or tuberculous pneumonia. Abscess formation also occurs frequently in aspiration or necrotizing pneumonia and, in this situation, characteristically develops in the midlung field, especially the superior segments of the lower lobes and the lingula.

Any intense inflammatory lesion of the lungs may be associated with marked edema of a lobe and lead to bulging of an interlobar fissure. This process is not unusual in Friedlander's pneumonia; however, bulging of the fissure also occurs in type III pneumococcal infection and may be observed rarely with other types of pulmonary infection.

Microbiologic Techniques in Diagnosis

The diagnostic work-up of patients with acute inflammatory disease of the lungs should include sputum smears for bacteria (and in some instances for tubercle bacilli or fungi), sputum culture, and one or two blood cultures. If pleural effusion is present, the fluid should be obtained and examined by appropriately stained smears and by culture.

Sputum can be obtained from almost all patients with pneumonia. In patients who are unable to produce sputum voluntarily, several techniques may prove helpful in obtaining a specimen: 1) deep breathing will sometimes be effective in evoking cough and sputum; 2) breathing aerosolized water for 5 to 10 minutes may lead to condensation of sufficient water on the respiratory mucosa to make a dry cough productive; 3) a nasal catheter inserted into the upper trachea will often cause a paroxysm of cough productive of sputum; or 4) transtracheal aspiration is virtually always effective in obtaining a sputum specimen, although this technique should not be employed routinely.

Although cultures of sputum, blood, and pleural fluid may provide definitive diagnostic evidence, these procedures will probably not yield useful information for 18 to 24 hours or even longer. Thus, as mentioned previously, initial antimicrobial therapy for patients with pneumonia must be based in large part on the findings in the Gram-stained smear of sputum and the evaluation of the clinical status of the patient. The presence of a preponderance of Gram-positive, lancet-shaped diplococci, clusters of Gram-positive cocci, or encapsulated Gram-negative rods would suggest pneumococcal, staphylococcal, or Friedlander's pneumonia, respectively, and antimicrobial therapy would be planned accordingly. Unfortunately, the findings on examination of the sputum smear are frequently equivocal; under these circumstances, if the patient is quite ill, it is sometimes advisable to plan relatively broad-spectrum antimicrobial therapy to cover the most likely etiologic possibilities until the results of the cultures become available.

Other Techniques Helpful in Diagnosis

Skin Tests

In many patients skin testing with tuberculin (intermediate strength) or fungus skin test antigens should be undertaken. Interpretation of results is discussed under each of the diseases in the preceding sections.

Serologic Tests

If the etiology of an acute pulmonary process is at all in doubt, an acute serum specimen should be obtained and stored. If it becomes evident that certain serologic tests might be helpful in diagnosis, such as those for *Mycoplasma* or virus pneumonia, a second specimen can be drawn later and studied in concert with the acute specimen.

Biopsy of Tissue

In some patients, usually as it becomes evident that the process is not responding to therapy and is becoming chronic, biopsy of a palpable lymph node, pleura, bone marrow, or liver for diagnostic purposes may be desirable. Percutaneous or open lung biopsy may be indicated in an occasional patient.

Bronchoscopy

Direct visualization of the larger radicles of the tracheobronchial tree may be indicated in certain instances to look for constrictions produced by tumor or other causes. Bronchial aspirates or washings should always be obtained at bronchoscopy and subjected to complete microbiologic and cytologic study.

Special Stains

Sputum should be stained with methenamine silver stain in patients suspected of *Pneumocystis* infection. Staining with specific antibody labeled with fluorescein may aid in detection of certain viruses (e.g., influenza) in the sputum, but these techniques are not available in most clinical laboratories. Sudan stains may reveal fat particles in the sputum.

398   EDWARD W. HOOK

TABLE 36

Sequence of Work-up of Patients with Acute Inflammatory Disease of the lungs

I. Make a presumptive diagnosis (including a presumptive microbiologic diagnosis if the process is considered to be microbial in origin) on the basis of
  A. History
  B. Physical examination
  C. Roentgenogram of chest
  D. Simple laboratory tests, including sputum smears and examination of pleural fluid, if present
II. Immediately initiate procedures required for definitive diagnosis
  A. Sputum culture for bacteria in all instances; also for tubercle bacilli, fungi, viruses, etc., in certain instances
  B. Blood cultures
  C. Pleural fluid cultures when possible
  D. Special stains, such as for fungi and *Pneumocystis*, if indicated
  E. Store acute serum if diagnosis is obscure
III. Initiate antimicrobial therapy, if appropriate
IV. Observe response; proceed with additional studies as indicated, especially if response to antimicrobials does not occur

Isolation of Viruses, Rickettsiae, and Mycoplasmas

Techniques are available for the isolation of these respiratory pathogens, but in general the methods are costly, slow, and unavailable in most clinical laboratories. At the present time the demonstration of a specific antibody response by serologic tests is a more practical approach to diagnosis.

The Sequence of Diagnostic Work-ups

The sequence of the diagnostic work-up is summarized in Table 36. If this approach is followed, rational therapy aimed at the most likely diagnosis can be initiated promptly in patients with acute inflammatory disease of the lungs. If all available diagnostic tests, including virus isolation and serologic techniques, were to be applied, a definitive diagnosis could be established in the large majority of such patients. A complete diagnostic work-up is not, of course, indicated in all patients, and the physician must decide on the extent of the work-up in each patient. Detailed virologic study is rarely indicated at the present time, except for research purposes.

BIBLIOGRAPHY

The bibliography is grouped according to the broad etiologic classification presented in Tables 26 and 27. References are not included for all entities that are discussed; standard texts should be consulted for more complete dissertations.

Bacteria—Frequently Encountered

1. Austrian, R., and Gold, J. Pneumococcic bacteremia with especial reference to bacteremic pneumococcic pneumonia. Ann. Internal Med. **60**:759, 1964.
2. Bernhard, W. F., Malcom, J. A., and Wylie, R. N. Lung abscess. Dis. Chest **43**:620, 1963.
3. Bizzozero, O. J., and Andriole, V. T. Tetracycline-resistant pneumococcal infection. Arch. Internal Med. **123**:388, 393, 1969.
4. Burmeister, R. W., Dreiling, B. J., Bazzano, G., and Brown, G. O. Pneumococcal pneumonia with leucopenia—the role of folic acid. Clin. Res. **14**:338, 1966.

5. Chomet, B., and Gach, B. M. Lobar pneumonia and alcoholism: an analysis of thirty-seven cases. Amer. J. Med. Sci. 253:300, 1967.
6. Cluff, L. E., and Reynolds, R. J. Management of staphylococcal infections. Amer. J. Med. 39:812, 1965.
7. Dines, D. E. Diagnostic significance of pneumatocele of the lung. J.A.M.A. 204:1169, 1968.
8. Epstein, M., Calia, F. M., and Gabuzda, G. J. Pneumococcal peritonitis in patients with postnecrotic cirrhosis. N. Engl. J. Med. 278:69, 1968.
9. Fekety, F. R., Jr., and McKaniel, E. The fever index in evaluation of the course of infectious diseases, with special reference to pneumococcal pneumonia. Yale J. Biol. Med. 41:282, 1968.
10. Hansman, D. Hospital infection with pneumococci resistant to tetracycline. Med. J. Aust. 1:498, 1967.
11. Hoffman, N. R., and Preston, F. S., Jr. Friedlander's pneumonia. A report of 11 cases and appraisal of antibiotic therapy. Dis. Chest 53:481, 1968.
12. Kabins, S. A., and Lerner, C. Fulminant pneumococcemia and sickle cell anemia. J.A.M.A. 211:467, 1970.
13. Kaye, D., and Hook, E. W. Acute bronchopulmonary infections. Mod. Treat. 1:240, 1964.
14. Kislak, J. W. Type 6 pneumococcus resistant to erythromycin and lincomycin. N. Engl. J. Med. 276:852, 1967.
15. Lampe, W. T., II. Klebsiella pneumonia: a review of forty-five cases and re-evaluation of the incidence and antibiotic sensitivities. Dis. Chest 46:599, 1964.
16. Louria, D. B., and Kaminski, T. The effects of four antimicrobial drug regimens on sputum superinfection in hospitalized patients. Amer. Rev. Resp. Dis. 85:649, 1962.
17. Mertz, J. J., Scharer, L., and McClement, J. H. A hospital outbreak of Klebsiella pneumonia from inhalation therapy with contaminated aerosol solutions. Amer. Rev. Resp. Dis. 95:454, 1967.
18. Pierce, A. K., Edmonson, E. B., McGee, G., Ketchersid, J., Loudon, R. G., and Sanford, J. P. An analysis of factors predisposing to Gram-negative bacillary necrotizing pneumonia. Amer. Rev. Resp. Dis. 94:309, 1966.
19. Rathbun, H. K., and Govani, I. Mouse inoculations as a means of identifying pneumococci in the sputum. Bull. Johns Hopkins Hosp. 120:46, 1967.
20. Rogers, D. E. Staphylococcal infections. Dis. Month (April 1958).
21. Schweppe, H. I., Knowles, J. H., and Kane, L. Lung abscess. N. Engl. J. Med. 265:1039, 1961.
22. Tillotson, J. R., and Lerner, A. M. Pneumonias caused by Gram-negative bacilli Medicine 45:65, 1966.
23. Tillotson, J. R., and Lerner, A. M. Characteristics of pneumonias caused by Escherichia coli. N. Engl. J. Med. 277:115, 1967.
24. Tillotson, J. R., and Lerner, A. M. Characteristics of pneumonias caused by Bacillus proteus. Ann. Internal Med. 68:287, 1968.
25. Tillotson, J. R., and Lerner, A. M. Characteristics of nonbacteremic Pseudomonas pneumonia. Ann. Internal Med. 68:295, 1968.

Bacteria—Infrequently Encountered

26. Basiliere, J. L., Bistrong, H. W., and Spence, W. F. Streptococcal pneumonia. Recent outbreaks in military recruit populations. Amer. J. Med. 44:580, 1968.
27. Black, P. H., Kunz, L. J., and Swartz, M. N. Salmonellosis—a review of some unusual aspects. N. Engl. J. Med. 262:811, 864, 921, 1960.
28. Blattner, R. J. Pneumonia caused by type B meningococcus. J. Pediat. 71:442 1967.
29. Brachman, P. S., Plotkin, S. A., Bumford, F. H., and Atchison, M. M. An epidemic of inhalation anthrax. II. Epidemiologic investigation. Amer. J. Hyg. 72:6, 1960.
30. Finegold, M. J. Pathogenesis of plague. A review of plague deaths in the United States during the last decade. Amer. J. Med. 45:549, 1968.
31. Gold, H. Anthrax: report of 117 cases. Arch. Internal Med. 96:387, 1955.
32. Gorfinkel, J. H., Brown, R., and Kabins, S. A. Acute infectious epiglottitis in adults. Ann. Internal Med. 70:289, 1969.

33. Hammett, J. B. Death from pneumonia with bacteremia due to Mimeae tribe bacterium. J.A.M.A. **206**:641, 1968.
34. Howe, C. Glanders. In *Oxford Medicine*, Christian, H. A., Ed. Vol. 5, Pt. 1, p. 185. Oxford University Press, New York, 1950.
35. Huckstep, R. L. *Typhoid Fever and Other Salmonella Infections.* E. & S. Livingstone, Ltd., Edinburgh, 1962.
36. Johnson, W. D., Kaye, D., and Hook, E. W. *Hemophilus influenzae* pneumonia in adults. Report of five cases and review of the literature. Amer. Rev. Resp. Dis. **97**:1112, 1968.
37. Paine, R. T., Jr., Garrard, D. L., Jr., and Walker, P. J. Meningococcal pneumonia. Arch. Internal Med. **119**:111, 1967.
38. Patterson, M. D., Darling, C. L., and Blumenthal, J. B. Acute melioidosis in a soldier home from South Vietnam. J.A.M.A. **200**:117, 1967.
39. Spink, W. W. *The Nature of Brucellosis.* University of Minnesota Press, Minneapolis, 1956.
40. Swartz, M. N., and Kunz, L. J. *Pasteurella multocida* infections in man. Report of two cases—meningitis and infected cat bite. N. Engl. J. Med. **261**:889, 1959.
41. Weber, D. R., Douglas, L. E., Brundage, W. G., and Stallkamp, T. C. Acute varieties of melioidosis occurring in U. S. soldiers in Vietnam. Amer. J. Med. **46**: 234, 1969.
42. Young, L. S., Bicknell, D. S., Archer, B. G., Clinton, J. M., Leavens, L. J., Feely, J. C., and Brachman, P. S. Tularemia epidemic: Vermont, 1968. Forty-seven cases linked to contact with muskrats. N. Engl. J. Med. **280**:1253, 1969.

Bacteria-like Agents (Mycoplasma Pneumonia and Psittacosis)

43. Capps, S. C., Allen, V. D., Sueltmann, A., and Evans, A. S. A community outbreak of Mycoplasma pneumonia. J.A.M.A. **204**:123, 1968.
44. George, R. B., Weill, H., Rasch, J. R., Mogabgab, W. J., and Ziskind, M. M. Roentgenographic appearance of viral and Mycoplasma pneumonia. Amer. Rev. Resp. Dis. **96**:1144, 1967.
45. Grayson, J. T., Kenny, G. E., Foy, H. M., Kronman, R. A., and Alexander, E. R. Epidemiological studies of *Mycoplasma pneumoniae* infection in civilians. Ann. N. Y. Acad. Sci. **143**:436–446, 1967.
46. Mogabgab, W. J. *Mycoplasma pneumoniae* and adenovirus respiratory illnesses in military and university personnel, 1959–1966. Amer. Rev. Resp. Dis. **97**:345, 1968.
47. Schaffner, W., Drutz, D. J., Duncan, G. W., and Koenig, M. G. The clinical spectrum of endemic psittacosis. Arch. Internal Med. **119**:433, 1968.
48. Smith, C. B., Friedwald, W. T., and Chanock, R. M. Shedding of *Mycoplasma pneumoniae* after tetracycline and erythromycin therapy. N. Engl. J. Med. **276**:1172, 1967.
49. Taylor, M. J., Burrow, G. N., Strauch, B., and Horstman, D. M. Meningoencephalitis associated with pneumonitis due to *Mycoplasma* pneumonitis. J.A.M.A. **199**:813, 1967.
50. Tyrrell, D. A. J. Clinical syndromes with Mycoplasma infections. Postgrad. Med. J. **43**:105, 1967.

Spirochetes

51. Alston, J. M., and Broom, J. C. *Leptospirosis in Man and Animals.* E. & S. Livingstone, Edinburgh, 1958.
52. Edwards, G. A., and Domm, B. M. Human leptospirosis. Medicine **39**:117, 1960.

Viruses

53. Andrews, C. H., and Tyrrell, D. A. J. Rhinoviruses. In *Viral and Rickettsial Infections of Man*, Horsfall, F. L., and Tamm, I., Eds., p. 546. J. B. Lippincott Co., Philadelphia, 1965.
54. Bryant, R. E., and Rhoades, E. R. Clinical features of adenoviral pneumonia in air force recruits. Amer. Rev. Resp. Dis. **96**:717, 1967.
55. Chanock, R. M., and Parrott, R. H. Para-influenza viruses. In *Viral and Rickett-*

sial Infections of Man, Horsfall, F. L., and Tamm, I., Eds., p. 741. J. B. Lippincott Co., Philadelphia, 1965.
56. Gwaltney, J. M., Jr., and Jordan, W. S., Jr. The present status of respiratory viruses. Med. Clin. N. Amer. 47:115, 1963.
57. Katz, S. L. Measles—its complications, treatment and prophylaxis. Med. Clin. N. Amer. 46:1163, 1962.
58. Kaye, D., Rosenbluth, M., Hook, E. W., and Kilbourne, E. D. Endemic influenza. II. The nature of the disease in the postpandemic period. Amer. Rev. Resp. Dis. 85:9, 1962.
59. Knyett, A. F. The pulmonary lesions of chickenpox. Quart. J. Med. 35:313, 1966.
60. Krugman, S., and Ward, R. Acute respiratory disease—etiology and clinical syndromes. In Infectious Diseases of Children, Krugman, S., and Ward, R., Eds., p. 221. C. V. Mosby Co., St. Louis, 1968.
61. Lepow, M. L., Balassanian, N., Emmerick, J., Roberts, R. B., Rosenthal, M. S., and Wolinsky, E. Interrelationships of viral, mycoplasmal and bacterial agents in uncomplicated pneumonia. Amer. Rev. Resp. Dis. 97:533, 1969.
62. Louria, D. B., Blumenfeld, H. L., Ellis, J. T., Kilbourne, E. D., and Rogers, D. E. Studies on influenza in the pandemic of 1957–1958. II. Pulmonary complications of influenza. J. Clin. Invest. 38:213, 1959.
63. Mufson, M. A., Chang, V., Gill, V., Wood, S. D., Romansky, M. J., and Chanock, R. M. The role of viruses, mycoplasmas and bacteria in acute pneumonia in civilian adults. Amer. J. Epidemiol. 86:526, 1967.
64. Pickard, R. E. Varicella pneumonia in pregnancy. Amer. J. Obstet. Gynecol. 101:504, 1968.
65. Rice, R. P., and Lada, F. A. Roentgenographic analysis of respiratory syncytial virus pneumonia in infants. Radiology 87:1021, 1966.
66. Rifkind, D. Editorial notes: cytomegalovirus mononucleosis. Ann. Internal Med. 69:842, 1969.
67. Schleissner, L. A., and Portnoy, B. Hepatitis and pneumonia associated with ECHO virus, type 9, infection in two adult siblings. Ann. Internal Med. 68:1315, 1968.
68. Triebwasser, J. H., Harris, R. E., Bryant, R. E., and Rhoades, E. R. Varicella pneumonia in adults. Report of seven cases and a review of the literature. Medicine 46:409, 1967.

Fungi

69. Louria, D. B. Fungus infections of the lungs. In Textbook of Pulmonary Diseases, Baum, G. L., Ed., p. 118. Little, Brown and Co., Boston, 1965.

Actinomycetes (Fungus-like Bacteria)

70. Neu, H. G., Silva, M., Hazen, E., and Rosenheim, S. H. Necrotizing nocardial pneumonia. Ann. Internal Med. 66:274, 1967.

Rickettsiae

71. Musher, D. M. Q fever. A Common treatable cause of endemic nonbacterial pneumonia. J.A.M.A. 204:111, 1968.

Protozoa and Other Parasites

72. Gelpi, A. P., and Mustafa, A. Ascaris pneumonia. Amer. J. Med. 44:377, 1968.
73. Moore, D. L., Carnahan, C. E., Mills, S. D., and Burgert, E. O. Pneumocystis carinii pneumonitis complicating leukemia. Mayo Clin. Proc. 44:162, 1969.
74. Rifkind, D., Faris, T. D., and Hill, R. B., Jr. Pneumocystis carinii pneumonia. Studies on the diagnosis and treatment. Ann. Internal Med. 65:943, 1966.

Cardiovascular Diseases

75. Fred, H. L. Bacterial pneumonia or pulmonary infarction? Dis. Chest 55:422, 1969.

Chemical and Physical Agents

76. Moskowitz, R. L., Lyons, H. A., and Cottle, H. R. Silo filler's disease. Clinical, physiologic and pathologic study of a patient. Amer. J. Med. 36:457, 1964.

77. Vishnevsky-Vysniauskas, C. Acute lipoid pneumonia. Dis. Chest **54**:475, 1968.
78. Volk, B. W., Nathanson, L., Losner, S., Slade, W. R., and Jacobi, M. The incidence of lipoid pneumonia in a survey of 389 chronically ill patients. Amer. J. Med. **10**:316, 1951.

Diseases of Presumed or Proven Immunologic Origin

79. Fiegenberg, D. S., Weiss, H., and Kirshman, H. Migratory pneumonia with eosinophilia associated with sulfonamide administration. Arch. Internal Med. **120**:85, 1967.
80. Fink, J. N., Sosman, A. J., Barboriak, J. J., Schlueter, D. P., and Holmes, R. A. Pigeon breeders' disease. A clinical study of a hypersensitivity pneumonitis. Ann. Internal Med. **68**:1205, 1968.
81. Korn, D. S., Florman, A. L., and Gribetz, I. Recurrent pneumonitis with hypersensitivity to hen litter. J.A.M.A. **205**:44, 1968.
82. Riddle, F. V., Channell, S., Blyth, W., Weir, D. M., Lloyd, M., Amos, W. M. G., and Grant, I. W. B. Allergic alveolitis in a maltworker. Thorax **23**:271, 1968.
83. Strauss, W. G., and Griffin, L. Nitrofurantoin pneumonia. J.A.M.A. **199**:765, 1967.
84. Wilson, E. S., Jr., and McCarty, R. J. Nitrofurantoin pneumonia. Amer. J. Roentgenol. **103**:540, 1968.

Neoplastic Diseases

85. Kirby, W. M. M., Waddington, W. S., and Francis, B. F. Differentiation of right upper lobe pneumonia from bronchiogenic carcinoma. N. Engl. J. Med. **256**:828, 1957.
86. Klatte, E. C., Yardley, J., Smith, E. B., Rohn, R., and Campbell, J. A. The pulmonary manifestations and complications of leukemia. Amer. J. Roentgenol. **89**:598, 1963.

Miscellaneous Diseases

87. Fraimow, W., Cathcart, R. T., Kirshner, J. J., and Taylor, R. C. Pulmonary alveolar proteinosis. A correlation of pathological and physiological findings in a patient followed up with serial biopsies of the lung. Amer. J. Med. **28**:458, 1960.
88. Larmi, T. K. I., and Dammert, K. Chronic idiopathic pneumonitis of the cholesterol type as a surgical problem. Scand. J. Thorac. Cardiovasc. Surg. **1**:127, 1967.
89. Padula, R. T., and Stayman, J. W. Chronic interstitial pneumonia: cholesterol type. Review of the literature and report of 2 cases. J. Thorac. Cardiovasc. Surg. **54**:272, 1967.
90. Reussi, C., Schiavi, J. E., Altman, R., Yussem, E. E., and Rauvier, J. Unusual complications in the course of anticoagulant therapy. Amer. J. Med. **46**:460, 1969.
91. Roseman, D. M., Kowlessar, O. D., and Sleisinger, M. H. Pulmonary manifestations of pancreatitis. N. Engl. J. Med. **263**:294, 1960.
92. Sapira, J. D. The narcotic addict as a medical patient. Amer. J. Med. **45**:555, 1968.
93. Schneider, R. M., Nevius, D. B., and Brown, H. Z. Desquamative interstitial pneumonia in a four year old child. N. Engl. J. Med. **277**:1056, 1967.
94. Soergel, K. H., and Sommers, S. C. Idiopathic pulmonary hemosiderosis and related syndromes. Amer. J. Med. **32**:499, 1962.
95. Stern, W. Z., Spear, P. W., and Jacobson, H. G. The roentgen findings in acute heroin intoxication. Amer. J. Roentgenol. **103**:522, 1968.
96. Wolfe, R. R., Adams, F. H., and Desilets, D. T. Pneumatoceles complicating hydrocarbon pneumonitis. J. Pediat. **71**:711, 1967.

Poorly Resolving Pneumonias

JAY S. GOODMAN and DAVID E. ROGERS

The majority of pulmonary infiltrates represent acute infections which are self-limited or clear rapidly with appropriate antibiotic therapy. Those initially diagnosed as "pneumonia" which fail to resolve in a reasonable period of time represent significant clinical problems. During the past 7 years, almost one-third of the patients seen by the infectious disease service at Vanderbilt University have had pulmonary disease initially believed to be infectious. One-half of these had poorly resolving infiltrates of diagnostic and/or therapeutic concern.

This chapter focuses on this particular group of patients, their disease processes, and the diagnostic considerations they provoked. Drawing primarily on our personal experience, we shall outline the etiologic possibilities to be considered when faced with a poorly resolving pneumonia, and indicate the features in the history and physical and laboratory examinations which we have found helpful in establishing an etiologic diagnosis. Finally, in an effort to give the reader an idea of the relative frequencies of different causes of prolonged pulmonary infiltrates, we have summarized our own experience with the more than 200 cases seen at this hospital which fitted our definition of "poorly resolving pneumonia." We have included in this group all patients with lobar or segmental infiltrates who continued to show roentgenographic densities after 30 days, or failed to show clinical improvement after 7 days of antimicrobial therapy. Short case histories are used throughout the chapter to illustrate points we wish to emphasize.

ETIOLOGY OF POORLY RESOLVING PNEUMONIAS

In the early 1900s "unresolved pneumonia" was considered an acceptable clinical diagnosis. This term most often reflected delayed resolution of pneumococcal pneumonia,[31] but infiltrates of many etiologies were undoubtedly included. Since the 1920s several authors have indicated that the factors responsible for poor resolution of pneumonic infiltrates can be determined in the majority of patients.[13, 37] In the mid 1940s Amberson[1] suggested that it should be the "inflexible rule" of the clinician never to make a diagnosis of poorly resolving pneumonia without searching for the cause. Because agents effective for treatment of many of the causes of poorly resolving pneumonias are now available, the need for accurate etiologic

JAY S. GOODMAN, M.D. Assistant Professor of Medicine, Vanderbilt University School of Medicine, Nashville, Tennessee. DAVID E. ROGERS, M.D. Professor of Medicine, Dean, and Vice President (Medicine), The Johns Hopkins University School of Medicine, and Medical Director, The Johns Hopkins Hospital, Baltimore, Maryland

TABLE 37

Etiologic Considerations in the Evaluation of Poorly Resolving Pneumonias

A. Specific microbial causes
> *Diplococcus pneumoniae*
> *Staphylococcus aureus*
> Gram-negative enteric bacilli
> Hemolytic and microaerophilic streptococci
> *Mycoplasma pneumoniae*
> *Pasteurella tularensis*
> *Chlamydia psittaci* (psittacosis)
> *Coxiella burnetii* (Q fever)
> Mycobacteria
> Fungi
> *Pseudomonas pseudomallei* (melioidosis)
> Viruses
> *Pneumocystis carinii*

B. Other causes of "Pneumonic" infiltration
> Bronchial tumors
> Alveolar cell carcinoma
> Lymphomatous and leukemic infiltrates
> Sarcoidosis
> Hamman-Rich disease
> Alveolar proteinosis
> Pancreatitis
> Pulmonary edema
> Cholesterol pneumonitis
> Metastatic carcinoma
> Pulmonary infarction
> Atelectasis
> Aspiration
> Pulmonary hemosiderosis
> Hypersensitivity reactions
> Collagen diseases
> Pneumoconioses
> Desquamative interstitial pneumonia

diagnosis of this syndrome has steadily increased. Indeed, in our experience, the majority of such patients have potentially reversible disease.

The possible etiologies which need consideration when a patient has a protracted pneumonic illness are shown in Table 37. Many of these disease processes can produce protean clinical pictures. In this chapter, however, they will be considered only in terms of their ability to produce poorly resolving pneumonias. The illnesses observed can be roughly grouped in four broad categories:

1. Pneumonias which are usually acute and self-limited, and behave atypically.

2. Pneumonias which are characteristically protracted because of the type of pathology produced by the infecting microorganism.

3. Pneumonias which are protracted because of failure to consider, recognize, or direct therapy at the etiologic agent.

4. Infiltrates believed to be "pneumonias" which are found to be produced by noninfectious processes masquerading as pulmonary infection.

The etiology of the majority of pulmonary infiltrates can be determined by thorough, detailed study. Success, however, is often determined by the sequence of various diagnostic techniques and how they are brought into play. Our own approach adheres to certain basic principles essential to evaluating patients with disease of any organ system. This entails retaking an adequate history, performing a thorough physical examination, carrying out certain basic laboratory tests, and, lastly, using special diagnostic procedures. It is surprising how often certain facets of this traditional approach are overlooked or short-circuited. Thus, we have seen severely ill patients who have been treated inappropriately because pertinent historical information was not obtained, because subtle physical findings were missed, or because remediable pulmonary infection was not appreciated until examination of a pneumonectomy specimen or autopsy material showed it to be present. The aspects of the clinical examination which have been particularly helpful to us are presented in the following sections.

HISTORY

In approaching the problem of the patient with a poorly resolving pneumonia, we have found it helpful to back away from data already recorded in the chart and to begin with a complete history and physical examination. In this way certain findings may come to light which were either missed or not awarded due significance on initial study.

An adequate history of the patient with a protracted pneumonia should include information relating to the illness and the associated host setting. An outline of helpful historical features is shown in Table 38. Regarding the pneumonia itself, it is helpful to know whether the onset was acute or indolent. Bacterial infections and pulmonary infarction are commonly dramatic in onset, while neoplasia and granulomatous disease generally have subtler beginnings. Systemic manifestations are often helpful in suggesting etiology. A history of a single shaking chill at the onset of the illness suggests pneumococcal pneumonia. When fever has been high and accompanied by chills, an infectious process is likely. A long history of night sweats in a patient with an otherwise indolent pulmonary infiltrate is more in keeping with a tuberculous or fungal pneumonia than neoplasia, although Hodgkin's disease involving the lung sometimes produces this picture.

The character of the cough and sputum should be noted. Psittacosis and mycoplasmal pneumonia are characteristically accompanied by a hacking, nonproductive cough. Patients with bronchiectasis, necrotizing pneumonias, and lung abscesses often produce large amounts of sputum with sedimenting layers of exudate and mucous. These individuals may complain of foul-tasting or foul-smelling sputum, signaling the presence of anaerobic strepto-

TABLE 38
Historical Information Helpful in Differentiating Protracted Pneumonias

A. The illness
   1. Type of onset (acute or indolent)
   2. Duration
   3. Systemic manifestations (fever, chills, night sweats, weight loss, fatigue)
   4. Pulmonary manifestations (cough, sputum, pleural pain, dyspnea)
   5. Extrapulmonary manifestations (periarticular pain, edema, pelvic pain, adenopathy)

B. The setting
   1. Age, race, geographic locale, travel
   2. Habits (tobacco, alcohol)
   3. Occupation (silica, asbestos, etc.)
   4. Exposure (animals, birds, old wood, etc.)
   5. Underlying disease (cardiopulmonary, neurologic, gastrointestinal)
   6. Predisposing conditions (blood dyscrasias, malignancy, corticosteroids, immunosuppressives, etc.)
   7. Family history (tuberculosis and other respiratory illnesses)

cocci or *Bacteroides* species. A history of a peculiar taste to the sputum provided the diagnosis in the following case.

Case 1. A 62-year-old woman was hospitalized with cough, fever, and a chronic left lower lobe infiltrate which was unresponsive to antibiotic therapy. An oleothorax had been performed 30 years earlier because of cavitary tuberculosis of the right upper lobe. On careful questioning the patient told us that her sputum tasted like "Wesson Oil." A positive fat (Sudan) stain of the sputum indicated the presence of a bronchopleural fistula on the right which had led to an oil aspiration pneumonia in the opposite lung.

Hemoptysis is common in tuberculosis, pulmonary infarction, bronchiectasis, and bronchial neoplasms. Pleural pain and dyspnea are characteristically severe with pulmonary infarction and staphylococcal pneumonia, but rare in viral or mycoplasmal pneumonias.

Certain extrapulmonary complaints may be helpful in pointing to particular diagnostic possibilities. Arthralgia or the periarticular pain of pulmonary hypertrophic osteoarthropathy makes suppurative lung disease or bronchogenic carcinoma likely. Arthralgia may also be part of the clinical picture of coccidioidal pneumonia ("desert rheumatism") and psittacosis. Arthritis, present in connective tissue diseases and sarcoidosis, may herald pulmonary disease of the same etiology. A history of calf pain, intermittent edema of an extremity, or pelvic pain may indicate venous disease underlying a pulmonary infarction. Recent localized lymphadenopathy should suggest tularemia.

The particular setting of an illness is of great diagnostic value and will support certain etiologic possibilities while making others unlikely. Age and race are important. An indolent lower lobe infiltrate in a 50-year-old man has different implications from the same lesion in a 15-year-old girl. In our experience advanced age has been associated most often with poorly resolving pneumococcal pneumonia, tuberculosis, aspiration pneumonia, and pulmonary embolism, the latter especially if the infiltrate emerges in a hospital setting. In Negroes, Puerto Ricans, and American Indians tuberculosis is a common cause of cryptic pulmonary infiltrates. Pulmonary histoplasmosis is rare in Negroes.

A particular geographic locale makes certain infections more likely. Coccidioidomycosis is a cause of acute pneumonia or chronic cavitary lung disease in the southwestern United States, where the fungus is harbored in the dry soil of the area. Histoplasmosis and North American blastomycosis are frequent in the central South. Tularemia and Q fever are more common in rural areas. A history of recent or remote travel to areas where certain diseases are endemic is also of importance. A chronic cavitary pneumonia resembling tuberculosis in a Viet Nam veteran could be melioidosis instead.[47]

Information about the patient's smoking and drinking habits should be obtained. Chronic pneumonia in a veteran heavy smoker suggests bronchogenic carcinoma. Pneumococcal, *Klebsiella*, and nonspecific aspiration pneumonias occur frequently in alcoholics.

A history of exposure to certain environmental factors (dust, animals, etc.) may help to unmask the etiology of a number of diseases which may present as poorly resolving pneumonias. Several helpful associations of this type are the following: silica (silicosis, silicotuberculosis); asbestos (bronchogenic carcinoma, pleural mesothelioma); old wood and soil (histoplasmosis, blastomycosis); sawmills (blastomycosis); birds, poultry, bird droppings (psittacosis, histoplasmosis, cryptococcosis); bats (histoplasmosis); wild rodents, ticks, deer flies (tularemia); and cattle and abattoirs (Q fever, brucellosis).

The following case illustrates the importance of an exposure history.

Case 2. An 8-year-old boy was admitted with a 4-day history of fever and chills and a right upper lobe pneumonia by x-ray (Fig. 43*A*). The white blood cell (WBC) count was 16,000/cu mm. He was at first believed to have pneumococcal pneumonia, but no pathogens were isolated from the sputum and there was no response to penicillin. Aspiration pneumonia, tuberculosis, and acute histoplasmosis were considered. After 1 week in the hospital his illness had progressed both clinically and radiographically (Fig. 43*B*). On careful re-evaluation, a history of recent exposure to ticks and a wild rabbit was obtained. The tularemia agglutinin titer was 1:1250; complete recovery followed streptomycin therapy.

The presence of an associated illness may provide a clue to the etiology of a protracted pulmonary infiltrate. Cardiac failure and arrythmias may

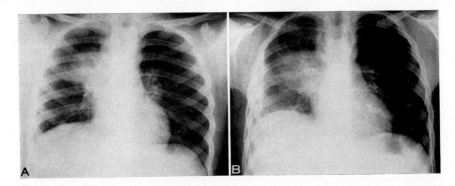

FIG. 43. Tularemic pneumonia (case 2). *A*. Chest film on admission to the hospital. *B*. Chest film 1 week later. Note accumulation of pleural fluid and progression of right upper lobe infiltrate.

underlie pulmonary embolism and infarction. Patients who are bedridden for long periods or whose extremities are immobilized in casts are similarly predisposed. Neurologic diseases interfering with deglutition or gag function, as well as conditions causing esophageal obstruction or gastroesophageal reflux, are frequently complicated by aspiration. The history of an old neck injury initially felt to be unimportant helped to clarify the etiology of a protracted pulmonary infiltrate in the following case.

Case 3. A 63-year-old woman with a 15-year history of recurrent pneumonias was admitted to the hospital with a right upper lobe infiltrate of 1 month's duration (Fig. 44*A*). She had a low-grade fever and a normal WBC count, and appeared chronically ill. Tuberculosis was considered probable,

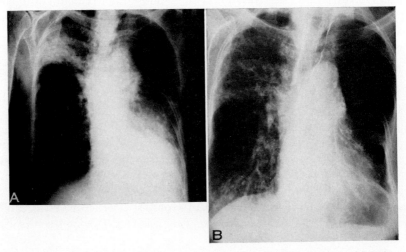

FIG. 44. Aspiration pneumonitis (case 3). *A*. Chronic right upper and left lower lobe infiltrates. *B*. Chest film following a barium swallow. Note barium within bronchi in the areas of infiltration.

and she was isolated and placed on isoniazid. Ten adequate sputum samples failed to reveal *Mycobacterium tuberculosis* or other pathogens. Serologic studies for psittacosis and histoplasmosis were negative. On careful re-evaluation the patient recounted the history of an automobile accident 20 years before, at which time she suffered a deep neck laceration. She also gave a history of frequent postprandial coughing since this injury. Chronic aspiration was then considered likely and was confirmed by a barium swallow (Fig. 44*B*). Cine-esophography revealed a defect of the right piriform sinus with overflow of contrast material into the trachea.

In the more acutely ill patient with a history suggestive of aspiration, one must consider the possibility of a necrotizing pneumonia due to staphylococci, Gram-negative bacilli, or anaerobic streptococci. Patients with severe chronic pulmonary disease are susceptible to staphylococcal and Gram-negative bacillary pneumonias. The latter infections can be induced by contaminated inhalation therapy equipment[39] and careless tracheal suction techniques.[48]

Infections of many types may be protracted and difficult because of a generalized depression in host resistance. Patients with diabetes mellitus, blood dyscrasias, cancer, agammaglobulinemia, collagen diseases, and hypercortisolism are at particular hazard. In such settings pulmonary infections produced by pneumococci, staphylococci, Gram-negative bacilli, and *M. tuberculosis* are common and severe. Furthermore, in many of these situations, invasion by opportunistic microbes, such as *Nocardia*, *Candida*, *Aspergillus*, *Pneumocystis*, and the cytomegalovirus is well known.[34] Therapy with corticosteroids, immunosuppressive agents, and antibiotics, alone or in combination, also greatly increases susceptibility to infection with unusual microorganisms. Such patients may be extremely ill, and their pneumonic illness not easily diagnosed. These difficulties are compounded by the ability of leukemias, lymphomas, other malignancies, and certain collagen diseases to involve the lung in a manner simulating pneumonia. As a practical point one should always approach this problem as if treatable infection is present. Even in patients with known leukemia the vast majority of pulmonary infiltrates represent infection.[25] An unusual diagnostic pitfall is illustrated by the following case.

Case 4. A 40-year-old man was admitted to the hospital because of a progressive infiltrate in the left lung (Fig. 45). He had noted the gradual onset of weakness for several months, during which time his face had become plethoric and rounded. Cushing's syndrome was diagnosed from urinary 17-hydroxycorticoid excretion of 50 mg/24 hours. Tuberculosis and opportunistic fungal disease were strongly considered as possible causes for the pulmonary infiltrate, but examination of sputum and bronchial washings was unrevealing. However, a bone marrow biopsy performed to search for pathogenic microorganisms revealed "oat cell carcinoma." It then became clear that the hypercortisolism in this case was due to ectopic

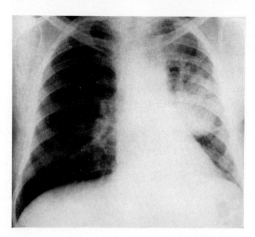

Fig. 45. Dense infiltrate with loss of volume in left lung due to oat cell carcinoma (case 4).

adrenocorticotropic hormone production by a bronchogenic carcinoma masquerading as pulmonary infection, and this syndrome was documented by appropriate studies.

Occasionally a therapeutic agent that a patient is receiving leads to the development of an "allergic" pneumonia which may be protracted, especially if this complication is not appreciated and the drug is not discontinued. p-Aminosalicylic acid, sulfonamides, nitrofurantoin, busulfan, and certain antihypertensive agents have been reported to cause such lesions.[10, 44, 46]

Finally, the family history may contain useful information. A poorly resolving pneumonia which began as an acute respiratory illness also affecting several members of the patient's household suggests a mycoplasmal or viral etiology. Recent or remote tuberculosis in the family may point to this disease in the patient.

PHYSICAL EXAMINATION

Because of the availability of the chest x-ray, physical examination in patients with pneumonic illnesses has tended to be downgraded by many physicians. When performed carefully and thoughtfully, however, it can sometimes reveal subtle but important findings which aid in etiologic diagnosis. Table 39 outlines those features of the physical examination which we have found helpful in these patients, stressing extrapulmonary clues.

The pattern of the recorded vital signs may suggest certain diagnoses. A pulse-temperature dissociation, with relative bradycardia, is seen more commonly in mycoplasmal pneumonia or psittacosis than in bacterial pulmonary infections. Tachycardia out of proportion to fever may indicate

TABLE 39

Features on Physical Examination Helpful in Differentiating
Persistent Pulmonary Infiltrates

1. Vital signs (temperature, pulse)
2. Chest (wheeze, rub, diaphragmatic movement, tracheal position)
3. Oropharynx (dental status, tongue lacerations, gag reflex, mucous membrane ulcers)
4. Lymph nodes (adenopathy—localized, generalized)
5. Extremities (clubbing, edema, varicosities)
6. Pelvis (tenderness, testicular or epididymal masses)
7. Neurologic signs (focal, diffuse, meningeal)
8. Cutaneous lesions (abscesses, ulcers, papules, etc.)

pulmonary embolism. A recurrent morning temperature elevation (typhus inversus) suggests tuberculosis.

Findings on chest examination are useful for following the course of an illness, but are relatively nonspecific and of little help in the differential diagnosis of a poorly resolving pneumonia. Classic signs of lobar consolidation, for example, may be present not only in pneumococcal pneumonia but also in mycoplasmal pneumonia, psittacosis, tularemia, tuberculosis, and pulmonary infarction. Some thoracic findings acquire meaning as the particular setting of the illness is taken into account. A chronic pneumonia accompanied by a localized wheeze or a paralyzed diaphragm in a patient who smokes excessively suggests bronchogenic carcinoma. A pleural friction rub in a postoperative patient with a protracted infiltrate from whom no pathogen has been isolated suggests pulmonary infarction. The position of the trachea may be helpful. When shifted toward an infiltrate, atelectasis is probable, suggesting the presence of bronchial obstruction or a Gram-negative bacillary pneumonia. A contralateral tracheal shift may occur in Friedlander's pneumonia.

Certain extrathoracic findings, when present, can be helpful diagnostic clues. Poor dental hygiene is frequently found in patients with necrotizing pneumonias and lung abscesses, implicating microorganisms commonly considered mouth saprophytes as responsible for pulmonary infection. A tongue laceration indicative of a generalized convulsion, or an abnormal gag reflex, suggests aspiration as the cause of a protracted pneumonia. Mucous membrane ulcers involving any portion of the mouth, pharynx, or larynx are seen frequently in disseminated histoplasmosis. The fungus can often be visualized on a hematoxylin-eosin or methenamine silver stain of the biopsied lesion, and can be cultured from this tissue on special media. Figure 46 shows a tongue ulcer, initially thought to be a carcinoma, which provided the diagnosis in a man with histoplasmosis. Palpable lymph nodes may indicate granulomatous disease or malignancy also involving the lung. The following case history illustrates the value of a good lymph node examination.

Case 5. A 45-year-old man was hospitalized because of a left upper lobe infiltrate of unknown duration (Fig. 47). He had a history of excessive cigarette smoking, but had had no weight loss or cough. Several examiners heard a wheeze over the left upper chest, but the remainder of the physical examination was negative. Sputum cultures, bronchoscopy, and bronchial washings were unrevealing. On the day prior to a scheduled diagnostic thoracotomy a careful physical examination revealed a single palpable right supraclavicular node. This was biopsied and revealed poorly differentiated carcinoma.

Asymmetry in the size of a thigh or calf which may be demonstrable only with the use of a measuring tape, or calf tenderness, may indicate the site

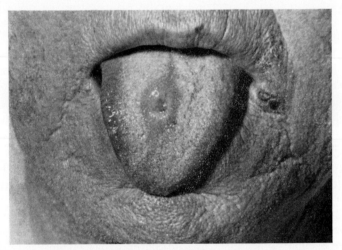

Fig. 46. Indurated ulcer of tongue due to disseminated histoplasmosis

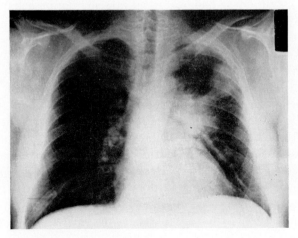

Fig. 47. Left upper lobe infiltrate due to oat cell carcinoma (case 5)

of origin of a pulmonary embolus. Varicosities and overt edema have the same significance. Clubbing of the fingers and toes, sometimes manifested only by sponginess of the nail beds, should suggest underlying suppurative lung disease or bronchogenic carcinoma. Clubbing is distinctly unusual in pulmonary tuberculosis. When clubbing is associated with the full-blown syndrome of pulmonary hypertrophic osteoarthropathy, primary bronchial carcinoma is probable and such lesions may still be resectable. Clubbing was an important finding in the following case.

Case 6. A 29-year-old man with a history of recurrent pulmonary infections was treated with penicillin for an episode of left lower lobe pneumococcal pneumonia. He improved, but a follow-up x-ray 4 weeks later showed a persistent infiltrate (Fig. 48*A*). The finding of clubbing of the fingers led to a bronchogram, which revealed sacular bronchiectasis localized to the left lower lobe (Fig. 48*B*). Resectional surgery was performed, and the patient has remained well.

A careful pelvic examination may reveal findings compatible with pelvic thrombophlebitis, a source of bland or septic pulmonary emboli. Examination of the scrotum for masses may uncover a primary testicular tumor which has metastasized to the lungs. Palpable epididymal masses suggest hematogenous tuberculosis or blastomycosis.

Subtle neurologic abnormalities may have diagnostic value in patients with protracted pneumonias. Changes in the mental state, especially if associated with focal neurologic signs, suggest metastatic tumor or brain abscess. Microorganisms which are likely to disseminate from the lung to the brain are *Nocardia asteroides*, anaerobic streptococci, and *Bacteroides*.

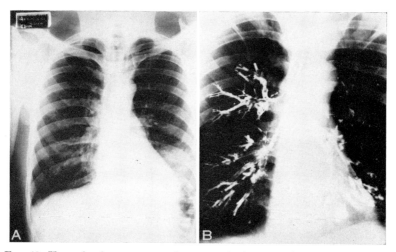

Fig. 48. Unresolved pneumococcal pneumonia (case 6). *A*. Left lower lobe infiltrate 4 weeks after adequate therapy. *B*. Bronchogram showing saccular bronchiectasis in the left lower lobe.

Diffuse muscle weakness, occasionally simulating myasthenia gravis, may be indicative of a neuromyopathy secondary to bronchogenic carcinoma. The appearance of meningeal signs in a patient with an indolent pneumonia suggests that the process may be cryptococcal or tuberculous.

Finally, certain cutaneous lesions may serve as extremely valuable diagnostic clues to the etiology of a poorly resolving pneumonia. Fever blisters are notably rare in tuberculosis and in mycoplasmal and staphylococcal pneumonia.[5] Viral infections such as varicella and rubeola may be associated with characteristic skin lesions and pulmonary involvement. Skin or mucosal ulcers are present in about 50 per cent of cases of pleuropulmonary tularemia. The presence of skin abscesses or pyoderma is suggestive of metastatic staphylococcal pulmonary infection. More frequently than appreciated, primary pulmonary infections are metastatic to the skin. Careful examination may turn up a small subcutaneous abscess which, on smear of its contents, shows branching forms of *Actinomyces* or *Nocardia*.[38] Draining sinuses of the chest wall may occur with these same two infections. Nocardial pneumonia was initially diagnosed from a skin lesion in the following case.

Case 7. A 62-year-old man was hospitalized with a 2-month history of fever, chills, and weight loss. Chest x-ray revealed a left lower lobe infiltrate with pleural reaction (Fig. 49*A*). No pathogens were found on initial sputum examination, and treatment with antibiotics for 1 week produced no clinical improvement. An obstructive bronchogenic carcinoma with a distal necrotizing pneumonia was considered most likely, but bronchoscopy

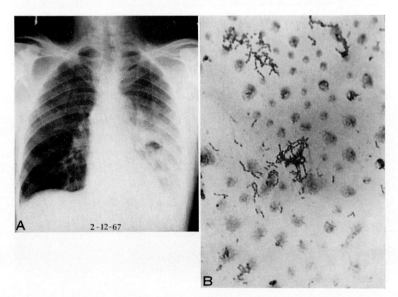

FIG. 49. Nocardiosis (case 7). *A*. Progressive left lower lobe pneumonia. *B*. Beaded branching rods on Gram-stained exudate from skin abscess.

was negative. A careful physical examination, however, revealed a small, tender nodule in the abdominal wall. Aspiration and smear of the exudate from this lesion revealed Gram-positive, weakly acid-fast, branching rods compatible with *N. asteroides* (Fig. 49*B*). This organism later grew on culture from the exudate and from bronchial washings, and the patient made a slow but uneventful recovery on sulfonamides.

Dissemination of organisms to the skin and mucous membranes also occurs in pneumonias caused by *Histoplasma, Blastomyces,* and *Crypto-coccus.* Large, crusted plaques or tiny, acne-like pustules are seen in disseminated blastomycosis. In the following case thoracotomy might have been avoided by attention to just such a lesion.

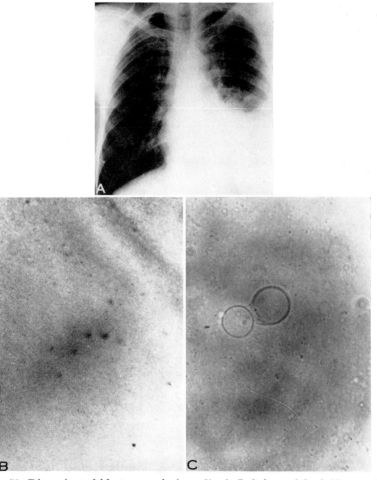

FIG. 50. Disseminated blastomycosis (case 8). *A.* Left lower lobe infiltrate with pleural reaction. *B.* Acneiform pustules on upper chest. *C.* Budding yeast of *Blastomyces dermatiditis* on wet mount of exudate from skin lesion.

Case 8. A 32-year-old former sawmill employee was hospitalized with a low-grade fever and left lower lobe pneumonia shown by x-ray (Fig. 50*A*). Because no pathogens were isolated from the sputum and the infiltrate failed to improve on antibiotic therapy, the patient underwent thoracotomy with resection of the left lower lobe. Culture of lung tissue revealed *Blastomyces dermatitidis.* Later, prior to the institution of amphotericin B therapy, the patient was questioned about several small, acneiform lesions over his upper chest and back, and indicated that these had been present since the beginning of his illness (Fig. 50*B*). A wet mount of one of these pustules with 10 per cent KOH showed a typical budding yeast of *B. dermatitidis* (Fig. 50*C*).

Acneiform lesions and skin ulcers may also be noted in cryptococcosis. Erythema multiforme and erythema nodosum, both probably hypersensitivity phenomena, are occasionally associated with histoplasmosis, coccidioidomycosis, sarcoidosis, tuberculosis, and mycoplasmal infection. Psittacosis is occasionally accompanied by erythema multiforme or by small macular lesions resembling rose spots (Horder's spots). Any of these cutaneous reactions may also reflect drug hypersensitivity in a patient who has received antibiotics for a pneumonic illness.

DIAGNOSTIC PROCEDURES

A large array of diagnostic procedures can be brought to bear on the patient with a poorly resolving pneumonia. The studies which have been most helpful in our experience are listed in Table 40. The specific studies performed should depend on the information obtained from the history and physical examination. In addition, the choice of diagnostic procedures should follow a logical sequence. Certain basic studies which involve little

TABLE 40

Laboratory Studies Helpful in the Diagnosis of Poorly Resolving Pneumonias

A. Basic procedures associated with little discomfort
  1. Sputum examination (Gram, acid-fast, and Wright's stains, wet mount, Sudan stain, cytology)
  2. Hematologic studies and blood chemistries
  3. Serologic studies (tularemia, psittacosis, histoplasmosis, etc.)
  4. Skin tests (tuberculin, histoplasmin, coccidioidin)
  5. Chest roentgenograms, tomograms, esophagrams

B. Special procedures associated with more discomfort and greater risk
  1. Thoracentesis and pleural biopsy
  2. Cervicomediastinal node biopsy, bone marrow, liver, and skin biopsies
  3. Bronchoscopy
  4. Bronchography
  5. Pulmonary angiography
  6. Phlebograms
  7. Percutaneous lung biopsy
  8. Thoracotomy

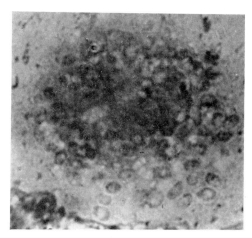

Fig. 51. Macrophage containing *Histoplasma capsulatum* on Wright-stained sputum smear.

patient discomfort or risk should be performed first. The more sophisticated and expensive studies, usually associated with greater risk to the patient, are reserved for clinical situations in which a diagnosis has not been forthcoming by other means and in which the patient's well-being is dependent on achieving a specific etiologic diagnosis.

An adequate sputum examination is essential for all patients with poorly resolving pneumonias. This includes a carefully performed Gram stain and acid-fast stain. Occasionally the diagnosis of pneumonia due to *Histoplasma*, *Cryptococcus*, or *Blastomyces* may be provided by a Wright stain of the sputum or a wet mount with potassium hydroxide. This simple maneuver is sometimes overlooked even in areas where these fungal infections are endemic. Figure 51 shows *Histoplasma capsulatum* within a macrophage found in a Wright-stained sputum smear from a patient with an upper lobe cavitating pneumonia. The importance of adequate sputum cultures is self-evident, but care must be taken that real sputum rather than saliva is sent to the bacteriology laboratory. Occasionally there is some question as to the significance of microorganisms grown from the sputum, especially Gram-negative bacilli, which may be representative of harmless sputum overgrowth in patients on antibiotic therapy. While Louria[27] has shown that quantitative sputum cultures may be helpful in such situations, we have not generally employed this procedure. Heavy growth of a pathogenic microbe from several sputum cultures suggests actual infection. Finding the same microorganism in a blood culture or pleural fluid culture is definitive. A fresh morning sputum is important for recovery of fungi, and is probably as good as a 24-hour collection for mycobacterial cultures. In the patient who is not producing sputum bronchial washings or transtracheal aspirates should be obtained. The latter procedure is carried out under local anesthesia by inserting a polyethylene catheter into the trachea through the cricothyroid membrane.[19] It is also helpful when routine sputum cultures show a mixed flora and there is doubt as to which microorganism may be causing infection. Fasting morning gastric aspirations are useful for culturing *M. tuberculosis* and pathogenic fungi. In the latter instance the material should not be subjected to concentration procedures. Cytologic examination of sputum for malignant cells should be routine in evaluating any protracted pneumonia, especially unilateral disease in veteran smokers over the age of 40.

Helpful diagnostic information can be obtained from the hematology and blood chemistry laboratories. A leukocytosis of more than 20,000/cu mm generally indicates bacterial rather than viral or mycoplasmal infection, although high leukocyte counts sometimes accompany pulmonary infarction. Persistent leukocytosis suggests an empyema, even when the x-ray does not show obvious pleural fluid. Leukopenia in a patient with pneumococcal pneumonia is often accompanied by delayed resolution. An elevated serum amylase level suggests that a left lower lobe infiltrate and pleural reaction may be an intrathoracic manifestation of pancreatitis. An elevated serum calcium level should suggest sarcoidosis or bronchogenic carcinoma. Elevations in bilirubin and lactic dehydrogenase are said to be helpful in separating pulmonary infarction and bacterial pneumonia, but in our experience are of little differential value. In puzzling pneumonias acute serum should be stored and convalescent sera should be obtained, so that appropriate studies can be carried out for *Mycoplasma pneumoniae*, psittacosis, tularemia, and certain fungi.

Skin testing can be helpful but not definitive in the diagnosis of tuberculosis, histoplasmosis, and coccidioidomycosis. A negative skin test for any of these diseases does not rule them out. Blastomycin is a poor antigen and frequently produces a negative result, even in proven cases of blastomycosis. Serum for complement fixation studies should be obtained *prior* to application of skin tests, since the latter may cause significant rises in serum complement-fixing antibodies. This is particularly important when histoplasmosis is suspected.[8] Antigens to both the mycelial and yeast phases of this fungus should be employed where possible in the complement fixation test. Antibodies to the yeast antigen are least affected by prior skin testing, and a titer of 1:16 or greater correlates well with active histoplasmosis.

While serial chest x-rays are helpful in following the course of poorly resolving pneumonias and in localizing pleural fluid, the x-ray pattern in many instances is not sufficiently specific to be of great diagnostic help. For instance, tuberculosis and histoplasmosis are generally upper lobe cavitary infections, but pulmonary infarction, aspiration pneumonia, and carcinoma may have an identical location and appearance. Specific roentgenographic patterns will be mentioned in a subsequent discussion of specific diseases. Specialized radiographic procedures are indicated in difficult cases. Tomography may reveal unsuspected cavitation, an endobronchial tumor, extrabronchial compression, or an eroded rib. An upper

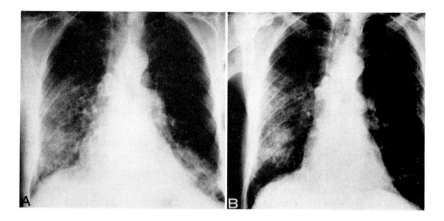

FIG. 52. Aspiration pneumonitis (case 9). *A*. Chest film showing bilateral lower lobe infiltrates of 6 weeks' duration. *B*. Roentgenogram obtained 5 weeks later, showing partial spontaneous clearing.

gastrointestinal series may demonstrate esophageal obstruction or gastro-esophageal reflux. A swallowing cine-esophagram may also be very helpful, as illustrated by case 3 and by the following case.

Case 9. A 65-year-old man was admitted because of persistent bilateral infiltration on chest x-ray following an apparent bacterial pneumonia (Fig. 52*A*). He had lost 15 pounds and was anemic, but his WBC count was normal. Cultures for mycobacteria and fungi, sputum cytology, serology, bronchoscopy, and bronchography were unrevealing. Alveolar cell carcinoma and desquamative interstitial pneumonia were considered as diagnostic possibilities. An open lung biopsy was scheduled, but was not performed because of spontaneous clinical and roentgenographic improvement (Fig. 52*B*). Five months after discharge from the hospital the patient had a recurrence of low-grade fever, weakness, and roentgenographic evidence of pneumonia. This time a history of postprandial coughing of several years' duration was obtained. A swallowing cine-esophagram showed persistent spillage of contrast material into the trachea. Examination of the larynx revealed dysfunction of the epiglottis and vocal cords of unknown etiology.

Other helpful procedures entail instrumental examination of the patient or surgical excision of tissue. While such studies are associated with a small but significant risk, they often yield a high return. If the physical examination and roentgenographic studies indicate the presence of pleural fluid, a diagnostic thoracentesis should be performed. We often perform such thoracenteses with a Cope needle so that a pleural biopsy may be obtained simultaneously. Pleural tissue may reveal a granuloma or carcinoma when studies of the pleural fluid itself are nonspecific. Pleural fluid and tissue should be subjected to the same laboratory studies as sputum. In addition, enumeration of the types of cells present in the fluid may be important. Large numbers of lymphocytes suggest tuberculosis, lymphoma, or carcinoma, and malignant cells have obvious significance. An elevated pleural fluid amylase level points to pancreatitis as the cause of a pleuropulmonary reaction. Liver, bone marrow, and skin biopsies have taught us that pulmonary diseases are frequently disseminated even when clinically focal. Scalene node or fat pad biopsy, even in the absence of palpable adenopathy, may be helpful when other studies have been unrevealing. However, in patients with bronchogenic carcinoma *without* palpable scalene nodes, this procedure is reported to have only a 12 per cent yield.[33] Pathogenic microorganisms or tumors found by scalene node biposy are generally diagnostic. Nonspecific granulomas, while suggestive of sarcoidosis, can also be found in scalene nodes from patients with tuberculosis, berylliosis, fungal pneumonias, and even carcinoma. Biopsy of mediastinal lymph nodes by mediastinoscopy is now being used in several centers.[53] This procedure, carried out under local anesthesia through a suprasternal incision, is particularly valuable when hilar adenopathy is shown by x-ray.

Healing of any pulmonary inflammatory lesion depends partly on the structural and functional integrity of the bronchi. Thus, careful consideration should be given the bronchial tree in the evaluation of protracted pneumonias, lest the presence of obstruction due to granulation tissue, stricture, or neoplasm go unrecognized. Bronchoscopy, a procedure which can be carried out with little morbidity in nearly all medical centers, can be therapeutic as well as diagnostic if an obstructing foreign body is discovered and removed. In addition, bronchial washings suitable for examination for mycobacteria, fungi, and malignant cells may be obtained. When bronchoscopic findings and bronchial washings are equivocal in patients with necrotizing pneumonias because of excessive inflammatory exudate, the procedure should be repeated at a later date. Bronchography, or contrast radiography of the bronchial tree by means of iodinated oil, is useful in documenting bronchiectasis or localized intrabronchial obstruction, and is probably an underused procedure.[16] We have seen three patients in whom a bronchogenic carcinoma was indicated by bronchography when the "diagnostic triad" of bronchoscopy, cytology, and scalene node biopsy was negative. The following case is illustrative.

Case 10. A 52-year-old man was admitted to the hospital because of a left upper lobe infiltrate of 3 months' duration which had failed to clear despite antibiotic therapy (Fig. 53*A*). He had a history of excessive cigarette smoking and a dry, hacking cough, but there had been no constitutional symptoms. Studies for tuberculosis and histoplasmosis, sputum cytology, bronchoscopy, and a scalene fat pad biopsy were unrevealing. A left bronchogram revealed a "cutoff" sign in the superior lingular bonchus (Fig. 53*B*). At thoracotomy an endobronchial carcinoma was discovered at this point and a left pneumonectomy was performed.

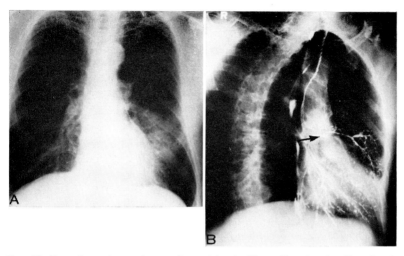

FIG. 53. Bronchogenic carcinoma (case 10). *A*. Chest film showing lingular infiltrate of 3 months' duration. *B*. Left bronchogram showing obstruction near origin of superior lingular bronchus (arrow).

When bronchiectasis is suspected in an individual with recurrent or protracted bacterial pneumonias bronchography is best delayed for 2 or 3 months after subsidence of an acute infection, which can itself cause transient bronchographic abnormalities (pseudobronchiectasis).

Pulmonary angiography, lung scintiscanning with radioactive iodinated macroaggregated albumin, and phlebography of the legs may be helpful in the diagnosis of pulmonary infarction. This disease, which has a protean clinical spectrum, may be extremely difficult to diagnose, especially if it is not accompanied by signs of venous or cardiac disease. The lung scintiscan is probably not as useful a differential tool as pulmonary angiography when there is obvious radiographic infiltration, since many types of pneumonia can produce an abnormal scan. However, when there are additional "cold areas" on the scan not corresponding to an area of radiographic infiltration or to bullae, pulmonary embolism is likely. Phlebograms showing filling defects in the femoral venous system support the diagnosis of pulmonary embolism and may serve as indirect evidence for this disease. All these procedures may yield negative results if performed late in the course of illness. The following case history illustrates the value of pulmonary angiography in the diagnosis of a cryptic pneumonia in a young man.

Case 11. A 31-year-old man was admitted to the hospital with a 2-week history of left-sided pleuritic pain and fever. Chest x-ray showed a left lower lobe infiltrate accompanied by atelectasis and pleural reaction (Fig. 54*A*). The WBC count was 15,000/cu mm. The patient was a heavy smoker but had a negative exposure history and appeared otherwise healthy. Sputum cultures revealed no pathogens; skin tests and serologic studies were negative, and bronchoscopy was unremarkable. He was initially be-

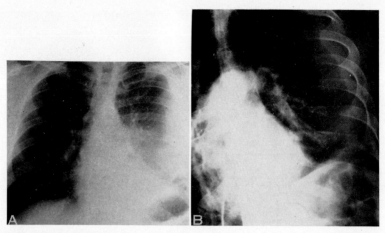

Fig. 54. Pulmonary infarction (case 11). *A*. Roentgenogram showing left lower lobe infiltrate with pleural reaction. *B*. Pulmonary angiogram demonstrating filling defects in left pulmonary artery.

lieved to have a bacterial pneumonia, but penicillin therapy for 2 weeks produced no change in his daily spiking fever or pulmonary infiltrate. Numerous thoracenteses were performed in an attempt to locate an empyema, but only small amounts of serous fluid were aspirated; these were negative on culture. Despite a normal electrocardiogram and the absence of any apparent underlying disease, pulmonary infarction was considered a likely possibility. A pulmonary angiogram (Fig. 54*B*) revealed striking filling defects in the left main pulmonary artery. Phlebograms of the lower extremities were normal. The patient made a slow recovery on anticoagulant therapy.

The use of percutaneous needle biopsy of the lung is being explored in several medical centers.[26] With this technique lung tissue can be obtained for culture and histopathology when more conservative methods have not yielded a diagnosis. The procedure is best performed under direct fluoroscopic control, and patients must have sufficient cardiopulmonary reserve to tolerate a substantial pneumothorax. The ideal lesion for biopsy in this manner is one with associated pleural reaction, so that the danger of pneumothorax is minimized. In the presence of certain types of lesions an open lung biopsy may be safer. The following case illustrates the value of a lung biopsy in uncovering a remediable disease that was not apparent by other means.

Case 12. A 68-year-old man with leukolymphosarcoma, who had been treated for disseminated histoplasmosis 8 months previously, was admitted to the hospital because of a progressive cavitary infiltrate involving the right upper lobe (Fig. 55*A*). He had a cough productive of large amounts of purulent sputum, which on culture revealed no pathogenic bacteria or

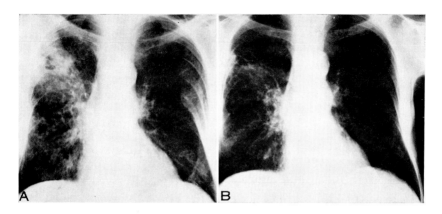

Fig. 55. Nocardiosis (case 12). *A*. Progressive cavitary infiltrate involving right upper lobe. *B*. Roentgenographic clearing 2 months following institution of sulfonamide therapy.

fungi. He had evidence of significant lymphomatous involvement of the nasopharynx, suggesting aspiration as a possible cause of his pulmonary lesion. A cervical lymph node biopsy revealed *Histoplasma capsulatum* on methenamine silver stain, but the organisms did not grow on culture. Amphotericin B was reinstituted along with antibiotics to cover the possibilities of active pulmonary histoplasmosis and aspiration pneumonia, respectively. There was no clinical or roentgenographic improvement, however, and several observers felt that the infiltrate was compatible with lymphomatous involvement of the lung. Percutaneous needle biopsy of the right upper lobe lesion revealed *Nocardia asteroides* both on histologic section and on culture; this organism had been sought without success in the patient's sputum and bronchial washings. Sulfonamide therapy was begun and the patient made a remarkable recovery (Fig. 55*B*). He expired 8 months later from his underlying malignancy.

Diagnostic thoracotomy is reserved for the patient in whom a diagnosis has not been forthcoming by other methods, and in whom treatable disease remains a possibility. Thoughtful selection of other diagnostic studies based on a careful history and physical examination has decreased the necessity for diagnostic thoracotomy in our institution.

VANDERBILT EXPERIENCE WITH POORLY RESOLVING PNEUMONIAS, 1961–1967

In the preceding sections we have outlined the approaches which have been useful to us in diagnosing protracted pneumonias. We now present an analysis of our experience with this syndrome at the Vanderbilt University Hospital. Obviously this represents highly selected clinical material. Consultation was requested on these patients by the physicians caring for them, either because their illnesses were of extreme interest, the anticipated response to therapy had not occurred, or an etiologic diagnosis had not been forthcoming. Furthermore, Vanderbilt University Hospital is a referral center located in an area where tularemia, histoplasmosis, and blastomycosis are relatively common, while some agents producing pulmonary disease in other areas are not. Despite these limitations, certain points emerge which help to define the problems involved in dealing with protracted pneumonias.

During the 7-year interval 1961–1967 our Infectious Disease Division was asked to see 1856 patients. Five hundred fifty patients were seen because of suspected pulmonary infection. Two hundred nine of these had illnesses which fulfilled our criteria for "poorly resolving pneumonia"; an etiologic breakdown of these cases is shown in Table 41.

Most of the poorly resolving pneumonias listed in Table 34 were manifestations of common disease processes. *More than half turned out to have an infectious etiology,* and the majority were due to well-known respiratory pathogens. Microorganisms such as the pneumococcus and *Mycoplasma pneumoniae,* which characteristically cause acute pneumonias responding rapidly to treatment, produced a significant amount of atypical disease. Other microbial agents, such as *M. tuberculosis,* staphylococci, and Gram-negative bacilli, did not usually present as diagnostic problems, but commonly produced protracted illness. Infections due to psittacosis, *Pasteurella tularensis,* and certain fungi were more difficult to diagnose and often were not considered in the initial evaluation of patients with these pneumonic illnesses. Unusual pulmonary pathogens such as *Candida* and *Aspergillus* species and the cytomegalovirus accounted for protracted pneumonias in a few patients with markedly altered host resistance. Finally, there was a sizable number of pneumonic infiltrates which were not due to recognized pulmonary pathogens. Infection with mouth saprophytes probably contributed to the clinical picture in most of the cases of aspiration pneumonia and some of the bronchial neoplasms. Pulmonary infarction and a variety of miscellaneous infiltrates which masqueraded as pneumonia did not appear to be associated with any microbial invasion. Diagnosis of the less common noninfectious infiltrates was difficult, and frequently required examination of lung tissue. A brief review of some of the important types of poorly resolving pneumonias with which we have had experience may help to elucidate the problems involved in dealing with patients who present with this syndrome.

Pneumococcal Pneumonia

The disease most commonly associated with poor resolution in our patients was pneumococcal pneumonia. Owing to the availability of penicillin and its ability to produce an almost immediate crisis, pneumococcal pneumonia has come to be considered a very limited illness. Therefore, persistent symptoms or delayed clearing of the chest roentgenogram despite antimicrobial therapy represents a worrisome problem for the clinician.[49]

TABLE 41

Poorly Resolving Pneumonias Seen at Vanderbilt University Hospital, Infectious Diseases Consultation Service, 1961–1967

Diagnosis	No. of Patients
Pneumonias due to specific pathogens	127
Pneumococcal pneumonia	41
Tuberculosis	18
Staphylococcal pneumonia	14
Gram-negative bacillary pneumonia	14
Histoplasmosis	9
Psittacosis	5
Tularemia	5
Blastomycosis	5
Mycoplasmal pneumonia	4
Nocardiosis	4
Cryptococcal pneumonia	3
Atypical mycobacteriosis	2
Aspergillosis	1
Candidiasis	1
Cytomegalovirus pneumonia	1
Infiltrates due to other causes	51
Aspiration pneumonia	15
Pulmonary infarction	12
Bronchogenic carcinoma	10
Miscellaneous	
Metastatic carcinoma	1
Alveolar cell carcinoma	1
Lymphoma	1
Leukemic infiltrates	1
Bronchial adenoma	1
Middle lobe atelectasis	1
Sarcoidosis	1
Hamman-Rich disease	1
Rheumatic disease	1
Systemic lupus erythematosus	1
Allergic eosinophilic pneumonia	1
Silicosis	1
Pulmonary hemosiderosis	1
Pulmonary edema	1
Infiltrates of unknown etiology	31
Total	209

Interestingly, the incidence of delayed resolution of pneumococcal pneumonia has actually increased from 4 per cent of cases early in this century to 15 per cent since the introduction of antibiotics.[18, 31, 35, 51] Some investigators have suggested that antibiotics might somehow interfere with the healing process.[2] However, it is likely that these agents do not impede resolution of pneumococcal pneumonia and that the apparent increasing incidence of delayed resolution reflects a shift in the type of patient admitted to the hospital with this disease. Young, robust individuals with straightforward lobar pneumonia are now rarely found on hospital wards.[42] Rather, the infection is seen frequently in individuals with significant underlying disease. Antimicrobial therapy considerably diminishes mortality, but rapid resolution of the pneumonic process may be thwarted either by local or constitutional pathology or by iatrogenic factors. Many of these conditions enhance susceptibility to and prolong the course of other pulmonary infections as well.

We have encountered 41 patients with pneumococcal pneumonia who manifested delayed resolution. These pneumonias were typical in onset and the majority showed a prompt clinical response to therapy, but thereafter pulmonary lesions persisted for an undue period of time. Nineteen of the 41 were older than 60 years, but all had some other associated condition or complication long recognized to be associated with delayed resolution, which appeared to provide a reasonable explanation for their protracted illness. These are outlined in Table 42. In 9 of the 41 patients two or more factors were present.

TABLE 42

*Conditions Associated with Poor Resolution of Pneumococcal Pneumonia in 41 Patients
(Vanderbilt University Hospital, 1961–1967)*

Condition	No. of Patients
Host conditions	
Chronic obstructive lung disease	7
Leukopenia	7
Bronchiectasis	5
Alcoholism	4
Leukemia	3
Neurologic disease	2
Diabetes mellitus	2
Tuberculosis	2
Aspiration	2
Metastatic carcinoma	1
Complications of pneumonia	
Empyema	5
Effusion	2
Atelectasis	2
Abscess	1
Iatrogenic factors	
Superinfection	
Staphylococci	1
Gram-negative bacilli	1
Inadequate therapy	1
Antibiotic resistance	1

Host Conditions

In 15 patients poor resolution appeared related to an underlying disease associated with abnormal bronchial drainage. Twelve individuals had chronic bronchitis and emphysema or bronchiectasis. These diseases impair normal ciliary action and the mobility and elasticity of the lung parenchyma. Two patients with incapacitating neurologic diseases (Guillain-Barré syndrome and myasthenia gravis) had ineffective bronchial drainage because of impaired cough and respiratory excursion. One patient with metastatic carcinoma to the lung had bronchial obstruction.

Seven patients had leukopenia associated with their pneumonia. It has long been recognized that when pneumococcal pneumonia is associated with an initial leukopenia delayed resolution is more common. Although the mechanisms involved have not been clarified, the suggestion that a disproportion between the number of leukocytes and other constituents in a consolidated lobe might be responsible for delayed resolution was put forth more than 30 years ago.[17] Theoretically, granulocyte deficiency within the early pneumonic lesion could result in decreased surface phagocytosis,[45] with spread of the infection. In addition, the lesion might contain insufficient lysosomal enzymes for rapid autolysis and liquefaction of the exudate. Pneumococcal pneumonia is known to be particularly virulent and destructive in patients with agranulocytosis.

Four patients with leukopenia were also chronic alcoholics. Leukopenic pneumococcal pneumonia is often seen in alcoholics, in whom it has been reported to result in greater mortality as well as a greater frequency of empyema, abscess, and delayed resolution.[9, 54] The clinical picture may mimic Friedlander's pneumonia. Kirby and associates[23] reported a series of 23 alcoholic patients with lobar pneumonia complicated by delayed resolution and atelectasis, most of whom had low white blood cell counts. A depressant effect of alcohol on marrow granulocyte reserves has been suggested to account for the leukopenia,[32] but in some alcoholic patients leukopenia can be reversed by folic acid administration.[6] A typical example of pneumococcal pneumonia in this setting is presented below.

Case 13. A 52-year-old chronic alcoholic man was admitted to the hospital with fever, cough, and chest pain of several days' duration. His temperature was 105°F, and dullness and rales were noted over the right anterolateral chest. Pneumococci (type XIX) grew from the sputum and blood. The white blood cell count was 2400/cu mm with a marked left shift. The WBC count rose to 15,900/cu mm on the seventh hospital day (after folic acid). Admission chest x-ray (Fig. 56A) showed consolidation of portions of the upper, middle, and lower lobes on the right side. The patient was treated with cephalothin because of a penicillin allergy, and improved clinically by the ninth hospital day. Subsequent x-rays (Fig. 56B–D) showed a slow but gradual clearing of the pneumonia. Diagnostic studies for tuberculosis and bronchial neoplasm were unrevealing.

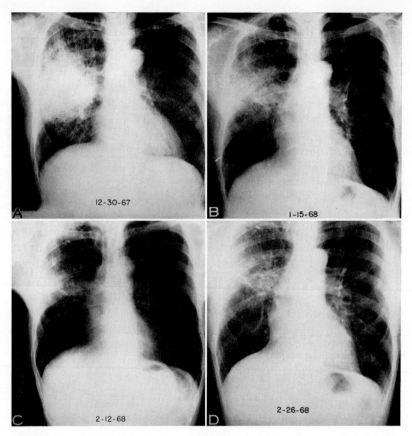

Fig. 56. Pneumococcal pneumonia (case 13). *A*. Chest film on admission to the hospital. *B–D*. Partial clearing of pneumonic infiltrate over a 2-month interval.

Of the three remaining patients with leukopenia, one had Hodgkin's disease, another had congestive splenomegaly, and a third had an unexplained admission WBC count of 3500/cu mm. Although not included in this category, two patients with chronic lymphocytic leukemia also had very low granulocyte counts, and one patient with chronic myelogenous leukemia may have had functionally abnormal granulocytes.

Diabetes mellitus has been reported to affect profoundly the speed of resolution of pneumococcal pneumonia.[18] This disorder was present in two of our patients, but was accompanied by chronic obstructive lung disease in one and by a type III pneumococcal infection in another. Type III pneumococci have enhanced resistance to phagocytosis and may be associated with necrosis of lung tissue and delayed resolution.

In two patients persistent infiltrates following therapy for pneumococcal pneumonia were due to concomitant active tuberculosis. In addition, one had chronic lymphocytic leukemia. The laboratory diagnosis of pulmonary tuberculosis is simple and inexpensive, and this possibility should be entertained in all patients with poorly resolving pneumonias, especially with upper lobe involvement.

Aspiration probably led to poor resolution of pneumococcal pneumonia in two patients. Both individuals were elderly, and pneumonia followed a convulsion in one and coma in the other. Although these pneumonias appeared to be primarily pneumococcal, mixed pulmonary infection with anaerobic mouth saprophytes may have been present.

Complications of Pneumonia

Certain complications of pneumococcal pneumonia, such as empyema, sterile effusion, atelectasis, or necrosis of lung tissue with abscess formation, may prolong the clinical illness and delay clearing of the chest roentgenogram.

Empyema was present in five patients. It was usually a complication of delay in therapy, and signs of pleural fluid were present on admission to the hospital. When interlobar in location, however, empyema sometimes simulated a dense infiltrate or even tumor on chest x-ray, and was difficult to locate with the thoracentesis needle. This situation is illustrated by the following case, in which a successful therapeutic trial with high doses of penicillin obviated surgical exploration of the chest. While this case is illustrative of the point we wish to make, it should be noted that satisfactory resolution of empyema without drainage is uncommon.

Case 14. A 76-year-old woman was admitted to the hospital 10 days following the onset of a febrile illness ushered in by a single chill. Her temperature was 101°F, and classic signs of consolidation were present over the right lower lobe area. The white blood cell count was 12,900/cu mm, and cultures of sputum and blood revealed pneumococci. Procaine penicillin, 600,000 units every 12 hours, was begun, but 72 hours later the patient's temperature was 103.8°F and her WBC count was 24,000/cu mm. Chest x-rays (Fig. 57) showed a persistent right lower lobe infiltrate and a "pseudotumor" effect, which probably was due to interlobar empyema. There were seven unsuccessful attempts at needle aspiration. Penicillin was increased to 20 million units/day intravenously, and the patient slowly improved, becoming afebrile by the 15th hospital day. She has remained well since discharge from the hospital.

Sterile effusions may be associated with persistent fever, and while they usually resolve without therapy, thoracentesis is necessary to distinguish effusion from empyema. Sterile effusion may become apparent late in the course of the illness (postpneumonic effusion). This complication was present in two of our patients.

Atelectasis occurring during the course of pneumococcal pneumonia probably accounted for delayed clearing of radiographic infiltrates in two patients. However, these cases did not resemble those with massive atelectatic collapse of the lung described by Finland and Loverud.[12] The single

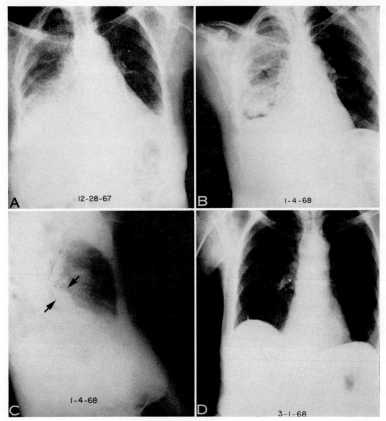

Fig. 57. Pneumococcal pneumonia (case 14). *A*. Admission chest x-ray. *B* and *C*. Roentgenograms after 1 week, showing collection of fluid in oblique fissure (arrows). *D*. Complete roentgenographic clearing 2 months later.

patient whose illness was complicated by abscess formation was an alcoholic with leukopenia and type IV pneumococcal pneumonia.

Iatrogenic Factors

Some of the problems associated with poor resolution of pneumococcal pneumonia did not exist prior to the advent of antimicrobial therapy. These include superinfection with other microorganisms, inadequate therapy, or antimicrobial resistance of the pneumococcus. It is our impression that clinical superinfection is more apt to occur in debilitated patients with underlying disease. The two superinfections in our series were associated with bronchiectasis and severe chronic obstructive lung disease, respectively. In one the organism involved was a *Staphylococcus aureus* which emerged after 5 days of tetracycline therapy for pneumococcal pneumonia. In our experience tetracycline has a peculiar association with staphylococcal infection, an observation which has experimental support.[43] The other patient developed an *Aerobacter aerogenes* superinfection while under therapy with 20 million units of penicillin per day. In addition, he received assisted ventilation with an intermittent positive pressure breathing apparatus, a procedure which has emerged as important in the genesis of Gram-negative pneumonias.[39]

Superinfection should be considered when a patient with pneumococcal pneumonia manifests a recurrence of fever by the fifth to seventh day of therapy. While such fever may be due to drug allergy, and change in the sputum flora to contain Gram-negative enteric bacilli or staphylococci is not unusual with antimicrobial therapy of pneumococcal pneumonia, this may represent new infection. Clinical superinfection is heralded by an increase in fever with a rise in leukocyte count, recrudescence of pulmonary symptoms, and/or an extension of the roentgenographic infiltrate. Louria and colleagues have shown that this complication is significantly enhanced by therapy with broad-spectrum antibiotics, unnecessarily large doses of penicillin, or combinations of the two.[29, 30] Most instances of superinfection can probably be prevented by using a single bactericidal drug in the lowest effective dosage whenever feasible in treating pneumococcal pneumonia. This therapy should not be altered because of a change in sputum flora if there are no signs of clinical deterioration.

Inadequate therapy is another preventable cause of poor resolution in pneumococcal pneumonia, and one patient in this series actually failed to receive appropriate therapy because of a nursing error. There is now evidence which indicates that occasional strains of pneumococci are resistant to certain broad-spectrum antibiotics which have been useful in treating pneumococcal pneumonia in penicillin-hypersensitive individuals. Our one instance of this occurrence, a fatal case of tetracycline-resistant pneumococcal pneumonia, has been reported.[41] Tetracycline-resistant pneumococci have been isolated with sufficient frequency to indicate that this drug should not be employed as initial therapy in pneumococcal pneumonia. In addition, a recent report indicates that erythromycin-resistant pneumococci exist, though they are probably not as common as tetracycline-resistant organisms.[24]

Several other conditions not encountered in this group of patients require comment because they might be expected to alter the course of pneumococcal pneumonia. One of these is bronchogenic carcinoma, which should be ruled out as a cause of delayed resolution, especially in patients who smoke. Bronchoscopy and cytologic studies were routine procedures in such patients in our series. Corticosteroid therapy has been alluded to as a possible cause of delayed resolution of pneumococcal pneumonia.[42] This association was not seen by us, nor was it notable in the studies of corticosteroids as therapeutic adjuncts in this disease.[20, 52] Individuals with defective antibody synthesis due to congenital hypogammaglobulinemia or multiple myeloma may have recurrent episodes of pneumococcal pneumonia. In our experience these infections resolve rapidly with adequate antibiotic therapy.

Penicillin-Resistant Pneumonias

Pneumonia caused by *Mycoplasma pneumoniae*, psittacosis, and tularemia may closely simulate pneumococcal pneumonia in x-ray pattern, physical signs, and constitutional symptoms, and penicillin therapy is often begun because pneumococcal pneumonia is suspected. Lack of response to this antibiotic is often the first clue that one is not dealing with an ordinary bacterial pneumonia. In our experience an unsuccessful therapeutic effort with penicillin so often preceded infectious disease consultation on these patients that we have chosen to group them in this manner. Common to our 14 cases of psittacotic, mycoplasmal, and tularemic pneumonia was their tendency to occur in otherwise healthy people, as well as failure to find pathogenic bacteria on routine sputum examination.

Severe headache and a dry, hacking cough were prominent features of mycoplasmal pneumonia and psittacosis. Pleural involvement was common in psittacosis and tularemia, but rare in mycoplasmal infection. One patient with mycoplasmal pneumonia presented with striking erythema multiforme, which was a helpful diagnostic clue. Three of five patients with tularemic pneumonia had the roentgenographic finding of a hilar "sentinel node." None of the patients with tularemic pneumonia had ulceroglandular lesions, but all had a history of contact with ticks, wild rabbits, or recent hunting or fishing trips. All patients with psittacosis had a history of bird contact, notably with parakeets. This history was often not elicited until late in the hospital course, the contact was often fleeting, and the birds did not necessarily appear ill. As emphasized in a recent review of this disease from our institution, such a history was the most important clue to the presence of psittacosis.[40]

Once the diagnosis of mycoplasmal pneumonia, tularemia, or psittacosis was suspected, it could usually be confirmed serologically. A cold agglutinin titer of 1:64 or greater was considered diagnostic of mycoplasmal infection in an adult. Titers tended to be elevated early in the illness. Because the cold agglutinin test shows significant titers in only 60 per cent of cases, the more sensitive and specific complement fixation test should be used where available. Although *M. pneumoniae* can be cultured from sputum or pharyngeal swabs on special media, this procedure is not yet widely available. Tularemia and psittacosis were diagnosed from agglutination and complement fixation reactions, respectively. Persistence in obtaining serial serum samples was important, since a diagnostic titer sometimes did not appear until late in convalescence, especially if tetracycline was administered early in the course. A therapeutic trial with streptomycin was occasionally employed in suspected tularemia, since the response of fever and constitutional symptoms is predictably rapid. Response of psittacosis to antibiotic therapy was often slow, and such a trial was of little value. Pulmonary infiltrates due to psittacosis and tularemia required considerable time for resolution, despite specific therapy. Mycoplasmal pneumonia sometimes followed a similar course, especially when pulmonary involvement was extensive, but most mycoplasmal infections we have seen have not resulted in poorly resolving pneumonias.

Hospital-Acquired Pneumonias

Infections caused by *Staphylococcus aureus, Escherichia coli, Proteus, Klebsiella-aerobacter,* and *Pseudomonas* species have emerged as serious clinical problems over the past 15 years. Staphylococcal pneumonia has been well studied as a sequel to Asian influenza.[28] More recently the frequency and clinical spectrum of pneumonias caused by Gram-negative bacilli have been appreciated.[50] Although pneumonia due to both these classes of microorganisms may arise outside the hospital, in our experience they have usually occurred in *hospitalized* individuals with serious underlying conditions. These pneumonias are frequently prolonged because of destruction of pulmonary tissue, formation of empyemas, and relative resistance to antimicrobial therapy. The 28 patients we have seen with protracted pneumonias due to these microorganisms, along with the major underlying conditions involved, are described in Table 43.

Both staphylococci and Gram-negative bacilli may reach the lungs from the bloodstream or by inhalation. Staphylococcal bacteremia, in contrast to the more commonly encountered Gram-negative bacteremias seen in our hospital, had a greater tendency to produce metastatic pneumonia. These infections were characterized by multifocal infiltrates, cyanosis, and tachypnea, with little cough or sputum production. Two infected cut-down sites, one wound infection, and a breast abscess were responsible for the bacteremias. Endocarditis, a well-recognized complication of staphylococcal sepsis, developed in one patient. The one hematogenous Gram-negative pneu-

TABLE 43

Major Underlying Condition in 28 Patients with Staphylococcal or Gram-Negative Bacillary Pneumonias

Underlying Condition	*Staphylococcus aureus* Pneumonia: No. of Patients	Gram-Negative Bacillary Pneumonia	
		No. of patients	Organism
Sepsis from extrapulmonary focus	4	1	*Bacteroides* species
Aspiration	4	4	*Escherichia coli* (2) *Aerobacter* species (2)
Postcardiac surgery	1	3	*Aerobacter* species (1) *Pseudomonas* species (2)
Hypercortisolism	0	2	*Pseudomonas* species
Chronic obstructive lung disease	1	2	*Proteus mirabilis* (1) *Escherichia coli* (1)
Pulmonary infarction	1	1	*Pseudomonas* species
Acute leukemia	1	0	
Bronchogenic carcinoma	1	1	
Superinfection	1	1	*Aerobacter* species

monia was caused by a *Bacteroides* species, following a postpartum infection of the uterus.

The remainder of the pneumonias were probably acquired by the respiratory route. Aspiration pneumonias complicated by secondary invasion with staphylococci or Gram-negative bacilli were not unusual in patients originally admitted with delirium tremens or coma due to neurologic or metabolic disease. These organisms probably colonized the respiratory passages of these patients after admission to the hospital. In the other cases predisposing conditions were multiple, and usually included prior antimicrobial therapy. Seven Gram-negative pneumonias were preceded by the use of mechanical ventilatory asistance with an intermittent positive pressure breathing machine. One patient with Cushing's disease and a tracheostomy developed *Pseudomonas* pneumonia which may have been due to use of a contaminated suction catheter. Another patient developed *Pseudomonas* pneumonia, bronchopleural fistula, and empyema while on high doses of adrenal corticosteroids for disseminated lupus erythematosus. Institution of appropriate antibiotic therapy for these infections was sometimes delayed because of initial failure to appreciate the kinds of microorganisms which are apt to take advantage of these particular situations. This was more common in the staphylococcal pneumonias, in which the organisms were often mistaken for pneumococci on sputum smears. The occurrence of spontaneous pneumothorax, pneumatoceles, and rapidly changing infiltrates with parafocal emphysema provided helpful clues to this diagnosis in several patients. Gram-negative pneumonias as a rule tended to be overdiagnosed, because these organisms are so often present in sputum cultures from patients on antibiotics. Interestingly, classical Friedlander's pneumonia due to *Klebsiella pneumoniae* was not observed during the 7-year interval involved.

Streptococcal Pneumonias

Group A β-hemolytic streptococci and microaerophilic streptococci each accounted for two poorly resolving pneumonias. Hemolytic streptococcal pneumonia has been well studied among military recruits. Although this infection has been considered rare, a recent report of 95 cases indicates that it can still be seen in an epidemic setting.[3] The clinical picture in our two sporadic cases was that of an acute febrile pneumonitis accompanied by "toxicity" and marked pleuritic chest pain, following mild upper respiratory tract symptoms in otherwise healthy individuals. Both patients had striking leukocytosis, but initial radiographic infiltrates were not extensive. The most remarkable feature of these cases, as well as those reported in the literature,[3, 7] was the rapid development of an extensive loculated pleural exudate. This complication ensued despite the early institution of penicillin therapy, and was responsible for a slow, tedious recovery. Although the causative organism was isolated from the pleural fluid and sputum of both patients, the diagnosis could have been difficult if antibiotics had been administered prior to hospitalization. In such cases elevated or rising antistreptolysin O titers may be diagnostically useful. Appreciation of the natural history of hemolytic streptococcal pneumonia enhances the likelihood of diagnosis and permits anticipation of a slow response to therapy.

Microaerophilic streptococci are commonly found in mixed pulmonary infections with other aerobic and anaerobic microorganisms. We have seen two patients in whom these organisms alone accounted for necrotizing pneumonias with pleural exudate. One patient with a known bronchogenic carcinoma developed an acute pneumonia, accompanied by empyema, distal to the bronchial obstruction. The other patient was a 26-year-old man with no apparent underlying pulmonary disease, poor dental hygiene, or history suggestive of aspiration. His initial pneumonic infiltrate cleared rapidly on penicillin therapy, but recurrent loculated empyemas containing a pure culture of microaerophilic streptococci eventually required surgical drainage. The pathogenesis of microaerophilic streptococcal infections in this type of patient is unknown, but similar examples have been reported by others.[11]

Tuberculosis and Other Mycobacterioses

Tuberculosis ranked as a common cause of poorly resolving pneumonias and was encountered in 18 patients. The clinical picture was generally one of subacute or chronic infection accompanied by an upper lobe infiltrate, sometimes bilateral, and often cavitary. Tuberculosis was suspected on initial clinical evaluation in many cases, but recovery of the organism from bronchial washings, urine, and lung, liver, or scalene node biposy was occasionally necessary for diagnosis in patients not producing sputum. Three negative sputum smears for acid-fast bacilli in the presence of cavitation were considered good evidence that the infiltrate was not due to active tuberculosis. About half the patients were elderly (greater than 60 years of age), and many were Negroes. Five patients had underlying hematologic or collagen diseases, and one had silicosis. Three patients were on corticosteroids without isoniazid (INH) prophylaxis. Although the prevalence, clinical picture, and course of tuberculosis are generally appreciated, certain potential diagnostic pitfalls are not. Some of these have been mentioned in the medical literature, and all, at one time or another, have been confirmed by our own experience with this disease.

1. Tuberculosis may occur in atypical pulmonary locations, (e.g., lower lobe), especially in patients with diabetes mellitus and hematologic malignancies.

2. Inactive tuberculous foci may be activated by corticosteroid administration, by the postgastrectomy state,[4] or by other pulmonary infections, such as histoplasmosis.[15]

3. The clinical response to antituberculous therapy may be very slow, and significant daily fever may persist for more than a month after beginning isoniazid. Thus, therapeutic trials with INH in patients with cryptic pulmonary disease are sometimes of little diagnostic value.

4. A negative skin reaction to purified protein derivative (PPD) or old tuberculin (OT) may be found in the presence of active tuberculosis in the following settings: a) in patients on corticosteroids; b) early in primary tuberculous infections; c) in patients with sarcoidosis, Hodgkin's disease, or other defects of the cellular immune mechanism; d) in severely ill patients with disseminated disease; and e) in a small percentage of elderly patients who are not seriously ill and have no obvious immunologic defect.[22]

Atypical mycobacteria caused pneumonias in two patients, both Caucasians. One patient had an upper lobe cavitary infiltrate caused by photochromogenic (group I) organisms. The other patient had a disseminated Battey bacillus infection (Group III) with extensive pulmonary involvement and a leukemoid reaction.

There is little clinical difference between atypical mycobacterial infections and tuberculosis. In addition, it is sometimes difficult to differentiate between actual infection and the casual discharge of atypical mycobacteria. Accurate etiologic diagnosis is imperative, however, since these organisms are often resistant to standard antituberculous therapy and may require treatment with relatively toxic drugs. It seems reasonable to consider actual infection to be present when the same organism is repeatedly isolated in large numbers from clinical material.[55] A negative tuberculin skin test or a positive reaction, limited to the 1:100 dilution of OT or second-strength PPD, in a patient who has acid-fast bacilli on smears of the sputum suggests that the infection is due to atypical mycobacteria. Specific skin test antigens for atypical mycobacteria are not yet commercially available.

Fungal Pneumonias

Twenty-three patients with poorly resolving pneumonias in our series were found to have pulmonary infiltrates caused by fungi. Histoplasmosis is endemic in our geographic area, and frequently entered the differential diagnosis of protracted pulmonary disease. Nine patients had poorly resolving pneumonia due to *Histoplasma capsulatum*. Their illnesses were subacute or chronic and were accompanied by upper lobe cavitary infiltrates closely simulating tuberculosis. Three patients had the early chronic form of the disease,[14] manifested by exudative-appearing pulmonary infiltrates which underwent roentgenographic changes, including healing, more rapidly than would be consistent with pulmonary tuberculosis. In the remainder differentiation from tuberculosis would have been difficult were it not for the fact that acid-fast bacilli were absent on multiple sputum smears, despite the presence of extensive cavitation. Three patients gave a history of heavy exposure to chicken manure in the recent past, and one each had been exposed to a starling roost or dust from a bird nest. The others may have had reactivation of an old pulmonary focus of histoplasmosis.

The diagnosis of histoplasmosis was confirmed in most patients by culture of sputum on Sabouraud's agar. Intraperitoneal injection of sputum into mice was sometimes necessary; organisms were cultured from the spleen when the animals were killed 4 weeks later.

North American blastomycosis accounted for five instances of poorly resolving pneumonia. Interestingly, three patients had previously worked in lumber yards or a sawmill. Two patients initially sought medical attention because of cutaneous lesions caused by *Blastomyces dermatitidis*. Roentgenographic lesions discovered in these patients consisted of "fibrotic" lower lobe infiltrates which, after diagnosis, showed definite clearing on amphotericin B therapy. Three patients entered the hospital because of cough, fever, and dense lower lobe infiltrates. In one, *Blastomyces* was seen on a sputum smear. The other two underwent diagnostic thoracotomy, and the organisms were grown from resected lung tissue.

Primary pulmonary cryptococcosis was diagnosed in three patients. Two were young men with dense, nummular lower lobe infiltrates which in one patient showed cavitation. Both were symptom-free except for a dry, hacking cough. Suspicion of metastatic tumor plus inability to isolate an infectious agent on cultures of gastric aspirates, bone marrow, or urine led to diagnostic lung biopsy in these patients. The third patient was a diabetic woman with a right upper lobe infiltrate simulating tuberculosis, from whose sputum *Cryptococcus neoformans* was readily isolated.

The foregoing cases of protracted pneumonia due to *Histoplasma capsulatum*, *Blastomyces dermatitidis*, and *Cryptococcus neoformans* did not present as severe toxic infections. On the other hand, patients with nocardiosis, candidiasis, and aspergillosis were more seriously ill. With the exception of two patients with nocardial pneumonia, all had underlying conditions which classically predispose to opportunistic infection. The problems encountered in the diagnosis and management of opportunistic infections have been recently reviewed.[34]

Aspiration Pneumonia, Pulmonary Infarction and Bronchogenic Carcinoma

These three major entities are common, and vary so much in their clinical and roentgenographic spectra that they frequently simulate one another as well as many other pulmonary diseases. The majority of the 37 patients in our series who had these illnesses came to our attention because they manifested atypical or bizarre clinical presentations. Thus, we now include the possibility of aspiration, bronchogenic carcinoma, or pulmonary infarction in our diagnostic considerations whenever faced with a cryptic unresolved pneumonia.

The clinical picture produced by aspiration varied considerably with the type of material entering the bronchial tree and the degree of resultant bronchial obstruction. In addition, the variable presence of anaerobic streptococci, *Bacteroides*, and fusospirochetal organisms from the oropharynx undoubtedly influenced the outcome. Aspiration in patients with poor dental hygiene often resulted in severe necrotizing pneumonias complicated by cavitation and abscess formation, especially if therapy had been delayed. However, identical clinical features occasionally masked an obstructing endobronchial tumor or a lung carcinoma which had necrosed and become secondarily infected. The absence of teeth and a history of smoking were helpful in indicating this diagnosis in several patients with necrotizing pneumonitis. Recurrent aspiration, either from clinically silent gastroesophageal reflux[21] or from subtle laryngeal defects (as in cases 3 and 9), may cause repeated episodes of poorly resolving pneumonia involving both lungs, and may result in chronic bronchopulmonary insufficiency. This type of illness mimics bacterial pneumonia, tuberculosis, alveolar cell carcinoma, and other miscellaneous pulmonary diseases.

Twelve cases of pulmonary infarction were encountered. The majority resembled bacterial or mycoplasmal pneumonias, except that they did not respond to antibiotics and were unduly prolonged. Daily fever in several individuals reached 103°F, or higher, and white blood cell counts over 20,000/cu mm were not unusual despite the apparent absence of infection. Pleural reaction and effusion were frequent, but examination of the pleural fluid, which was usually serous, yielded no helpful findings. Two patients developed cavitation within upper lobe pulmonary infarctions, a complication which has been reported by others[36] and which further confused the picture.

All of the 10 individuals with bronchogenic carcinoma were heavy cigarette smokers and over 40 years of age. Most of these patients presented with a localized, indolent unresolving pneumonia. Partial atelectasis of a segment or lobe was present by x-ray. A dry cough and a history of weight loss were frequent, but other symptoms were rare. Failure to find an explanation for such an infiltrate in this type of patient was an indication for thoracotomy.

Infiltrates of Unknown Etiology

Thirty-one of our 209 poorly resolving pneumonias defied adequate explanation, despite all efforts to establish an etiologic diagnosis. This is a larger percentage of diagnostic failures than our foregoing discussion suggests is inevitable. The principal reason for this group in the present series deserves comment. In certain patients, steady recovery from a poorly resolving pneumonia led to the decision to forgo more uncomfortable or hazardous diagnostic procedures, despite the lack of diagnosis with simpler studies. Slow resolution of an infiltration over several months of observation, in the absence of significant symptomatology or evidence suggesting serious disease, was considered an acceptable outcome. Thus, some of these infiltrates were probably due to aspiration or pulmonary infarction which could not be documented, or to a systemic disease that was being adequately treated. Other pneumonias may have been due to viral, mycoplasmal, or other self-limited infections in which the etiologic agent was not isolated nor adequate serologic studies performed. Several patients with chronic obstructive lung disease or bronchiectasis had acute pulmonary illnesses presumed to be bacterial, in which specific microbial pathogens were not isolated although slow recovery occurred on antimicrobial therapy. Three patients with poorly resolving pneumonias who were subjected to thoracotomy because of suspected serious pulmonary lesions were assigned a pathologic diagnosis of "organizing pneumonia" (of unknown etiology).

SUMMARY

Failure of a pneumonia to resolve within a reasonable period of time represents a common and worrisome clinical problem. In the present chapter we have attempted to outline and discuss the causes of pneumonias which do not clear within 30 days, or fail to show clinical improvement after 7 days of attentive medical care. There are several groups of diseases which may produce this clinical picture. Bacterial pneumonias of known etiology may pursue an atypical course. These cases frequently stimulate concern regarding some underlying host condition, such as a bronchial carcinoma. Pneumonias produced by other pathogens may resolve slowly because their intrinsic pathology is not conducive to rapid healing of the lung parenchyma. Such infections may present as diagnostic problems, and correct therapy is often delayed. Lastly, a variety of primarily noninfectious conditions can mimic pneumonias caused by many infectious agents.

Drawing primarily from our own experience as infectious disease consultants, we have tried to present a diagnostic framework useful in approaching the patient with a poorly resolving pneumonia. We have emphasized certain kinds of information which should be obtained, in a logical progression, through a careful history, physical examination, and series of laboratory studies. Specific clues which were helpful in explaining some of our own cases have been stressed.

An etiologic diagnosis can be arrived at for the majority of poorly resolving pneumonias. Potentially treatable or reversible diseases are frequently present. It is hoped that the approach outlined in this chapter will be useful to others in the diagnosis of such cases. At the same time it is anticipated that an awareness of the conditions likely to be associated with poorly resolving pneumonias will help make needless surgery and misdirected therapy uncommon in these patients.

REFERENCES

1. Amberson, J. B. Significance of unresolved, organizing, or protracted pneumonia. J. Mich. Med. Soc. **42**:599, 1943.
2. Auerbach, S. H., Mims, O. M., and Goodpasture, E. W. Pulmonary fibrosis secondary to pneumonia. Amer. J. Pathol. **28**:69, 1951.
3. Basiliere, J. L., Bistrong, H. W., and Spence, W. F. Streptococcal pneumonia. Recent outbreaks in military populations. Amer. J. Med. **44**:580, 1968.
4. Befeler, B., and Baum, G. L. Active pulmonary tuberculosis after upper gastrointestinal surgery. Amer. Rev. Resp. Dis. **96**:977, 1967.
5. Bennett, I. L., and Nicastri, A. Fever as a mechanism of resistance. Bacteriol. Rev. **24**:16, 1960.
6. Burmeister, R. W., Dreiling, B. J., Bazzano, G., and Broun, G. O. Pneumococcal pneumonia with leukopenia—the role of folic acid. Clin. Res. **14**:338, 1966.
7. Burmeister, R. W., and Overholt, E. L. Pneumonia caused by hemolytic streptococcus. Arch. Internal Med. **111**:367, 1963.
8. Campbell, C. C. Serology in the respiratory mycoses. Sabouraudia **5**:240, 1967.
9. Chomet, B. Lobar pneumonia and alcoholism: an analysis of 37 cases. Amer. J. Med. Sci. **253**:300, 1967.

10. Fiegenberg, D. S., Weiss, H., and Kirshman, H. Migratory pneumonia with eo-sinophilia associated with sulfonamide administration. Arch. Internal Med. **120**:85, 1967.
11. Finegold, S. M., Smolens, B., Cohen, A. A., Hewitt, W. L., Miller, A. B., and Davis, A. Necrotizing pneumonia and empyema due to microaerophilic strepto-cocci. N. Engl. J. Med. **273**:462, 1965.
12. Finland, M., and Loverud, H. I. L. Massive atelectatic collapse of lung com-plicating pneumococcus pneumonia. Ann. Internal Med. **10**:1828, 1937.
13. Gleichman, T. K., Leder, M. M., and Zahn, D. W. Major etiological factors pro-ducing delayed resolution in pneumonia. Amer. J. Med. Sci. **218**:369, 1949.
14. Goodwin, R. A., Snell, J. D., Hubbard, W. W., and Terry, R. T. Early chronic pulmonary histoplasmosis. Amer. Rev. Resp. Dis. **93**:47, 1966.
15. Goodwin, R. A., Snell, J. D., Hubbard, W. W., and Terry, R. T. Relationships in combined pulmonary infections with *Histoplasma capsulatum* and *Myco-bacterium tuberculosis*. Amer. Rev. Resp. Dis. **96**:990, 1967.
16. Greene, R. E. Unresolving pneumonia. J.A.M.A. **203**:287, 1968.
17. Heffron, R. *Pneumonia, with Special Reference to Pneumococcus Lobar Pneu-monia*, p. 96. Commonwealth Fund, New York, 1939.
18. Israel, H. L., Weiss, W., Eisenberg, G. M., Strandness, D., and Flippin, H. F. Delayed resolution of pneumonias. Med. Clin. N. Amer. **40**:1291, 1956.
19. Kalinske, R. W., Parker, R. H., Brandt, D., and Hoperich, P. D. Diagnostic usefulness and safety of transtracheal aspiration. N. Engl. J. Med. **276**:604, 1967.
20. Kass, E. H., Ingbar, S. H., and Finland, M. Effects of adrenocorticotropic hor-mone in pneumonia: clinical, bacteriological, and serological studies. Ann. Internal Med. **33**:1081, 1950.
21. Kennedy, J. H. "Silent" gastroesophageal reflux: an important but little known cause of pulmonary complications. Dis. Chest. **42**:42, 1962.
22. Kent, D. C., and Schwartz, R. Active pulmonary tuberculosis with negative tuberculin skin reactions. Amer. Rev. Resp. Dis. **95**:411, 1967.
23. Kirby, W. M. M., Waddington, W. S., and Francis, B. F. Differentiation of right-upper-lobe pneumonia from bronchogenic carcinoma. N Engl. J. Med. **256**:828, 1957.
24. Kislak, J. W. Type 6 pneumococcus resistant to erythromycin and lincomycin. N. Engl. J. Med. **276**:852, 1967.
25. Klatte, E. C., Yardley, J., Smith, E. B., Rohn, R., and Campbell, J. A. The pul-monary manifestations and complications of leukemia. Amer. J. Roentgenol. **89**:598, 1963.
26. Krumholz, R. A., Manfredi, F., Weg, J. G., and Rosenbaum, D. Needle biopsy of the lung. Report on its use in 112 patients and review of the literature. Ann. Internal Med. **65**:293, 1966.
27. Louria, D. B. Uses of quantitative analyses of bacterial populations in sputum. J.A.M.A. **182**:1082, 1962.
28. Louria, D. B., Blumenfeld, H. L., Ellis, J. T., Kilbourne, E. D., and Rogers, D. E. Studies on influenza in the pandemic of 1957–1958. II. Pulmonary com-plications of influenza. J. Clin. Invest. **38**:213, 1959.
29. Louria, D. B., and Brayton, R. G. The efficacy of penicillin regimens with ob-servations on the frequency of superinfection. J.A.M.A. **186**:987, 1963.
30. Louria, D. B., and Kaminski, T. The effects of four antimicrobial drug regimens on sputum superinfection in hospitalized patients. Amer. Rev. Resp. Dis. **85**:649, 1962.
31. McCrae, T. Delayed resolution in lobar pneumonia. Johns Hopkins Med. J. **15**:277, 1910.
32. McFarland, W., and Libre, E. P. Abnormal leukocyte response in alcoholism. Ann. Internal Med. **59**:865, 1963.
33. Morgan, S. W., and Scott, S. M. A critical reappraisal of scalene fat pad biopsies. J. Thorac. Cardiovasc. Surg. **43**:548, 1962.
34. Murray, J. F., Haegelin, H. F., Hewitt, W. L., Latta, H., McVickar, D., Ras-mussen, A. F., and Rigler, L. G. Opportunistic pulmonary infections. Ann. Internal Med. **65**:566, 1966.

35. Musser, J. H., and Norris, G. W. Lobar pneumonia. In *Modern Medicine*, Osler, W., Ed., p. 537. Lea Brothers and Co., Philadelphia, 1907.

36. North, L. B. Cavitary pulmonary infarction. Amer. Rev. Resp. Dis. 96:1056, 1967.

37. Pickhardt, O. C. Unresolved pneumonia. A surgical analysis. Arch. Surg. 16:192, 1928.

38. Raich, R. A., Casey, F., and Hall, W. H. Pulmonary and cutaneous nocardiosis. Amer. Rev. Resp. Dis. 83:505, 1961.

39. Reinarz, J. A., Pierce, A. K., Mays, B. B., and Sanford, J. P. The potential role of inhalation therapy equipment in nosocomial pulmonary infection. J. Clin. Invest. 44:831, 1965.

40. Schaffner, W., Drutz, D. J., Duncan, G. W., and Koenig, M. G. The clinical spectrum of endemic psittacosis. Arch. Internal Med. 119:433, 1967.

41. Schaffner, W., Schrieber, W. M., and Koenig, M. G. Fatal pneumonia due to a tetracycline-resistant pneumococcus. N. Engl. J. Med. 274:451, 1966.

42. Shulman, J. A., Phillips, L. A., and Petersdorf, R. G. Errors and hazards in the diagnosis and treatment of bacterial pneumonias. Ann. Internal Med. 62:41, 1965.

43. Simon, H. J. Epidemiology and pathogenesis of staphylococcal infection. I. An experimentally induced attenuated staphylococcal infection in guinea pigs and its modification by tetracycline. J. Exp. Med. 118:149, 1963.

44. Smalley, R. V., and Wall, R. L. Two cases of busulfan toxicity. Ann. Internal Med. 64:154, 1966.

45. Smith, M. R., and Wood, W. B., Jr. An experimental analysis of the curative action of penicillin in acute bacterial infections. II. The role of phagocytic cells in the process of recovery. J. Exp. Med. 103:499, 1956.

46. Sollaccio, P. A., Ribaudo, C. A., and Grace, W. J. Subacute pulmonary infiltration due to nitrofurantoin. Ann. Internal Med. 65:1284, 1966.

47. Spotnitz, M., Rudnitzky, J., and Rambaud, J. J. Melioidosis pneumonitis. Analysis of nine cases of a benign form of melioidosis. J.A.M.A. 202:950, 1967.

48. Sutter, V. L., Hurst, V., Grossman, M., and Colonje, R. Source and significance of *Pseudomonas aeruginosa* in sputum. Patients requiring tracheal suction. J.A.M.A. 197:854, 1966.

49. Tillett, W. S., McCormack, J. E., and Cambier, M. J. Treatment of lobar pneumonia with penicillin. J. Clin. Invest. 25:589, 1945.

50. Tillotson, J. R., and Lerner, A. M. Pneumonias caused by gram-negative bacilli. Medicine 45:65, 1966.

51. Van Metre, T. E., Jr. Pneumococcal pneumonia treated with antibiotics. The prognostic significance of certain clinical findings. N. Engl. J. Med. 251:1048, 1954.

52. Wagner, H. N., Bennett, I. L., Lasagna, L., Cluff, L. E., Rosenthal, M. B., and Mirick, G. S. The effect of hydrocortisone upon the course of pneumococcal pneumonia. Johns Hopkins Med. J. 98:197, 1956.

53. Ward, P. H., Stephenson, S. E., and Harris, P. F. Exploration of the mediastinum under local anesthesia. Ann. Otol. Rhinol. Laryngol. 75:368, 1966.

54. Witt, R. L., and Hamburger, M. The nature and treatment of pneumococcal pneumonia. Med. Clin. N. Amer. 47:1257, 1963.

55. Yamamoto, M., Ogura, Y., Sudo, K., and Hibino, S. Diagnostic criteria for disease caused by atypical mycobacteria. Amer. Rev. Resp. Dis. 96:773, 1967.

Polycythemia

RICHARD T. SILVER

INTRODUCTION

A standard textbook description of the patient with polycythemia vera includes ruddy cyanosis of the face and extremities, ecchymoses, bloodshot eyes, engorged mucous membranes, significant splenomegaly, hyperplastic bone marrow, and elevated red and white blood cell counts, hemoglobin concentration, hematocrit, and platelet count. This easily recognized constellation usually does not present too difficult a diagnostic problem; nor, for that matter, does the diagnosis of secondary polycythemia in the wheezing, emphysematous coal miner with a hematocrit of 60 per cent who gasps that he has smoked two packs of cigarettes a day for years. Unfortunately, these examples represent extremes of the clinical spectrum of polycythemia and, of course, the majority fall between them.

How does one diagnose "polycythemia"? How may primary and secondary polycythemia be distinguished? What are the limitations of the available diagnostic procedures? What are reasonable guidelines for the diagnosis?

This chapter will concern itself with answering these questions in a discussion of the clinical diagnosis of polycythemia.

DEFINITION

Polycythemia may be defined as an increase in the volume of circulating red blood cells per kilogram of body weight or, equivalently, as an increase in the red blood cell mass. Clinically this is expressed as an absolute increase in the number of red cells, usually, but not always, accompanied by corresponding increases in hemoglobin and hematocrit values.

Polycythemia may occur as a primary disease of unknown cause, polycythemia vera (p. vera), or as a secondary manifestation of other illnesses, which will be discussed subsequently.

Some writers use the terms erythremia and erythrocytosis to refer to primary and secondary polycythemia, respectively. Others use erythremia as a classification for patients whose only abnormality is an increased red cell volume. Both terms are superfluous and confusing, and are therefore not recommended.

The term "relative" polycythemia is also a misnomer, and its use should

RICHARD T. SILVER, M.D. Clinical Associate Professor of Medicine, Cornell University Medical College, Associate Attending Physician, The New York Hospital, New York, New York; Director, Chemotherapy Service, Division of Hematology, New York Hospital–Cornell Medical Center; Member, Polycythemia Vera National Study Group under the auspices of the National Cancer Institute, National Institutes of Health, Bethesda, Maryland.

be discontinued. A better term is "false" polycythemia. False polycythemia is not polycythemia, because red cell volume per kilogram of body weight is normal. In this instance the elevated hematocrit relates to a decrease in plasma volume. In true polycythemia plasma volume may be increased, normal, or decreased. Other terms referring to false or relative polycythemia include stress polycythemia, stress erythrocytosis, pseudopolycythemia, benign polycythemia, and probably some of the cases designated as Gaisbock's syndrome.

For emphasis, it is worth repeating that the determination of red cell volume per kilogram of body weight separates both primary and secondary polycythemia from false polycythemia. Primary polycythemia (p. vera) can be differentiated from secondary polycythemia by other means to be described, but not by blood volume determination, as has sometimes been implied.[24]

Some hematologists[27, 52] consider that polycythemia is characterized by an abnormal increase in hemoglobin concentration, rather than by an increase in the volume of red blood cells. This is because an abnormal increase in hemoglobin concentration is invariably accompanied by an increase in erythrocyte number, although the converse is not always so. Polycythemia as defined here, however, refers to an *absolute* increase in red cell mass and not to an increased *concentration* of either red cells or hemoglobin. Polycythemia is also more appropriately related to red cell mass (volume per kilogram of body weight) because of historical facts, the derivation of the term, and the evidence that in both primary and secondary polycythemia red cell production relates to the number of circulating red cells and not to hemoglobin concentration.[62]

Considerations Pertaining to the Interpretation of Some Laboratory Tests

Hematocrit

In many laboratories the hematocrit, the volume of packed red cells, is the commonly used test from which the diagnosis of polycythemia is first suspected. The extensive reliance upon the hematocrit for the *diagnosis* of polycythemia is, however, the source of much confusion, both at the bedside and in published texts. It is not widely appreciated that, although there is a reasonably good correlation between the hematocrit and the circulating total red blood cell volume over a wide range of hematocrit determinations, the value of a single measurement of the hematocrit for *predicting* total red cell volume is poor. For hematocrits ranging from 50 to 60 or 65 per cent, the total red cell volume may range from normal to a maximum of twice normal. Thus, Berlin et al.[5] have shown that at a hematocrit of 60 per cent red cell volume can range from 30 to 65cc/kg of body weight. Furthermore, red cell volume cannot be accurately predicted indirectly from measuring plasma volume. Hence, red cell volume must be measured directly in order to determine whether it is increased.

In order to compare total red cell volume from one individual to another, it is best to express it in terms of cubic centimeters per kilogram of body weight, since the use of volume alone does not provide for a comparison between individuals of different body mass. Even expressing red cell volume per kilogram of body weight is not unequivocally precise, since the amount of blood associated with lean body mass is larger than that associated with adipose tissue. Red cell volume can also be compared by employing body surface area or some function of one or another determinant of body composition. In view of present techniques, however, and the practical aspects of the problem, red cell mass expressed as cubic centimeters per kilogram of body weight is satisfactory for the great majority of cases.[4]

The most satisfactory and widely used method for determining red cell volume is direct tagging of red cells with radioactive chromium (Cr^{51}). This method is easy to perform and is reproducible;[51] the coefficient of variation is 1.5 to 1.8 per cent if two determinations are performed within 24 hours of each other.

The red cell mass in the normal man differs from that in the normal woman. As measured by Cr^{51}-labeled red cells, a red cell mass greater than 36 cc/kg of body weight is considered increased in a man, and greater than 32 cc/kg is considered increased in a woman.[4, 5]

Since it is clear that an increased hematocrit determination does not necessarily signify an increased red blood cell mass, it may be legitimately inquired if, on the other hand, polycythemia vera might be diagnosed more often if red cell volume were measured in patients with unexplained splenomegaly, even in the presence of normal hematocrit values. The probability of finding an elevated red cell volume in such a patient is small, but presumably this could occur. There are no published data on this point.

Arterial Oxygen Saturation and Erythropoietin Levels

Only within the last decade or two has polycythemia been categorized in terms of its underlying pathophysiologic mechanisms. The causes of secondary polycythemia can be simply classified for clinical use according to 1) those related to inadequate oxygen delivery to tissues with respect to need and 2) those that are not so related.

Before considering this further, it will be helpful to define the following terms. *Hypoxia* means inadequate tissue oxygenation. It may result from an increased demand for or a decreased supply of oxygen. *Hypoxemia* refers to decreased oxygen content in the blood. It implies decreased arterial oxygen tension, decreased arterial oxygen saturation, or both. *Arterial oxygen tension* (pO_2) is the partial pressure of oxygen in arterial blood, measured in millimeters of mercury. Because of the shape of the oxyhemoglobin dissociation curve, arterial oxygen tension may be reduced without any reduction in arterial oxygen saturation. *Arterial oxygen saturation* is the percentage of hemoglobin saturated with oxygen in arterial blood.

ARTERIAL OXYGEN SATURATION

Customarily an arterial oxygen saturation of 92 per cent or more has been considered characteristic of polycythemia vera, whereas a lower saturation has been regarded as strong evidence of polycythemia related to hypoxemia.[4, 70] Recent investigations have cast doubt on the usefulness of arterial oxygen saturation measurements in differentiating primary and secondary polycythemia, even when the latter is related to impaired arterial oxygen supply.[44, 45]

Many patients with certain lung diseases have respiratory alkalosis due to hyperventilation. Because of the influence of pH on the oxyhemoglobin dissociation curve, oxygen saturation in these patients may be normal, even though arterial oxygen tension is significantly reduced. To illustrate, at pH 7.40 an abnormal oxygen tension (po_2) of 65 mm Hg results in an abnormal saturation of about 91.5 per cent. At pH 7.45, however, the saturation is 93.5 per cent for the same po_2. Changes in pH of this magnitude may result even from hyperventilation induced by an arterial puncture, particularly of the "single stick" type.[59]

The frequency with which misleading normal arterial oxygen saturation determinations are recorded is unknown. Smith reviewed the records of 110 patients with severe bronchitis and emphysema seen at The New York Hospital[59] and found that 49 of them had venous hematocrits above 55 per cent. In the majority of these 49 patients the mean arterial saturation was 89 per cent. In seven (14 per cent), however, the arterial saturation was 92 per cent or more, and the mean hematocrit for these seven patients was 58 per cent. All seven had a high normal pH and a low or borderline arterial oxygen tension (po_2). In all, however, exercise measurements unmasked significant hypoxemia.

It is even less well known and appreciated that polycythemia vera, uncomplicated by cardiac or pulmonary disease, may in itself cause arterial oxygen undersaturation. The frequency of this abnormality has also been estimated by Smith,[59] who compiled data from four large series of patients with p. vera.[12, 40, 44, 70] Among 112 patients the arterial saturation was less than 94 per cent in 52 (46 per cent) and less than 92 per cent in 26 (23 per cent).

The cause of hypoxemia in polycythemia uncomplicated by cardiac or pulmonary disease is not well understood. There is no evidence to indicate that the arterial unsaturation in p. vera is related to abnormal hemoglobin function, to the high hematocrit, or to increased blood volume per se. It is generally agreed that, as a group, patients with polycythemia vera have normal ventilatory function, alveolar ventilation, and distribution of ventilation. Controversy still exists, however, about diffusion measurements and ventilation-perfusion relationships. It is still unknown whether hypoxemia is an integral feature of the disorder or a nonspecific finding. In p. vera hypoxemia may represent the combined effects of age, associated and unrelated lung disease, and possibly vascular abnormalities of the pulmonary microcirculation.

In essence, then, the conclusions drawn concerning the usefulness of an arterial oxygen saturation determination in the differential diagnosis of polycythemia revolve about its lack of discriminatory value except in those cases associated with moderately severe arterial unsaturation, i.e., less than 90 per cent. Mild unsaturation (90 to 94 per cent) is commonly found in primary and some varieties of secondary polycythemia.

ERYTHROPOIETIN

Although determination of the humoral substance erythropoietin currently has limited use as a diagnostic test for clinical application, the polycythemias should be examined in relation to it.

Based upon abundant evidence in animals and man, a decrease in arterial oxygen tension will result in an increase in red cell production, presumably mediated via erythropoietin. Thus, in six patients with polycythemia secondary to hypoxemia, Adamson and Finch,[2] employing a polycythemic mouse assay system, found increased or normal urinary erythropoietin values. If normal values were found there was an exaggerated urinary erythropoietin response to phlebotomy, for urinary erythropoietin values exceeded normal levels at any given hematocrit level.

A major exception to the generality relating falling oxygen tension to rising red cell mass is that group of patients with emphysema who have diminished arterial oxygen tension but normal red cell mass. An increase in erythropoietin has nevertheless been demonstrated in a few of these individuals, implying that the absence of polycythemia is not dependent upon an inability to produce erythropoietin.[62] Chronic infections, seen commonly in obstructive pulmonary disease, has been offered as one explanation for the suboptimal increase in red cell mass observed in these hypoxemic patients.

In contrast to the observations in polycythemia secondary to anoxia, many studies of patients with p. vera have indicated that this type of polycythemia is not oxygen-dependent and is not associated with increased erythropoietin in plasma or urine.[23] In fact, erythropoietin output is probably less than normal,[23] implying both that red cell production by the marrow is autonomous and that erythropoietin output has been suppressed by the increased red cell mass.

Polycythemia unrelated to tissue hypoxia or to p. vera may be seen as a reflection of autonomous erythropoietin production by benign and malignant tumors. Biologically active erythropoietic substances, which have been demonstrated in some instances in plasma, urine, and tissue extracts from such patients,[9, 29] are not subject to physiologic control mechanisms and are independent of the red cell mass. The causal relationship between polycythemia and tumor is indicated by the fact that, in many cases, remission of the former has occurred following removal of the latter.[9, 17, 19, 29, 61] This type of polycythemia has been most frequently associated with renal abnormalities, especially neoplasms and benign cysts. It has been possible to demonstrate erythropoietin in cyst fluid or kidney extracts in some instances, but elevated levels of erythropoietin have not been consistently observed in plasma or urine. Whether the tumor or cyst is directly related to the increased production of erythropoietin has not been demonstrated. Thus, for example, the tumor or cyst may cause local changes in the kidney by compressing blood vessels, and may thus lead to increased elaboration of erythropoietin.[26, 64] In any case, the infrequent and inconsistent ability to demonstrate increased erythropoietin probably reflects the relative insensitivity of current bioassay techniques and/or the relatively low level of erythropoietin production.

The probable relation between erythropoietin and the polycythemias may be summarized as follows:

1. Increased but regulated erythropoietin production proportional to the stimulus in secondary hypoxemic polycythemia.

2. Autonomous erythropoietin production irrespective of red cell mass in the secondary polycythemia accompanying tumors.

3. Autonomous erythropoiesis by the marrow irrespective of erythropoietin levels in p. vera.

Vitamin B_{12} and Leukocyte Alkaline Phosphatase

Two biochemical tests have assumed some importance in the diagnosis of polycythemia vera. These are the levels of serum vitamin B_{12} and its binding proteins and the leukocyte alkaline phosphatase score.

VITAMIN B_{12} AND ITS BINDING PROTEINS

Recent evidence which indicates that vitamin B_{12} metabolism is affected in the myeloproliferative diseases includes abnormalities of the serum level of vitamin B_{12}, total vitamin B_{12}-binding capacity (TBBC), and unsaturated vitamin B_{12}-binding capacity (UBBC). Measurements of these parameters are proving valuable in differential diagnosis and in assessing response to therapy.

In polycythemia vera and in chronic granulocytic leukemia levels of serum B_{12} and vitamin B_{12}-binding capacity are elevated above normal, parallel to the degree of white cell proliferation. Serum vitamin B_{12} tends to be modestly increased above normal in polycythemia vera[28] and greatly increased in chronic granulocytic leukemia.[22] A similar but more striking relative increase occurs in the UBBC. In 15 normal adults average values for serum B_{12} and UBBC were 700 and 1800 pg/ml, respectively. In 31 patients with polycythemia vera the value of serum B_{12} was 900 pg/ml, and the UBBC approximately 3000 pg/ml. In 20 patients with chronic granulocytic leukemia the average serum B_{12} level was 3200 pg/ml, and the UBBC, 8400 pg/ml.[28]

Elevation of the UBBC can aid in the differential diagnosis of polycythemia vera and false (relative) polycythemia. In one series[21] UBBC was more than 2000 pg/ml in 24 of 27 patients with active polycythemia vera, but in only 4 of 28 normal patients and 3 of 17 with false polycythemia. The mean UBBC values in the three groups were 3516, 1667, and 1857 pg/ml, respectively. Corresponding mean serum B_{12} levels were 894, 472, and 305 pg/ml.

LEUKOCYTE ALKALINE PHOSPHATASE

Since some patients with polycythemia vera may have a significant elevation of the white blood cell count, the leukocyte alkaline phosphatase (LAP) stain can be of value in distinguishing these cases of polycythemia vera from chronic granulocytic leukemia.

Briefly, the principle of the LAP staining method is based upon the amount and staining intensity of a precipitated dye at presumed sites of enzyme activity within mature and band-forming neutrophils, the only granulocytes with significant LAP activity in the peripheral blood or bone marrow. Usually peripheral blood is scored semiquantitatively; 100 neutrophils are graded 0 to 4+. The total score may thus range from 0 to 400.

Abnormally low or absent LAP activity is observed in chronic granulocytic leukemia and in some cases of myelofibrosis with myeloid metaplasia.[14] A marked increase both in LAP activity and in the number of neutrophils showing such activity may be seen in polycythemia, idiopathic thrombocytopenia, leukemoid reactions, and other cases of myelofibrosis with myeloid metaplasia.

The normal LAP score ranges from 25 to 50. In leukemoid reactions and in polycythemia vera it may rise above 200, whereas in chronic granulocytic leukemia it is usually below 25.

Although the LAP stain can be helpful in distinguishing many cases of chronic granulocytic leukemia from polycythemia vera (and other diseases in the myeloproliferative group), a low level per se should not be considered an unequivocal criterion for chronic granulocytic leukemia or against polycythemia vera. In one study of polycythemia vera[1] the LAP score was high in eight patients, within the normal range in 11, and reduced in one. This last patient, however, had had "severe polycythemia vera" for 3 years and then developed typical chronic granulocytic leukemia, including demonstration of the Philadelphia chromosome. On the other hand, a few cases of seemingly bona fide chronic granulocytic leukemia, including the finding of the Philadelphia chromosome, have yielded relatively normal LAP scores.[6]

In general, LAP values in uncomplicated secondary polycythemia are normal. However, since so many factors may cause an elevation in the LAP (e.g., infection, fever, hemorrhage), and since the LAP may be normal in primary polycythemia, this test may lose its discriminatory value in the individual case.

CLINICAL POLYCYTHEMIA

For reasons which will be discussed some cases of polycythemia vera must be diagnosed as such by excluding all potential causes of secondary polycythemia. Hence, the secondary polycythemias will be discussed first (Table 44).

Secondary Polycythemia

From a clinical standpoint the causes of secondary polycythemia (Table 44) may be divided into a more common group, related to arterial hypoxemia, and a less common group, which is not. In this latter category polycythemia is associated with a number of benign and malignant conditions of various organs, especially the kidney, cerebellum, liver, and uterus.

Secondary Polycythemia Related to Inadequate Oxygen Delivery with Respect to Need

Oxygen delivery depends upon the arterial oxygen tension, blood flow to the tissues, and the amount of active hemoglobin available for combination with oxygen. The majority of causes of secondary polycythemia related to inadequate oxygen delivery are readily apparent at the bedside. As a general rule, the severity of the polycythemia may be correlated with the degree of hypoxia.

INADEQUATE OXYGEN DELIVERY DUE TO DECREASED ARTERIAL OXYGEN TENSION

With Anatomic or Physiologic Cardiopulmonary Abnormalities. Chronic obstructive pulmonary disease (emphysema and bronchitis) and some neuromuscular disorders, such as poliomyelitis, amyotrophic lateral sclerosis, and myasthenia gravis, may be complicated by alveolar hypoventilation and hypoxemia. This is characterized by arterial oxygen un-

TABLE 44
Clinical Classification of Polycythemia

I. Secondary polycythemia
    A. Related to inadequate oxygen delivery to tissues with respect to need
        1. Due to decreased arterial oxygen tension
            a. With physiologic or anatomic cardiopulmonary abnormalities
                (1) Abnormalities of lungs, chest bellows, or ventilatory control mechanism
                (2) Right-to-left vascular shunts
            b. Without physiologic or anatomic cardiopulmonary abnormalities
                (1) Low oxygen tension, i.e., high altitudes
                (2) Impaired oxygen-carrying capacity of hemoglobin
        2. Due to decreased blood flow: congestive heart failure
    B. Unrelated to inadequate oxygen delivery and need and associated with benign or malignant lesions of
        1. Kidney: cysts, hydronephrosis, adenoma, hypernephroma, sarcoma
        2. Cerebellum: hemangioblastoma
        3. Uterus: myoma
        4. Liver: hepatoma, hamartoma
        5. Other: adrenal (pheochromocytoma), lung
II. Primary polycythemia (polycythemia vera)

saturation, CO_2 retention, and a low or normal arterial pH. Alveolar hypoventilation is distinguished from both a simple diffusion defect and an uncomplicated right-to-left shunt by the presence of CO_2 retention in association with oxygen unsaturation.

A rare form of secondary alveolar hypoventilation and polycythemia, the so-called Pickwickian syndrome,[11] has been recognized as an unusual complication of extreme obesity. In this condition obesity imposes a mechanical burden on the bellows action of the chest and abdominal wall. In its most severe form there are accompanying cyanosis, right-sided heart failure, and central nervous symptoms, including headache, somnolence, and muscle twitching.

Alveolar hypoventilation may occur in the absence of obesity or of diseases of the lungs or musculoskeletal apparatus of the chest in the rare primary hypoventilation syndrome, attributed to an intrinsic disorder of the respiratory control center in the medulla.[55] The most prominent feature of patients with this syndrome is polycythemia. Unless arterial oxygen saturation studies are carried out, cases of the primary hypoventilation syndrome in which the presenting picture is that of secondary polycythemia may be misdiagnosed as instances of primary polycythemia. When the diagnosis of secondary polycythemia has been established by the presence of arterial oxygen unsaturation, other causes of arterial oxygen unsaturation must also be excluded.

Other types of lung disease, such as pulmonary sarcoidosis and fibrosis, are often accompanied by arterial unsaturation and polycythemia, but not by alveolar hypoventilation. These diseases are characterized by diffuse interstitial fibrosis with thickening of the alveolar-capillary membrane, resulting in impaired diffusion of oxygen from the alveolus into the pulmonary capillary, and by derangement in ventilation-perfusion relationships. The radiographic appearance of the lungs in these patients is usually suggestive. Differential diagnosis is also facilitated by the observation that there is no concomitant elevation of the arterial CO_2 tension or decrease of the blood pH. This is because CO_2 is 20 times more diffusible than oxygen, and death usually occurs from hypoxia long before there is CO_2 retention.

In chronic congestive heart failure thickened alveolar membranes and disturbances in ventilation-perfusion ratios may also give rise to a low arterial oxygen tension. In addition, low cardiac output causes reduction in blood flow and may promote additional polycythemia.

Polycythemia also occurs when there is partial shunting of blood from the pulmonary circuit into the systemic circulation, without opportunity for adequate oxygenation in the normally functioning pulmonary capillary bed. The most common defects producing this are pulmonary stenosis with a defective ventricular or atrial septum, all causes of the Eisenmenger complex, patent ductus arteriosus with reversal of flow, pulmonary arteriovenous fistula, persistent truncus arteriosus, complete transposition of arterial trunks, and the tetralogy of Fallot. An intracardiac right-to-left shunt is almost always associated with other abnormalities which point to its presence. Occasionally a pulmonary arteriovenous fistula will be associated with a minimum of other findings. The presence of a shunt can usually be established by failure to achieve an oxygen tension of more than 600 mm Hg in the arterial blood after administration of 100 per cent oxygen for 30 minutes. Unsaturation due either to a diffusion defect or to alveolar hypoventilation is corrected by this procedure.

Without Physiologic or Anatomic Cardiopulmonary Abnormalities.

Inadequate Oxygen in Inspired Air. Even without physiologic or anatomic abnormality of the lungs, chest bellows, or ventilatory control mechanisms, reduced arterial oxygen tension may develop when there is inadequate oxygen in the inspired air. The association of polycythemia and life at high altitudes has been known for years, and is similar in pathogenesis to that seen in any cardiopulmonary disorder resulting from insufficient oxygenation of the arterial blood. The studies of Hurtado et al.[31] on high-altitude polycythemia clearly show the inverse relationship between atmospheric oxygen saturation at various altitudes and hemoglobin concentration in the peripheral blood. In general, the level of polycythemia is directly proportional to the degree, duration, and continuity of the hypoxic stimulus, although the hematologic response to anoxia has finite limits.

Impaired Oxygen-Carrying Capacity of Hemoglobin. A reduction in the amount of effective circulating hemoglobin available for combination with oxygen should cause compensatory polycythemia whenever tissue hypoxia develops. This could occur if the hemoglobin combines with a substance, such as carbon monoxide, for which it has more affinity than oxygen; if an irreversible chemical reaction occurs and alters the hemoglobin molecule (e.g., sulfhemoglobin); if the ferrous porphyrin complex is oxidized to the ferric form (e.g., methemoglobin); or if a structurally abnormal hemoglobin with impaired oxygen-carrying capacity is present (e.g., hemoglobins M and Chesapeake).

Carbon monoxide fortunately reacts reversibly with hemoglobin, and thus does not severely reduce oxygen transport for long periods. In two series of patients with sulfhemoglobinemia[8, 54] total hemoglobin concentration was normal. Thus, polycythemia has not been observed clinically in either of these circumstances.

Many drugs which cause the oxidation of hemoglobin from the ferrous to the ferric state result in the formation of methemoglobin. These include, for example, nitrites, chlorates, quinones, and aminophenols.[7] However, polycythemia is ordinarily not found in acquired methemoglobinemia, since the poisoning is usually of short duration.

Two fundamentally different types of congenital methemoglobinemia have been identified. One type is related to an abnormality in the metabolism of the erythrocyte, resulting in inability to reconvert methemoglobin to hemoglobin.[32] The majority of these cases are probably due to a deficiency of reduced diphosphopyridine nucleotide (DPNH)–methemoglobin reductase activity. Although the homozygous subject may be slightly polycythemic, the recessive mode of inheritance, the cyanosis manifested at birth, and the unusually dark color of the blood should hardly present a diagnostic problem.

The second type of congenital methemoglobin is due to the inheritance of one of a group of abnormal hemoglobins capable of forming a stable methemoglobin derivative, the M hemoglobin. As with other hemoglobinopathies, the pattern of inheritance is dominant in type. Cyanosis is the only clinical manifestation. Mild polycythemia in hemoglobin M disease has been reported in at least one case. In addition to hemoglobin electrophoresis, hemoglobin M can be distinguished from other forms of methemoglobin by spectrophotometric differences.[32]

Another abnormal hemoglobin, hemoglobin Chesapeake, has been found to be associated with elevated hematocrit levels both in an affected individual and in heterozygous carriers.[13] In the homozygous individual there was low arterial oxygen tension, and no leukocytosis, thrombocytosis, or splenomegaly. No increase in erythropoietin activity could be demonstrated.

Other recently discussed abnormal hemoglobins associated with familial polycythemia are hemoglobins J Capetown, Yakima, Kempsey, Rainier, and Ypsi.[72] The clinical findings in these instances are similar to those described for hemoglobin Chesapeake. Secondary polycythemia is produced in individuals with these hemoglobinopathies because the oxygen dissociation curves are shifted toward the left. These shifts reflect an increased affinity of whole blood for oxygen. Thus, for any specific decrease in the partial pressure of oxygen, the fall in oxygen saturation of hemoglobin is less than normal; therefore, the red blood cells of an affected individual yield relatively less oxygen to the tissues, and the resulting anoxia leads to increased erythropoiesis.

DECREASED BLOOD FLOW WITH NORMAL ARTERIAL OXYGEN DELIVERY

Decreased arterial blood flow without a corresponding change in oxygen content or in oxygen demand has been associated with an increase in red cell mass, presumably resulting from local tissue hypoxia. This can occur with low cardiac output, usually seen in patients with congestive heart failure.[18] Correction of the congestive failure has been associated with return of the red cell values toward normal.

Some patients with congestive heart failure have mild arterial hypoxemia because of coexisting pulmonary abnormalities, not because of changes in cardiac output. These patients, however, have an increase in red cell mass exceeding the volume predicted by the degree of hypoxemia. Hence, other factors must also be influencing erythrocyte production; these may be related to reduced blood flow. As yet there is no substantial clinical evidence that diminished renal blood flow causes polycythemia, although increased erythropoietin activity has been observed in experimental renal ischemia.[26, 64]

Polycythemia Unrelated to Inadequate Tissue Oxygen Delivery and Need

This type of polycythemia has been associated with benign and malignant conditions of the kidney, cerebellum, uterus, liver, adrenal, lung, and other organs.

KIDNEY

Diseases of the kidney have been the commonest causes of this type of secondary polycythemia, although in only a small proportion of the various renal conditions does polycythemia develop. The frequency ranges from approximately 0.5 to 4 per cent. Polycythemia has been associated with benign lesions, including renal adenoma, unilateral or bilateral hydronephrosis, and cysts, including solitary cysts, multiple cysts, and polycystic kidneys. Cystic renal disease has been associated with polycythemia 2 to 3 times more frequently than has renal carcinoma.[15, 33, 35, 46] The male predominance in renal polycythemia has been noted.[33]

It is incorrect to assume that all patients with polycythemia secondary to renal lesions lack elevations of the white blood cell count or platelet count or do not have hepatosplenomegaly. In a retrospective study of 91 patients thought to have polycythemia vera (as diagnosed by stringent criteria), eight patients had significant renal lesions.[33] Of these eight, seven had two or three abnormalities, which consisted of an increased white blood cell count, platelet count, or splenomegaly.

Considering, furthermore, the 20 per cent of patients with polycythemia vera who do not have hepatosplenomegaly or an increased white blood cell count or platelet count, it is readily apparent that in any case of polycythemia a coexisting renal lesion must be excluded by appropriate study.[4, 33]

POSTERIOR FOSSA TUMORS

A number of posterior fossa tumors, mainly cerebellar hemangioblastomas, have been reported in association with polycythemia. In one series of 106 patients with posterior fossa tumors, hemoglobin values greater than 18 g/100 ml were found in 11.[61] In only a few instances had red blood cell volume studies been performed. However, elevated peripheral red cell values returned to normal after corrective surgery. From 9 to 20 per cent of other series of patients with cerebellar hemangioblastomas have had polycythemia.[69] In these cases the mean age of the patients was 37 years. This contrasts with a mean age of 56 years for patients with polycythemia and kidney tumors.[69] Cerebellar hemangioblastoma with polycythemia is more likely to occur in men, as is the polycythemia associated with kidney tumors.

OTHER TUMORS ASSOCIATED WITH SECONDARY POLYCYTHEMIA

Polycythemia has been found in 10 per cent of 176 patients with hepatoma.[43] It has also been found in association with uterine fibroids.[58] It is striking that, despite the frequency of fibroids in women, the association with polycythemia is rare indeed.[30] With this tumor, as with others, the polycythemia usually remits following removal of the fibroids. In one unusual case[19] only the tip of the spleen was palpable and the patient had an elevated platelet count. Postoperatively, physical and laboratory examinations became unremarkable.

Review of the literature indicates that polycythemia has been associated with a number of other malignant and benign tumors, including undifferentiated carcinoma of the lung,[17] carcinoma of the stomach with metastases to the liver,[29] adrenal gland adenoma[42] and carcinoma,[44] Wilms' tumor,[66] multiple myeloma,[16] pheochromocytoma,[68] an ovarian tumor associated with Cushing's syndrome,[38] atrial myxoma,[41] and hamartoma of the liver.[36]

The important clinical point ascertained from review of these cases is that, although the predominant proliferative component is erythroid, in some instances there may be leukocytosis and thrombocytosis as well. In fewer instances there has been splenomegaly; these findings have been reported most frequently in patients with polycythemia secondary to renal disease. In the individual case, therefore, leukocytosis, thrombocytosis, and even slight splenomegaly do not exclude secondary polycythemia. Thus, a diligent search for any kind of tumor must be made in the patient initially evaluated for polycythemia unless the findings are obviously and grossly those of p. vera.

MISCELLANEOUS CAUSES OF POLYCYTHEMIA

A number of chemical and physical agents, such as coal tar derivatives, aniline, phosphorus, gum, shellac, cobalt, and batyl alcohol, have been implicated, mainly in experimental polycythemia[45, 62] and rarely in isolated clinical reports, but these are not of importance in the clinical differentiation of polycythemia.

There is also much experimental evidence citing the erythropoietic effect of naturally occurring hormones, including the corticosteroids, adrenocorticotropin, growth hormone, testosterone, and thyroid hormone.[45, 62] Except for Cushing's syndrome, they do not have much significance in the differential diagnosis of clinical polycythemia. Patients with Cushing's syndrome with atypical presenting manifestations, but with an increased red cell mass,[48] should be distinguished by high plasma cortisol levels, lack of diurnal plasma cortisol variation, and increased urinary 17-hydroxycorticoid excretion.

A special comment should be made about the entity that has been described as "benign polycythemia" or "stress polycythemia." This term derives from several reports[37, 39, 57] describing increased hematocrit values in patients of early middle age (thus younger than patients with p. vera) with stocky builds and plethoric complexions. Many of the patients smoked cigarettes and were thought to be anxious. They had a high frequency of hypertension and vascular disease. In one series[57] the highest hematocrit values ranged between 55 and 65 per cent. Progressive increase in the hematocrit, white count, platelet count, and spleen size did not occur during prolonged periods of observation. Review of these reports indicates that the majority of the patients had normal red cell masses, and thus the designation "polycythemia" in naming the condition is inappropriate. The false polycythemia was related to a decrease in plasma volume with a normal total red cell volume.[39] The increased frequency of hypertension in these patients may have been related to the referral of some of the patients from a hypertension clinic.[20] Although there is an implied relationship between blood pressure and blood volume, no correlation between these parameters in polycythemia has been observed in detailed studies.[49] Although false polycythemia has been related to emotional stress, no proper psychologic studies have been performed to justify the conclusion that tense, anxious personalities are more frequent in patients with false polycythemia than in other subjects in a control population.[20]

Another explanation for the selected high hematocrit values relates to the absence of a rigid, arbitrary value for the upper limit of normal for the volume of packed red cells. The hematocrit values now generally accepted as normal at sea level (males, 47 ± 5 per cent; females, 42.0 ± 5 per cent) represent the mean ± 2 standard deviations.[73] This implies that on the basis of the normal distribution curve of the hematocrit the values of 4.6 per cent of the normal population lie beyond this range. It can be argued, of course, that those measurements of physiologic parameters which levels are at the extremes of the distribution curve may be of pathologic significance when they stand in appropriate quantitative and temporal relationship to other disease determinants. Before importance is ascribed to them, however, assurance should be sought that they do not reflect an arbitrary definition of abnormality. This is a good example of the designation of a disease state at one end of the spectrum of polycythemia, when none exists in fact.[73]

Polycythemia Vera

The disease is more common in men than in women, the ratio being approximately 2:1. Polycythemia vera is usually diagnosed in middle life. Its peak age incidence is in the late forties and fifties, and its range from 20 to 50 years. Polycythemia vera is rare in children.[25]

Polycythemia vera has been reported rarely in Negroes and is said to occur with increased frequency in Jews.[15] Whether the latter observation is related to selection by virtue of specific hospital populations is not clear.

Although not specifically hereditary, polycythemia vera has been reported as a familial condition in isolated instances.[1, 60, 63] Its transition and relation to other diseases of the myeloproliferative group have been discussed in detail.[14, 50] The author has observed the development of chronic granulocytic leukemia, myelofibrosis with myeloid metaplasia, and polycythemia vera in one or another member of three generations of the same family.

Clinical Manifestations of Polycythemia Vera

Polycythemia vera presents a panorama of hematologic signs and symptoms; the findings in each case depend upon the severity of the clinical and hematologic stage which the disease has reached.

In general, the development of symptoms of polycythemia vera is insidious. Symptoms include easy fatigue, weakness, shortness of breath, dizziness, tinnitus, visual disturbances, headache, and pruritus. The pruritus increases in intensity after taking a tub bath and less often after showering. It is worse when the temperature of the water is warm rather than cool. (The association of pruritus with the basophil count will be discussed subsequently.) Burning or throbbing pain in the legs, feet, or hands, accompanied by a mottled redness, may occur.

Minor wounds may provoke unusual loss of blood. Other episodes of minor bleeding into the skin or mucous membranes are not infrequent. The most common source of major hemorrhage is the upper gastrointestinal tract.[71] Of importance in this regard is the increased incidence of peptic ulcer, seen in about 10 per cent of patients with p. vera.[67] Thus, iron deficiency may distort the over-all picture because of anemia, hypochromia, and microcytosis. Sometimes iron deficiency occurs in a previously polycythemic woman, owing to menometrorrhagia, and produces the same distorted picture. In these instances the nature of the underlying polycythemia is manifested only when hemorrhage is controlled, and after the anemia has been treated with iron.

The same incompletely understood abnormalities of coagulation responsible for the hemorrhagic tendency paradoxically contribute to thrombotic episodes, which may also cause the presenting manifestations of p. vera. Patients referred because of vascular thromboses of unknown cause in small vessels in the hands or feet may, upon hematologic evaluation, be shown to be suffering from polycythemia and, in particular, thrombocythemia. Thromboses of larger vessels may involve the arterial and venous circulations of the heart, brain, liver, spleen, and lung, and produce related symptoms. Thrombophlebitis is common.

In a typical florid case of classical p. vera the complexion, as first reported by Osler,[47] is dusky red-purple. This discoloration is most noticeable over the face, lips, hands, legs, and feet. Ecchymoses are common. The scleral and conjunctival vessels are engorged. Early in the disease the liver is slightly enlarged in about 50 per cent of the cases. The spleen is enlarged in over 75 per cent of patients. Its size depends upon the stage of the illness, and ranges from being barely palpable below the left costal margin to filling the left half of the abdomen. Spleen size is not a simple function of blood volume.[49] Extremely large spleens may herald the future development of myelofibrosis with myeloid metaplasia.

Hematologic Manifestations

Commonly observed ranges of values include red cell counts of 7,000,000 to 10,000,000/cu mm, hematocrits of 55 to 70 per cent, and hemoglobin concentrations of 18 to 24 g/100 ml. Often the hemoglobin is not increased as much as the red cell count, and thus the hematocrit may be slightly reduced in proportion to the red blood cell count. If there has been hemorrhage, the hemoglobin content of the red blood cells is reduced more than their size, and the red cells may appear hypochromic and microcytic. In general, however, the individual erythrocytes appear normocytic and normochromic. A rare normoblast may be found. Reticulocytes are usually normal in number except after a hemorrhage.

In about half the cases there is a moderate increase in the peripheral white blood cell count, ranging between 10,000 and 30,000/cu mm. Values greater than 50,000/cu mm have been reported.[56] Metamyelocytes may be seen in the peripheral blood smear. An increase in the absolute basophil count was found in 70 per cent of the patients reported by Wasserman and Gilbert.[71] They suggested that the increase in the number of these cells, known to be rich in histamine, may be related to certain features of polycythemia vera, such as peptic ulcer and pruritus.

Blood platelets are increased in number in about one-third of the cases at the time of diagnosis. Generally the degree of elevation is modest, the platelet count ranging between 500,000 and 1,000,000/cu mm. In some patients the initial platelet count may be more than 1,000,000/cu mm, accompanied by only a modest elevation of the hematocrit. Of great importance is the fact that the platelet count may increase substantially after spontaneous bleeding or phlebotomy. The association of increased platelet counts and hemorrhage or thromboses usually occurs at a level of 1,000,000 to 2,000,000/cu mm.

The bone marrow in patients with polycythemia vera is hypercellular, and marrow fat is reduced. This is particularly well recognized in biopsy sections (Figs. 58 and 59). Usually each of the three developmental series participates in the hyperplasia, although erythroid hyperplasia is paramount. (In contrast, the hyperplasia in secondary polycythemia is confined typically to the erythroid series.) There is no abnormality in maturation. Orthochromic normoblasts predominate. There may be a slight shift to the left in the neutrophilic series. Eosinophils and basophils may also be common.

In the writer's opinion, primary and secondary polycythemia cannot be distinguished unequivocally solely on the basis of bone marrow findings, although an increase in megakaryocytes and immaturity and hyperplasia of the granulocytic series favor p. vera. Recent reports have suggested that marrow iron stores are depleted in primary but not in secondary polycythemia. This difference, it has been implied, may be of diagnostic importance. However, since secondary iron deficiency is so common in women, it is doubtful that the absence of marrow iron can be of significant differential value, at least in the female patient.

The nature of the reticulin network in the marrow in polycythemia has not received sufficient attention. Normally reticulin fibers extend throughout the marrow and provide a supporting stroma for hematopoietic tissue.

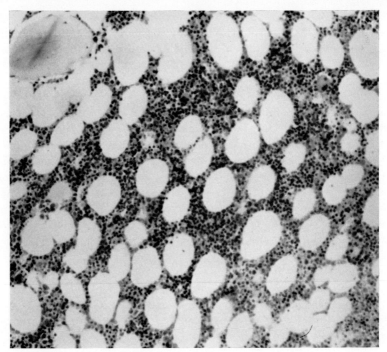

Fig. 58. Normal bone marrow biopsy (10× objective)

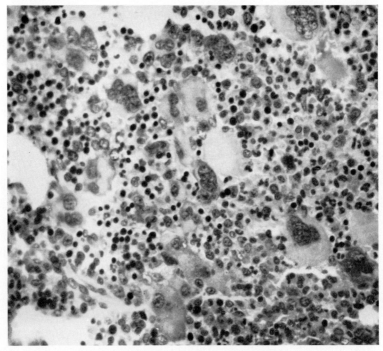

Fig. 59. Hyperplastic bone marrow as seen in polycythemia vera. Megakaryocytes appear in particular profusion. Biopsy (16× objective).

Generally the network is varied in appearance, sometimes more complete in one area than in another.

In disease states two different patterns of the reticulin network can be recognized.[10] The first consists of an increased prominence of the normal network, which probably occurs in response to an increase in functioning hematopoietic tissue. It is a nonspecific change, since it is found in a variety of hematologic disorders. The second, the "fibroblastic" pattern, consists of coarsening of the network, which becomes composed of fibers which are thicker than normal. These thick fibers tend to form bundles or fascicles and follow a waving or swirling course. The fibroblastic pattern has been seen in patients with polycythemia vera and other myeloproliferative diseases. Whether or not the amount of reticulin and its nature will help in the differential diagnosis of primary and secondary polycythemia remains to be determined.

Hyperuricemia

Hyperuricemia, a characteristic of all the myeloproliferative diseases, occurs in the majority of patients with p. vera. No good correlation between serum uric acid levels and red and white cell values has been demonstrated. The incidence of gout in patients with p. vera has ranged from 5 to 10 per cent.[65] This figure will probably be lowered in the future because of the use of allopurinol. Although gout may precede the development of p. vera, it usually occurs 5 or 10 years after the onset of the polycythemia. Thus, gout and excessive uric acid excretion appear in the later stages of p. vera, and often when there is evidence of myelofibrosis and myeloid metaplasia.

Increased urate production and excretion may result in the precipitation of uric acid in the kidneys, causing stones or uric acid nephropathy. Renal colic is an unusual presenting manifestation of patients with p. vera, but it has been observed.

Although serum uric acid may be increased in secondary polycythemia, it is rare to find the same high levels which occur in the primary disease.

Kinetic Studies

Erythrokinetic studies are not particularly useful in the clinical diagnosis of polycythemia vera. Many studies indicate that the life span of the erythrocyte in p. vera is not prolonged.[34] Thus, the increase in number of red cells is related to increased erythropoiesis. As shown by ferrokinetic studies, iron utilization is maximal and compatible with the increased total hemoglobin mass.[53]

Natural History

Although this chapter is concerned primarily with diagnosis, an appreciation of the natural course of p. vera is necessary, since a patient may be observed during a stage when the disease is in transition.

Polycythemia vera is an illness of reasonably long duration, usually ranging between 10 and 20 years. Although the influence of chemotherapy

and radioactive phosphorus on the disease is still not clear, in some of
these patients, after a number of years, the hemoglobin level gradually falls
and anemia develops. The spleen (and sometimes the liver) progressively
enlarges, and may fill the entire abdomen. Splenic infarcts, causing mild
to severe left upper quadrant pain, may mimic an acute abdominal crisis
or renal colic. On rare occasions the enormous spleen may cause large
bowel obstruction. Erythrocytes of variable size and shape, teardrop forms,
nucleated red cells, and immature granulocytes appear in the peripheral
blood. The white blood cell count, often normal or moderately elevated
throughout the early phase of the illness, continues to rise further. Blood
platelets may increase or decrease in number. Bone marrow examination
at this time reveals a prominent "fibroblastic" reticulin network, myelofibrosis (Fig. 60), and osteosclerosis. Although the degree of extramedullary
hematopoiesis (myeloid metaplasia) generally is proportional to the duration of the disease, some patients present features of it early in the course
of the illness, and even relatively early during the polycythemic phase.
Without an antecedent history of polycythemia vera it may appear that
the patient is suffering from primary myelofibrosis with myeloid metaplasia
(MMM). Sometimes the clinical and hematologic picture resembles chronic
granulocytic leukemia. Nevertheless the histochemical, biochemical, and
cytogenetic findings remain more consistent with polycythemia vera than
with typical chronic granulocytic leukemia. (But remember that some
patients with early chronic granulocytic leukemia may have an increased

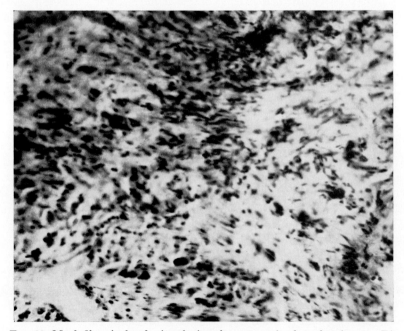

Fig. 60. Myelofibrosis developing during the course of polycythemia vera. Biopsy
(16× objective).

red cell count and hemoglobin value.) Many of the cases reported as terminating in chronic granulocytic leukemia may in fact have been persistent p. vera with overtones of MMM. Whether or not there are chromosomal and leukocyte alkaline phosphatase changes in those few patients with p. vera who do develop bona fide chronic granulocytic leukemia is a point of great interest, but one not definitively answered as yet. In other patients the terminal picture is indistinguishable from that seen in acute leukemia (Fig. 61), with or without an intervening period, of variable duration, of MMM or apparent chronic granulocytic leukemia.

Differential Diagnosis of Polycythemia Vera

To return to the comments in the introduction, the diagnosis of florid polycythemia vera in the absence of causes known to produce secondary polycythemia is relatively easy. The diagnosis of less obvious cases of polycythemia vera is difficult, and in the past has been based in part upon the fancy and experience of the individual hematologist and his own prerequisites for the diagnosis. For example, there are patients who have been followed for years without therapy, whose only hematologic abnormality is an unexplained increase in red cell volume.[45] It is possible that some of these patients may have a disorder comparable to polycythemia vera, which has affected only erythrocyte formation, or perhaps some variety

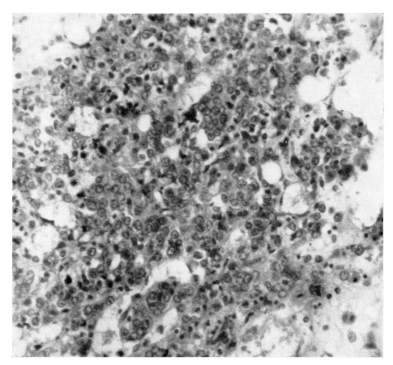

Fig. 61. Terminal acute leukemia developing during the course of polycythemia vera. Bone marrow biopsy (40× objective).

of incompletely manifested secondary polycythemia. Should this "illness" be considered a special type of polycythemia or should it be included at one end of the spectrum of the disease known as polycythemia vera? The writer prefers the latter, since it emphasizes the spectrum of the disease, although the fewer the characteristics of p. vera present in any patient, the less secure is the diagnosis.

In the majority of cases of secondary polycythemia due to hypoxemia the structural abnormalities of the heart and lung are sufficiently apparent to indicate the underlying cause of the polycythemia. Exceptions to this relate perhaps to obscure lung or neuromuscular disease or to an inapparent right-to-left shunt. In these last instances reduced arterial oxygen saturation can be of great help in diagnosis. Furthermore, other abnormalities of primary polycythemia, such as splenomegaly, deranged serum B_{12} levels and LAP values, or increased platelet and white cell counts, usually do not occur. In the rare case of a possible hemoglobinopathy, hemoglobin electrophoresis should be performed.

It is again emphasized that moderate arterial unsaturation does not rule out the diagnosis of p. vera. On the other hand, if arterial saturation is above 94 per cent, the clinician can confidently exclude hypoxemic polycythemia, though not the secondary polycythemia associated with tumors or p. vera. It is worth repeating that in the polycythemia accompanying tumors there may be increases in the platelet and white cell counts, and even splenomegaly, and that some cases of primary polycythemia may not be associated with some or most of the expected characteristics in addition to the increased red cell mass. To confound the situation even more, the coexistence of primary and secondary polycythemia (e.g., p. vera and chronic lung disease) is not at all uncommon.

Although it is easy to list the common characteristics that occur in groups of patients with various types of polycythemia, the clinician at the bedside, faced with a *single* patient with an increased red cell mass, cannot rely on group statistics or a fixed set of criteria which need be satisfied to

TABLE 45

Evaluation of the Patient with Polycythemia

1. History
2. Physical examination, including neurologic and pelvic examinations
3. Complete blood count, reticulocyte count, platelet count
4. Urinalysis
5. Red blood cell volume
6. Leukocyte alkaline phosphatase determination
7. Hemoglobin electrophoresis
8. Serum uric acid and potassium determinations
9. Plasma cortisol determination
10. Serum B_{12} and B_{12}-binding capacity
11. Arterial oxygen tension and saturation determinations
12. Bone marrow biopsy with stains for iron, reticulin, and collagen
13. Chest x-ray and intravenous pyelogram

help him arrive at a diagnosis for an *individual*. What this all means, therefore, is that *each* case of polycythemia must be evaluated thoroughly with the biochemical and laboratory studies previously outlined and summarized in Table 45. The results must then be interpreted within the limitations discussed. Clearly, the diagnosis of "mild" polycythemia vera must be made only after ruling out all known possible causes of secondary polycythemia.

In its broadest sense, the diagnosis of p. vera in many instances is a diagnosis of exclusion, initiated first by the finding of an increased red cell mass.

The author gratefully acknowledges the advice and criticism of James P. Smith, M.D., Assistant Professor of Medicine, Division of Pulmonary Diseases, Department of Medicine, New York Hospital- Cornell Medical Center.

REFERENCES

1. Abildgaard, C. F., Cornet, J., and Schulman, I. Primary erythrocytosis. J. Pediat. **63**:1072, 1963.
2. Adamson, J. W., and Finch, C. A. Erythropoietin and the polycythemias. Ann. N. Y. Acad. Sci. **149**:560, 1968.
3. Anstey, L., Kemp, N. H., Stafford, J. L., and Tanner, R. K. Leucocyte alkaline-phosphatase activity in polycythaemia rubra vera. Brit. J. Haematol. **9**:91, 1963.
4. Berlin, N. I. Differential diagnosis of the polycythemias. Seminars Hematol. **3**:209, 1966.
5. Berlin, N. I., Lawrence, J. H., and Gartland, J. Blood volume in polycythemia as determined by P-32 labeled red blood cells. Amer. J. Med. **9**:747, 1950.
6. Block, J. B., Carbone, P. P., Oppenheim, J. J., and Frei, E. The effect of treatment in patients with chronic myelogenous leukemia. Ann. Internal Med. **59**:629, 1963.
7. Bodansky, O. Methemoglobinemia and methemoglobin producing compounds. Pharmacol. Rev. **3**:144, 1951.
8. Brandenburg, R. O., and Smith, H. L. Sulfhemoglobinemia: a study of 62 clinical cases. Amer. Heart J. **42**:582, 1951.
9. Brandt, P. W. T., Dacie, J. V., Steiner, R. E., and Szur, L. Incidence of renal lesions in polycythemia. Brit. Med. J. **2**:468, 1963.
10. Burston, J., and Pinniger, J. L. The reticulin content of bone marrow in haematological disorders. Brit. J. Haematol. **9**:172, 1963.
11. Burwell, C. S., Robin, E. D., Whaley, R. D., and Bickelmann, A. G. Extreme obesity associated with alveolar hypoventilation—a Pickwickian syndrome. Amer. J. Med. **21**:811, 1956.
12. Cassels, D. E., and Morse, M. The arterial blood gases, the oxygen dissociation curve and the acid base balance in polycythemia vera. J. Clin. Invest. **32**: 52, 1953.
13. Charache, S., Weatherall, D. J., and Clegg, J. B. Polycythemia associated with a hemoglobinopathy. J. Clin. Invest. **45**:813, 1966.
14. Dameshek, W., and Gunz, F. Leukemia and the myeloproliferative disorders. In *Leukemia*, 2nd ed., p. 363. Grune and Stratton, New York, 1964.
15. Damon, A., and Holub, D. A. Host factors in polycythemia vera. Ann. Internal Med. **49**:43, 1958.
16. Dittmar, K., Kochwa, S., Zucker-Franklin, D., and Wasserman, L. R. Coexistence of polycythemia vera and biclonal gammopathy (γGK and γAL) with two Bence Jones proteins (BJK and BJL). Blood **31**:81, 1968.
17. Donati, R. M., McCarthy, J. M., Lange, R., and Gallagher, N. I. Erythrocythemia and neoplastic tumors. Ann. Internal Med. **58**:47, 1963.
18. Eichna, L. W., Farber, S. J., Berger, A. R., Earle, D. P., Rader, B., Pelligrino, E., Albert, R. E., Alexander, J. D., Taube, H., and Youngwirth, S. Cardio-

vascular dynamics, blood volumes, renal functions and electrolyte excretions in the same patients during congestive failure and after recovery of cardiac compensation. Circulation 7:674, 1953.

19. Engel, H. W., and Singer, K. Polycythemia with fibroids. J.A.M.A. 159:190, 1955.
20. Fessel, W. J. Odd men out. Arch. Internal Med. 115:736, 1965.
21. Gilbert, H. S., Krauss, S., Herbert, V., and Wasserman, L. R. Value of serum unsaturated B_{12}-binding capacity (UBBC) in differentiating polycythemia vera (PV) from relative polycythemia and as a parameter in evaluating effects of therapy, Clin. Res. 15:278, 1967.
22. Gottlieb, C. W., Retief, F. P., Pratt, P. W., and Herbert, V. Correlation of B_{12}-binding proteins with disorders of B_{12} metabolism: relation to hypo- and hyper-leukocyte turnover. J. Clin. Invest. 45:1016, 1966.
23. Gurney, C. Erythropoietin and erythropoiesis. Ann. Internal Med. 65:377, 1966.
24. Haden, R. L. The red cell mass in polycythemia in relation to diagnosis and treatment. Amer. J. Med. Sci. 196:493, 1938.
25. Halbertsma, T. Polycythemia in childhood. Amer. J. Dis. Child. 46:1356, 1933.
26. Hansen, P. Polycythemia produced by constriction of the renal artery in a rabbit. Acta Pathol. Microbiol. Scand. 60:465, 1964.
27. Harris, J. W. Polycythemia. In The Red Cell, Chap. 10, p. 313. Harvard University Press, Cambridge, Mass., 1963.
28. Herbert, V. Diagnostic and prognostic values of measurement of serum B_{12}-binding proteins. Blood 32:305, 1968.
29. Hertko, E. Polycythemia (erythrocytosis) associated with uterine fibroids and apparent surgical cure. Amer. J. Med. 34:288, 1963.
30. Horwitz, A., and McKelway, W. P. Polycythemia associated with uterine myomas. J.A.M.A. 158:1360, 1955.
31. Hurtado, A., Merino, C., and Delgado, E. Influence of anoxemia on the hemopoietic activity. Arch. Internal Med. 75:284, 1945.
32. Jaffe, E. R., and Heller, P. Methemoglobinemia in man. Progr. Hematol. 4:48, 1964.
33. Jawerski, Z. F., and Hirte, W. E. Polycythemia (erythrocytosis) and non-neoplastic renal disease. Can. Med. Ass. J. 84:1421, 1961.
34. Johnson, P. C., Hughes, W. L., Bird, R. M., and Patrick D. Diagnosis of hemolysis by a simplified Cr^{51} determination. Arch. Internal Med. 100:415, 1957.
35. Jones, N. F., Payne, R. W., Hyde, R. D., and Price, T. M. L. Renal polycythemia. Lancet 1:299, 1960.
36. Josephs, B. N., Robbins, G., and Levine, A. Polycythemia secondary to hamartoma of the liver. J.A.M.A. 179:867, 1962.
37. Kaung, D. T., and Peterson, R. E. Relative polycythemia or pseudopolycythemia, Arch. Internal Med. 110:456, 1962.
38. Kepler, E. J., Dockerty, M. B., and Priestly, J. T. Adrenal-like ovarian tumor associated with Cushing's syndrome. Amer. J. Obstet. Gynecol. 47:43, 1944.
39. Lawrence, J. H., Berlin, N. I., and Huff, R. L. The nature and treatment of polycythemia. Medicine 32:323, 1953.
40. Lertzman, M., Frome, B. M., Israels, L. G., and Cherniak, R. M. Hypoxia in polycythemia vera. Ann. Internal Med. 60:409, 1964.
41. Levinson, J. P., and Kinkaid, O. W. Myxoma of the right atrium associated with polycythemia. Report of successful excision. N. Engl. J. Med. 264:1187, 1961.
42. Mann, D. L., Gallagher, N. I., and Donati, R. M. Erythrocytosis and primary aldosteronism. Ann. Internal Med. 66:335, 1967.
43. McFadzean, A. J. S., Todd, D., and Tsang, K. C. Polycythemia in primary carcinoma of the liver. Blood 13:427, 1958.
44. Murray, J. F. Arterial studies in primary and secondary polycythemic disorders. Amer. Rev. Resp. Dis. 92:435, 1965.
45. Murray, J. F. Classification of polycythemic disorders. Ann. Internal Med. 64:892, 1966.
46. Nixon, R. K., O'Rourke, W., Rupe, C. E., and Korst, D. B. Nephrogenic polycythemia. Arch. Internal Med. 106:797, 1960.
47. Osler, W. Chronic cyanosis with polycythemia and enlarged spleen: a new clinical entity. Amer. J. Med. Sci. 126:187, 1903.
48. Plotz, C. N., Knowlton, A. I., and Ragan, C. The natural history of Cushing's syndrome. Amer. J. Med. 13:597, 1952.

49. Prentice, T. C., Berlin, N. I., and Lawrence, J. H. Effect of therapy on blood volume, blood pressure, and spleen size in polycythemia vera. Arch. Internal Med. 89:584, 1952.
50. Randall, D. L., Reiquam, C. W., Githens, J. H., and Robinson, A. Familial myeloproliferative disease. Amer. J. Dis. Child. 110:479, 1965.
51. Read, R. C. Studies of red cell volume and turnover using radiochromium. N. Engl. J. Med. 250:1021, 1954.
52. Reinhard, E. H. Polycythemia. In Cecil-Loeb Textbook of Medicine, Beeson, P. B., and McDermott, W., Eds., 12th ed., p. 1055. W. B. Saunders Co., Philadelphia, 1967.
53. Reynafarje, C., Lozano, R., and Valdivieso, J. The polycythemia of high altitudes: iron metabolism and related aspects. Blood 14:433, 1959.
54. Reynolds, T. B., and Ware, A. G. Sulfhemoglobinemia following habitual use of acetanilid. J.A.M.A. 149:1538, 1952.
55. Rodman, T., and Close, H. P. The primary hypoventilation syndrome. Amer. J. Med. 26:808, 1959.
56. Rosenthal, N., and Bassen, F. A. Course of polycythemia. Arch. Internal Med. 62:903, 1938.
57. Russel, R. P., and Conley, C. L. Benign polycythemia: Gaisbock's syndrome. Arch. Internal Med. 114:734, 1964.
58. Singmaster, L. Uterine fibroids associated with polycythemia. J.A.M.A. 163:36, 1957.
59. Smith, J. P. Personal communication.
60. Spodaro, A., and Forkner, C. E. Benign familial polycythemia. Arch. Internal Med. 52:593, 1933.
61. Starr, G. F., Stroebel, C. S., Jr., and Kearns, T. P. Polycythemia with papilledema and infratentorial vascular tumors. Ann. Internal Med. 48:978, 1958.
62. Stohlman, F. Pathogenesis of erythrocytosis. Seminars Hematol. 3:181, 1966.
63. Szur, L., Lewis, S. M., and Goolden, A. W. G. Polycythemia vera and its treatment with radioactive phosphorus. Quart. J. Med. 28:397, 1959.
64. Takaku, F., Hirashima, K., and Nakao, K. Studies on the mechanism of erythropoietin production. Effect of unilateral constriction of the renal artery. J. Lab. Clin. Med. 59:815, 1962.
65. Talbott, J. H. Gout and blood dyscrasias. Medicine 38:173, 1959.
66. Thurman, W. G., Grabstald, H., and Lieberman, P.H. Elevation of the erythropoietin levels in association with Wilms' tumor. Arch. Internal Med. 117:280, 1966.
67. Videbaek, A. Polycythemia vera. Course and prognosis. Acta Med. Scand. 138:179, 1950.
68. Waldmann, T. A., and Bradley, J. E. Polycythemia secondary to a pheochromocytoma with production of an erythropoiesis stimulating factor by the tumor. Proc. Soc. Exp. Biol. Med. 108:425, 1961.
69. Waldmann, T. A., Levine, E. H., and Baldwin, M. The association of polycythemia with a cerebellar hemangioblastoma, the production of an erythropoiesis stimulating factor by the tumor. Amer. J. Med. 31:318, 1961.
70. Wasserman, L. R., Dobson, R. L., and Lawrence, J. H. Blood oxygen studies in patients with polycythemia and in normal subjects. J. Clin. Invest. 28:60, 1949.
71. Wasserman, L. R., and Gilbert, H. S. Complications of polycythemia. Seminars Hematol. 3:199, 1966.
72. Weatherall, D. J.: Polycythemia resulting from abnormal hemoglobins. N. Engl. J. Med. 280:604, 1969.
73. Wintrobe, M. M. In Clinical Hematology, 6th ed., Chap. 2, The Erythocyte, p. 86, Lea and Febiger, Philadelphia, 1967.

Purpura

RALPH L. NACHMAN

The purpuric syndromes include those clinical conditions characterized by capillary hemorrhages located chiefly in the skin and mucous membranes. Excessive bleeding may follow significant trauma; however, the typical lesions are spontaneous petechiae and ecchymoses which result from a breakdown in the anatomic and physiologic integrity of small blood vessel walls. Recent advances in our understanding of the platelet–blood vessel wall interaction afford an insight into the pathogenesis of these disorders.

The first step in the primary hemostatic defense mechanism involves the adhesion of circulating platelets to denuded collagen in the vicinity of damaged endothelial surfaces (Fig. 62). Adherent platelets release adenosine diphosphate (ADP), which leads to aggregation and eventual platelet plug formation.[31] This phenomenon, acting in concert with the generation of small amounts of thrombin in the vicinity of the platelet aggregate, leads to retraction and consolidation of the plug and eventual sealing of the disrupted vessel. It should be noted that the coagulation mechanism—the blood-clotting factors—plays only a minimal role in this primary hemostatic process.

These considerations allow a reasonably accurate clinical and diagnostic approach to the classification of hemorrhagic diatheses into two main groups, 1) the coagulation disorders and 2) the purpuric syndromes. This differentiation is important in the initial evaluation of any major hemorrhagic problem, and can usually be defined at the bedside with only a minimum of laboratory procedures.

The major clinical and diagnostic features in these two groups of disorders are outlined in Table 46. These, of course, will vary from patient to patient, depending upon the severity of the individual disorder.

The history in a patient with purpura will usually reveal the spontaneous onset of cutaneous petechiae and ecchymoses not associated with trauma; deep hematoma and hemarthroses are not features. Many females, particularly blondes, will admit to "bruising easily" most of their lives, and in such individuals the onset of purpura is difficult to pinpoint. It is important to note the relationship of any significant hemorrhage to previous surgery, such as tonsillectomy or tooth extraction; prolonged bleeding for 2 to 3 days or more is usually a sign of an underlying coagulation disorder. The Rumpel-Leede vascular fragility test is a useful bedside procedure, particularly in those purpuric syndromes which wax and wane and in which the history

RALPH L. NACHMAN, M.D. Associate Professor of Medicine and Chief, Division of Hematology, Department of Medicine, New York Hospital-Cornell Medical Center, New York

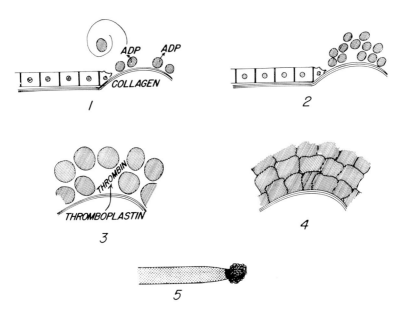

FIG. 62. Summary of the hemostatic reaction. Damaged vessel (*1*) with denuded collagen. Platelet adhesion is associated with release of intracellular adenosine diphosphate (ADP), which leads to the cohesion of platelets (*2*). Tissue thromboplastin induces thrombin formation in periplatelet atmosphere (*3*). A compact platelet plug is formed (*4*), leading to sealing of the vessel (*5*). (Reprinted, with permission, from Spaet, T. H. The platelet in hemostasis. Ann. N. Y. Acad. Sci. **115**:39, 1964.)

TABLE 46

Major Differential Features in Coagulation Defects and Purpuric Disorders

Feature	Coagulation Defects	Purpuric Syndromes
Type of bleeding	Intramuscular and deep hematomas	Cutaneous and mucosal petechiae with ecchymoses
Trauma	Frequent	Rare
Hemarthroses	Frequent	None
Duration	Usually life-long	Recent in onset
Family history	Frequently positive	Usually negative
Sex	More common in males	More common in females
Bleeding time	Normal	Usually abnormal
Tourniquet test	Negative	Usually positive

is vague. The procedure is superfluous in patients with overt diffuse petechiae and ecchymoses. The Duke bleeding time is also a valuable bedside test which may differentiate those patients with platelet or vascular disorders from those with underlying coagulation defects. The rebleeding phenomenon should not be confused with a prolonged primary bleeding time. Patients with severe hemophilia may rebleed 1 to 2 hours following a Duke or Ivy bleeding time procedure. This breakdown of the clot at the injured site does not reflect a defect in the platelet–blood vessel wall inter-action, but rather indicates the formation of a poorly formed friable clot because of deficiency of a circulating procoagulant.

Any consideration of the purpuric disorders must take into account the fact that platelets are probably intimately involved in the maintenance of the functional integrity of the blood vessel wall under normal physiologic circumstances. Vascular endothelium and platelets share to a large extent contractile properties, and may actually contain similar intracellular smooth muscle-like proteins.[5] These shared structural and biochemical features may render the endothelial cell and the platelet similarly susceptible to injurious stimuli. Despite these relationships it is still not clear why certain patients bleed at a given level of impairment of the primary hemostatic process. Some patients may have significant hemorrhagic symptoms at a platelet count of 40,000/cu mm while others are apparently asymptomatic at a level of 10,000/cu mm. Obviously many variables yet to be defined influence the fundamental integrity of the vessel wall. In fact, certain purpuric syndromes are characterized by an apparent disorder of the endothelial cell and/or the blood vessel wall in the absence of any overt platelet defect. These condi-tions, known as vascular or nonthrombocytopenic purpura, together with the thrombocytopenias and the thrombocytopathies, constitute the major categories of the purpuras.

THROMBOCYTOPENIA

Certainly the most common causes of the purpuric syndromes involve the thrombocytopenic state in one form or another. In fact, many physi-cians do not think of purpura in any frame of reference other than that of thrombocytopenia. As will be seen, this is not always wise, but certainly the first diagnostic evaluation of a patient with purpura involves a con-sideration of the platelet count. Experienced observers can estimate with reasonable accuracy the approximate level of the platelet count by careful perusal of a peripheral blood smear. In general there should be approxi-mately 5 to 10 platelets seen per oil immersion field. This, of course, will vary with the individual observer, the microscope, and the technique used in making the peripheral smear. Fewer than 100 platelets per 100 oil im-mersion fields usually indicates moderate to severe thrombocytopenia. Actual platelet-counting techniques vary from laboratory to laboratory; however, the phase method is probably the most accurate, with an average normal value in most hands of 250,000/cu mm. Purpuric lesions are usually not seen until the platelet count falls below 50,000/cu mm.

It is useful to categorize the multiple and varied causes of thrombocyto-penia in the framework of decreased production, excessive destruction or utilization, intravascular dilution, and sequestration (Table 47). The diagnostic distinctions emphasized in this classification are to a certain extent arbitrary and artificial. The pathogenetic mechanisms are not mutually exclusive, and multiple factors may influence the development of a specific form of thrombocytopenia. It is clear from the classification

TABLE 47
Causes of Thrombocytopenia

I. Decreased production
   Drugs, radiation, chemicals
   Hypoplastic anemia
   Congenital syndromes
   Bone marrow replacement
   Megaloblastic anemias
   Renal disease
II. Decreased survival
   A. Immunologic disorders
      ITP
      Drug purpura
      Neonatal purpura
      Post-transfusion purpura
      Secondary
   B. Increased consumption
      Defibrination
      Thrombotic thrombocytopenia
      Hemangioma
      Acute infections
III. Dilutional
IV. Sequestration (splenomegalic states)

in Table 47 that the diagnostic dilemma which a thrombocytopenic patient presents mimics, in a large sense, the problem which is faced in the patient with severe anemia. Thus, the major pathogenetic categories in the anemic patient are similar to those outlined above in relation to thrombocytopenia.

Considerations at the bedside may rapidly allow an approach to a reasonable differential diagnosis in the purpuric patient. The presence of primary disorders such as uremia, malignancy, or cirrhosis with significant splenomegaly may immediately point to an offending mechanism. In addition to these possibilities, an extensive drug history should always be obtained from any patient with a purpuric syndrome, despite what appears to be an obvious clinical cause. Once thrombocytopenia has been documented, a bone marrow examination is almost always indicated in these patients.

Thrombocytopenia Due to Disorders of Platelet Production

Multiple anatomic as well as biochemical restrictions may impair the integrity of the functioning megakaryocyte. In these situations the erythroid and myeloid cellular elements of the marrow may also be involved to varying degrees. Bone marrow failure may occur in the setting of aplastic or hypoplastic anemia, uremia, and megaloblastic anemia. Megakaryocytic depression from bone marrow replacement may also result from leukemia, myeloma, carcinoma, lymphoma, or myelofibrosis. Drugs, chemical agents, and ionizing radiation may similarly cause marrow injury and megakaryocytic depletion.

A few rare congenital causes of impaired blood platelet production have been reported. Familial aplastic anemia (Fanconi's anemia) with thrombocytopenia is a fatal childhood disease associated with multiple congenital defects, such as dwarfism, hypogonadism, skeletal abnormalities, and mental retardation.[12] Congenital megakaryocytic hypoplasia, another rare syndrome of infancy, is associated with bilateral absence of the radii and cardiac abnormalities.[25] An unusual and fascinating congenital thrombocytopenia was reported by Shulman et al. in 1960.[26] The thrombocytopenia in this patient was reversible following the administration of normal human plasma. The defect has been considered as representing a deficiency of a factor in normal plasma required for normal megakaryocyte maturation and platelet production.

It is apparent that numerous systemic disorders may secondarily affect the functional integrity of marrow cellular elements; thrombocytopenia with purpura in many of these conditions may reflect only one component of a pancytopenia. For reasons that are not altogether clear, megakaryocytes appear to be more sensitive than red and white cell precursors to certain marrow-suppressive agents, such as various forms of chemotherapy and ionizing radiation. In these clinical circumstances thrombocytopenia may be the earliest manifestation of a myelotoxic effect. The bone marrow examination is clearly the most definitive diagnostic tool in delineating the various etiologic possibilities in this group of disorders. The bone marrow biopsy has been particularly helpful in delineating the aplastic and hypoplastic anemias as well as extrinsic invasion by tumor cells (Fig. 63).

It is of utmost clinical importance that these particular causes of thrombocytopenic purpura be clearly defined and differentiated from those clinical entities characterized by decreased platelet survival, as the fundamental approach to therapy differs significantly. Thus, platelet concentrates, which are now becoming more generally available, are particularly useful in treating patients with severe thrombocytopenia who are suffering from disorders characterized by impaired platelet production. Repeated transfusions may tide these patients over severe hemorrhagic episodes, such as those occurring in drug-induced aplastic anemia. In contrast, the administration of platelet concentrates to patients who are destroying cells peripherally, as in immunologic purpura, is usually ineffective and in fact contraindicated except in the most critical circumstances.

Thrombocytopenia—Decreased Platelet Survival

Immunologic Disorders

Approximately 50 years ago Bedson first demonstrated that thrombocytopenia could be produced by heterospecific antisera directed against an animal's platelets.[6] Since then a convincing body of evidence has been accumulated that clearly demonstrates the participation of the platelet in immunologic reactions. The platelet membrane is particularly capable of adsorbing nonspecifically certain antibody-drug complexes.[17, 18, 27, 28] In this setting the platelet acts as an "innocent bystander" with which an

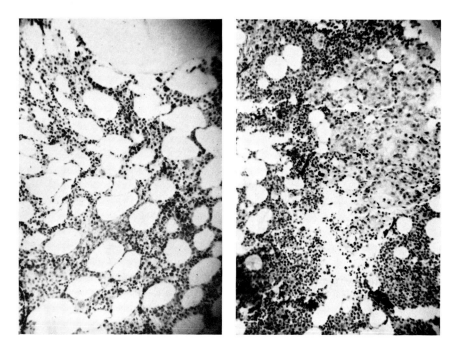

FIG. 63. Bone marrow biopsy of a normal individual (left) and a patient with metastatic carcinoma (right). The nest of tumor cells is seen in the upper right-hand portion of the biopsy on the right. ×16.

extrinsic immune complex interacts. The most convincing direct evidence of antiplatelet activity has been demonstrated by the production of marked platelet depression in normal recipients following the infusion of isolated γ-globulin fractions from the blood of some patients with idiopathic thrombocytopenic purpura.[30] The major thrombocytopenic diseases which are primarily associated with immunologic mechanisms include idiopathic thrombocytopenic purpura, post-transfusion purpura, neonatal thrombocytopenia, and drug purpura. Immunologic thrombocytopenia may occur as a secondary phenomenon in a number of disorders, such as systemic lupus erythematosus,[21] chronic lymphocytic leukemia,[10] Evans' syndrome,[11] and infectious mononucleosis.[15]

IDIOPATHIC THROMBOCYTOPENIC PURPURA

Acute. Acute idiopathic thrombocytopenic purpura (ITP) is primarily a disease of young children, affecting males and females equally. The sudden onset of acute purpura in an otherwise healthy child frequently follows 1 to 2 weeks after a viral or bacterial infection, not infrequently an ordinary cold or sore throat. The clinical syndrome is usually characterized by extensive purpura and ecchymoses in the absence of a palpable spleen, with severe thrombocytopenia and megakaryocytic hyperplasia of the bone marrow. In well over 90 per cent of the patients the disorder is self-limited, clearing

spontaneously within 10 to 14 days. A small percentage of patients may go
on to develop chronic thrombocytopenia.

Chronic. Chronic ITP is predominantly a disease of young adults, affecting women 3 to 4 times as frequently as men. The disease is generally
insidious in onset, with a relatively long history of easy bruising and
menorrhagia. Many patients give a history of mild to moderate bleeding
manifestations following trauma or minor surgery, such as tooth extractions.
Usually the explosive onset of severe purpura and thrombocytopenia in an
otherwise healthy individual should direct the attention of the physician
toward other considerations, such as drug or post-transfusion purpura.

The thrombocytopenia in chronic ITP is frequently in the range of 50,000
to 100,000 platelets/cu mm. The megakaryocytes are usually markedly
increased in the marrow, with a relative predominance of early young forms
(Fig. 64).

The physical findings at the bedside, except for the associated petechiae
and ecchymoses, are minimal. There is no characteristic pattern of distribution of the hemorrhagic lesions. The spleen in practically all cases is
not palpable. In fact, the presence of a large, palpable spleen should direct
attention away from an idiopathic immunologic disorder. It is true that a
rare patient with ITP may have a spleen enlarged to one to two finger-
breadths below the left costal margin; however, this is clearly the exception.

The disease may be present for a number of years, and may undergo
periodic remissions and relapses. Generally the hemorrhagic complications
are not life-threatening. In some patients the disorder appears to have

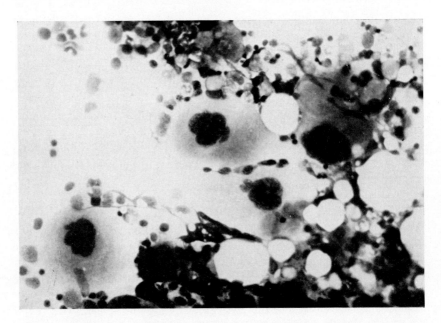

FIG. 64. Bone marrow aspirate from a patient with chronic ITP. There is a prominence of young megakaryocytes. ×25.

cyclical characteristics, with striking exacerbations of the systemic hemorrhagic symptoms with the menses. These women are really hemorrhagic cripples 4 or 5 days out of the month.

The differential diagnosis of chronic ITP, as can be deduced from its very name, remains in large part an exercise in clinical exclusion. This is primarily due to the fact that there exists no good test system *in vivo* to demonstrate the presence of circulating antiplatelet activity in the suspect patient. Numerous tests *in vitro* have been used without any consistent reliability, and include platelet agglutinins, complement fixation, inhibition of clot retraction, platelet factor 3 release, inhibition of labeled serotonin uptake, and anti-γ-globulin consumption tests.[4, 9] Tests *in vivo* have clearly demonstrated the presence in some patients of species-specific γ-globulin which causes significant thrombocytopenia when infused into normal recipients.[30] Unfortunately these transfusion experiments, although of great pathogenetic significance, have no practical applications at the present time with respect to differential diagnosis. Thus, the diagnosis is essentially made by a consideration of the major clinical laboratory hallmarks as outlined above, the relative paucity of physical findings, the absence of associated primary disorders, the exclusion of other primary immunologic thrombocytopenic conditions, and finally, the response to therapy. In most patients perhaps the most significant diagnostic differential now involves the exclusion of primary drug purpura. The details of these considerations will be elaborated below; however, a good rule of thumb to follow in the initial approach to all these patients is to remove or replace all drugs for at least 2 or 3 weeks. Thrombocytopenia which persists beyond this period is almost surely not drug-related.

Therapeutic Considerations. In view of the fact that much of the diagnosis of chronic ITP is based on a series of clinical exclusions, the response to therapy is usually followed as a characteristic parameter of the disorder. Adrenal cortical steroids in a fairly high dose range, e.g., 60 mg of prednisone daily, are usually employed initially in an attempt to promote a significant rise in the platelet count. Most patients with chronic ITP who respond to steroids do so within 2 to 3 weeks. The majority of patients will relapse within a few weeks to months after discontinuation of steroids. In general, following an initial trial of steroids, splenectomy remains the treatment of choice in chronic ITP. Approximately 70 per cent of the patients will achieve long-term and even permanent remissions. Most of the patients who go into remission following splenectomy show significant rises in the platelet count, often up to normal, within a few days. It should be remembered, however, that up to 10 per cent of patients may require weeks or even months before a significant remission develops.

Post-splenectomy failure with severe bleeding may respond to high doses of steroids, even if the patients had previously proven to be refractory to the steroid effect. Immunosuppressive agents have not, in general, been very successful. Particular attention should be paid to a characteristic group of these ITP patients, namely women who do not respond to splenectomy and who show systemic exacerbations of the hemorrhagic disease during the menses. Hormonal components probably play an important role in these patients; a few women have shown significant improvement following suppression of the menses with agents such as Enovid.

DRUG PURPURA

Drug hypersensitivity must be considered a possible cause in practically every adult with thrombocytopenic purpura. Individuals with this syndrome may develop hemorrhagic symptoms after months or even years of symptom-free use of a drug. Thrombocytopenia may develop within minutes to hours after administration of a drug to a sensitized patient. The duration of purpura is variable, and to a large extent is dependent on the metabolism of the drug. Thrombocytopenia, in the great majority of cases, will clear within a few days following removal of the offending agent. As previously noted, purpura which persists for more than 2 to 3 weeks after drug exposure is terminated should not be considered drug purpura, and other conditions, such as ITP, should be seriously considered.

In this pharmaceutical era many patients must be carefully and extensively questioned regarding drug intake. Many individuals forget that they have been chronically taking aspirin, sedatives, and/or various tranquilizing agents. A large number of drugs have been implicated in this syndrome. Table 48 lists some compounds which have been documented as causative agents in drug purpura. Particularly frequent offenders include quinine, quinidine, sulfonamides, chlorothiazide, and hydrochlorothiazide. One should have a high level of suspicion of drug sensitivity when purpura develops in a patient receiving any of these drugs. A large number of reports have incriminated aspirin, penicillin, phenacetin, and phenobarbital. This probably reflects the extraordinarily wide use of these drugs. It should be noted, however, that, in effect, any drug taken by a patient is a possible cause of drug purpura.

This distribution of the purpuric and ecchymotic lesions in this syndrome does not significantly differ from that observed in ITP or other immunologic purpuric syndromes.

Ackroyd, in his classic studies of Sedormid purpura, provided the first direct evidence that this disease is an immunologic disorder.[1] An immune mechanism has been identified for many of the drugs listed in Table 48, group A. A number of test systems have subsequently been utilized clinically to demonstrate drug, platelet, and antibody interactions as a proof of drug purpura. These include test dosing *in vivo*, complement fixation *in vitro*, platelet factor 3 release, α-amino nitrogen generation, clot retraction inhibition, and platelet agglutination.[14] Many of these tests are based on the premise that the probable mechanism responsible for the pathogenesis of immunologic drug purpura involves the adsorption by platelets of immune complexes consisting of drug and antibody, with secondary damage to the cell.[28] Test dosing *in vivo*, although perhaps the most accurate, is also

TABLE 48
Drugs Implicated in Thrombocytopenic Purpura*

A. Etiologic relationship clearly shown

Acetazolamide	Hydroxychloroquin
Allylisopropylcarbamide (Sedormid)	Novobiocin
Antazoline phosphate	Quinidine
Chlorothiazide	Quinine
Digitoxin	Ristocetin
Diphenylhydantoin sodium	Stibophen
Hydrochlorothiazide	Sulfamethazine

B. Etiologic relationship frequently suspected but not confirmed by tests in vitro or in vivo

Aminopyrine	Meprobamate
Amobarbital	Penicillin
Aspirin	Phenacetin
Carbutamide	Phenobarbital
Chloramphenicol	Phenylbutazone
Chlorpheniramine maleate	Prednisone
Chlorpromazine	Prochlorperazine
Chlorpropamide	Promethazine
Codeine	Reserpine
Dextroamphetamine sulfate	Streptomycin
Digitalis	Sulfadiazine
Digoxin	Sulfamethoxypyridazine
Gold	Sulfisoxazole
Erythromycin	Tetracyline
Isoniazid	Tolbutamide
Meperidine	

* Modified from Horowitz and Nachman.[14]

the most dangerous test, and in general should not be done, in view of the potential hazard of intracerebral bleeding. The clot retraction inhibition test, although not the most sensitive, is the most simple test to perform in vitro, and an example is shown in Figure 65. A mixture of drug, antibody, and platelets is incubated and clot retraction is measured. The inhibition of clot retraction observed is a manifestation of platelet damage secondary to an antigen-antibody reaction. Another, more sensitive in vitro system is based on the platelet factor 3 release mechanism. The test consists of incubation of intact, platelet-rich plasma, containing antibody and drug in appropriate concentrations, at 37°C for 1 hour. Samples of the incubation mixture are taken at fixed intervals and tested for platelet factor 3 activity, using a clotting test system in which the only variable is the amount of available lipid. Control incubations lacking platelets, drug, or antibody are tested at the same time. Immunologic damage leads to platelet factor 3 release, which in turn causes more rapid clotting of the indicated test system. An example of a positive result is shown in Figure 66.

No single test is capable of detecting all cases of drug purpura. Complement fixation is probably the most sensitive in vitro test available; however, it is not easy to perform and usually requires an expert laboratory facility.

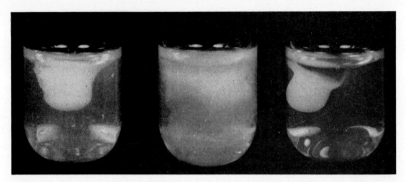

FIG. 65. Clot retraction inhibition studies, using the platelet-rich plasma from a patient with digitoxin purpura. Left, the patient's recalcified platelet-rich plasma in the presence of saline. Center, inhibition of clot retraction in the presence of digitoxin and the patient's recalcified platelet-rich plasma. Right, control, using recalcified normal platelet-rich plasma in the presence of digitoxin. (Reprinted, with permission, from Young, R. C., Nachman, R. L., and Horowitz, H. I. Thrombocytopenia due to digitoxin. Demonstration of antibody and mechanism of action. Amer. J. Med. 41:605, 1966.)

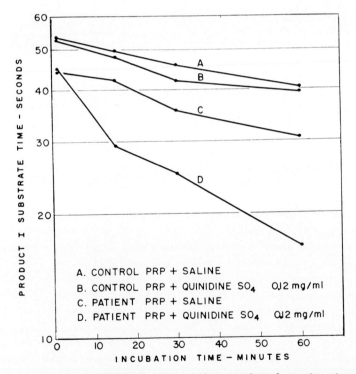

FIG. 66. Augmentation of platelet factor 3 (measured as shortening of product I substrate time) in the presence of platelet-rich plasma (PRP) from a patient with quinidine purpura. A significant increase of platelet factor 3 can be seen in mixture D, but not in control mixtures. The more platelet factor 3 available, the shorter the clotting time. (Reprinted, with permission, from Seminars in Hematology 2:298, 1965.)

We routinely utilize clot retraction and platelet factor 3 test systems for screening of potential drug purpura *in vitro*.

The most rational approach to management of suspected drug thrombocytopenia should begin with a careful evaluation of the history of drug ingestion. It is best to discontinue all drugs, replacing those that are absolutely indicated with pharmacologically equivalent but chemically different preparations.

POST-TRANFUSION PURPURA

Post-transfusion purpura is a relatively rare form of immunologic purpura which must be distinguished from drug purpura and ITP.[29] The syndrome is characterized by the sudden, rather explosive onset of purpura, usually developing within 7 days of a transfusion. The disease develops because of the mismatching of an inherited platelet antigen and subsequent development of a complement-fixing antiplatelet isoantibody which produces marked thrombocytopenia in a sensitized individual. The disorder is self-limited; however, purpura may last up to 3 weeks. Diagnosis rests on the serologic demonstration of platelet antigen mismatching. The disorder should be suspected in any individual who develops sudden purpura without any overt underlying reason shortly after a blood transfusion.

SECONDARY IMMUNOLOGIC PURPURA

Autoimmune hemolytic anemia may be accompanied by idiopathic thrombocytopenic purpura, a complex referred to as Evans' syndrome.[11] The diagnostic highlights of the disorder include a direct positive Coombs test with hemolysis, marked thrombocytopenia, and the absence of a palpable spleen.

Thrombocytopenia presenting in a manner mimicking that of classic ITP occurs in approximately 10 per cent of patients with systemic lupus erythematosus. ITP may present as the only significant clinical feature of an early stage of lupus. Thus, immunologic studies for lupus should be performed on all patients who present with ITP.

A clinical picture identical with that of chronic ITP can be observed during the course of chronic lymphocytic leukemia and lymphosarcoma, although it should be emphasized that the great majority of cases of thrombocytopenia associated with these diseases are secondary to marrow involvement.[10] The clinical and pathologic aspects of the underlying lymphoma are usually self-evident during this stage. The thrombocytopenia which occasionally complicates infectious mononucleosis may in some instances result from circulating cold agglutinins which react with intrinsic platelet antigens.

Thrombocytopenia Due to Increased Consumption of Platelets

Defibrination

Defibrination states, such as are seen in generalized intravascular coagulation, or in the more restricted process of giant hemangioma (Kassabach-

Meritt syndrome), are generally associated with significant degrees of thrombocytopenia. The thrombocytopenia results from the excessive utilization of platelets at multiple sites in association with increased formation of procoagulants in the circulating blood.

Defibrination states generally imply the removal of circulating fibrinogen and other coagulation factors. The process has been regarded as a "consumption coagulopathy." [23] The syndrome varies in intensity, and may be associated with catastrophic hemorrhage or multifocal thrombotic disease without overt hemorrhage. The disorder has been observed in many clinical states, including purpura fulminans, leukemia, carcinomatoses, drug reactions, hemorrhagic shock, and following snakebite or transfusion of mismatched blood. An acute form of defibrination may be observed in association with abruptio placentae or septic abortion.[16]

Thrombotic Thrombocytopenic Purpura

Thrombotic thrombocytopenic purpura is usually an acute disease which presents with a clinical spectrum including fever, microangiopathic hemolytic anemia, thrombocytopenia, kidney disease, and transient neurologic symptoms.[2] Diagnosis may be difficult, owing to the variability of involvement of several organ systems. The most frequently noted complaints are related to neurologic abnormalities and hemorrhagic phenomena. The anemia is usually brisk, and it is not unusual to observe hematocrits below 20 per cent on the initial examination. Hemorrhagic complications are severe, and 80 per cent of the patients die within 1 month of onset. An important diagnostic feature is the microangiopathic peripheral blood picture, which is always seen, and presents as increased numbers of schistocytes, burr cells, and helmet-shaped red cell fragments (Fig. 67). There is no good evidence that this disease represents a true defibrination syndrome. Thus, except for the platelet count, the clotting parameters are usually normal. Diagnostic confirmation of this syndrome requires the histologic demonstration of the characteristic pathologic lesion, consisting of widespread hyaline occlusion of terminal arterioles and capillaries. These lesions are probably composed of aggregates of agglutinated degenerating platelets. It is best to consider the disease as an unknown disorder of the blood vessel wall with secondary deposition and utilization of circulating platelets.

Acute Infection

Thrombocytopenia occasionally complicates an acute infectious process such as typhus, bacterial endocarditis, and various childhood exanthems. Direct platelet damage due to cell-bacterium or cell-virus interaction is probably a significant factor in the development of the thrombocytopenia. Experimental evidence suggests that the extracellular toxins of both the staphylococcus and the streptococcus, as well as the endotoxin of Gramnegative organisms, may cause platelet damage and aggregation.[22] The platelet depression in most of these disorders is self-limited, clearing spontaneously with the improvement in the infectious process. Platelet phago-

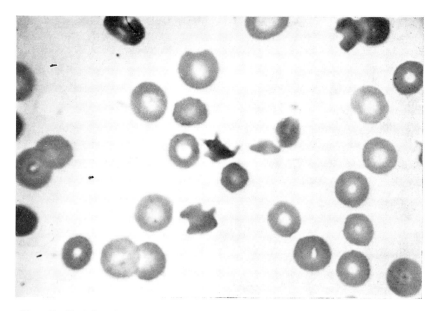

Fig. 67. Peripheral smear from a patient with thrombotic thrombocytopenic purpura. The fragmented schistocytes are conspicuous.

cytosis may be an important component of the thrombocytopenia of these conditions.

Dilution Thrombocytopenia

Massive blood transfusions, extracorporeal circulation, and exchange transfusions are associated with moderate degrees of thrombocytopenia due to replacement with platelet-poor blood.

Sequestration Thrombocytopenia—Splenomegalic States

Thrombocytopenia may develop in any condition associated with an enlarged spleen. Normally about one-third of the body platelet mass is concentrated in the spleen.[3] This splenic platelet pool exchanges with the remaining two-thirds of the circulating platelets. In splenomegaly due to many causes the splenic platelet pool may be greatly increased, so that up to 90 per cent of platelets are sequestered in the spleen at any one time. Thus, a redistribution of platelets occurs, leading to peripheral thrombocytopenia despite normal platelet production and normal platelet survival. Among the frequent causes of splenomegalic thrombocytopenia in the United States are cirrhosis, lymphoma, and systemic lupus erythematosus.

THROMBOCYTOPATHIC PURPURA: DISORDERS OF PLATELET FUNCTION

Thrombocytopathic purpura represents a group of separate clinical disorders which present with a relatively characteristic clinical triad: 1) hemorrhagic history in the absence of any overt aberration of the coagulation mechanism, 2) normal platelet count, and 3) abnormal platelet function.[7] Patients with these qualitative disorders of platelet function usually have bleeding of the mucosal type, generally manifested by epistaxis and menorrhagia, and mild purpura. The hemorrhagic disease is usually mild, and many patients give only a minimal history of bleeding. However, some of these patients develop significant hemorrhagic difficulty with surgical procedures.

Thrombocytopathic diseases can usually be identified by measurement of platelet factor 3 activity. Platelet factor 3 represents surface phospholipoprotein activation, which is necessary for the coagulation mechanism and eventual formation of the fibrin clot. A simple screening test for this activity involves the measurement of the prothrombin content of serum after blood has been allowed to clot at 37°C for 1 hour under standard conditions, with and without normal platelets or platelet substitutes. Under normal circumstances less than 20 per cent of the prothrombin originally available in the plasma will be found in the serum. An abnormal amount of prothrombin in the serum, corrected by the addition of a platelet substitute to whole blood before clotting, in the presence of a normal platelet count, is suggestive of a thrombocytopathy. The test remains abnormal if the basic defect involves a circulating clotting factor.

Thrombocytopathy may occur secondarily in a number of different diseases, such as liver disease, scurvy, uremia, macroglobulinemia, and systemic lupus. In these situations platelet factor 3 is either not available or intrinsically deficient.

Other physiologic parameters of platelet function may be altered in thrombocytopathic states. These may include aberrations of platelet adhesiveness as well as abnormalities in clot retraction. Certain drugs, such as aspirin, may induce a secondary thrombocytopathic condition primarily affecting the ability of platelets to release intracellular ADP.[20]

Thrombasthenia (Glanzmann's disease) is a rare congenital disorder of platelet function associated with a prolonged bleeding time and defective clot retraction.[8] The disease probably represents an intrinsic defect of the plasma membrane of the platelet. In some patients the platelet fibrinogen is significantly decreased.[19] Characteristically thrombasthenic platelets exhibit a marked defect in aggregation following the addition of ADP or thrombin. The platelets on the peripheral smear may appear enlarged and isolated, and clumping is usually absent. Purpura is not ordinarily a feature of the disease.

NONTHROMBOCYTOPENIC PURPURA

A varied group of clinical syndromes are characterized by intrinsic abnormalities of the blood vessel wall with subsequent mucosal and skin hemorrhages, in the absence of platelet or plasma procoagulant defects. These disorders, vascular or nonthrombocytopenic purpuras, are listed in Table 49. It should be noted that many otherwise healthy women complain of frequent bruising, usually life-long and familial. This condition, referred

TABLE 49
Causes of Nonthrombocytopenic Purpura

Senile purpura
Drugs
Henoch-Schönlein purpura
Dysproteinemia
Scurvy
Autoerythrocyte sensitivity

to as "purpura simplex," is essentially of only cosmetic importance. It is, however, important to distinguish this benign condition from the more serious purpuric states.

Senile Purpura

This is a frequent syndrome, occurring in the seventh and eighth decades of life in both sexes. Purpuric hemorrhages are usually localized over the dorsa of the hands and the extensor surfaces of the forearms. Superficial large ecchymotic areas may develop following mild trauma. The lesions occur in thin, parchment-like, atrophic skin, and are probably related to degeneration of elastic tissue.[24] They are essentially of no clinical significance.

Nonthrombocytopenic Drug Purpura

Some of the drugs listed in Table 48 may produce purpura in the absence of thrombocytopenia. In these conditions the vascular endothelium itself serves as the target organ instead of the circulating platelet, presumably involving different receptor sites. The bleeding disorder is generally mild, and the only indicated therapy is removal of the suspected offending agent.

Henoch-Schönlein Purpura

This hypersensitivity vasculitis occurs most frequently in children, usually following a streptococcal infection or occasionally a sensitizing food or drug. Extensive purpuric ecchymotic lesions are scattered over the skin of the extensor surfaces of the extremities. Many of the hemorrhagic lesions are edematous, and are thus palpable. Typically the rash occurs in successive crops and the face is frequently involved. Hemorrhagic lesions may also involve the joints and gastrointestinal tract, and nephritis is a common feature. Abdominal complications include gastrointestinal intramural hematoma and gross mucosal hemorrhage. Hematuria is seen in 50 per cent of the patients.

The disease is ordinarily self-limited, subsiding usually within 1 month of onset. Fatalities may result from renal failure or massive intestinal hemorrhage.

Dysproteinemia

Abnormal elevations of the serum globulins may be associated with vascular purpura. These syndromes are seen in macroglobulinemia, cryoglobulinemia, diffuse hyperglobulinemia, and multiple myeloma. The non-thrombocytopenic purpura probably develops from coating of the platelet surface, with interference with normal membrane function, as well as from coating of the endothelial surfaces, leading to impairment in blood vessel integrity. It is probable that the elevated globulins interact with the coagulation factors and grossly retard the clotting mechanism. Sludging of the red cells also contributes to significant capillary anoxia. Purpuric lesions may occasionally be elicited at the bedside in cryoglobulinemia by exposing an extremity to ice water for a short period of time.

Hyperglobulinemic purpura (Waldenström) primarily affects middle-aged women, and is characterized by successive crops of lower extremity petechiae occurring at variable intervals, leading to eventual pigmentary changes.[32] There is usually an associated polyclonal elevation of γG-globulins. This condition is benign and no therapy is indicated.

Scurvy

Scurvy is a rare disease in the Western world. Chronic vitamin C deprivation is primarily a disease of the very young and the very old. Epistaxis, hematuria, and gastrointestinal bleeding are seen in infants. Confluent extensive ecchymoses are seen in adults, with associated deep muscle hematomas. There is some evidence which suggests that, in addition to the blood vessel wall defect, qualitative platelet defects are important in the pathogenesis of the bleeding.

Autoerythrocyte Sensitization

This rare condition, confined to women, is characterized by a peculiar response to bruising, with the development of painful ecchymoses. Characteristically the lesions occur over the anterior aspects of the upper and lower extremities, and tend to spread superficially. The trunk is only rarely involved. In general ecchymoses appear only over areas easily subject to superficial trauma. The fundamental nature of the illness is not known; however, there is evidence which suggests that some of these women become sensitive to their own red cells.[13] Most of these patients have profound emotional difficulties, and it has been considered that this represents in part a psychosomatic disorder. It is difficult to separate these patients from severely disturbed individuals suffering from factitious purpura.

REFERENCES

1. Ackroyd, J. F. The cause of thrombocytopenia in Sedormid purpura. N. Engl. J. Med. 24:1301, 1966.
2. Amorosi, E. L., and Ultmann, J. E. Thrombotic thrombocytopenic purpura: report of 16 cases and review of the literature. Medicine 45:139, 1966.
3. Aster, L. H. Splenic platelet pooling as a cause of "hypersplenic" thrombocytopenia. Trans. Ass. Amer. Physicians 78:362, 1965.
4. Baldini, M. Idiopathic thrombocytopenia. N. Engl. J. Med. 24:1301, 1966.
5. Becker, C. G., and Nachman, R. Contractile protein of platelets and endothelial cells. J. Clin. Invest. 48:7a, 1969.
6. Bedson, S. P. Blood platelet antiserum, its specificity and role in the experimental production of purpura. J. Pathol. Bacteriol. 25:94, 1922.

7. Bowie, E. J. W., Thompson, J. H., Jr., and Owen, C. A., Jr. The blood platelet (including a discussion of the qualitative diseases). Mayo Clin. Proc. **40**:625, 1965.
8. Caen, J. P., Castaldi, P. H., Leclerc, J. S., Incerman, S., Larreu, M. J., Probst, M., and Bernard, J. Congenital bleeding disorders with long bleeding time and normal platelet count. Amer. J. Med. **41**:4, 1966.
9. Corn, M., and Upshaw, J. D., Jr. Evaluation of platelet antibodies in idiopathic thrombocytopenic purpura. Arch Internal Med. **109**:157, 1962.
10. Ebbe, S., Wittels, B., and Dameshek, W. Autoimmune thrombocytopenic purpura ("ITP" type) with chronic lymphocytic leukemia. Blood **19**:33, 1962.
11. Evans, R. S., Takahashi, K., Dhave, A. B., Payne, R., and Lui, C. K. Primary thrombocytopenia and acquired hemolytic anemia. Evidence for a common etiology. Arch. Internal Med. **87**:48, 1951.
12. Fanconi, G. Familiae infantile pevizioseortize anamie (peviiziisea blutbid und kenstitution). Jahrb. Kinderheilk **117**:257, 1927.
13. Groch, G. S., Finch, S. C., Rogoway, W., and Fischer, O. S. Studies in the pathogenesis of autoerythrocyte sensitization syndrome. Blood **28**:19, 1966.
14. Horowitz, H. I., and Nachman, R. L. Drug purpura. Seminars Hematol. **2**:287, 1965.
15. Lalezari, P., Bernard, J., and Murphy, G. Cold reacting leukocyte agglutinins and their significance. In *Histocompatibility Testing*. Curtoni, E. S., Mattina, P. L., and Tosi, R. M., Eds, p. 421. The Williams & Wilkins Co., Baltimore, 1967.
16. Merskey, C., Johnson, A. J., Kleiner, G. J., and Wohl, H. The defibrination syndrome: clinical features and laboratory diagnosis. Brit. J. Haematol. **13**:528, 1967.
17. Miescher, P., and Cooper, N. The fixation of soluble antigen-antibody complexes upon thrombocytes. Vox Sang. **5**:138, 1960.
18. Miescher, P., and Gorsten, F. Mechanisms of immunogenic platelet damage. In *Blood Platelets*, Johnson, S. A., Monto, R. W., Reback, J. W., and Horn, R. C., Jr., Eds., p. 1071. Little, Brown and Co., Boston, 1961.
19. Nachman, R. L., and Marcus, A. J. Immunological studies of proteins associated with the subcellular fractions of thrombasthenic and afibrinogenaemic platelets. Brit. J. Haematol. **15**:181, 1968.
20. O'Brien, J. Effects of salicylates on human platelets. Lancet **1**:779, 1968.
21. Rabinowitz, Y., and Dameshek, W. Systemic lupus erythematosus after idiopathic thrombocytopenic purpura. Ann. Internal Med. **52**:1, 1960.
22. Rahal, J. J., Jr., MacHahon, H. C., and Weinstein, L. Thrombocytopenia and symmetrical peripheral gangrene associated with staphylococcal and streptococcal bacteremia. Ann. Internal Med. **69**:35, 1968.
23. Rodriguez-Erdmann, F. Bleeding due to increased intravascular blood coagulation; hemorrhagic syndromes caused by consumption of blood clotting factors (consumption-coagulopathies). N. Engl. J. Med. **273**:1370, 1965.
24. Schuster, S., and Scarborough, H. Senile purpura. Quart. J. Med. **30**:33, 1961.
25. Shaw, S., and Oliver, R. A. M. Congenital hypoplastic thrombocytopenia with skeletal deformities in siblings. Blood **14**:374, 1959.
26. Shulman, I., Pierce, M., Laker, S., and Cuvanbhoy, Z. Studies on thrombopoiesis. I. A factor in normal human plasma required for platelet production; chronic thrombocytopenia due to its deficiency. Blood **16**:943, 1960.
27. Shulman, N. R. Immunoreactions involving platelets. I. A steric and kinetic model for formation of a complex from a human antibody, quinidine as a haptene and platelets, and for fixation of complement by the complex. J. Exp. Med. **107**:665, 1958.
28. Shulman, N. R. Mechanism of blood cell damage by adsorption of antigen antibody complexes. In *Immunopathology, 3rd International Symposium*, Grabar, P., and Miescher, P., Eds., p. 338. Grune and Stratton, New York, 1963.
29. Shulman, N. R., Aster, R. H., Leitner, A., and Hiller, M. C. Immunoreactions involving platelets. V. Post-transfusion purpura due to a complement fixing antibody against a genetically controlled platelet antigen. A proposed mechanism for thrombocytopenia and its relevance in "autoimmunity." J. Clin. Invest. **40**:1597, 1961.

30. Shulman, N. R., Marder, V. J., and Weinnach, R. S. Similarities between known antiplatelet antibodies and the factor responsible for thrombocytopenia in idiopathic purpura. Physiologic, serologic and isotopic studies. Ann. N. Y. Acad. Sci. **424**:499, 1965.
31. Spaet, T. H., and Zucker, M. B. Mechanism of platelet plug formation and role of adenosinediphosphate. Amer. J. Physiol. **206**:1267, 1964.
32. Waldenström, J. Clinical methods for the determination of hyperproteinaemia and their practical value for diagnoses. Nord. Med. **20**:2288, 1943.

Diffuse Demineralization
of Bone

PAUL D. SAVILLE and
W. P. LAIRD MYERS

INTRODUCTION

In clinical medicine the first hint that a patient has a skeletal disorder is often the radiologist's comment that the bones visualized in a radiographic study, usually done for another purpose, appear demineralized. This information may be dismissed by the clinician unless the findings are striking, and the patient's problem may not receive the attention it deserves unless the demineralization has led to a fracture.

It is our intent in this chapter to present a clinical approach to the problem of the demineralized skeleton. For purposes of this presentation, demineralization will be defined in radiographic terms, since neither densitometry nor chemical analysis of mineral per unit volume of bone gives information that forms the basis of the clinical presentation. Demineralization of bone in radiographic terms usually exists when the radiologist notes one or more of several radiologic features:

1. The bones look less dense than they should.

2. Vertebral endplates stand out in relation to the rest of the vertebral body.

3. There is increased prominence of vertical trabeculae of the vertebrae.

4. Deformities of architecture are noted: fractures, pseudofractures, decreased vertebral height relative to width (normal height-to-width ratio is 0.8 to 0.9), and vertebral biconcavity (normally the interspace is about 25 to 33 per cent of the vertebral height).

5. A combination of the absence of osteophytes and the presence of calcification of the aorta is often an attendant radiographic feature of the commonest demineralizing disease, osteoporosis.

A radiographic diagnosis of demineralization based only on the first sign is open to sources of error, such as the subjective interpretation of the radiologist and technical factors incident to exposure, film development, etc. The need for a more objective approach has long been realized, but, even with new radiographic techniques, it must be recognized that defining demineralization in radiographic terms has clear limitations, since skeletal

PAUL D. SAVILLE, M.D. Professor of Medicine, Creighton University School of Medicine, Omaha, Nebraska.   W. P. LAIRD MYERS, M.D. Professor of Medicine, Cornell University Medical College, New York, New York; Chairman, Department of Medicine, Memorial Hospital for Cancer and Allied Diseases, New York, New York.

tissue may be demineralized and yet this may not be radiographically apparent. It is usually stated that about 30 per cent of the mineral content of the skeleton must be lost before the change can be noted radiographically.[28]

Despite these limitations, radiography of bones has obvious clinical practicality and simplicity and will continue to form the basis on which most patients will come to medical attention for demineralizing bone disease. It should be emphasized that this chapter will concern itself with diffuse demineralization rather than localized disease. "Diffuse" implies a systemic disorder and, although not all bones will show demineralization to the same degree, the changes seen are usually sufficient to suspect a generalized disorder of bone metabolism rather than a localized one.

MEASUREMENT OF BONE DENSITY

The difficulties in accurate densitometry are surprisingly great. Essentially, judgment of bone density depends upon measurement of the attenuation of an x-ray beam by bone. Soft tissues also produce some effect, and the attenuation by soft tissue relative to bone varies with changes in beam energy as well as change in the composition of the soft tissues. Clinical x-rays are polychromatic, and the proportions of the different wavelengths vary according to electrical adjustments made by the radiologist; they may also vary with fluctuations in line voltage. In addition, film quality and processing affect judgment. As a result of all these factors, assessment of mineral density of bones surrounded by appreciable soft tissue is imprecise, even when aluminum wedges and similar devices are used for comparison, since these are not accurate models for bone surrounded by soft tissue. On the other hand, for bones not surrounded by large amounts of soft tissue, such as those of the hands and wrists and the os calcis, significant advances have been made in radiodensitometry by several investigators.

There are three general methods that can be applied to regional bone density measurements: radiogrammetry, radiodensitometry, and photon source densitometry.

Radiogrammetry

This is the direct measurement from standard radiographs of the thickness of bone cortex at various sites.

Cortex of the Second Metacarpal

Garn and his co-workers[24] have made extensive studies using this technique. The width of the cortex may be expressed as such or as the ratio of the cortical thickness to the total bone width. With this technique these investigators have shown that men as well as women lose bone in their early forties. They have also shown that Asians, even when born in this country, have thinner cortices than Caucasians. The changes in males and females with age are shown in Figure 68.

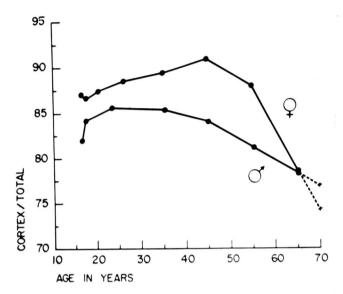

Fig. 68. Cortex thickness of the second metacarpal, expressed as a percentage of total metacarpal diameter for men and women between 10 and 70 years of age. (Reprinted, with permission, from *Relations of Development and Aging*. Charles C Thomas, Springfield, Ill., 1964.)

Cortical Thickness of the Femoral Shaft

Nordin and Smith[40] have described a method for measuring the thickness of the cortex of the femoral midshaft and then expressing it as a fraction of the total shaft width. They have shown how this femoral index changes with age in normal individuals and also in osteoporotic individuals (Fig. 69).

Cortical Thickness of the Radial Shaft Just below the Tuberosity

Meema and Meema[33] have demonstrated that a short length of radial cortex just below the tuberosity is roughly circular in cross-section, and that the cortex here is easy to measure, as illustrated in Figure 70. The changes in cortical thickness of the radial shaft with age found among a group of normal women and women with spine fractures due to osteoporosis are shown in Figure 71. A good correlation has been found between cortical thickness of the radius measured directly from radiographs in cadavers and the fat-free dry weight of samples of iliac crest bone. Furthermore, if a plug of bone of constant volume is taken from the iliac crest, the fat-free dry weight of this plug will be a function of its mineral content.[45]

Radiodensitometry

This is the combination of radiographs and some additional measuring device to judge density of the bone. Doyle[19] measures the density of the lower end of the ulna by submerging the wrist in a Perspex tank of water which also contains an aluminum wedge. The wrist and wedge are radio-

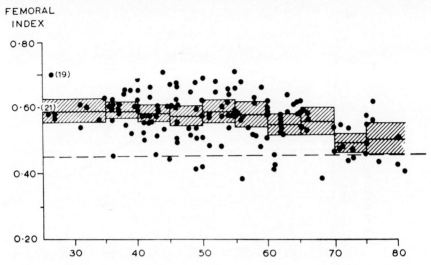

FIG. 69. Femoral cortex index: femoral cortex thickness expressed as a fraction of femoral diameter of the midshaft for women between 20 and 80 years of age. (Reprinted, with permission, from *Diagnostic Procedures in Disorders of Calcium Metabolism.* Little, Brown and Co., Boston, 1965.)

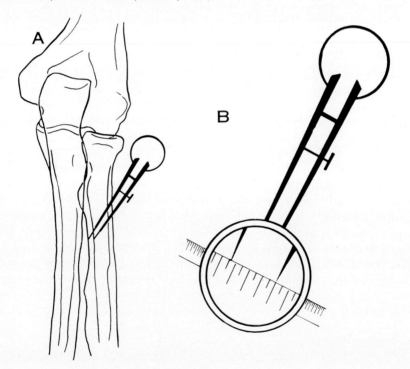

FIG. 70. *A.* Cortex thickness of the radial shaft below the tuberosity measured with a pair of calipers combining both medial and lateral cortices into one measurement. *B.* Calipers are then examined using a Bausch and Lomb magnifying lens with tenths of a millimeter engraved on its surface.

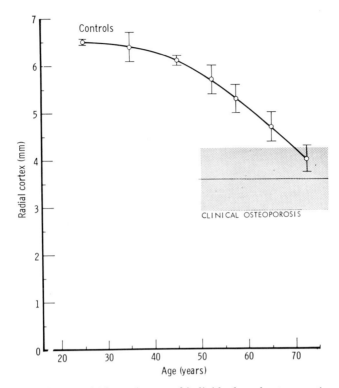

FIG. 71. Radial cortex thickness in normal individuals and osteoporotics suffering from spinal compression fractures. The hatched area for osteoporotics is ±1 standard deviation. Circles and vertical bars for normal persons gives mean ± 1 standard error.

graphed under standard conditions, and density of the ulna at various distances up the shaft is measured by feeding the images of the step wedge and the ulna through a recording densitometer and comparing one with the other. Bone density is expressed in millimeters of aluminum, and this figure, when multiplied by 130, is converted into milligrams of bone mineral per cubic centimeter of bone. This method is sufficiently precise to demonstrate changes in bone mineral content in a single individual with time. Barnett and Nordin[3] have reported similar densitometric studies for the accurate assessment of vertebral density. Although these techniques have greatly increased our knowledge, they require special equipment and training and, in general, are not presently suitable for routine clinical use.

Photon Source Densitometry

In this method direct measurements are made of the absorption of a monochromatic beam of radiation by bone. Methods have been described which use iodine 125 or americium 241 as sources of monochromatic gamma rays. The reports by Sorenson and Cameron[54] seem highly promising in this regard for the precise measurements of bone mineral *in vivo*, at least in bones not surrounded by large amounts of soft tissue.

Clinical Approach to Bone Density

Dotter et al.[18] found a good correlation between their clinical judgment of spine radiographs and autopsy estimates of bone ash content. Since the *thoracic spine* is overlapped on either side by the lungs and has many air-tissue interfaces, densitometry is not practical. However, a lateral view of the *lumbar spine*, when taken under standard clinical conditions, may be used to grade spine density with a reasonable degree of reproducibility.[54] A convenient scale for grading bone density is noted below and illustrated in Figures 72 through 76.

Grade 0 = normal bone density.

Grade 1 = minimal loss of density; endplates begin to stand out, giving a stenciled effect.

Grade 2 = increased prominence of vertical trabeculae; endplates are thinner.

Grade 3 = more severe loss of bone density than grade 2; endplates become less visible, and vertebral biconcavity is evident.

Grade 4 = ghostlike vertebral bodies; density is no greater than soft tissue; no trabecular pattern is visible (when the vertebral outline is covered, the body is invisible).

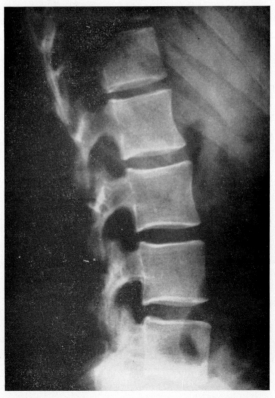

FIGS. 72–76. Various grades of spine density. Figure 72 shows normal bone density

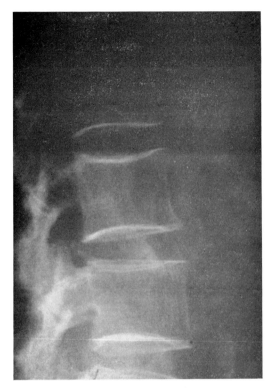

FIG. 73. Grade 1 demineralization

When comparing spine grades, judged by eye on standard radiographs of the lumbar spine, with cortical thickness of the radius measured directly from radiographs of the left elbow, it has been found that, as spine density decreases, cortical thickness decreases significantly, even though there is considerable overlap between the grades.[47] Although this holds true for women with the postmenopausal type of osteoporosis and for men and women with rheumatoid arthritis, we have noted that, in men with idiopathic osteoporosis and spine fractures, the long bones are commonly of normal thickness. Thus, there may be certain disorders in which there is no correspondence between demineralization of the vertebrae and cortical thickness of long bones, and for this reason the use of more than one parameter of skeletal density may give a more complete picture.

CALCIUM AND PHOSPHORUS METABOLISM

Between 400 and 1000 mg of calcium are ingested daily by adults in Western countries, and of this about 25 per cent is absorbed—more in children. The fraction absorbed decreases with increasing intake; absorption occurs in the duodenum and jejunum, and is mediated by calcium-binding protein in the intestinal mucosa.[53] Despite wide fluctuations in calcium intake, serum levels are remarkably constant. The skeleton acts as an enormous reservoir of calcium (1200 g) with a turnover in adults of

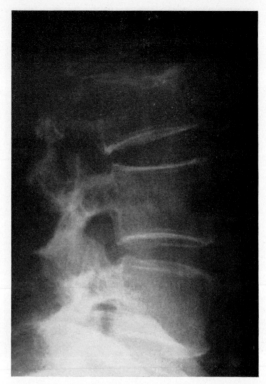

FIG. 74. Grade 2 demineralization

about 300 to 500 mg daily. When necessary, parathyroid hormone and calcitonin can change the absolute bone resorption rate considerably. When an imbalance between bone formation rate and resorption rate has occurred over a prolonged period of time, clinically detectable changes may appear in the skeleton. Pure calcium deficiency leads to smaller body size in young animals and osteoporosis in mature animals and, presumably, in humans as well. Vitamin D is necessary both for transport of calcium across the intestinal mucosa[56] and to permit parathyroid hormone to exert its action on bone resorption. Vitamin D also seems necessary for normal formation of bone collagen as well as normal mineralization of the preformed matrix. Lack of vitamin D leads to impaired absorption of calcium, alterations in the calcium-phosphorus ionic product, undermineralization of the organic matrix, and changes in the total amount of organic matrix.

Unlike calcium, most ingested phosphorus is absorbed from the intestine, and that which is not utilized for calcium or nitrogen metabolism is excreted in the urine. Thus, while urinary calcium has rather narrow limits, urinary phosphorus excretion varies widely in normal individuals.

Values for serum and urinary calcium and phosphorus as well as serum alkaline phosphatase activity in health and disease are listed in Table 50. With newer techniques serum calcium can be determined with much

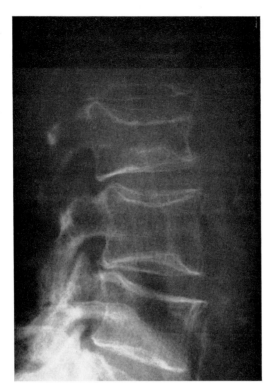

FIG. 75. Grade 3 demineralization

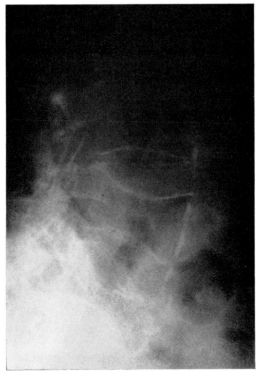

FIG. 76. Grade 4 demineralization

TABLE 50

Biochemical Changes in Various Diseases Affecting Bone

Disease	Serum Calcium	Serum Phosphorus	TRP*	Urinary Calcium†
	mg/100 ml		%	
Normal values	9.5 ± 0.3	3.7 ± 0.4	85 ± 10	100–300 mg/24 hr (men) 80–250 mg/24 hr (women) 50–270 mg/g creatinine
Idiopathic osteoporosis	9.5 ± 0.3	3.7 ± 0.4	85 ± 10	100–300 mg/24 hr (men) 80–250 mg/24 hr (women) 50–270 mg/g creatinine
Phosphate deprivation	May be slightly raised	<3	>95	Raised slightly
Primary hyperparathyroidism‡	>10.5	<3	<75	>270 mg/g creatinine >300 mg/24 hr in absence of renal failure
Osteomalacia‡	Low or normal	<3	<75	<50 mg/g creatinine
Uremic bone disease‡	Low	>5	<75	Very low, ∼10 mg/24 hr
Metastatic bone disease (lytic)§	Normal or high	Normal or high	Normal	High, e.g., up to 500 mg/24 hr or more, depending on level of serum calcium
Metastatic cancer with syndrome of ectopic hyperparathyroidism	High	<3	<75	High, depending in part on level of serum calcium
Multiple myeloma	High in 10%	Normal or high	Normal or low	High

* TRP = tubular reabsorption of phosphorus, expressed as a percentage.
† On unrestricted calcium intake.
‡ Serum alkaline phosphatase activity is elevated.
§ Serum alkaline phosphatase activity may be elevated if lesions are mixed lytic and blastic.

greater precision and accuracy than previously. In most laboratories the normal level of serum calcium ranges from 8.8 to 10.5 mg/100 ml, while those who use automated methods may find normal values as low as 8.5 mg/100 ml. Therefore, physicians utilizing these newer methods should consider hypercalcemia as being present with values somewhat lower than the more traditional 11 mg/100 ml.

Urinary calcium determinations present a different problem. Until the last few years urinary calcium determinations were among the least precise of the tests performed in most laboratories. Among the problems encountered was a tendency for calcium to precipitate from the urine with standing. This difficulty can be overcome by strongly acidifying the urine with concentrated hydrochloric acid and agitating the specimen well before an aliquot is removed for analysis. Even when urinary calcium can be accurately determined, there remain problems of interpretation. The renal excretion of calcium tends to vary somewhat with dietary intake and also with body size. Some physicians prescribe a 200-mg calcium diet for 3 days before determining urinary calcium excretion, and under these conditions normal values range from 50 to 150 mg/24 hours in adults. In contrast, on self-selected diets, normal values for 24-hour urinary calcium excretion in adults range from 80 to 250 mg in women and from 100 to 300 mg in men.[26] The distribution for 24-hour urinary calcium excretion is skewed to the right because there are, among normal individuals, a few who have a very high urinary calcium excretion, while the majority fall into a lower range, around 150 to 200 mg/24 hours. A useful technique for normalizing urinary calcium data is to measure calcium and creatinine in the same sample and then express either the calcium-to-creatinine ratio or calcium in milligrams per gram of creatinine. In normal individuals urinary calcium content is 50 to 270 mg of calcium per gram of creatinine, with a mean of 160 mg/g. We have found that the calcium-to-creatinine ratio in a morning random sample is highly correlated with that of a 24-hour sample taken from the same patient on a metabolic ward ($r = 0.86$). Therefore, we consider that a random sample of urine passed in the morning, while the patient is on his usual diet, can be used to evaluate urinary calcium excretion without the inconvenience of collecting a 24-hour sample. With rapid and accurate methods for measuring urinary calcium, the Sulkowitch test should now be abandoned. Hypercalciuria will commonly be missed by the Sulkowitch test because these patients usually have polyuria and pass a large volume of dilute urine, giving a rather weakly positive reaction.

The concentration of serum phosphorus varies between the sexes and with age. In adults serum phosphorus values below 3.0 mg/100 ml should be considered abnormal, while in children values below 4.0 mg/100 ml are usually considered abnormal. The level of serum phosphorus may vary considerably during the day, so that measurement should be made on serum samples obtained in the fasting state. The urinary excretion of phosphorus varies within very wide limits according to the intake. These values are usually between 300 and 1200 mg/24 hours. Amounts below 300 mg suggest phosphorus deprivation.[30] A more useful parameter of phosphorus metabolism is to consider the renal handling of phosphorus in relation to the serum level. Since calcium and creatinine are determined in a random morning urinary sample, measurements of phosphorus can be made on the same sample and on a fasting blood sample. With these values determined, the renal tubular reabsorption of phosphorus (TRP) can be calculated as follows. The phosphorus-to-creatinine clearance (C_p/C_{cr}) ratio is first calculated as

$$\frac{\text{Urinary P (mg/100 ml)}}{\text{Serum P (mg/100 ml)}} \times \frac{\text{serum creatinine (mg/100 ml)}}{\text{urinary creatinine (mg/100 ml)}}.$$

Then TRP $= (1 - C_p/C_{cr}) \times 100$. The normal values for each are, respectively, 0.13 ± 0.01 and $87 \pm 10\%$. Serum phosphorus concentration may be low because of inadequate ingestion of phosphate due, for example, to starvation, dieting, vomiting, or surgery, or because the ingested phosphate is precipitated in the intestinal lumen with antacids containing aluminum gels.[30] It may also be low because of a renal tubular "leak," as occurs in vitamin D-resistant rickets, primary or secondary hyperparathyroidism, the Fanconi syndrome, renal acidosis, and Wilson's disease.

Fasting serum phosphorus concentrations may be high normally in young children, in some cases of gigantism and acromegaly, in severe degrees of renal failure, in hypoparathyroidism, and in some patients with metastatic cancer, notably mammary carcinoma. It should be emphasized that the 24-hour excretion of urinary phosphorus is *not* increased in disorders with "phosphate leaks," but rather the urinary phosphorus is high *relative* to the serum levels. Table 50 emphasizes the relationships among serum calcium, phosphorus, and TRP in several conditions.

Alkaline phosphatase activity in serum is due to the presence of a number of nonspecific phosphomonoesterases which have a pH optimum of 8.6 to 9.4. These enzymes are thought to be derived primarily from bone, liver, kidney, and intestinal mucosa. Bone alkaline phosphatase is thermolabile and can be inactivated by heating to 56°C for 20 minutes, while liver phosphatase is thermostable.[23] Human intestinal alkaline phosphatase can be distinguished from both bone alkaline phosphatase and hepatic phosphatase because the activity of the former is almost completely inhibited by L-phenylalanine. There are several methods for measuring alkaline phosphatase activity and several different types of units used in reporting results. Furthermore, when different laboratories use the same method, there may be considerable variation in the results. Despite this, within any given laboratory there is ordinarily no difficulty in obtaining consistent results or in distinguishing normal from abnormal. Clinicians should obtain the range of normal values in their particular laboratory from the laboratory director.

In addition to the high values seen in rapidly growing children, the following bone diseases are usually associated with increased activity of alkaline phosphatase in the serum: 1) fractures of large bones or multiple fractures; 2) rickets and osteomalacia; 3) hyperparathyroidism with bone disease; 4) primary or metastatic bone cancer, especially osteogenic sarcoma and osteoblastic metastases from breast and prostate; and 5) Paget's disease of bone—the values in this disease may be extremely high. Alkaline phosphatase activity is usually normal in myelomatosis, hypoparathyroidism, hyperparathyroidism without bone disease, and osteoporosis.

The activity of alkaline phosphatase in the serum may be affected not only by bone disease but also by disease of extraskeletal sites, notably the hepatobiliary system, where excretion of the enzyme into the bile may be prevented. In addition, in pregnant women the serum alkaline phosphatase activity may be increased because of contributions of isoenzymes from the placenta and, perhaps, from the fetus. High serum alkaline phosphatase activity resulting from hepatobiliary disease may be distinguished from that due to bone disease, in that in the former levels of 5'-nucleotidase activity are usually increased as well, whereas in the latter these levels are normal.[17] Of course, in patients who have disease of the skeleton and the liver, such as metastatic cancer, the activities of both alkaline phosphatase and 5′-nucleotidase are often elevated.

CLINICAL APPROACH TO THE PATIENT WITH A DEMINERALIZED SKELETON

With the above background information regarding the major methods of evaluating bone density and some aspects of calcium and phosphorus metabolism, one may outline a reasonable clinical approach to the patient who has a demineralized skeleton. For the purposes of this analysis we shall consider that the condition has been so diagnosed on the basis of radiographs, and semiquantitatively assessed according to the method outlined above. It is assumed that the evidence is that of a generalized disease rather than simply localized demineralization, such as that encountered with immobilization of an extremity. The following questions should be answered in order.

1. *Do the radiographs of the skeleton, including long bones and hands, reveal any characteristic features that might suggest the nature of the underlying disease?* As will be noted below in a discussion of some examples of demineralizing diseases, there are radiographic features that favor a diagnosis of osteitis fibrosa, or of osteoporosis, or of certain infiltrative diseases of the skeleton which, if present in addition to the general finding of demineralization, may provide important clues to the correct diagnosis. An example of such a feature would be the subperiosteal resorption of osteitis fibrosa (Fig. 77).

2. *Is the patient sick, or does he just have demineralized bones with no other clinical findings?* The "nonsick" patient with a demineralized skeleton is most likely to have idiopathic osteoporosis. By "nonsick" is meant that the patient is asymptomatic except, possibly, for the presence of localized pain due to a collapsed vertebra. On the other hand, a sick patient with radiolucent bones is apt to have either osteoporosis in association with some other disease (collagen disease, endocrine disease, etc.), osteomalacia, or an infiltrated marrow. Patients with osteitis fibrosa may be symptomatic or not, and, if so, the symptoms are usually directed to the genitourinary tract (i.e., renal lithiasis), not to the skeleton.

3. As a corollary to question 2 above, *has the patient taken a diet, or does he have an underlying disease, or has he received treatment that might have produced skeletal demineralization?* Obviously, a patient whose diet is deficient in calcium and vitamin D may have demineralized bones, as may one who has been on long-term adrenal corticosteroids, so that these historical facts must be known when evaluating radiolucent bones. Prior ovariectomy may be an important factor, but it should be noted that osteoporosis is not by any means an invariable result of ovariectomy.

4. *Is there any abnormality of serum calcium, phosphorus, or alkaline phosphatase activity?* Characteristically osteoporosis is a disease marked by

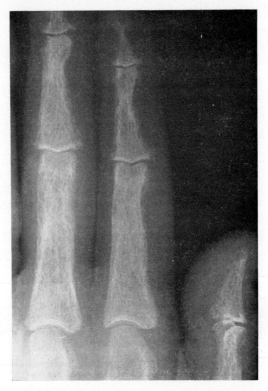

FIG. 77. Subperiosteal erosion of bone seen on the radial side of the phalanges in a patient with a large parathyroid adenoma.

normal levels of serum calcium, phosphorus, and alkaline phosphatase activity, whereas osteomalacia, osteitis fibrosa, and neoplastic disease involving the skeleton usually produce changes in one or more of these biochemical parameters. These determinations are basic to any laboratory investigation of demineralized bones.

5. *Is there laboratory evidence of an endocrine disturbance (notably thyroid, adrenal, and gonadal) or dysproteinemia?* As is well known (and as will be illustrated below), diseases of the thyroid (both hyper- and hypothyroidism), adrenals (notably Cushing's syndrome), and hypogonadism may lead to skeletal demineralization, and therefore it is obviously important to identify these conditions. The same can be said of dysproteinemias, the best known of which are multiple myeloma and Waldenström's macroglobulinemia.

The systematic answers to these questions should provide important clues to a correct diagnosis. A summary approach to the work-up of a patient with a demineralized skeleton is shown in Table 51. Of course, not all of the studies listed need be done in each instance, and one should try to arrive at a diagnosis using the minimum number of studies. These studies have been listed in three stages of increasing complexity and, in the major-

TABLE 51

Suggested Studies for Investigation of Demineralizing Diseases of the Skeleton. These studies are listed in three stages of increasing complexity. In the majority of instances the diagnosis can be arrived at with the first two levels of studies.

Stage	Blood	Urine	X-rays	Other
I	Calcium × 2 Phosphorus × 2 Alkaline phosphatase × 2 Blood urea nitrogen Creatinine CO_2, chloride Total protein with serum albumin and globulin	Ca (24-hr urinary Ca or Ca/creatinine ratio on random morning sample) Creatinine	Bone survey, including long bones, hands, skull, and acromioclavicular joints Chest x-ray and flat film of abdomen	Complete blood count Urinalysis
II	Protein-bound iodine Serum protein electrophoresis Uric acid Na, K, Mg	P (this plus the data above permits calculation of tubular reabsorption of phosphate, TRP, and phosphate clearance) Urinary 17-hydroxycorticosteroids	Spot views of symptomatic bones Intravenous pyelogram X-rays of esophagus, stomach, and small bowel	Marrow aspiration Bone biopsy (to include cortical bone) Vaginal smear for estrogenic activity Tests for malabsorption
III	Serum Ca (after 10 days of cortisol 120 mg/day if patient is hypercalcemic)	Ca (after dietary P deprivation) P (after Ca infusion) Hydroxyproline	Special x-rays as indicated by patient's history or clinical findings	Ca kinetics and bone scan, utilizing Ca^{47}, Sr^{85}, or F^{18} Parathyroid scan with Se^{75}-selenomethionine Radioimmunoassay for parathyroid hormone

ity of instances, the diagnosis can be determined without proceeding to level III. Level I includes the blood and urinary determinations noted. At least two determinations of serum calcium, phosphorus, and alkaline phosphatase activity should be done to avoid incorrect decisions due to possible laboratory error, since these three are central to the analysis of any patient with demineralization. The presence of hypercalcemia should make one consider that the patient's demineralization is most likely due to hyperparathyroidism or malignancy. The serum bicarbonate and chloride levels are included because of possible alterations in certain bone diseases (decreased CO_2 and increased chloride occasionally seen in hyperparathyroidism, increased CO_2 in milk-alkali syndrome, etc.). The serum protein analysis is important for the full interpretation of the serum calcium level (since calcium is approximately 50 per cent protein-bound) and for the detection of dysproteinemias. Urinary calcium, as discussed above, may be measured on a 24-hour collection or on a morning random sample, calculating the calcium-to-creatinine ratio. The x-ray films noted are those most likely to show the changes of hyperparathyroidism (hands and acromioclavicular joints for resorptive changes; flat film of the abdomen for renal stones).

If the above studies fail to lead to a diagnosis, additional studies should be undertaken as noted at level II. Some patients with hyperthyroidism may show diffuse demineralization—hence the protein-bound iodine determination. Serum protein electrophoresis will permit more exact analysis of the possibility of dysproteinemia. Serum uric acid concentration may be increased in hyperparathyroidism as well as in marrow-infiltrative disorders (notably the lymphomas). Potassium and magnesium are included, not because they will aid in the differential diagnosis, but because their concentrations may be altered in certain patients with skeletal demineralization, notably those with hypercalcemia. Serum sodium concentration may give an indication of a salt depletion state, which, if present, may lead to spuriously low values for urinary calcium. Urinary phosphorus (total as well as TRP) is highly dependent on dietary intake, and this must be known to interpret these data. Table 50 shows alterations of TRP in various bone disorders, but it should be noted that these alterations are nonspecific and serve only to complete the analysis of a particular case of demineralization. The urinary steroid excretion (17-hydroxycorticosteroids) may provide information suggesting that the demineralization has an adrenal basis. The gastrointestinal x-rays are taken to determine the presence of extrinsic pressure (shift of esophagus due to parathyroid adenoma, Fig. 78) or intrinsic disease that might lead to malabsorption. Microscopic study of the bone marrow may prove to be decisive in making a diagnosis. Referring to Sutton's law, which is defined elsewhere in this volume, it should be kept in mind that marrow aspiration with bone biopsy is often "where the money is." The vaginal smear will help to establish the presence or absence of estrogens in the analysis of female patients with demineralized bones.

Level III lists studies which are ordinarily not necessary but may be helpful at times in unraveling a complicated skeletal disorder. Response to cortisol has been cited as useful in the differential diagnosis of hypercalcemia,[16] in that patients with sarcoidosis usually respond with a reduction in serum calcium concentration, patients with malignancy respond in a variable fashion, and patients with hyperparathyroidism usually do not respond. Measurements of urinary calcium and phosphorus, after phosphate deprivation and calcium infusion, respectively, have certain usefulness in hyper-

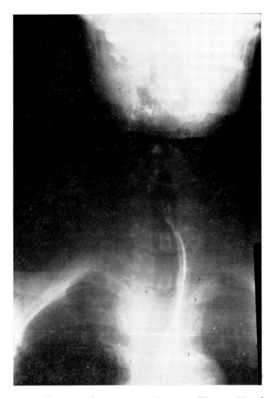

FIG. 78. Barium swallow in the same patient as Figure 77, showing displacement of the esophagus (but not trachea) by the parathyroid adenoma.

parathyroidism, in that phosphate deprivation makes manifest hypercalciuria in these patients and calcium infusion usually fails to suppress hyperphosphaturia. Excretion of hydroxyproline serves as an indicator of increased bone turnover[4, 20, 49] but has no specificity in terms of differential diagnosis. Finally a word about radionuclides. The bone-seeking nuclides Ca[47], Sr[85], and F[18] are gamma emitters and therefore permit detection of their localization in the skeleton by external means. Increased uptake may occur in a variety of bone lesions, and hence such uptake is not diagnostic per se. Nevertheless, in a clinical setting where one suspects malignant disease as the cause of a demineralized skeleton, a search scan of the skeleton may reveal areas of increased uptake before localizing changes are evident on the skeletal radiographs.[25] Under these circumstances biopsy of such an area may yield the diagnosis. Also it has been found that, if a patient has a collapsed vertebra due to osteoporosis, although the uptake of a bone-seeking isotope is high initially it usually returns to normal within 5 to 6 months. Thus, if a collapsed vertebra is known to have been present for more than 6 months, and the uptake over it is high, suspicion of a nonosteoporotic lesion, such as a neoplasm, should be heightened. The kinetics of bone-seeking radionuclides have revealed differences among them[57] and some suggestive differences between hyperparathyroidism and cancer simulating hyperparathyroidism,[36] but in general the influence of demineralizing bone disease on the kinetics is nonspecific in terms of differential diagnosis. The use of Se[75]-selenomethionine to localize hyperfunctioning parathyroid tissue may be helpful in certain cases, although it is not perfected for routine clinical use. In one series[44] preoperative localization was accomplished in two-thirds of 25 patients with surgically proven hyperparathyroidism. Immunoassay for parathyroid hormone has been developed, and although some observations have been reported on its use on blood samples from human subjects,[42] it is not yet generally available. Even when it is, high levels of circulating hormone may not be specific for parathyroid disease, since some nonparathyroid tumors appear to be capable of synthesizing parathyroid hormone or a closely related analogue.[36] Studies such as serum ionized calcium or citric acid concentrations and cerebrospinal fluid calcium concentration have been the subject of a variety of investigations, but at this time have no established place in the differential diagnosis of the demineralized skeleton.

SOME EXAMPLES OF DISEASES CHARACTERIZED BY SKELETAL DEMINERALIZATION

Osteitis Fibrosa

When hyperparathyroidism presents with radiographic changes, the diagnosis is usually fairly straightforward. Radiographic changes may be pathognomonic or nonspecific. The former include subperiosteal bone resorption, best seen on the radial borders of the phalanges (Fig. 77), the femoral necks, and the ischiopubic rami. "Granular" demineralization of the skull is also typical, and sometimes destruction of the outer ends of the clavicles, as well as bone cysts and trabeculation of bone cortices, may be seen. Resorption of the lamina dura, once thought typical, is now regarded as of little value because of the inconstancy of this radiographic finding and because other disorders may lead to it. Nonspecific changes consist of generalized increased radiolucency of the skeleton. Primary hyperparathyroidism is also commonly associated with nephrocalcinosis or nephrolithiasis, or both. Sometimes a parathyroid adenoma is large enough to displace the esophagus (Fig. 78); unlike thyroid nodules, it does not usually cause tracheal displacement. Thyroid nodules are commonly found in association with parathyroid adenomas, and are often mistaken for the latter on physical examination and sometimes at surgery. Hyperparathyroidism is most often due to a parathyroid adenoma,[7] although primary chief cell hyperplasia has been described in recent years.[12]

When specific radiographic changes in the skeleton are accompanied by hypercalcemia and hypophosphatemia, and especially when nephrolithiasis is present, the diagnosis of primary hyperparathyroidism is as certain as medical diagnoses can be, and surgery is indicated. Other investigations will usually reveal a low TRP level and a *moderate* degree of hypercalciuria, which, however, may come into the normal range if dietary calcium is low (either by design or by accident, such as vomiting) or if renal failure supervenes. When specific radiographic changes are present, but the serum calcium is low or normal, secondary hyperparathyroidism should be suspected. Indeed, the severest bone changes usually occur with disease secondary to chronic renal failure, in which the glomerular filtration rate may be less than 15 per cent of normal for many years. In this setting the urinary calcium is always very low and the serum phosphorus is high, often 10 mg/100 ml or more. A rare diagnostic difficulty occurs when chronic renal failure due to nephrolithiasis results in secondary hyperparathyroidism, which may be mistaken for primary hyperparathyroidism associated with secondary nephrolithiasis and renal failure. Even under these conditions the concentration of serum calcium is usually the clue to the diagnosis. In primary hyperparathyroidism the levels of serum calcium are almost always greater than 10 mg/100 ml, whereas in renal failure with secondary hyperparathyroidism they are usually less than 10 mg/100 ml. Although parathyroid tumors have been described in the presence of a normal serum calcium concentration,[58] if a patient's serum calcium is normal there is no indication for urging immediate surgical exploration, since he is in no imminent danger from the adenoma, even if present. It is more likely, in the presence of a repeatedly normal level of serum calcium, that the patient does not have hyperparathyroidism. Thus, in any suspected case, it is well to observe the patient carefully until persistent hypercalcemia clarifies the diagnosis.

When radiographic changes are nonspecific, and simply show generalized demineralization of the skeleton, the diagnosis of osteitis fibrosa becomes more difficult. The level of serum alkaline phosphatase activity is usually not of great help, though if there is severe demineralization and the alkaline phosphatase is normal, the diagnosis is more likely to be a nonparathyroid disorder, such as osteoporosis. The main differential diagnosis in a patient with hypercalcemia and a demineralized skeleton lies between true hyperparathyroidism and pseudohyperparathyroidism—a term used to designate the hypercalcemic syndrome of cancer that mimics hyperparathyroidism.

Osteitis fibrosa commonly causes generalized aching pain throughout the skeleton. Hypercalcemia leads to headache, constipation, nausea, anorexia, muscle weakness, and hyporeflexia. Polyuria and polydipsia are due to the hyposthenuria associated with hypercalciuria. Acute arthritis, occasionally seen in the course of hyperparathyroidism, may be due to coexistent pseudogout[31] or true gout.[51] Punctate calcium deposits on the cornea around the limbus may be seen with a slit lamp or even with the naked eye in severe cases. The latter sign may be seen with any cause of chronic hypercalcemia and, in addition, in the hypocalcemia of secondary hyperparathyroidism, when the calcium-phosphorus ionic product is very high, owing to a high serum phosphorus concentration. Extensive calcification of the media of medium-sized arteries may be noted on radiographs, and, of course, nephrolithiasis and/or nephrocalcinosis are commonly seen in primary hyperparathyroidism.

Osteoporosis

Most cases of osteoporosis are idiopathic in the sense that the cause(s) are not known. Most patients presenting with symptomatic osteoporosis are women over the age of 50. Rarely, a disease known to be associated with osteoporosis may be found on work-up, but even then the patient is often a woman over the age of 50. Below are listed some of the conditions which can aggravate or produce osteoporosis:

A. Idiopathic osteoporosis
    1. Postmenopausal women (common)
    2. Congenital: osteogenesis imperfecta (50 per cent autosomal dominant; 50 per cent sporadic)
    3. Young people (rare)
    4. Peripartum women (rare)
B. Secondary osteoporosis
    1. Endocrinopathies
        a. Thyroid (hypersecretion–hyperthyroidism)
        b. Pituitary (hypersecretion–acromegaly)
        c. Adrenal (hypersecretion–Cushing's syndrome)
        d. Ovary (hyposecretion–ovarian agenesis and castration)
        e. Testis (hyposecretion–eunuchoidism)
    2. Nutritional
        a. Alcoholism
        b. Starvation
        c. Impaired calcium absorption due to surgery, e.g., gastrectomy, small bowel resection
        d. Scurvy
    3. Systemic disease
        a. Rheumatoid arthritis
        b. Ulcerative colitis
        c. Malabsorption syndromes
    4. Immobilization
        a. With fractures
        b. Without fractures

Idiopathic Osteoporosis

Albright et al.[1] postulated the concept of postmenopausal osteoporosis and the hormonal deficiency theory of the disease. These investigators found that 80 per cent of their patients were women who had passed the menopause but were not really senile, and, in general, these findings have been confirmed. In our experience, the average age of women when they presented at our metabolic bone disease clinic with symptoms of osteoporosis was 65 years;[46] this was also the average age of all women 50 and over seen at our hospital, which suggests that the age of presentation of symptoms merely reflects the distribution of age of the population at risk, rather than any relation to the menopause. Of interest was the finding that the average age at the menopause was 46.7 years in osteoporotics and 46.6 years in controls matched for age. Finally, a small group of women castrated between the ages of 18 and 36 also presented with osteoporosis at an average age of 62.[46]

In a consecutive series of 80 women with idiopathic osteoporosis, the most frequently fractured vertebra was the 12th thoracic.[48] The frequency of fractures decreased with each vertebra above and below the 12th thoracic. No fractures affecting the first or second thoracic vertebra were observed in this series. Multiple fractures occurred in about half the patients, and 20 per cent of the patients developed new fractures between 1 and 10 years after coming under observation, whether they were treated with estrogens or not. Strontium 85 scintimetry revealed a count rate over the fractured vertebra between 3 and 13 times that of the normal vertebrae. Similar values are also found with other causes of fracture, such as metastatic malignant disease. The difference between the fractured and nonfractured vertebrae was greatest when the fracture was fresh, and decreased rapidly after the time of fracture until it was undetectable by 5 months, in contrast to pathologic fractures of the spine. Therefore, strontium 85 scintimetry of the spine may be useful in distinguishing osteoporotic fractures from pathologic fractures if the age of the lesion is known to be 5 months or more. A compression fracture of an isolated vertebra in the presence of other normal-appearing vertebrae should, of course, raise the suspicion of a neoplasm, but at times osteoporosis and neoplastic disease of the spine coexist, a situation which can be clarified only by biopsy.

In osteoporosis radiographs of the spine show lack of mineralization, which is best viewed on the lateral view of the lumbar region. Of note are the lack of osteophytes and of senile spondylosis so commonly seen in elderly people, and the presence of usually well-marked and premature calcification of the aorta. There may be wedge fractures or expansion of the discs, giving biconcavity or so-called "codfish" vertebrae. Since horizontal trabeculae are resorbed first, there is a tendency to vertical striation in the vertebral bodies.

Pain from the spinal fractures is the symptom that causes an osteoporotic patient to seek medical attention. Osteoporosis without fractures does not cause symptoms. Furthermore, the spinal fractures occur with little or no trauma, and although the pain comes on suddenly in the classical case, it comes gradually, over a period of hours or days, in about one-third of the patients. This atypical presentation in so many cases probably accounts for the fact that many such patients consider themselves to have "lumbago." It is well known that routine radiographs of the spine in elderly women will reveal unsuspected compression fractures with a frequency which rises with age to around 20 per cent by the age of 75.

Osteogenesis Imperfecta Tarda

All physicians are aware of the syndrome of osteogenesis imperfecta and its classical presentation. However, less well appreciated is the patient who has rather mild bone disease and who presents in later childhood or in adult life with spinal osteoporosis. Figure 79 illustrates the spine radiographs of a 36-year-old woman who never had multiple long bone fractures; indeed, her long bones were radiographically normal. However, she was

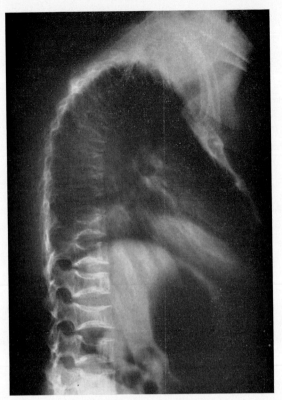

FIG. 79. Spine of patient with osteogenesis imperfecta (see text)

deaf, presumably from otosclerosis, and had blue sclerae and lax ligaments (Fig. 80). Furthermore, she gave a family history strongly suggestive of a dominant autosomal genetic trait.

Fifty per cent of cases of osteogenesis imperfecta are sporadic, and the patients give no family history of the disease; many are not deaf, and some do not have blue sclerae. Under these conditions a diagnosis cannot be made with certainty. Helpful signs include multiple Wormian bones in skull radiographs, while a bone biopsy taken from cortical bone in an area *that has not been fractured* may show the presence of primitive fibrous bone (instead of lamellar bone), which is always abnormal in older children and adults, and would strongly support a diagnosis of osteogenesis imperfecta.

Peripartum Osteoporosis

This rare syndrome presents between the 9th month of pregnancy and the first 2 months of the postpartum period.[39] We have seen it in patients who have lactated as well as those who have not. One of us has followed one young woman from the time of presentation with spine fractures, at the end of her first pregnancy, through her next pregnancy 1 year later. The second pregnancy was quite uneventful and was not associated with

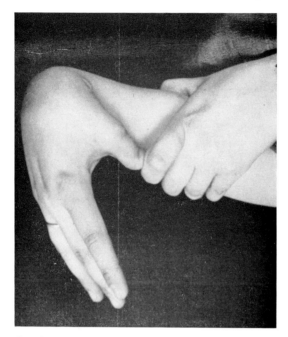

FIG. 80. Lax ligaments in a patient with osteogenesis imperfecta

any new fractures. Thus, great caution is indicated in advising these patients regarding therapeutic abortion at the time of subsequent pregnancies.

Osteoporosis and Myasthenia Gravis

We have seen two patients, both young women, who developed severe incapacitating generalized osteoporosis and classical, mild myasthenia gravis. In each case the myasthenia was well controlled with drugs. Figure 81 illustrates a radiograph of one of the cases. The onset of fractures occurred around 16 years of age, and she fractured her tibiae and femora on many occasions in the first 5 years of this disease, most of which were spent in the hospital. In the last 5 years, the patient has had neither fractures nor bone pain. The second patient presented at 32 years of age with a fracture of her sternum and several thoracic vertebrae. These fractures followed an episode of sneezing and were accompanied by a loss of 5 inches in height. The patient went into positive balance for calcium and phosphorus when stilbestrol, 1 mg daily, was administered by mouth, even though she had normal menses. Because of this odd finding, both patients have been maintained for years on estrogens, which may have contributed to a lack of further symptoms.

Hyperthyroidism

Patients with hyperthyroidism are commonly in negative calcium balance with poor calcium absorption and hypercalciuria, the latter often extreme.[11]

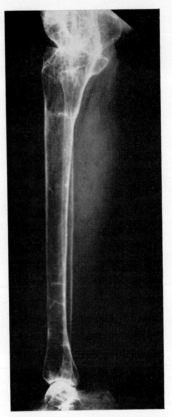

Fig. 81. Extreme osteoporosis of the tibia in a young woman with idiopathic osteoporosis and myasthenia gravis.

However, although bone demineralization occurs, symptoms on this basis are exceedingly uncommon.

Cushing's Syndrome

Patients with Cushing's syndrome, especially the naturally occurring disease, commonly have osteoporosis and may have pain from vertebral fractures. Rib fractures are not infrequent. Unlike idiopathic osteoporosis, the skull may be radiographically demineralized and may even demonstrate areas that mimic lytic neoplastic lesions. In children, surgical cure of Cushing's syndrome results in new bone formation, but in adults this does not occur.

Hypogonadism

The skeletons of women with ovarian agenesis are less dense than those of normal women, but we have no data to indicate that this leads to skeletal symptoms. On the other hand, women castrated between 18 and 36 years of age do not present with *symptomatic* osteoporosis any earlier than do normal women.[46] In men, eunuchoidism leads to vertebral compression fractures, and this exaggerates the disproportion between trunk length and leg length; the resultant striking appearance will lead the physician to the correct diagnosis without too much difficulty.

Nutritional Factors

The role of dietary calcium has not been clearly established in demineralizing bone diseases. Smith and Frame[53] found no clear-cut relation between spine density and calcium consumption in a large number of normal women. Chalmers et al.[9] have shown that elderly women living alone are frequently malnourished, and may have osteomalacia due to inadequate diets coupled with lack of sunlight. Chronic alcoholics under 45 years of age who come to autopsy have been found to have diminished bone density, similar to that of normal individuals over the age of 70.[45] Alcohol causes a brisk diuresis of the divalent cations magnesium and calcium.[27] Thus, heavy drinking probably contributes to osteoporosis by combining dietary inadequacy with increased calcium excretion. While osteomalacia is the classical bone disease that occurs in the malabsorption syndromes, osteoporosis is at least as common.[38] Both diseases may coincide. We have found that men who have been subjected to partial gastrectomy tend to present with osteoporosis, while women tend to have osteomalacia.

Osteoporosis in Men

Symptomatic osteoporosis in men is uncommon. However, 50 cases were seen by one of us in a metabolic bone disease clinic over a period of 10 years. The ages of these men were normally distributed, with a mean ± standard deviation of 59 ± 10 years. Seven of these patients had had partial gastrectomy, five had rheumatoid spondylitis, and three had hypogonadism. In the remainder no obvious contributing factors were found. The syndrome of rheumatoid spondylitis presenting with osteoporosis and spinal fractures is not widely appreciated, even among rheumatologists. In addition to the male patients mentioned here, we have also had one woman presenting with rheumatoid spondylitis and osteoporosis, plus associated regional enteritis.

Rheumatoid Arthritis and Osteoporosis

Patients with rheumatoid arthritis (men, women, and children) commonly have osteoporosis whether or not they have been treated with corticosteroid drugs.[32] Although the administration of corticosteroids can aggravate osteoporosis, age, sex, and severity of the disease are more important factors.[50] In children, osteoporosis is especially troublesome in girls who develop rheumatoid arthritis before the age of 5. In these children long bone fractures may occur during physiotherapy or manipulation of contractures. There is no proof that the administration of corticosteroids to these children aggravates the osteoporosis or the tendency to fractures.[6]

Osteomalacia

Vitamin D Deficiency

Vitamin D_3 is formed in the skin and sebaceous secretions by activation of the provitamin 7-dehydrocholesterol by actinic rays in a narrow spectrum between 290 and 320 mμ. Irradiation of the plant sterol ergosterol forms vitamin D_2 (calciferol). Either vitamin is effective in human beings and in rats, but calciferol is ineffective in chicks and less effective than D_3 in higher primates. There is very little vitamin D in natural foods, even in milk, and what there is fluctuates seasonally. Only halibut liver oil and cod liver oil have a high vitamin D content. In the United States, but not in Western Europe, milk is supplemented with calciferol, 400 IU/quart (10 μg). Recently the identification of 25-hydroxycholecalciferol as the active metabolite of vitamin D has been reported,[14] giving promise of benefit to patients who may be unable to convert vitamin D to this metabolite.

Because milk is supplemented with vitamin D and because the United States in general is a rather sunny nation relative to Northern Europe, deficiency rickets is extremely rare in this country. When it occurs it usually presents between 6 months and 2 years of age, and the rapidly growing epiphyses at the wrists and knees are those most often affected.[49] Osteomalacia in adults is rare, but has been reported from Scotland in elderly women living alone and consuming diets deficient in vitamins.[9] It is also seen among people who practice purdah, e.g., among Bedouins, but most cases of osteomalacia and rickets due to deficiency of vitamin D result from malabsorption syndromes.

In infancy and childhood there may be skeletal deformities including those of the skull (craniotabes) and bowing of the legs. Recognition of the disease often occurs when the child first begins to walk. Although adults may show the skeletal sequelae of childhood rickets, if the disease develops in adult life it is usually characterized radiographically by pseudofractures (ischial and pubic rami, borders of scapulae, femoral neck). In addition to skeletal deformities, rickets produces a typical lesion at the ends of long bones: there are fraying, cupping, and broadening of the bone at the juncture of the shaft and the cartilage. Ordinarily a generalized decrease in skeletal density is not a radiographic feature of osteomalacia; thus, if diffuse demineralization is present in association with the typical signs of rickets and osteomalacia, a coexistent disease such as osteoporosis should be considered. Bone biopsy should help to clarify the situation, since widened osteoid seams characterize osteomalacia, whereas thin trabeculae with normal osteoid seams are present in osteoporosis.

Children with simple deficiency rickets, unlike those with malabsorption syndromes and azotemic renal disease, will show chemical and radiographic evidence of healing within 8 weeks following therapy with 1000 IU of calciferol daily. These *physiological* doses of calciferol have no beneficial effect in the malabsorption syndromes or azotemic renal disease, in which chemical and radiographic healing may require from 10,000 to 200,000 units of calciferol daily. Thus, the therapeutic response to vitamin D is a useful clue to the etiology.

Azotemic Renal Disease

There are three components of the bone disease associated with renal failure: 1) osteomalacia (rickets), 2) osteitis fibrosa, and 3) osteosclerosis. Usually they occur together, in proportions varying from individual to individual and in the same individual from time to time. The mechanisms responsible for the bone disease are believed to be somewhat as follows: renal failure leads to hyperphosphatemia, which, in turn, depresses serum calcium concentration and also decreases intestinal absorption of phosphorus against a gradient. As a result of the high intestinal phosphate content, calcium is poorly absorbed, since it is precipitated with the phosphate, thus further aggravating the tendency to hypocalcemia. The latter, in turn, stimulates the parathyroids. Parathyroid hormone now mobilizes calcium from bone, thus partially correcting the tendency to hypocalcemia, but producing osteitis fibrosa. It is also probable that there is an abnormality of vitamin D metabolism, so that the vitamin is not hydroxylated to the active metabolite 25-hydroxycholecalciferol. It will be appreciated that, as a result of these mechanisms, osteomalacia and osteitis fibrosa usually occur together. Precisely why osteosclerosis may occur in some cases is not understood.

Renal Tubular Dysfunction

There are several renal tubular dysfunctions which may give rise to bone disease; some of them are hereditary, others acquired. There may be a defect in the renal tubular reabsorption of phosphate, glucose, and amino acids, alone or in combination. The phosphate (or, rarely, phosphate plus glucose) reabsorptive defect is associated with the clinical syndrome of vitamin D-resistant rickets. This is an inherited disease associated with an X-linked dominant gene. Because of excess phosphaturia, the serum inorganic phosphorus concentration is always low; consequently the ionic product of calcium and phosphorus is inadequate for proper precipitation of calcium phosphate into the growing organic matrix, so that rickets and osteomalacia result. Clinically and radiographically, the rickets and osteomalacia are similar to the findings produced by simple deficiency of vitamin D.

The Fanconi syndrome[15] usually includes reabsorptive defects for phosphate, glucose, bicarbonate, and amino acids. This syndrome may appear as a congenital disorder, but it may also occur from the toxic effects of tetracyclines which have been stored for long periods at high temperatures. Wilson's disease, in which copper deposits damage the renal tubules, may give rise to the Fanconi syndrome,[22, 43] as may cystine storage disease and cadmium and lead poisoning. It has also been described with multiple myeloma. Finally, chronic pyelonephritis occasionally causes metabolic acidosis with a low renal tubular reabsorption of phosphorus, which leads to osteomalacia. In all the above conditions the bone disease can be healed, rendering the patient free from bone pain, even though the underlying renal or gastrointestinal disease is incurable.

Neoplastic Diseases

Patients with neoplastic diseases may have a variety of bone disorders characterized by demineralization. These may be categorized as those directly related to the neoplasm (ectopic hyperparathyroidism, osteomalacia secondary to tumor-induced malabsorption, infiltration by extrinsic cells, etc.), those related to the effects of treatment of the cancer (osteoporosis secondary to corticosteroids, osteomalacia secondary to postsurgical malabsorption, etc.), and those independent of and coexisting with the neoplasm. It is not our intention to review all of these, but rather to cite examples of the first category, namely those skeletal disorders primarily related to the neoplasm.

Solid Tumors

Invasion of the skeleton by tumors is an all-too-frequent manifestation of a wide variety of cancers, notably those of the breast, prostate, and lung. The invasion usually gives rise to discrete, destructive lesions which are either osteolytic, osteoblastic, or mixed; the radiographic appearance is often characteristic. However, at times tumors may infiltrate the marrow cavity in sheets of extrinsic cells, giving rise to the radiographic appearance of a diffusely demineralized skeleton. Under these circumstances the diagnosis of an unsuspected cancer may be delayed—a delay which can be avoided by keeping in mind the value of marrow aspiration and biopsy. Many problem cases have been solved by this simple procedure.

For many years it was considered that tumors cause havoc with the skeleton only by physical displacement of bone by tumor tissue. Although this is still the most common way, in 1956 cases were described for the first time in which patients had hypercalcemia associated with cancer but without evidence of tumor invasion of the skeleton, either on biopsy or at postmortem examination.[34, 41] These observations have been confirmed repeatedly, and have formed the basis of the syndrome termed ectopic hyperparathyroidism (or pseudo*hyper*parathyroidism—not to be confused with pseudo*hypo*parathyroidism as described by Albright).[2] Its cardinal features include the biochemical changes of hyperparathyroidism, normal parathyroid glands, absence of invasion of bone by tumor, and correction of the hypercalcemic state by antitumor measures, such as surgical resection of the tumor. These patients may present with demineralization of the skeleton on x-ray; microscopically osteoclastic resorption has been observed. Some 50 cases have been collected from the literature in a review by Lafferty.[29] As Lafferty points out, this syndrome, once regarded as rare, actually may account for as many cases of hypercalcemia as does primary hyperparathyroidism. This assessment may have to be changed, as multiple automated blood tests in asymptomatic patients appear to be uncovering many unrecognized cases of hyperparathyroidism, but the evidence at present emphasizes that cancer must be considered in the differential diagnosis when one is presented with what appears to be hyperparathyroidism. It would appear that some of these tumors are able to secrete parathyroid hormone, or a substance closely akin to it. Consistent with this hypothesis is the demonstration of immunologic cross-reactivity of certain of these tumors in a radioimmunoassay system for bovine parathyroid hormone.[52] Ectopic hormone production by nonendocrine tumors has been the subject of a number of reviews.[5, 37]

Differentiation of ectopic and true hyperparathyroidism may present substantial difficulties for the clinician, but the following points have been helpful: 1) Clinically evident nephrolithiasis does not occur in ectopic hyperparathyroidism in our experience (nephrocalcinosis, however, does). 2) The typical changes of subperiosteal resorption (Fig. 77) as of this time have been described only in true hyperparathyroidism. 3) Levels of urinary calcium are usually lower in hyperparathyroidism than in cancer, for comparable degrees of hypercalcemia. Special tests, including the hydrocortisone test,[16] have not been of value in our hands in differentiating ectopic from true hyperparathyroidism.[35] Problems in differentiation become even greater when it is realized that cancer and hyperparathyroidism due to a parathyroid adenoma may coexist in the same patient. In a series of 50 patients with primary hyperparathyroidism seen at Memorial Hospital, 12 had coexistent active cancer and 7 of these 12 had breast cancer.[21]

Leukemia

Skeletal lesions are rare in chronic myelogenous and chronic lymphoid leukemias, but are common in patients with acute leukemia, particularly children. Craver and Copeland[13] called attention to these lesions some 35 years ago and noted that "in general, osteoporosis predominated in all of the bones showing changes roentgenographically." In a review of the skeletal lesions of acute leukemia in adults and children, Thomas et al.[55] cited the following radiographic findings: juxtaepiphysial radiolucent bands, growth arrest lines (in children), generalized osteoporosis, osteolytic lesions, and periosteal defects. All these changes, as illustrated in Figure 82 are usually to be found in children, although adults may have some of them. In chronic granulocytic leukemia, destructive bone lesions have been described as heralding the onset of blastic transformation.[8] Occasionally osteosclerosis may be a feature of leukemic involvement of the skeleton. Patients with leukemia usually do not present with symptoms suggesting a primary skeletal disorder, but rather with anemia, bleeding, splenomegaly, and at times, protracted fever. These symptoms frequently lead to a correct hematologic diagnosis on blood smear and marrow aspiration, but at times children with acute leukemia may present with articular complaints (due to periosteal or osseous lesions), which, together with fever and anemia, suggest acute rheumatic fever. These complaints usually lead to diagnostic x-rays which may reveal demineralization of the long bones, and it is in this

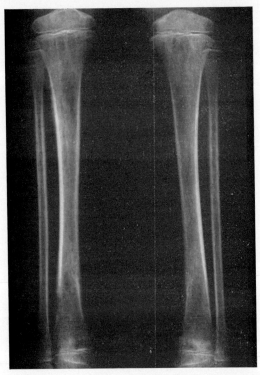

FIG. 82. X-rays of tibiae in a child with acute leukemia. Note zone of rarefaction at the distal end of each tibia with a growth arrest line proximal to it. Note also periosteal elevation and destructive lesions of the cortex.

setting that the special radiographic features noted above may be helpful in differential diagnosis. It should also be remembered that hypercalcemia may occur in acute and chronic leukemia just as in other neoplastic diseases that may infiltrate the skeleton.

Multiple Myeloma

Patients with this disorder may be discovered by chance, following investigation of diffusely demineralized bones detected on radiographs done for some other purpose. Myeloma with diffuse demineralization is rare, however; in general patients present with bone pain and anemia and, when studied, are found to have lytic bone lesions and an abnormal protein in the serum or urine or both, as well as abnormal plasma cells in the marrow aspirate. The dysproteinemia may persist for a number of years before metabolic and infectious consequences ensue; these may include renal disease (with azotemia or tubular defects), hypercalcemia, para-amyloidosis, and bacterial infections, especially pneumonia. Skeletal x-rays usually reveal osteolytic lesions with no surrounding bony reaction. Consistent with this, we have observed absence of uptake of Ca^{47} in areas surrounding the lytic lesions of myeloma. In addition to these punched-out lesions, destruction of

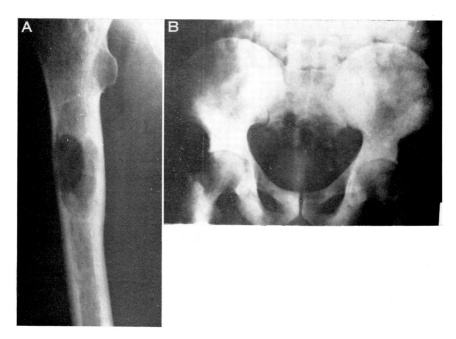

FIG. 83. *A*. Osteolytic defect in the proximal femur in a patient with Hodgkin's disease. *B*. Osteosclerosis of pelvic bones in a patient with Hodgkin's disease. Osteolytic defects are more common in this disease, but occasionally osteosclerosis is striking. Note absence of demineralization of unaffected bone.

the endosteal surface of cortical bone over a considerable distance has been cited as suggestive evidence of myeloma.[10]

Lymphomas

Patients with Hodgkin's disease, lymphosarcoma, and reticulum cell sarcoma usually present with one or more of the following: lymphadenopathy, anemia, fever, and splenomegaly. These symptoms usually lead to a lymph node biopsy and a correct diagnosis; rarely has a lymphoma been discovered through changes detected in bones in the course of radiography done for another purpose. Commonly these lesions are osteolytic, but occasionally, notably in Hodgkin's disease, osteosclerosis is the major radiographic finding. These changes are shown in Figure 83 for purposes of illustration; it will serve to emphasize that in these patients generalized demineralization is usually *not* seen, in contrast to patients with acute leukemia and some with multiple myeloma.

CONCLUDING REMARKS

This chapter has been written at a time when our knowledge regarding bone diseases is unfolding at a rapid rate. In particular, efforts to quantitate bone density are increasingly successful, and it should not be long before we have accurate methods that have widespread clinical applicability. Until then we must rely on radiographs, and it is with this in mind that we have presented a clinical approach to the patient with radiolucent bones. No attempt has been made to review all the diseases which might possibly lead to skeletal demineralization, but it is felt that the approach discussed represents a useful way in which to proceed, regardless of the nature of the underlying disease.

REFERENCES

1. Albright, F., Blumberg, E., and Smith, P. H. Postmenopausal osteoporosis. Trans. Ass. Amer. Physicians 55:298, 1940.
2. Albright, F., and Reifenstein, E. *The Parathyroid Glands and Metabolic Bone Disease.* The Williams & Wilkins Co., Baltimore, 1948.
3. Barnett, E. S., and Nordin, B. E. C. Radiological assessment of bone density. 1. The clinical and radiological problem of thin bones. Brit. J. Radiol. 34:683, 1961.
4. Bonadonna, G., Merlino, M. J., Myers, W. P. L., and Sonenberg, M. Urinary hydroxyproline and calcium metabolism in patients with cancer. N. Engl. J. Med. 275:298, 1966.
5. Bower, B. F., and Gordan, G. S. Hormonal effects of nonendocrine tumors. Annu. Rev. Med. 16:83, 1965.
6. Bradley, B. W., and Ansell, B. M. Fractures in Still's disease. Ann. Rheum. Dis. 19:135, 1960.
7. Castleman, B., and Mallory, T. B. Pathology of parathyroid gland in hyperparathyroidism. Study of 25 cases. Amer. J. Pathol. 11:1, 1935.
8. Chabner, B. A., Haskell, C. M., and Canellos, G. P. Destructive bone lesions in chronic granulocytic leukemia. Medicine 48:401, 1969.
9. Chalmers, J., Conacher, W. D. H., Gardner, D. L., and Scott, P. J. Osteomalacia: a common disease in elderly women. J. Bone Joint Surg. 49B:403, 1967.
10. Commissie voor Beentumoren. *Radiological Atlas of Bone Tumors.* The Williams & Wilkins Co., Baltimore, 1966.
11. Cook, P. B., Nassim, J. R., and Collins, J. The effects of thyrotoxicosis upon the metabolism of calcium, phosphorus, and nitrogen. Quart. J. Med. 28:505, 1959.
12. Cope, O., Keanes, W. M., Roth, S. I., and Castleman, B. Primary chief cell hyperplasia of parathyroid glands: new entity in surgery of hyperparathyroidism. Ann. Surg. 148:375, 1958.
13. Craver, L. F., and Copeland, M. M. Changes of the bones in the leukemias. Arch. Surg. 30:639, 1935.
14. De Luca, H. F. 25-Hydroxycholecalciferol. The probable metabolically active form of vitamin D3: its identification and subcellular site of action. Arch. Internal Med. 124:442, 1969.
15. Dent, C. E. Rickets and osteomalacia from renal tubule defects. J. Bone Joint Surg. 34B:266, 1952.
16. Dent, C. E., and Watson, L. The hydrocortisone test in primary and tertiary hyperparathyroidism. Lancet 2:662, 1968.
17. Dickson, T. F., and Purdom, M. Serum 5' nucleotidase. J. Clin. Pathol. 7:341, 1954.
18. Dotter, W. E., Baylink, D. J., and Hurxthal, L. M. Two methods for the study of osteoporosis and other metabolic bone disease. III. X-ray signs for visually estimating vertebral bone density. The Lahey Clin. Found. Bull. 13:217, 1964.
19. Doyle, F. H. Ulnar bone mineral concentration in metabolic bone diseases. Brit. J. Radiol. 34:698, 1961.
20. Dull, T. A., and Henneman, P. H. Urinary hydroxyproline as an index of collagen turnover in bone. N. Engl. J. Med. 268:132, 1963.
21. Fahey, T. J., Jr., and Myers, W. P. L. Unpublished data, 1969.
22. Finby, N., and Bearn, A. G. Roentgenographic abnormalities of the skeletal system in Wilson's disease (hepato-lenticular degeneration). Amer. J. Roentgenol. 79:603, 1958.
23. Fitzgerald, M. X. M., Fennelly, J. J., and McGeeney, K. The value of differential

alkaline phosphatase thermostability in clinical diagnosis. Amer. J. Clin. Pathol. 51:194, 1969.
24. Garn, S. M., Rohmann, C. G., and Nolan, P. The developmental nature of bone changes during aging. In *Relations of Development and Aging*, Birren, J. A., Ed., p. 41. Charles C Thomas, Springfield, Ill., 1964.
25. Greenberg, E. J., Weber, D. A., Pochaczevsky, R., Kenny, P. J., Myers, W. P. L., and Laughlin, J. S. Detection of neoplastic bone lesions by quantitative scanning and radiography. J. Nucl. Med. 9:613, 1968.
26. Hodgkinson, A., and Pyrrah, L. N. The urinary excretion of calcium and inorganic phosphate in 344 patients with calcium stone of renal origin. Brit. J. Surg. 46:10, 1958.
27. Kalbfleisch, J. M., Lindeman, R. D., Ginn, H. E., and Smith, W. O. Effects of ethanol administration on urinary excretion of magnesium and other electrolytes in alcoholic and normal subjects. J. Clin. Invest. 42:1471, 1963.
28. Lachmann, E., and Whelan, M. The roentgen diagnosis of osteoporosis and its limitations. Radiology 26:165, 1936.
29. Lafferty, F. W. Pseudohyperparathyroidism. Medicine 45:247, 1966.
30. Lotz, M., Zisman, E., and Bartter, F. Evidence for a phosphorus depletion syndrome in man. N. Engl. J. Med. 278:409, 1968.
31. McCarty, D. J. Crystal-induced inflammation; syndromes of gout and pseudogout. Geriatrics 18:467, 1963.
32. McConkey, B, Fraser, G. M., and Bligh, A. S. Osteoporosis and purpura in rheumatoid disease. Prevalence and relations to treatment with corticosteroids. Quart. J. Med. 31:419, 1962.
33. Meema, H., and Meema, S. Measurable roentgenologic changes in some peripheral bones in senile osteoporosis. J. Amer. Geriat. Soc. 11:1170, 1963.
34. Myers, W. P. L. Hypercalcemia in neoplastic disease. Cancer 9:1135, 1956.
35. Myers, W. P. L. Studies of serum calcium regulation. Advan. Internal Med. 11:163, 1962.
36. Myers, W. P. L., Rothschild, E. O., Carney, V., Kaplan, N., Greenberg, E. J., Dimich, A., and Weber, D. Tumor-induced hypercalcemia: radiocalcium and bone culture studies. Calcified Tissue Res. 2: (Suppl.): 68, 1968.
37. Myers, W. P. L., Tashima, C. K., and Rothschild, E. O. Endocrine syndromes associated with nonendocrine neoplasms. Med. Clin. N. Amer. 50:763, 1966.
38. Nordin, B. E. C. Effect of malabsorption syndrome on calcium metabolism. Proc. Roy. Soc. Med. 54:497, 1961.
39. Nordin, B. E. C., and Roper, A. Post-pregnancy osteoporosis syndromes. Lancet 1:431, 1955.
40. Nordin, B. E. C., and Smith, D. A. *Diagnostic Procedures in Disorders of Calcium Metabolism*. Little, Brown and Co., Boston, 1965.
41. Plimpton, C. H., and Gellhorn, A. Hypercalcemia in malignant disease without evidence of bone destruction. Amer. J. Med. 21:750, 1956.
42. Reiss, E., and Canterbury, J. M. Primary hyperparathyroidism; application of radioimmunoassay to differentiation of adenoma and hyperplasia and to preoperative localization of hyperfunctioning parathyroid glands. N. Engl. J. Med. 280:1381, 1969.
43. Rosenoer, V. N., and Mitchell, R. C. Skeletal changes in Wilson's disease (hepatolenticular degeneration). Brit. J. Radiol. 32:805, 1959.
44. Rothschild, E. O. Unpublished data, 1970.
45. Saville, P. D. Changes in bone mass with age and alcoholism. J. Bone Joint Surg. 47:492, 1965.
46. Saville, P. D. Osteoporosis and the menopause. Clin. Orthop. Related Res. 55:43, 1967.
47. Saville, P. D. A quantitative approach to simple radiographic diagnosis of osteoporosis: its application to the osteoporosis of rheumatoid arthritis. Arthritis Rheum. 10:416, 1967.
48. Saville, P. D. When to hospitalize for osteoporosis. Hosp. Practice 4:60, 1969.
49. Saville, P. D., and Alderman, M. H. Deficiency rickets in New York: dissociation between urinary hydroxyproline and glycylproline with treatment. Arch. Internal Med. 125:341, 1970.

50. Saville, P. D., and Kharmosh, O. Osteoporosis with rheumatoid arthritis. Influence of age, sex, and corticosteroids. Arthritis Rheum. 10:423, 1967.
51. Scott, J. T., Dixon, A. S., and Bywaters, E. G. L. Association of hyperuricemia and gout with hyperparathyroidism. Brit. Med. J. 1:1070, 1964.
52. Sherwood, L. M., O'Riordan, J. L. H., Aurbach, G. D., and Potts, J. T., Jr. Production of parathyroid hormone by nonparathyroid tumors. J. Clin. Endocrinol. Metab. 24:140, 1967.
53. Smith, R. W., and Frame, B. Concurrent axial and appendicular osteoporosis: its relation to calcium consumption. N. Engl. J. Med. 272:73, 1965.
54. Sorenson, J. A., and Cameron, J. R. A reliable *in vivo* measurement of bone-mineral content. J. Bone Joint Surg. 49A:481, 1967.
55. Thomas, L. B., Forkner, C. E., Jr., Frei, E., Besse, B. E., and Stabeman, J. R. The skeletal lesions of acute leukemia. Cancer 14:608, 1961.
56. Wasserman, R. H., and Taylor, A. N. Vitamin D-dependent calcium-binding protein. Response to some physiological and nutritional variables. J. Biol. Chem. 243:3987, 1968.
57. Weber, D. A., Greenberg, E. J., Dimich, A., Kenny, P. J., Rothschild, E. O., Myers, W. P. L., and Laughlin, J. S. Kinetics of radionuclides used for bone studies. J. Nucl. Med. 10:8, 1969.
58. Wills, M. R., Pak, C. Y. C., Hammond, W. G., and Bartter, F. C. Normocalcemic primary hyperparathyroidism. Amer. J. Med. 47:384, 1969.

Index

Hurler syndrome, 63
Morquio syndrome, 63
Scheie's syndrome, 63
Mucormycosis
  development in patients with underlying disease, 373
  pulmonary, 373
Muscle
  disease
    acromegaly, 274
    Addison's disease, 274
    effect of aging: senile muscular wasting, 239
    electromyography, 204
    endocrine disease, 243
    endocrine disorders, 272
    hypoadrenalism, 274
    hypopituitarism, 274
    hypothyroidism, 272
    infectious, 276
      bacterial, 277
      parasitic, 277
      trichinosis, 277
      viral, 276
    infections, chronic, 238
    infiltrative disease, 238
    inflammatory disease which may be related to autoimmunity, 239
    laboratory studies, 219
      creatine excretion, 219
      electromyogram, 219
      muscle biopsy, 219
      nerve conduction velocity, 219
      serum levels enzymes from muscle, 219
    malabsorptive disease, 238
    muscular dystrophy, 251
    neoplastic disease, 238
    rare myopathies, 256
    weakness with atrophy, 218
  disorder
    electrolyte disorders, 260
    hypercalcemia, 263
    hyperkalemia, 262
    hypermagnesemia, 264
    hypernatremia, 264
    hypokalemia, 260
    hyponatremia, 264
    weakness without atrophy, 260
  papillary. See Papillary muscle
  rigidity and spasms, 247
  serum enzymes (table), 202
  skeletal; electromyography, 203
Murmur. See under Aortic regurgitation
  cardiomyopathy, 85
Muscular
  disease
    episodic

peripheral arterial insufficiency, 293
    weakness following recovery, 292
  dystrophy
    Duchenne type, 252
    electromyography, 251
    Erb type, 254
    facioscapulohumeral (fig.), 251
    facioscapular type, 253
    incidence, 251
    intermediate limb-girdle type, 254
    Landouzy-Déjerine type, 253
    levator palpebrae, biopsy of (fig.), 253
    mild, restricted, slowly progressive type, 253
    muscle biopsy, 252
    myotonic form, 254; (figs.), 255, 256
    ocular, 254; (fig.) 252
    pseudohypertrophic type, 252
    severe, generalized, rapidly progressive
      creatine excretion, 252
      enzymes, serum levels, 253
    types, 251
    vitamin E deficiency, similarity, 255
de Musset's sign, 26
Myalgia, epidemic
  pleurodynia and, 276
Myasthenia gravis, 248
  diagnosis, 269
  electromyography, 271
  incidence, 264
  laboratory studies, 271
  manifestations, 265
  neonatal, 267
  neostigmine methylsulfate effects (fig.), 265
  osteoporosis and. See under Osteoporosis
  serologic reactions, 270
  triple fissured tongue (fig.), 267
Mycobacterioses
  poorly resolving pneumonias, 435
Mycobacteria
  pulmonary tuberculosis, 359
Mycoplasma
  isolation in diagnosis of inflammatory lung disease, 398
Myeloma
  multiple
    dysproteinemia, 514
    para-amyloidosis (fig.), 239
Myers, W. P. Laird. See Saville and Myers, 485–518
Myocardial disease, primary, 79–101
  biventricular enlargement (fig.), 84
  chest x-ray, 86
  circulatory failure, 82
  classification, 79; (table), 80
  clinical presentation, 81